THE **Complete History** AND **Physical Exam** GUIDE

THE **Complete History** AND **Physical Exam** GUIDE

ERIC H. HANSON, MD, MPH
Headquarters United States Air Force,
Office of the Surgeon General,
Directorate of Modernication,
Science and Technology Division,
Chief, Science and Technology
and Operational Biotechnology,
Bolling Air Force Base,
Washington, D.C.

THOMAS S. NEUHAUSER, MD
Staff Pathologist,
Medical Directory of Hematology,
Wilford Hall Medical Center,
Lackland Air Force Base,
San Antonio, Texas

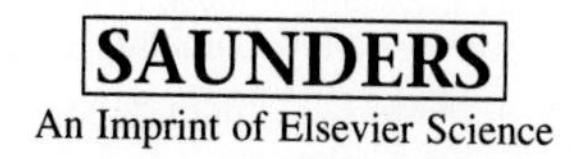

SAUNDERS
An Imprint of Elsevier Science

The Curtis Center
Independence Square West
Philadelphia, Pennsylvania 19106

The Complete History and Physical Exam Guide ISBN 0-7216-8712-1
Copyright © 2003, Elsevier Science (USA). All rights reserved.

No part of this publication may be reproduced or transmitted in any form or by any means, electronic or mechanical, including photocopying, recording, or any information storage and retrieval system, without permission in writing from the publisher. Permissions may be sought directly from Elsevier's Health Sciences Rights Department in Philadelphia, PA, USA: phone: (+1) 215 238 7869, fax: (+1) 215 238 2239, e-mail: healthpermissions@elsevier.com. You may also complete your request on-line via the Elsevier Science homepage (http://www.elsevier.com), by selecting "Customer Support" and then "Obtaining Permissions."

NOTICE

Medicine is an ever-changing field. Standard safety precautions must be followed, but as new research and clinical experience broaden our knowledge, changes in treatment and drug therapy may become necessary or appropriate. Readers are advised to check the most current product information provided by the manufacturer of each drug to be administered to verify the recommended dose, the method and duration of administration, and contraindications. It is the responsibility of the licensed prescriber, relying on experience and knowledge of the patient, to determine dosages and the best treatment for each individual patient. Neither the publisher nor the author assumes any liability for any injury and/or damage to persons or property arising from this publication.

International Standard Book Number 0-7216-8712-1

Acquisitions Editor: William Schmitt
Developmental Editor: Anne-Marie Shaw
Publishing Services Manager: Pat Joiner
Project Manager: Keri O'Brien
Senior Designer: Mark A. Oberkrom
Cover Designer: Christine Hoog

Printed in the United States of America.

Last digit is the print number: 9 8 7 6 5 4 3 2 1

Preface

"Learn to see, learn to hear, learn to feel, learn to smell, and know that by practice alone can you become expert. Medicine is learned by the bedside and not in the classroom. Let not your conceptions of the manifestations of disease come from words heard in the lecture room or read from the book. See, and then reason and compare and control. But see first."

Sir William Osler [1919]

Source: Osler, William. In Thayer LS. Osler, the teacher. *Johns Hopkins Hosp Bull.* 1919; 30:198-200.

What remains unchanged in contemporary clinical practice from the artful era of the giants of medicine (Hippocrates, Galen, Osler)? An accurate and complete history and physical examination (H&P). Throughout the centuries, the art of practicing medicine has always relied heavily on obtaining a thorough and accurate H&P.

The goal of *The Complete History and Physical Exam Guide* is to provide you, the health care practitioner, with a systematic and efficient tool for developing and refining your H&P skill set.

"There is no more difficult art to acquire than the art of observation, and for some men it is quite as difficult to record an observation in brief and plain language."

Sir William Osler [1903]

Source: Osler, William. On the educational value of the medical society. *Boston Med Surg J.* 1903; 148:275-9.

The Complete History and Physical Exam Guide is designed to cultivate the skill of observation and to emphasize the diagnostic importance of the H&P. Nobody wants to miss critical specialty H&P information, especially when in a specialty setting for training. This book was written to help ensure that all vital pertinent information is brought to bear in the evaluation and treatment of patients. Forty-nine specialty-trained physicians collaborated in the production of this pocket-sized clinical book whose unique primary focus *is the development of H&Ps for specialty- and topic-focused settings. Their efforts culminated in the present compilation of specialty-focused H&Ps, which may be used by all practitioners in the health care field.*

Chapters 1 through 6, in Section I, present the essential elements of a thorough H&P. Then, in Section II, 28 specialty-focused chapters demonstrate how to obtain accurate specialty H&Ps using a consistent, concise, comprehensive, and yet detailed approach. Proceeding in a logical, stepwise fashion, from chief complaint to sample write-up, each chapter provides the questions to ask and how to ask them, the tests to order, and the diagnoses to consider.

Other features that make this easy-to-follow book unique are found in every specialty-focused chapter and include three different approaches to each review of systems, expanded emphasis on health maintenance and psychosocial histories, and specialty-focused definitions, abbreviations, acronyms, and eponyms. Sample write-ups end each chapter and offer a starting point for each specialty. The book concludes with 5 chapters devoted to important but often overlooked topics.

The information presented in this guide book pertains to adult medicine (except for that contained in the Pediatrics chapter) and is intended as a practical supplement to comprehensive medical and *physical examination textbooks in the various medical fields.*

There are many ways to approach an H&P, *especially a specialty-focused H&P, and we hope our efforts provide you with a guide that proves helpful in* your clinical training and medical practice.

Disclaimer

The conclusions and opinions expressed in this document are those of the authors. They do not reflect the official position of the U.S. Government, Department of Defense, or the United States Air Force.

Acknowledgments

This book is dedicated to all physicians, physician assistants, nurse practitioners, nurses, and other health care providers who have volunteered to confront the sometimes overwhelming, but always gratifying task of providing health care.

The editorial and production assistance provided by Anne-Marie Shaw, Bill Schmitt, and Keri O'Brien has been greatly appreciated.

We would especially like to thank our families, parents, and friends—Lynene; John, Ruth, James, Julie, Nikolai, and Gabriel; MJ, Mike, Troy, Ted, Robb; Katerina, and Tasha—for their unwavering support.

Contents

I

ESSENTIALS OF THE HISTORY AND PHYSICAL EXAMINATION

1

HISTORY AND PHYSICAL EXAMINATION (H&P) ESSENTIALS

Eric H. Hanson, MD, MPH

H&P ESSENTIALS

I. Chief complaint
II. History of present illness
III. Past medical and surgical history
IV. Medications, allergies, and adverse reactions
V. Health maintenance
VI. Family history
VII. Psychosocial history
VIII. Review of systems
IX. Physical examination

Chapter 18, Internal Medicine and Family Practice, contains an expanded version of the history and physical examination presented in this chapter.

I. CHIEF COMPLAINT

A. Chief Complaint

1. Describe, using patient's own words, in one or two sentences.
2. Include chronology and temporality of symptoms: Onset (acute, subacute, or chronic), duration (minutes, hours, days, weeks, months, or years), frequency, and progression.

B. Patient Information

1. Record patient's name, age, gender/sex, race, and ethnicity.
2. Acknowledge source of history and source's reliability (e.g., J. L., patient's daughter, who appears reliable).
3. Note admission date, time, site (e.g., emergency department, direct admit, or transfer), and type (elective, urgent, or emergent).

II. HISTORY OF PRESENT ILLNESS (HPI)

A. Symptoms, Conditions, and Disorders: Note responses to following characteristics.

1. Chronology and temporality: Onset, duration, frequency, and progression.
2. Quality of symptoms (e.g., sharp, dull, stabbing, or bandlike pain).

3. Quantity of symptoms: Indicate severity on a scale from 1 to 10 and a comparison value (e.g., a traumatically amputated extremity = 10).
4. Aggravating factors: Setting or context.
5. Alleviating factors: Setting or context.

B. **Medications, Treatments, and Reactions:** Inquire about and note the following information:
1. Current medications, treatments, and therapies.
2. Responses to interventions, recent regimen changes, and allergic and other adverse reactions to past treatments.

C. **Review of Systems:** Record pertinent positives and negatives.

III. **PAST MEDICAL AND SURGICAL HISTORY**

A. **Past Medical History for Adult Illnesses (PMH or PMHx)**
1. Record active and inactive medical problems. Differentiate acute, subacute, and chronic problems. Acute diagnoses are usually included in the HPI (see previous section).
2. Describe serious adult medical illnesses, including dates, diagnoses, degrees, durations, physicians, hospitals, treatments, medications, complications and sequelae, and responses to interventions.

B. **Past Surgical History (PSH or PSHx):** Take a surgical history, noting dates, diagnoses, procedures, responses to interventions, hospitals, operative and postoperative complications and sequelae, anesthesia types (local, spinal, or general), and anesthetic complications.

C. **Emergency and Trauma History**
1. Record hospitalizations. Include dates, diagnoses, degrees or severities, durations, physicians, hospitals, treatments, medications, and complications and sequelae.
2. Report transfusions. Include dates, total number, and known complications (e.g., HIV, hepatitis).
3. Describe any trauma and injuries.
   a. Fractures: Limitations of range of motion (ROM), deformities, disabilities, or weaknesses.
   b. Motor vehicle accidents (MVAs): Types of injury, types of vehicle, positions in vehicle, speeds of vehicle, deceleration forces, and uses of restraints, seat belts, or other protective measures (e.g., air bags).

D. **Childhood History**
1. Inquire about and note any serious childhood illnesses and injuries, such as respiratory infections, urinary tract infections, cardiac disorders (e.g., congenital, rheumatic fever), seizures, and trauma.
2. Describe social history, in particular, any behavioral, learning, and school problems.
3. Describe childhood health maintenance, noting especially whether patient received immunizations and regular medical checkups.

IV. MEDICATIONS, ALLERGIES, AND ADVERSE REACTIONS

A. Medications

1. Record patient's current prescription medications. Include indications, last doses, and consistency and duration of use.

HPI MEDICATION INFORMATION SAMPLE.

Medication	Dose and Route	Frequency	Indication
Aspirin	Two 325-mg tabs per os (PO)	As needed (prn) (once a day [qd], twice a day [bid], three times a day [tid], once every night [qhs])	Headache
Cimetidine (Tagamet)	400 mg PO	bid (before each meal [qac] and qhs)	Dyspepsia

2. Note over-the-counter (OTC) medications used by patient, including analgesics, laxatives, sleeping medications, vitamins or supplements, herbal preparations, and diet pills.
3. Inquire about and note any alternative medicine therapies the patient is using.

B. Allergies

1. Report any known allergic reactions to substances (e.g., medications, pollens, particulates, metals, envenomations).
2. Describe types of reactions (e.g., respiratory or neurologic manifestations). Distinguish such reactions from possible adverse medication affect (e.g., nausea after taking a pill).
3. Record types of treatment the patient has received for an allergic reaction. Note medications, routes of administration (e.g., PO, IV, SQ), hospitalization, intubation, and response/outcome.

V. HEALTH MAINTENANCE

A. Prevention

1. Inquire about and note what periodic health assessments, exams, and screenings the patient received.
2. Include information about the following immunizations:
   a. Childhood immunizations: Diphtheria; pertussis; tetanus, usually given as diphtheria and tetanus toxoids and acellular pertussis (DTaP); inactivated polio vaccine (IPV); measles, mumps, and rubella vaccine (MMR); varicella vaccine;

Hemophilus influenza type b (Hib) conjugate vaccine; hepatitis B (Hep B); and heptavalent pneumococcal conjugate (PCV) vaccine. Hepatitis A vaccine (Hep A): Recommended in selected states and regions and for certain high-risk populations. Influenza vaccine: Recommended for children 6 months of age or older who have certain risk factors. Pneumococcal polysaccharide vaccine (PPV): Recommended in addition to PCV for certain high-risk groups.

b. Adult immunizations: Tetanus-diphtheria toxoid vaccine; influenza vaccine (50 years of age and older and certain high-risk groups); pneumococcal vaccine (65 years of age and older and certain high-risk groups); Hep B (adults at risk); MMR; and varicella vaccine.

B. Diet: Describe patient's typical diet (e.g., what was eaten during the last 24 hours, dietary restrictions, and caffeine use).

C. Exercise: Describe exercise regimen (e.g., type of exercise, frequency, duration, and intensity).

D. Social Habits

1. Record patient's use of alcohol, including type (beer, wine, or hard liquor); number of drinks per day or per week; size of glass (amount per drink); and number of years used.
2. Record any use of tobacco, including type (chew, snuff, cigarettes, cigars); amount (e.g., packs, cigars, or snuff containers per day); and number of years used (pack-years).
3. Include any illicit or recreational drug use, noting type, route, frequency of use, and duration of use.

VI. FAMILY HISTORY

Ask patient about the health and illnesses of first-degree relatives (i.e., father, mother, siblings, and children). Note, in particular, the presence or absence of hypertension (HTN); atherosclerotic disease (e.g., coronary artery disease [CAD], cerebrovascular accidents [CVA]); stroke; diabetes; cancer; and neuropsychologic disorders. Also record age and cause of death, when applicable.

VII. PSYCHOSOCIAL HISTORY

A. Personal History

1. Record patient's place of birth (city and country).
2. Inquire about patient's religious preference and note possible medical implications.
3. Record patient's race, ethnicity, and cultural background, and possible health implications.
4. Record patient's marital status and number/gender of children.
5. Ask patient to describe and record current residence and living conditions (e.g., three bedrooms, one bath, eight occupants).

B. Current Illness Effects on the Patient

1. Ascertain and note patient's perception of the severity of the illness.

2. Address death and dying issues, as applicable.
3. Inquire about and note whether patient has established advanced directives (e.g., Living Will or Durable Power of Attorney for Health Care [DPAHC]).

C. **Family Support**

1. List family members, significant others, and additional sources of support.
2. Ascertain and note family's awareness of present illness.
3. Determine and note physical proximity of family and other support persons.
4. Record important contact phone numbers.

VIII. **REVIEW OF SYSTEMS AND PHYSICAL EXAMINATION**

A. **Review of Systems:** Question patient about each of the following symptoms and conditions. Record all positive responses and significant negative responses.

REVIEW OF SYSTEMS.	
1. General	11. Gastrointestinal
2. Head	12. Genitourinary
3. Eye	13. Gynecologic
4. Ear	14. Hematopoietic
5. Nose	15. Endocrine
6. Throat	16. Lymphatic
7. Neck	17. Musculoskeletal
8. Respiratory	18. Skin
9. Chest wall/breasts	19. Neurologic
10. Cardiovascular	20. Psychiatric

1. **General:** Appetite, fatigue, weakness, insomnia, night sweats or chills, and recent weight changes.
2. **Head:** Headaches and head trauma.
3. **Eyes:** Glasses, vision changes, diplopia, redness or inflammation, discharge, blind spots or blurring, photophobia, scotomata, glaucoma, and date of last exam.
4. **Ears:** Hearing changes, ringing in the ears (i.e., tinnitus), vertigo, earaches, and otitis media or externa.
5. **Nose:** Diminished smell (olfaction), congestion, obstruction, runny nose (e.g., rhinorrhea), or nosebleeds (i.e., epistaxis).
6. **Mouth:** Problems with teeth or gums, dentures, sore throats, hoarseness, or difficulty swallowing.
7. **Neck:** Pains, decreased ROM, swollen glands, masses, or goiter.

8. **Respiratory:** Cough, sputum (color and quantity), hoarseness, coughing up blood (i.e., hemoptysis), shortness of breath, pneumonia, reactive airway disease (RAD) or asthma, wheezing, bronchitis or emphysema, pulmonary embolus, pain with breathing (i.e., pleurisy), tuberculosis (TB), and history of a positive purified protein derivative (PPD)/TB skin test.
9. **Chest wall and breasts:** Clinical and breast self-exams (BSE), breast masses or lumps, discharge from the nipples (i.e., galactorrhea), nipple inversion, pain, masses, fibrocystic disease (FCD), breast cancer, and frequency of mammograms.
10. **Cardiovascular:** Chest pain, palpitations, murmurs, rheumatic heart disease (RHD), hypertension (HTN), stroke or transient ischemic attacks (TIAs), orthopnea (propping up in bed to sleep; assess number of pillows used), paroxysmal nocturnal dyspnea (PND), dyspnea on exertion (DOE), edema, leg pain or cramps, claudication, varicose veins, intermittent attacks of ischemia of fingers, toes, ears or nose (i.e., Raynaud's phenomenon), previous electrocardiograph (ECG).
11. **Gastrointestinal (GI):** Nausea, vomiting, hematemesis, diarrhea, change in stools or pattern of bowel movements, dysphagia, heartburn, abdominal pain, cholecystitis, hernias, constipation, hemorrhoids, melena, hematochezia or bright red blood per rectum (BRBPR), and appendicitis.
12. **Genitourinary (GU):** Dysuria, unusual urine smell or color, sexually transmitted diseases (STDs), hematuria, frequency of urination, nocturia, reduced caliber or force of stream, flank pain, kidney stones, benign prostatic hyperplasia (BPH).
13. **Obstetrics and gynecology (OB/GYN):** Number of pregnancies and outcomes (i.e., full-term, premature, aborted, and live birth); types of pregnancies (e.g., gravida, para, and twins); first day of last normal menstrual period (LNMP); last Pap smear; menstruation characteristics (e.g., frequency, regularity, amount of flow, and dysmenorrhea); age at menarche; age at menopause; miscarriages; spontaneous abortions (i.e., less than 20 weeks gestation); postmenopausal bleeding; hot flashes; vaginal dryness; contraception methods; and vulvar, cervical, or endometrial disorder.
14. **Hematology:** Bleeding or bruising, coagulopathy, anemia, thalassemia, operations, transfusions, and transfusion reaction.
15. **Endocrine:** Polyphagia, polydipsia, polyuria, enlarged thyroid, heat or cold intolerance, sweating, hyperlipidemia, dyslipidemia (e.g., low high-density lipoproteins [HDL]), changes in hair or skin texture or growth, and changes in hat, glove, or shoe sizes.

16. **Lymphatics:** Enlarged lymph nodes and tenderness.
17. **Musculoskeletal:** Joint pain, stiffness, swelling, soreness or inflammation, bone diseases, bony deformity, muscle tenderness, and muscle weakness.
18. **Skin:** Rashes, lesions, pallor, jaundice, itching (i.e., pruritus), pigmentation changes, moles, and bruises.
19. **Neurologic:** Numbness, tingling, burning, prickling or hyperesthesia (e.g., paresthesias), unpleasant abnormal sensations (i.e., dysesthesias), involuntary movements, ataxia, tremors, vertigo (e.g., external world revolving around patient [objective vertigo] or patient revolving in space [subjective vertigo]), dizziness, loss of consciousness (syncope), seizures, epilepsy, memory loss, and strokes.
20. **Psychiatric:** Reaction to illness, use of medications, psychotherapy, tension, anxiety, bizarre thoughts, paranoia, phobias, violent tendencies, insomnia, sexual dysfunction, and depression.

Depression screening tool mnemonic ("SIG E CAPS"): **S** = sleep; **I** = interests; **G** = guilt; **E** = energy; **C** = concentration; **A** = appetite (food and sex); **P** = psychomotor; **S** = suicide screen.

B. Physical Examination

1. **Vital signs:** Record the following results of physical examination.

PHYSICAL EXAMINATION.	
1. Vital Signs	11. Lungs
2. General Appearance	12. Cardiovascular
3. Head and Neck	13. Abdomen
4. Eyes	14. Genitalia
5. Ears	15. Rectum/Prostate
6. Nose	16. Back/Spine
7. Mouth	17. Extremities
8. Throat	18. Skin
9. Teeth	19. Lymphatics
10. Chest	20. Neurologic

a. Temperature: Tympanic membrane (TM), rectal or oral. <100.4°F = low-grade fever; >100.4°F = fever. Document maximum temperature in last 24-72 hours (Tmax/24 hours).
b. Respiratory rate (RR): Age-dependent range (Table 1-1).

Table 1-1. AGE-DEPENDENT RANGES OF RESPIRATORY RATES.

Newborns/ Neonates	1-6 Months of Age	6 Months-1 Year of Age	1-2 Years of Age	3 Years of Age	5 Years of Age	Above 5 Years of Age and Adult
35-45	25-35	25-35	20-30	16-24	14-24	14-20

- **c.** Pulse: Rate; regular or irregular (if irregular note the apical impulse). Rate = normal >60 to <100 beats per minute (bpm), bradycardic <60 bpm or tachycardic >100 bpm. If pulse is irregular note the apical impulse.
- **d.** Blood pressure (BP): Extremity tested, time intervals used with orthostatics, supine, sitting or standing.
- **e.** Height, weight, and body mass index (BMI).

2. General appearance and mental status

- **a.** Age, gender/sex, race, and ethnic background.
- **b.** Body habitus and hygiene, nutrition, and state of health.
- **c.** General description of comfort level (e.g., ill-appearing, mild discomfort, despondent, cooperative).

3. Head and neck

- **a.** Head.
  - **(1)** Scalp, distribution and texture of hair, and loss or thinning of hair (e.g., alopecia).
  - **(2)** Skull and facies abnormalities or tenderness to palpation (TTP).
- **b.** Neck.
  - **(1)** ROM and suppleness.
  - **(2)** Lymph nodes: Greater than 1 cm is considered abnormal. Specify location, number, size, whether fixed or mobile, and tenderness.
  - **(3)** Thyroid size, texture, and consistency. Presence of thyroid bruits, masses, or nodules.
  - **(4)** Carotid pulse (regular or irregular) or carotid bruits.
  - **(5)** Jugular venous distention (JVD) or hepatojugular reflex (HJR).

4. Eyes

- **a.** Lids, conjunctivae, and sclerae.
- **b.** Pupils equally round and reactive to light (PERRL), accommodation (PERRLA), and direct and consensual (PERRLADC).
- **c.** Extraocular muscles intact (EOMI).
- **d.** Visual fields: Normal to direct confrontation.
- **e.** Visual acuity: Jaegher chart with standard-size letters, viewed at 12 inches; Snellen chart with standard letters, normally viewed at a distance of 20 feet.
- **f.** Ophthalmoscopic exam: Lenses, media, discs (normal cup-to-disc ratio <0.5), vessels, and macula. Presence of abnormalities (e.g., hemorrhages, exudates, microaneurysms, arteriovenous [A-V] nicking of retinal vessels, copper wiring, and arteriolar narrowing).

5. Ears

- **a.** Auricles and canals.
- **b.** Tenderness to tragus traction.

   c. Tympanic membranes (TMs): Color, landmarks, light reflex, and mobility with insufflation.
   d. Hearing by rustling fingers or whispered voice.
   e. Differentiation of conductive versus sensorineural hearing loss (e.g., Weber tests lateralization of sound and Rinne test for air and bone conduction).
6. **Nose**
   a. Patency and appearance of mucosa (e.g., boggy or congested, normal, dry).
   b. Septum midline: Absence of polyps, exudate, or discharge.
   c. Sinus tenderness of maxillary and frontal sinuses to palpation.
7. **Mouth**
   a. Lips, buccal mucosa, and salivary ducts and glands appearance.
   b. Tongue: Symmetry, size, texture, and side-to-side motion (cranial nerve XII).
8. **Throat:** Tonsils, pharynx, uvula, and palate appearance. Absence of erythema or exudate.
9. **Teeth and gums**
   a. Dentition status, missing or carious teeth, and bleeding or inflamed gums.
   b. If applicable, ask patient to remove dentures or bridges and examine under dental plates.
10. **Chest**
   a. Thorax.
      (1) Symmetry, anterior-posterior (AP) diameter, movement with respiratory excursion.
      (2) Abnormal veins or pulsations.
      (3) Gynecomastia (males).
   b. Breasts (men and women).
      (1) Contour, symmetry, or retractions.
      (2) Masses or tenderness.
      (3) Nipple inversion or discharge.
      (4) Lymph nodes.
11. **Lungs**
   a. Clear to auscultation and percussion (CTAP); breath sounds equal bilaterally.
   b. Equal diaphragmatic excursion in the posterior midscapular line.
   c. Voice transmission tests: Tactile fremitus, whispered pectoriloquy, and egophony. (See Chapter 18, Internal Medicine and Family Practice, for explanations of tests.)
   d. Note adventitious (extra) lung sounds: Wheezes, rales or crackles, stridor, rhonchi, and rubs. Diagram their locations.

12. **Cardiovascular**
    a. Neck.
        (1) Carotid pulses (regular or irregular) or carotid bruits.
        (2) Jugular venous distension (JVD) or hepatojugular reflex (HJR).
    b. Heart.
        (1) Intercostal space (ICS) of the point of maximal impulse (PMI) at apex.
        (2) Location and character of lifts, heaves, thrills, and rubs.
        (3) Quality and splitting of first (S1) and second (S2) heart sounds.
        (4) S3 gallop: Third heart sound or "ventricular gallop." Low volume and frequency (pitch). Best heard with the bell at the apex in the early diastolic period and is normal in children.
        (5) S4 gallop: Fourth heart sound or "atrial gallop." Low volume and frequency. Best heard with the bell at the apex in the end-diastolic period.
        (6) Murmurs: Loudness (I-VI/VI); location and transmission; timing and duration (systolic or diastolic); components (e.g., opening snap, knocks); character and pitch (Is the murmur best heard with bell or diaphragm?); position of patient for eliciting or accentuating murmurs.
13. **Abdomen**
    a. Inspection: Distended, scars, striae, or dilated veins.
    b. Auscultation of bowel sounds and bruits.
    c. Palpation.
        (1) Abdomen: Tenderness or masses. Rebound tenderness, rigidity, or guarding. Fluid wave (positive or negative).
        (2) Hernia: Palpation with Valsalva or cough; bulge in abdominal wall versus palpable bowel in inguinal, femoral, or umbilical areas. (Direct or indirect hernia.)
        (3) Aorta: Tenderness, size, bruits.
        (4) Liver: Size and position (centimeters [cm] below the right costal margin [RCM] at the midclavicular line [MCL]); texture; hepatojugular reflux (HJR).
        (5) Gallbladder: Tenderness to palpation (TTP); Murphy's sign—pain with inspiration).
        (6) Spleen: Palpable or percussable, size, and position.
        (7) Kidneys: Size, bruits.
        (8) Bladder: Suprapubic tenderness.
14. **Genitalia**
    a. Men.
        (1) External appearance. Circumcised?
        (2) Penile lesions or discharge.

(3) Testicles: Descended bilaterally, tenderness, masses, consistency, varicocele, hydrocele.

b. Women.

(1) Bartholin's glands, Skeen's glands, urethral meatus, vulva (BSUV).

(2) Vaginal mucosa, masses, discharge. Cul-de-sac visualization.

(3) Rectocele, cystocele.

(4) Cervix: Parity, position, cervical motion tenderness, discharge, Pap smear.

(5) Uterus: Size, position (anteverted or retroverted), and masses.

(6) Adnexa: Ovarian sizes if palpable, position, masses, tenderness.

15. **Rectum/Prostate**

a. External appearance. Specify absence of fissures, fistulas, hemorrhoids. Diagram abnormalities using a clock designation.

b. Sphincter tone (normal or lax).

c. Guaiac test (positive or negative).

d. Prostate: Size, shape, and consistency (S/S/C). Specify absence of masses, nodules, and enlargement (i.e., 1.5, 2, or 2.5 times normal size).

16. **Back/Spine**

a. Symmetry, kyphotic and lordotic curvatures.

b. ROM.

c. Sacral edema, scars, or birthmarks/nevi.

d. Spinous processes sacroiliac (SI) joint tenderness.

e. Costovertebral angle tenderness (CVAT).

f. Muscle atrophy or tenderness, straight leg raise (SLR).

17. **Extremities**

a. Inspection: Bilateral symmetry, deformity, or weakness.

b. ROM: Active ROM, passive ROM, and specific joints.

c. Bone, joint, or muscle tenderness; swelling or inflammation; varicosities.

d. Vascular.

(1) Pulses 0 to 4+ (0 = absent; 1+ = difficult to palpate, weak; 2+ = normal; 3+ = easily palpable, increased; 4+ = bounding).

(2) Capillary refill (CR). Less than 2 seconds is considered normal.

(3) Clubbing, cyanosis, or edema (C/C/E); pitting edema: Bilateral measurement in millimeters (mm), documenting location.

(4) Lymphatics.

18. **Skin**

a. Texture, temperature, and turgor (e.g., cool/warm, moist/dry).

b. Pigmentation, nevi, or nail abnormalities.
c. Location of petechiae, rashes, nevi, birthmarks, jaundice, telangiectasias, C/C/E.

19. **Lymphadenopathy**
    a. Occipital, auricular, submental, tonsillar, cervical (anterior and posterior), supraclavicular, axillary, epitrochlear, or inguinal lymph nodes.
    b. Lymph nodes: Abnormal >1 cm diameter. Specify location, number, size, fixed or mobile, and tenderness.
20. **Neurologic** (See Chapter 21, Neurology, for detailed explanations.)
    a. Mental status exam: Attitude, reliability, general appearance, emotion (mood and affect), speech and language, thought processes, thought content, cognition, intelligence, insight, and judgment.
    b. Cranial nerves (CN) to direct confrontation. CN I = olfactory (smell), CN II = optic (vision), CN III = oculomotor (levator palpebrae, superioris, superior, medial and inferior recti muscles), CN IV = trochlear (superior oblique), CN V = trigeminal (muscles of mastication), CN VI = abducens (lateral rectus), CN VII = facial (facial expression, taste anterior two thirds of the tongue), CN VIII = vestibulocochlear (hearing and balance), CN IX = glossopharyngeal (stylopharyngeus), CN X = vagus (pharynx and larynx muscles), CN XI = spinal accessory (trapezius and sternocleidomastoid), CN XII = hypoglossal (tongue muscles except palatoglossal).
    c. Motor: Strength (0/5 absent, 1/5 trace, 2/5 weak, 3/5 fair, 4/5 good, 5/5 normal); ROM; and pronator drift.
    d. Sensory: Light touch, pin prick, proprioception, vibratory.
    e. Deep tendon reflexes (DTRs): Grading (0 = no response, 1+ = diminished, 2+ = normal, 3+ = increased, 4+ = hyperactive). Biceps C5-6, triceps C6-7, knee L2-4, ankle S-1.
    f. Babinski's sign: Extension of the great toe and abduction of the other toes instead of the normal flexion reflex to plantar stimulation. Down going bilateral great toes is a "normal" test.
    g. Cerebellar: Gait, station, and coordination (e.g., rapid alternating movements [RAM], finger-to-nose [F → N] and heel-to-shin [H → S] tests).

IX. SAMPLE PHYSICAL EXAMINATION WRITE-UP WITHOUT ABNORMALITIES

A. Exam Categories By System

1. **Vital Signs**
    a. Temperature: T = 98.6°F, afebrile over the last 24 hours. Maximum temperature (T_{max}) = 100°F in last 72 hours.
    b. Respiratory rate (RR): 16.

c. Pulse: 72.
d. Blood pressure: Sitting, 124/84 in left arm and 126/86 in right arm.
e. Height and weight: Ht = 73 inches, Wt = 187 pounds.

2. **General Appearance:** Well-nourished 23-year-old (yo) married white female (MWF), A&O x 4 (oriented to person, place, time, and condition) in no apparent distress (NAD). Another example with abnormalities: 23 yo MWF, A&O x 4 in moderate/severe discomfort and diaphoretic; sitting with arms clutching epigastrium, but still cooperative with questioning and examination.
3. **Head and Neck:** Normocephalic/atraumatic (NC/AT). Neck—full range of motion (FROM), no lymphadenopathy. Trachea midline. Thyroid smooth without nodules or bruits. No carotid bruits. No jugular venous distension (JVD) or hepatojugular reflux (HJR).
4. **Eyes:** Lids normal, conjunctivae clear (nonhyperemic) and sclerae nonicteric, pupils equally round and reactive to light and accommodation (PERRLA), extraocular muscles intact (EOMI), full visual fields by confrontation. Visual acuity (VA) Right (OD) __/__ Left (OS) __/__ (Jaegher chart at 12 inches; with or without glasses). Fundoscopic exam reveals sharp disk margins, cup-to-disk (C/D) ratio less than 0.5, normal macula and venous pulsations.
5. **Ears:** No tragus traction tenderness. No discharge noted, canals patent bilaterally (AU). TM's normal landmarks, light reflex and mobility. Acuity to whispered voice grossly intact. Weber midline, Rinne test air conduction greater than bone conduction (AC > BC).
6. **Nose:** No discharge noted. Nasal mucosa moist and pink. Septum midline and turbinates without polyps, congestion, or inflammation. No frontal or maxillary sinus TTP.
7. **Mouth:** Lips, buccal mucosa and gingiva; oropharynx (O/P) moist and pink, without erythema, ulcerations, or petechiae. Tongue symmetrical without fissures or ulcerations.
8. **Throat:** Tonsils without erythema or exudate.
9. **Teeth:** Normal dentition (no dentures or bridges; if present remove for exam).
10. **Chest:** Symmetrical with equal expansion. No pain, tenderness, or masses upon palpation. No gynecomastia (males). Breasts and axilla without pain, tenderness, or masses upon palpation. No nipple retraction or inversion, erythema, or discharge. No axillary lymph nodes palpable.
11. **Lungs:** Lungs clear to auscultation and percussion (CTAP), breath sounds equal bilaterally. Normal chest symmetry/AP

diameter without use of accessory muscles. No wheezes, rales (crackles), or rhonchi. No dullness to percussion. Diaphragmatic excursion is approximately __cm in the midscapular line. Tactile fremitus normal.

12. **Cardiovascular:** Normal S1 and S2. Normal S2 splitting with inspiration. S3 and S4 absent. Regular rate without murmurs, rubs, heaves, or thrills. Point of maximal intensity (PMI) __cm in the __th intercostal space (ICS)/left midclavicular line (MCL). Peripheral pulses symmetric and 2+ throughout.
13. **Abdomen:** Soft, nontender, nondistended, normal active bowel sounds (S, NT, ND, NABS) without hepatosplenomegaly (HSM). Liver edge not palpable and (normal 6 to 12 cm) at the right MCL by percussion. No masses palpable. No abnormal aortic pulsations. No peritoneal signs. No dilated veins, bruits, shifting dullness, or fluid wave. No suprapubic tenderness. No hernia palpable with Valsalva/cough/straining.
14. **Genitalia**
    a. Male: Normal male external genitalia without lesions, circumcised/uncircumcised, testes descended bilaterally and normal size, shape, and consistency (S/S/C).
    b. Female: Normal external female genitalia. Normal Bartholin's glands, Skeen's glands, and urethra (B/S/U) and vaginal mucosa (BSUV). Introitus without lesions or discharge. Nulliparous cervix without erythema, lesions, or discharge. Bimanual exam: Anteverted uterus normal S/S/C; nulliparous cervix, cervical motion tenderness (CMT) absent, normal adnexa without mass or tenderness.
15. **Rectum/Prostate:** No external anal lesions. Normal sphincter tone, no fissures, fistulas, or palpable hemorrhoids. Heme or guaiac negative. Prostate normal S/S/C without nodules or masses.
16. **Back/Spine:** Straight and symmetrical. No abnormal spinal curvatures. No costovertebral angle tenderness (CVAT).
17. **Extremities:** Upper extremities (UE) and lower extremities (LE) symmetrical, full range of motion (FROM) without joint tenderness, swelling, or deformity. No clubbing/cyanosis/edema (C/C/E). Pulses 2+ bilaterally.
18. **Skin:** Warm and dry. Normal turgor. No lesions, rashes, or petechiae.
19. **Lymphatics:** No cervical, axillary, or inguinal adenopathy.
20. **Neurologic:** Alert and oriented times four (A&Ox4); person, place, time, and condition). Mini-mental status examination (MMSE) unremarkable. Cranial nerves II to XII intact by direct confrontation. Motor 5/5 strength throughout with good tone.

Sensory intact throughout to pain, light touch, two-point discrimination, vibratory, and proprioception. Cerebellar function intact by finger-to-nose (F → N), heel-to-shin (H → S), and RAM. Gait is symmetrical and balanced (broad-based). Station: No drift, Romberg negative. Reflexes 2+ symmetrical. Babinski negative (down going). No asterixis.

2

RECORDING LABORATORY VALUES AND DIAGNOSTIC INFORMATION, AND CONVERSION TABLES

Eric H. Hanson, MD, MPH, and Sam Galvagno, DO

I. LABORATORY VALUES

A. Notation for Standard Blood Tests

1. Compare abnormal lab values with past records, past admission records, or computer files.
2. Use shorthand notation (see following examples) for recording laboratory and study values.

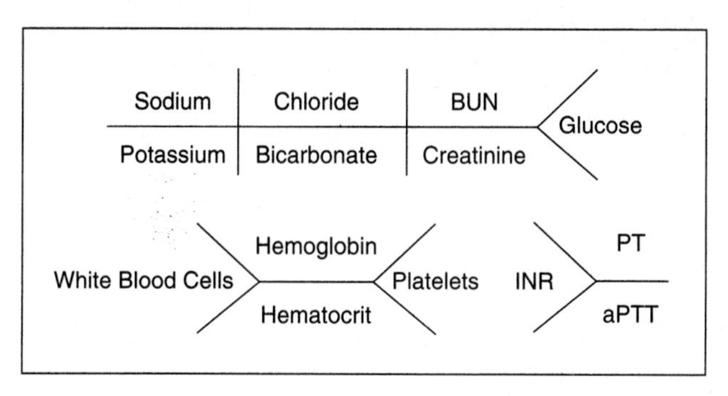

3. Record additional information (e.g., mean corpuscular volume [MCV], percent neutrophils) next to the shorthand notation.

B. Arterial Blood Gas Notation

1. Report blood gases as follows:

pH/CO_2/Bicarbonate/SPO_2/Base excess
Example: 7.40/40/28/100%/-1

2. Record the anion gap next to the serum chemistry values or next to the arterial blood gas values.
3. In the assessment portion of the report, identify the primary acid-base disorder identified and describe differential diagnosis discussed. Always correlate the arterial blood gas results with the patient's condition.

II. SUPPLEMENTARY DIAGNOSTIC INFORMATION

A. Electrocardiogram (ECG)

1. Record rate, rhythm, axis, and intervals after a systematic analysis.

2. Record evidence for infarction, ischemia, or chamber abnormalities.
3. Seek previous ECGs and compare to present ECG.

B. **Chest Radiograph:** Identify abnormality first, then provide a systematic analysis of the film.

C. **Pulmonary Function Tests**

1. Report results of spirometry, expiratory flow-volume curves, and flow-volume interpretation.
2. Include results from other studies, such as diffusion capacities (DL_{CO}) or bronchial provocation tests.

D. **Other Diagnostic Tests:** Note diagnostic information from tests such as computed tomographic (CT) studies, magnetic resonance imaging (MRI), and other studies.

III. EQUIVALENTS AND CONVERSION TABLES (Tables 2-1 and 2-2)

Table 2-1. APPROXIMATE HOUSEHOLD, APOTHECARY, AND METRIC VOLUME EQUIVALENTS.

Household	Apothecary	Metric (Milliliters)
1 teaspoon (t or tsp)	<1 fluid dram	4 mL
1 teaspoon, medical	1 fluid dram	5 mL
1 dessert spoon	>1/4 fluid ounce	8 mL
1 tablespoon (T or Tbsp)	1/2 fluid ounce	15 mL
2 tablespoons	1 fluid ounce	30 mL
1 teacup	4 fluid ounces	120 mL
1 measuring cupful	8 fluid ounces	240 mL
1 pint (pt)	16 fluid ounces	473 mL
2 pints (1 quart)	32 fluid ounces	946 mL
1 quart (qt)	32 fluid ounces	946 mL
4 quarts (1 gallon)	128 fluid ounces	3785 mL
1 gallon (gal)	128 fluid ounces	3785 mL

Table 2-2. APOTHECARY WEIGHTS AND VOLUMES.

Apothecary Weight	Apothecary Volume
20 drops (gtts)	1 mL
12 ounces	1 pound (lb)
16 fluid ounces	1 pint (pt)
2 pints	1 quart (qt)
4 quarts	1 gallon (gal)

A. Formulas for Converting Degrees Fahrenheit and Degrees Celsius (Box 2-1)

1. To convert °F to °C:

(Degrees Fahrenheit − 32) ÷ 1.8 = Degrees Celsius

2. To convert °C to °F:

(Degrees Celsius × 1.8) + 32 = Degrees Fahrenheit

Box 2-1. TEMPERATURE CONVERSIONS (CELSIUS TO FAHRENHEIT).

37.0 = 98.6	38.6 = 101.4	40.1 = 104.2
37.1 = 98.8	38.7 = 101.6	40.2 = 104.4
37.2 = 99.0	38.8 = 101.8	40.3 = 104.6
37.3 = 99.2	38.9 = 102.0	40.4 = 104.8
37.4 = 99.4	39.0 = 102.2	40.6 = 105.0
37.6 = 99.6	39.1 = 102.4	40.7 = 105.2
37.7 = 99.8	39.2 = 102.6	40.8 = 105.4
37.8 = 100.0	39.3 = 102.8	40.9 = 105.6
37.9 = 100.2	39.4 = 103.0	41.0 = 105.8
38.0 = 100.4	39.6 = 103.2	41.2 = 106.0
38.1 = 100.6	39.7 = 103.4	41.3 = 106.2
38.2 = 100.8	39.8 = 103.6	41.4 = 106.4
38.3 = 101.0	39.9 = 103.8	41.5 = 106.6
38.4 = 101.2	40.0 = 104.0	41.6 = 106.8

B. Miscellaneous Calculations and Conversions

1. Intravenous flow rate (drops or gtts/min) calculation. Volume (mL) to be infused × Drip factor (i.e., number of drops equal to one mL; Mini-drip is 60 gtts/mL, Maxi-drip is 10 gtts/mL, Blood administration is 10 gtts/mL) ÷ Administration time (minutes).
2. Volume and intravenous rate conversion formulas:

mg/100 mL = (mEq/L ÷ 10) × Equivalents/weight
mEq/L = mg/100 mL × 10 ÷ Equivalent weight
mg/mL = mg/mL × 1000
mL/min = mL/hr ÷ 60
mg/kg/min = (mg/mL × mL/min) ÷ wt(kg)
mL/hr = (wt(kg) × mg/kg/min) ÷ mg/mL × 60

3. Concentration conversions: Example: 20% KCl solution = 20 grams KCl per deciliter (g/dL).

4. Miscellaneous metric conversions:

$$\text{cm}\,\text{II}_2\text{O} \times 0.735 - \text{mm}\,\text{IIg}$$
$$\text{mm Hg} = 1.36 = \text{cm}\,H_2O\ (1\ \text{mm Hg} = 1.36\ \text{cm}\,H_2O)$$
$$1\ \text{inch} = 2.54\,\text{cm}$$
$$1\ \text{pound} = 0.454\,\text{kg}$$
$$2.204\ \text{pounds (lb)} = 1\ \text{kg} = 1\ \text{liter fluid}$$
$$1\,\text{cm} = 0.3973\ \text{inch}$$
$$4\ \text{quarts} = 1\ \text{gallon}$$

3

ASSESSMENT AND PLAN FORMULATION

Sam Galvagno, DO, and Eric H. Hanson, MD, MPH

I. ASSESSMENT AND PLAN (A&P) OVERVIEW

After the patient's history, review of systems, physical examination, and initial labs and studies have been completed, all of this information must be compiled and interpreted. The assessment and plan formulation provides a useful summary of the patient's problems and recommended diagnostic and therapeutic approaches for consultants, attending physicians, medical students, nurses, dietitians, social workers, and other health care personnel who will view the patient's medical record or chart.

II. INPATIENT A&P FORMULATIONS

A. **Combined or Traditional Approach:** This approach is commonly used with a patient who has a known diagnosis or when an etiology appears highly likely. It is also a useful way to approach any differential diagnosis or internal medicine write-up. Describe by focusing on the characteristics of the disorder.

1. Anatomy involved.
2. Symptoms and signs.
3. Pathophysiology.
4. Etiology.

B. **Problem-Oriented Medical Record (POMR)**

1. The problem list is created using any symptoms and objective findings from the physical examination (PE) or laboratory values that require further evaluation.
2. The problems listed do not all have to be diagnoses.
3. List problems in order of importance.
4. Designate each problem as active or inactive and acute or chronic. State the duration.

C. **Traditional and POMR Approach:** A combination of these approaches is often used. Although the process will be cumbersome at first, these guidelines provide a logical and organized approach.

III. FOUR-STEP APPROACH TO A&P FORMULATION

A. **Four-Step Approach to A&P Formulation**

1. Gather clinical information.
   a. "Diagnoses You Can't Miss." Begin thinking of the "diagnoses you can't miss" as soon as you start gathering clinical information. The primary questions to ask yourself when you evaluate a patient for the first time on the ward,

in the clinic, or as a physician in the emergency department are as follows:

(1) Does this patient (or will this patient) need resuscitation? If the answer is yes, then focus immediately on airway, breathing, and circulation (ABCs).

(2) Can we provide care here (e.g., on the ward) or do we need to transfer the patient to the ICU?

b. Problem list. Correlate the information from the history of present illness (HPI) and PE into a problem list. A problem list is a useful way to organize your thoughts and convey clear, concise information to others. Think about the symptoms described by the patient (with additional information gathered from the HPI) and the objective findings and signs elicited on the PE. Assessment and plan for each problem will then be discussed after the problem list.

c. Compilation of the problem list occurs in an additive, step-by-step mental process.

(1) Add the date and chronology of the diagnoses and indicate whether they are acute or chronic.

(2) Include complications associated with the disorder.

(3) Indicate past and current therapies.

2. Construct a differential diagnosis list.

a. Consider serious "diagnoses you can't miss" (rule out [r/o] any life-threatening disorders first) and minor disorders capable of producing the current signs and symptoms.

b. Construct a differential diagnosis, placing disorders with the highest probability at the top of the list.

c. Diagnostic testing.

(1) Early stages of the work-up will consist of commonly ordered tests or studies (e.g., complete blood count [CBC], electrolytes, blood urea nitrogen/creatinine [BUN/Cr], urinalysis [UA], prothrombin time/partial thromboplastin time [PT/PTT], electrocardiogram [ECG], chest x-ray [CXR]. When considering further testing, ask yourself, "How will this change the patient's management plan?"

(2) Weigh the risks and benefits of each therapeutic or lab/study intervention.

(3) Unexpected test results that are markedly abnormal and require prompt evaluation or treatment should be repeated for confirmation while preparation is made for possible treatment, if the results are true.

(4) Spurious factors, such as human or equipment errors, account for a high proportion of unexpected results. If possible, r/o lab error before engaging unsuspected disorders as the etiology.

3. Refine the differential diagnosis.
   a. Provide a brief summary before identifying and discussing each individual problem.
   b. Evaluate each problem using the following format:
      (1) Anatomy involved.
      (2) Pathophysiology.
      (3) Possible etiologies.
4. Select a tentative diagnosis. Consider the disease process in terms of anatomy, pathophysiology, and possible etiologies.

B. A&P Outline for the HPI and PE Write-Up

1. Continue with a brief discussion of each active problem.
   a. Pertinent positive symptoms and signs (symptoms, PE objective data, lab data, studies).
   b. Pertinent negative symptoms and signs not seen with the patient upon presentation.
   c. Differential diagnosis list with "diagnoses you can't miss" at the top.
   d. Diagnostic and therapeutic plans.
   e. Patient education and counseling about the disorder and treatment plan.
   f. General outline for a medicine write-up.
      (1) Summary of chief complaint(s).
      (2) Positive factors: Signs and symptoms to justify a diagnosis.
      (3) Negative factors: Signs and symptoms associated with the disorder(s) but not present at the time of patient presentation.
      (4) Problem list.
      (5) Laboratory tests: Reasons for ordering, sensitivity, specificity, and likelihood considerations.
      (6) Clinical studies.
      (7) Anatomy involved.
      (8) Pathophysiology.
      (9) Possible etiologies, differential diagnosis.
      (10) Incidence/prevalence and other epidemiologic information.
      (11) Risks and complications, morbidity and mortality of the disorder(s).
      (12) Treatment and side effects.
      (13) Patient education.
      (14) Prognosis/determinants of survival.
2. Identify areas of insufficient data (e.g., fever of unknown origin [FUO] with illness of more than three weeks' duration and lack of specific diagnosis/etiology after 1 week of inpatient investigation).
3. Discuss any further possible work-up or treatment options.

IV. A&P SAMPLE WRITE-UP

J.R. is a 19-year-old male presenting to the emergency department for the chief complaint of headache, vomiting, and general malaise. Mr. R.'s medical history is significant for insulin-dependent diabetes mellitus, opioid dependence, polysubstance abuse, and recent PPD conversion. Mr. R is lethargic during the interview but relates a history of diffuse headache, myalgia, malaise, and vomiting for 2 days. He vomited three times before arriving to the emergency department. Mr. R states he has been coughing for the past day with production of greenish phlegm. He admits to noncompliance with his insulin for 1 day; he was "too sick" to administer his morning injection. He does not relate any recent history of polyuria, polydipsia, or visual disturbances. His medications include isoniazid (INH) and vitamin B_6, Humulin® insulin 70/30 (45 units in AM and 20 units before dinner), and methadone, 35 mg each day. He tested HIV negative 2 months ago. He continues to use marijuana regularly but denies any additional intravenous drug abuse or tobacco use. He admits to occasional binge drinking. Initial vitals upon admission to the emergency department are as follows: HR 104, BP 154/84, SPO_2 98% (room air), T (oral) = 103.2°F.

Upon examination, the patient is lethargic and irritable but conversant when prompted. He is a thin Hispanic male who appears well-developed but dehydrated. No odors of alcohol or acetone are detectable on the breath. His breathing appears to be nonlabored at a rate of 24-25/minute. Perioral skin flaking is noted as well as dry mucous membranes. Auscultation of the lungs fails to reveal any adventitious sounds. The heart has a regular rate and rhythm without any murmurs or rubs. Bowel sounds are present in all quadrants, and no tenderness is produced with palpation. The neurologic exam does not reveal either Brudzinski's or Kernig's sign. Skin turgor is normal and no rash is present.

Laboratory tests are significant for the following: glucose: 467 mg/dL; serum osmolality: 29 mOsm/kg; anion gap: 16; serum sodium: 421 mg/dL; serum potassium: 4.2 mEq/L; serum acetone: positive; chest radiograph: left lateral basilar infiltrate; arterial blood gas: 7.30/36/16/100%; urinalysis: 3+ glucose, 3+ ketones; serum alcohol level: 0; white blood cell count: 16.9 with 88% neutrophils.

Summary: This is a 19-year-old male with a history of insulin-dependent diabetes and a positive PPD test presenting with fever, cough, dehydration, and laboratory data supporting the tentative diagnosis of diabetic ketoacidosis (DKA), possibly caused by the physiologic stress of a community-acquired pneumonia.

#1. Metabolic acidosis with increased anion gap (normal osmolar gap)

Anatomy: Insufficient production of insulin by beta-cells of the islets of Langerhan's in the pancreas.

Pathophysiology

Generation of ketones; produced by incomplete oxidation of fatty acids.

Glycolysis inhibited; gluconeogenesis stimulated by lack of insulin.

Etiology: Given previous history of DM: diabetic ketoacidosis (DKA). Possibly exacerbated by underlying infection (pneumonia versus active pulmonary tuberculosis versus medication noncompliance).

Treatment

Insulin infusion, aggressive rehydration with 0.9% saline, potassium correction as needed.

Insulin bolus of 0.15 U/kg; will monitor glucose every 2 to 4 hours after first 2 hours (goal: decrease glucose by 80 mg/dL/hr).

Address underlying cause: pneumonia (see following section).

ICU admission indicated for close observation of blood glucose levels.

#2. Hypovolemia

Anatomy: Osmotic diuresis in the kidney; action of insulin opposed in the liver by counterregulatory hormones (e.g., catecholamines, glucagons).

Pathophysiology

Elevated glucose and serum ketones; osmotic diuresis.

Catecholamine release stimulated also in response to insulin deficiency.

Etiology: DKA most likely.

Treatment

Calculate fluid deficit and replace with 0.9% saline until blood pressure and organ perfusion restored. Gradually decrease infusion rate and transition to hypotonic saline (0.45%) for next 12 hours.

Continue fluids until glucose below 300 mg/dL then change to 5% dextrose in water to prevent hypoglycemia.

Replace electrolytes accordingly; anticipate potassium and phosphate deficits caused by intracellular osmotic shifts; and obtain baseline ECG and follow serum chemistries.

#3. Pulmonary infiltrate

Anatomy: Left lower basilar segment of lung affected.

Pathophysiology: Inflammation and edema of the lung parenchyma, most likely secondary to infection. Infection would explain fever (normal host response) and elevated white blood cell count, as well as underlying cause of DKA.

Etiology: Pneumonia; most likely community-acquired; *S. pneumococcus* most likely. Consider further diagnostic testing and blood cultures to identify organism. Tuberculosis must also be considered.

Treatment

Initiate intravenous antibiotics (beta-lactam and macrolide or fluoroquinolone) for both community-acquired and atypical pneumonia coverage.

Blood cultures: Consider invasive (bronchoscopy) measures as needed for diagnostic purposes.

Isolation until results of previous work-up for PPD positively known.

HIV testing indicated given history of polysubstance abuse; will attempt to obtain consent.

#4. PPD positive

Anatomy: Local immune reaction in the dermis and epidermis.

Pathophysiology: Gell & Coombs Type IV, cell-mediated delayed hypersensitivity reaction. Reaction caused by sensitized lymphocytes, killer T-cells, and macrophages.

Etiology: Active tuberculosis or old tuberculosis infection. Positive PPD only means exposure, not active infection.

Treatment

Attempt to obtain old medical records for previous work-up.

Collect three sputum specimens for acid-fast staining to rule out active pulmonary TB.

Maintain INH therapy with Vitamin B_6. Isolation until pulmonary TB ruled out.

#5. Opioid dependence

Anatomy: Opioid receptors in brain and nervous system.

Pathophysiology: Down regulation of receptors; requiring maintenance levels of opioid to prevent withdrawal.

Etiology: Possible intravenous drug use because of social circumstances/environment.

Treatment

Continue methadone dosage once confirmed by methadone maintenance program.

Psychiatric and social consultation may be of benefit once patient stabilized.

4

CHARTWORK GUIDELINES

Eric H. Hanson, MD, MPH

I. CHART ORDERS

A. Admission Orders (ADC VAAN DISSEL)

1. **A**dmit to:
2. **D**iagnosis:
3. **C**ondition:
4. **V**ital signs:
5. **A**llergies:
6. **A**ctivity:
7. **N**ursing: Specify parameters for ambulation, chest percussion (i.e., pulmonary toilet), incentive spirometry, daily weights, monitoring inputs and outputs (I&Os), dressing changes, wound care, patient precautions, guaiac stools, etc. Notify for:
   - **a.** Temp > 100.5°F.
   - **b.** HR > 120 or < 50.
   - **c.** BP < 100/60 or > 180/100.
   - **d.** RR > 40.
   - **e.** Urine output (U/O) <0.5–1.0 mL/kg/hour.
   - **f.** Bright red blood saturating dressing.
8. **D**iet: Regular, dental soft, clear, liquid, fortified clear, cardiac diet, renal diet.
9. **I**nputs and outputs (I&Os): IV fluid, type, rate, heplock, strict I&O record.
10. **S**pecial medications.
    - **a.** Incoming medications.
    - **b.** Therapeutic medications.
11. **S**ymptomatic medications: For pain, sedation, constipation, sleep, anxiety, etc.
12. **E**xams: Electrocardiograph (ECG), chest x-ray (CXR), intravenous pyelogram (IVP) with appropriate preparations.
13. **L**abs: CBC, electrolytes, BUN/Cr, Ca/Mg/Phos, LFTs, urinalysis (UA), drug levels, type and cross (T&C), PT/PTT, arterial blood gas (ABG).

B. Preoperative (Preop) Orders

1. Nothing by mouth, or nil per os (NPO), after midnight.
2. Intravenous (IV) orders.
3. Meds: Preoperative antibiotics, etc.
4. Labs: T&C, CBC, PT/PTT, electrolytes, BUN/CR.

5. Prep and shave as needed (prn), antiseptic shower.
6. Void (have patient urinate) on call to operating room (OR).
7. Premedicate with __________ (usually ordered by anesthesia).

II. CHART NOTES

A. Preop Note

1. Preop diagnosis.
2. Procedure.
3. Indications.
4. Labs.
5. CXR.
6. ECG.
7. Consent discussed and signed. Explained risks, benefits, expected results, and alternatives to the patient.
8. Evaluated by anesthesia (date and time).

B. Procedure Note

1. Procedure.
2. Indications.
3. Informed consent discussed and signed (see Chapter 37, Ethical Considerations). Indications, adverse reactions, complications, expected results, and alternatives discussed with patient.
4. Describe procedure.
5. Anesthesia and pain control.
6. Specimens.
7. Complications.
8. Condition after procedure.
9. CXR (if applicable).

C. Night-of-Surgery Note

1. Procedure.
2. Level of consciousness (LOC).
3. Vital signs (VS).
4. I&O.
5. Physical exam.
6. Labs.
7. Assessment.
8. Plan.

D. Off-Service Note

1. Date of admission.
2. Diagnosis or diagnoses.
3. Hospital course.
4. Past medical history.
5. Discharge medications.
6. Physical exam.
7. Labs.
8. Assessments.
9. Follow-up plan.

E. Operative Note

1. Preop diagnosis.
2. Postop diagnosis.
3. Procedure.
4. Surgeons.
5. Anesthesia and pain control.
6. Findings.
7. Specimens/frozens sent to Pathology.
8. Drains/tubes/IVs.
9. Estimated blood loss (EBL) in milliliters.
10. Fluids used in the procedure.
11. Tourniquet time (orthopedic cases).
12. Complications.
13. Condition/disposition.

F. Postop Check

1. Notify attending or provider on call if no urine output 6 to 8 hours postprocedure.
2. Pain assessment and treatment.
3. Incentive spirometer 10 times per hour.
4. Antiembolic stockings and pillows.
5. NPO until no nausea and positive flatus with active bowel sounds.
6. Ambulation and turning instructions.

G. Intensive Care Unit (ICU) Note

1. 24-hour events.
2. Indwelling lines.
3. Oxygen (O_2) status.
4. Medications.
5. Vital signs.
6. Physical exam.
7. I&Os.
8. Labs.
9. Radiology.
10. Studies.

H. ICU Assessment and Plan by Systems

1. Central nervous system (CNS).
2. Respiratory.
3. Cardiovascular.
4. Gastrointestinal (GI)/nutrition.
5. Renal/metabolic.
6. Genitourinary (GU).
7. Infectious disease (ID).

I. Discharge Summary Note

1. Admission date.
2. Discharge date.
3. Admitting diagnosis.

4. Discharge diagnosis.
5. Attending and service caring for patient.
6. Referring physician: Provide address and telephone number, if available.
7. Procedures: Minor surgeries, surgeries, and invasive diagnostic procedures (e.g., thoracentesis, lumbar punctures).
8. Brief history: Pertinent history, physical, and lab data. Summarize the most important points about the admission.
9. Hospital course: Summarize the evaluation, treatments, and progress.
10. Condition at discharge: Note qualitative and quantitative, subjective and objective improvements at discharge.
11. Disposition: Location to where the client was discharged (e.g., home, another hospital, nursing home). Try to give specific information and accepting physician if transferred to another medical institution.
12. Discharge medications: List medications, number of refills, side effects of medications discussed with the patient.
13. Discharge instructions and follow-up: (e.g., clinic return date, diet instructions, activity restrictions).
14. Problem list: Listing of active and past (chronic) medical problems.

J. Delivery Note

______-year-old (married or single) (state race/ethnicity) gravida (G) ______ now para (P) ______, abortion (Ab). Admitted to ______ (clinic vs. other). Estimated date of confinement (EDC) ______, and a prenatal course (uncomplicated or describe any problems, infections, tobacco, drug, or alcohol use). Labor course and complications (pitocin induced, premature rupture) and draped in the usual sterile fashion. Under controlled conditions delivered a ______ lb ______ oz (______ gram) viable male or female infant under ______ (general, spinal, pudendal) anesthesia. Delivery was via spontaneous vaginal delivery (SVD) with midline episiotomy (or forceps or cesarean section). APGARs were ______ at 1 minute and ______ at 5 minutes (state delivery date and time). Cord blood sent to lab and placenta expressed with trailing membranes intact. Uterus explored. Lacerations of the ______ degree repaired by standards method with good hemostasis and restoration of normal anatomy.

1. Estimated blood loss (EBL).
2. Maternal blood type (MBT).
3. Hematocrit (HCT): Predelivery and postdelivery.
4. Rubella titers (RT).
5. VDRL test.
6. Condition of mother.

K. Sign-Out Note

SAMPLE SIGN-OUT NOTE.		
Date, Name, Age, Gender	**Diagnoses and Medical History**	**To Do**
Orientation to Person/Place/Time	**Meds (Dose & Frequency)**	**Concerns**
07 SEP 2002/1930 Robbins, Gerald 71-yo WM Deaf and combative Alert and oriented to person only	CRF CHF IDDM HTN Digoxin Lasix Insulin Lisinopril	1. Check K^+ level, Tx PRN 2. BP, Tx as needed 3. Check blood culture if temperature >102°F, start antibiotics 4. If bleeding occurs; check CBC; transfuse PLT, FFP or NTD

L. SOAP(P) Note

Date. Medical Student Third-year (MS III) Note or Medical Student Progress Note (MSPN).

Time. Hospital Day (HD) #1, Antibiotic Day #1, Postop Day (POD) #2.

S: Patient c/o "right side of my stomach hurting." He complained of sporadic throbbing pain and nausea, but denies vomiting, diarrhea, hematochezia, chills, dysuria, chest pain, or SOB.

O: VS (0600 hrs): T = 99.6°F, T_{max} 24 hrs = 100.5°F, R = 22, P = 100, BP = 120/80.

PE: Gen: 20-yo obese male. In distress, writhing in bed secondary to pain.

HEENT: No change from prior exam.

Lungs: Clear to auscultation and percussion (CTAP).

CV: RR with I/VI SEM best at LLSB. No change from prior exam.

Abd: Obese, no bowel sounds audible. Positive rebound, shake and jar tests. Involuntary guarding of RLQ.

Ext: No C/C/E.

LAB: CBC (23 Mar 94, 0620): WBC = 11.2 K, hemoglobin/hematocrit (H/H) = 12/36.

I&Os: Record for all drains and Foley catheter. Call if urine output <30 mL/hour.

A: Acute abdomen. Rule out appendicitis.

P: Consulted General Surgery. Scheduled for laparoscopic evaluation and probable appendectomy at 1200. Continue NPO and intravenous fluids (IVFs). Type and cross two units.

P (Prevention): Postoperative education on preventing infection at the surgical site.

M. ICU Progress Note Format

1. Date:
2. Hospital/unit day:
3. **Physical exam vital signs:** T: ______, BP: ______, HR: ______, RR: ______, oxygen saturation (percentage of hemoglobin carrying oxygen [SaO_2]): ______.
4. 24-hour events:
5. **Neuro:** Mental status/Glasgow Coma Scale (MS/GCS): ______, deep tendon reflexes (DTRs): ______, focal deficits: ______.
6. **Respiratory (Resp):** Physical Exam (Exam or PE): ______, ventilator mode: ______, fraction of inspired oxygen (FIO_2): ______, rate (R): ______, tidal volume (TV): ______, peak end-expiratory pressure (PEEP): ______, minute volume (MV): ______, peak inspiratory pressure (PIP): ______, hydrogen ion concentration (pH): ______, partial pressure (tension) of carbon dioxide (PCO_2): ______, partial pressure (tension) of oxygen (PO_2): ______, oxygen saturation (SAT): ______, bicarbonate dissolved in blood (HCO_3^-): ______, CXR: ______, weaning parameters (from the ventilator): ______.
7. **Cardiovascular (CV):** Exam: ______, HR: ______, mean arterial pressure (MAP): ______, central venous pressure (CVP): ______, PAP: ______, pulmonary capillary wedge pressure (PCWP): ______, cardiac output (CO): ______, systemic vascular resistance (SVR): ______, peripheral vascular resistance (PVR): ______, alveolo-arterial oxygen gradient (A-a DO_2): ______, oxygen delivery (DO_2): ______, oxygen consumption or uptake (VO_2): ______, electrocardiograph (ECG): ______, cardiovascular medications (CV meds): ______.
8. **Nutrition/Metabolic:** Electrolytes: ______, calcium (Ca): ______, magnesium (Mg): ______, phosphorus (Phos): ______, albumin (Alb): ______, cholesterol (Chol): ______, triglycerides (TG): ______, glucose range: ______, 24-hr insulin: ______, nitrogen balance: ______, diet: ______, basal energy expenditure (BEE): ______, calories (Kcal): ______, protein: ______, dextrose/fat ratio (Dex/fat): ______.
9. **Fluids/Lines:** Arterial (A), tracheostomy (T), nasogastric tube (NG), Foley (F), preop weight: yesterday: ______, today: ______, exam: ______, edema: ______.

   Inputs: Total parenteral nutrition (TPN): ______, intravenous (IV): ______, per os or by mouth (PO): ______ = total.

   Outputs: Urine: ______, nasogastric tube (NG): ______, drains: ______ = total.

   Net fluid balance =

10. **Renal:** Blood urea nitrogen (BUN): ______, creatinine (Cr): ______, hourly urine output (UOP): ______, urine electrolytes: Sodium (Na): ______, potassium (K): ______, chloride (Cl): ______, serum/urine osmolarity (S/U Osm): ______, creatinine clearance (Cr clearance): ______.
    Urinalysis (UA): Specific gravity (Sp gr), Protein (Pr), and list other parameters.
11. **GI/Hepatic:** Exam: ______, serum aspartate aminotransferase (ALT), serum alanine aminotransferase (AST), (ALT : AST ratio or SGPT/SGOT ratio): ______, alkaline phosphatase (alk phos): ______. Total/direct bilirubin (T/D Bili): ______, Albumin (Alb): ______. Total protein (TP): ______.
12. **Heme:** White blood cells (WBC): ______. Hemoglobin and hematocrit (H/H): ______, platelets (PLT): ______, prothrombin time/partial thromboplastin time (PT/PTT): ______, thrombin time (TT): ______, reticulocytes (Retic): ______, fibrin (Fib): ______, fibrin split products (FSP): ______ Blood products: ______.
13. **Skin:** Exam: ______, decubiti: ______, dressings: ______.
14. **ID:** Temperature (Temp): ______, WBC: ______, cultures/Gram stains: ______, antibiotics (dose and day): ______.
15. Radiology:
16. Other studies:
17. Medications:

III. PRESCRIPTION WRITING

Name______________	Age______________
Address______________	Date______________
Claritin 10 mg.	Tylenol #3.
Sig: 1 tab po once a day (qd)	Sig: 1 tab po every six hours prn pain.
Disp: #30.	Disp: # 6 (Six).*
Refill: 2.	Refill: 0 (Zero—Do Not Refill).

Sig = directions.
Disp = total quantity to dispense.

*For all controlled substances, always write out the number to dispense and number of refills to prevent tampering. Include DEA# on prescriptions for all controlled substances. A pharmacist may call you someday asking if you really wanted to give out 6 or 60 tablets. There are three things to remember when writing a prescription: Write legibly, write legibly, write legibly.

5

PRESENTATION OF MEDICAL CASES

Sam Galvagno, DO, and Eric H. Hanson, MD, MPH

I. PRESENTATION OF MEDICAL CASES

A. Tips to Think About

1. Average attention span is 30 seconds.
2. Bullet presentations are short, concise 1- to 2-minute presentations to quickly update people who are unfamiliar with the case.
3. Formal presentations follow the format below and should last 5 to 7 minutes (cases with "multiple medical problems" must be prioritized to fall under the 7-minute mark). Superfluous information and data must be filtered to give the pertinent information about your diagnosis (or differential diagnosis) and, simultaneously, present your team with a clear assessment and plan.
4. Understanding, control, and preparation provide confidence. Practice one more time after you have it down. Concise, organized, positive, and memorable are important descriptors to strive for with each presentation. Speak clearly, decisively, and loud enough so that no one is straining to hear what you say.
5. Open with a greeting, maintain eye contact (or look right above their heads), smile, try to look awake, and free up your hands (try not to read directly off cards or notes).
6. Remember, there are only two types of questions:
   - **a.** Those you don't want to be asked.
   - **b.** Those you would love to be asked and never are.
7. Think of your own medical questions to ask the Attendings before you enter the room.
8. Utilize each presentation as a chance to improve your presentation skills, as well as a chance to learn by experience.

B. Preparation for Presentations

1. History and Physical (H&P) information.
   - **a.** Photocopy the H&P sheets. Highlight the pertinent information that you want to convey about this patient to your colleagues. Consolidate the information to allow placement in an outline format on a notecard.
   - **b.** Practice, practice, practice . . . until the notecards are not required, if possible. Use the notecards before the presentation or to jog your memory during the presentation. Each practice should require only 2 to 7 minutes.

C. **Notecard Information**
1. Patient information.
2. Chief complaint (CC) and duration.
3. History of present illness (HPI).
   a. Logical progression of signs and symptoms.
   b. Significant positives and negatives from the review of systems.
   c. Other pertinent information (e.g., family history, cardiac risk factors, tobacco use, alcohol use).
4. Medical history: Significant active medical problems.
5. Surgical history: Significant or contributory to the chief complaint.
6. Medications: Dosing, duration of use, missed or last doses, adverse or allergic reactions.
7. Physical exam findings.
   a. Always include vital signs: "Vital signs are stable" is acceptable only if true.
   b. General description of appearance and/or condition.
   c. Pertinent positives only.
8. Lab tests: Tests ordered and pertinent abnormalities.
9. Problem list: Include differential diagnosis if further evaluation is required.
10. Assessment and plan for each problem: Have a plan ready.

D. **"Bullet Presentations"**
1. Patient information: Name, age, and sex.
2. Chief complaint.
3. Medical history. Multiple medical problems including . . .
4. History of present illness. Include only the most important facts to "paint a picture."
5. Medications.
6. Physical exam: Statement of general condition, vital signs, and exam findings.
7. Lab findings.
8. Problem list: Current treatment and plan for all active medical problems.
9. Summary: Two sentences. Practice this every day on rounds.

Sample Bullet Presentation: J.R., 41-year-old female. Fairly reliable historian.

Chief Complaint: Shortness of breath; cough.

PMHx: Multiple medical problems including pulmonary embolism during last pregnancy, duodenal ulcer, hypertension, tuberculosis. Social history remarkable for heavy smoking (2 ppd × 20 years). Recent cocaine use 3 days ago.

HPI: 2-day history shortness of breath with dry, unproductive cough. Chills for 2 days with pain in left upper chest worsening over 2 days. No fever, no hemoptysis, no orthopnea, no paroxysmal nocturnal dyspnea.

Meds: INH, B_6, rifampin, labetalol, warfarin (off warfarin for 3 days-prescription ran out).

PE: Profoundly diaphoretic African-American female in severe respiratory distress. Able to speak in full sentences but occasionally requiring pause to catch her breath.

Vitals: HR 96, BP 130/84, R 28, SPO_2 93% on room air, T 97.7°F.

Oropharynx nonerythematous; submandibular lymph nodes tender on right; remainder of HEENT exam unremarkable.

Thorax symmetrical; breath sounds decreased bilaterally but no adventitious sounds.

Remainder of physical exam unremarkable.

Pertinent lab findings:

ABG: 7.39/40/223/23.7/100% (on 9 L/minute oxygen; repeat ABG off O_2 was normal).

CBC and Chem7: No abnormalities.

Coagulation studies (Coags): PTT 20.4, PT 12.4, INR 1.2.

CXR: Moderate cardiomegaly; right cavitary lesion in right middle lobe; infiltrates resolved from comparison study 1 month ago.

EKG: NSR at 90 bpm. LAE. LVH. T-wave inversions in V_{4-6}.

Cardiac enzymes: No abnormalities.

Helical CT scan of thorax: Large right-sided pulmonary embolus.

Problem list:

1. Pulmonary embolus: Initiate heparin with early transition to p.o. warfarin; will follow coagulation studies; continuous pulse oximetry.
2. Likely hypercoagulable state: Initiate appropriate laboratory work-up; obtain old chart for results of previous work-up(s).
3. Tuberculosis with stable right middle lobe lesion: Continue INH, B_6.
4. Hypertension, stable: Continue labetalol.
5. Duodenal ulcer, stable: Carafate and proton-pump inhibitor I.V. until p.o. tolerated.

Summary: This is a 41-year-old female with a pulmonary embolism that was most likely caused by noncompliance with warfarin therapy for a presumed underlying hypercoagulable state.

E. Formal Presentations

FORMAL PRESENTATION FORMAT.
1. Opening remarks and patient information
2. Chief complaint and chronology
3. History of present illness
4. Physical examination findings
5. Labs and studies
6. Therapy to date
7. Problem list or differential diagnosis list
8. A&P for each problem
9. Discussion and presentation summary

1. Opening remarks and patient information: Name, age, sex, race/ethnicity, occupation.
   a. Add brief mention of reliability/source.
   b. Limit to age, sex, and reason for presentation.
2. Chief complaint and chronology: Avoid using the patient's own words in the formal presentation (e.g., use hematuria instead of red urine).
3. History of present illness (HPI):
   a. Diagnosis, duration, degree, aggravating/alleviating factors:
      (1) Acute versus insidious?
      (2) Mild, moderate, severe?
      (3) Progressive or diminishing in severity?
      (4) Factors exacerbating/relieving?
      (5) Degree of disability caused at present time?
   b. Significant active medical problems. Medical history contributory to the overall current state of health.
   c. Surgical history.
   d. Medications: Dosing, duration of use, missed or last doses. Adverse or allergic reactions. Medication and resultant reaction, and treatment.
   e. Health maintenance issues.
   f. Psychosocial history pertinents.
   g. Significant positives and negatives from the review of systems.
   h. Other pertinent information (e.g., family history, cardiac risk factors).
4. Physical exam findings:
   a. Always include vital signs: BP, P, RR, and temperature.
   b. General description of appearance and/or condition.
   c. Pertinent exam findings: Tailor to the presentation situation, attending and/or resident requests.
5. Lab tests: CBC, urinalysis, chemistries, ECG, ABGs, chest x-ray, CT scan, MRI, etc. Usually in this order. State the values that are in the range of normal if pertinent to active problems.
6. Therapy to date.
7. Problem list or differential diagnosis:
   a. Delineate signs and symptoms as well as the time relationship to the present.
   b. Make note of the effect of treatment with respect to the chief complaint.
8. Assessment and plan for each problem. Have a plan ready (may be covered in the discussion).
9. Discussion and presentation summary:
   a. Two-sentence statement outlining age, sex, condition, and active medical problem(s). Make it clear you are finished and wait or ask for questions regarding the assessment and plan. Prepare for anticipated questions on anatomy,

pathophysiology, etiology, differential diagnosis, treatment, and prognosis.

b. Practice this statement every day with rounds and adjust with current status of the patient.

II. SAMPLE FORMAL PRESENTATION

J.R. is a 41-year-old female brought to the ED by EMS for the complaint of shortness of breath and cough. Mrs. R., a patient with a medical history significant for tuberculosis (currently on INH and rifampin after being diagnosed in April), duodenal ulcer, hypertension, and a previous pulmonary embolism diagnosed during her last pregnancy, relates a 2-day history of shortness of breath, a dry, unproductive cough, and pain in her left upper chest when she coughs forcefully. She denies any fever but has had chills for the past 2 days, a pain that is worse with coughing. She denies any history of hemoptysis, orthopnea, or paroxysmal nocturnal dyspnea. Further review of systems fails to reveal any additional positive findings.

The patient's social history is significant for heavy tobacco use: 2 packs per day for 20 years. She admits to recent cocaine use 3 days ago. She denies any other illicit drug use. Current medications include INH, B_6, rifampin, labetalol, and coumadin, all of which she takes daily with the exception of the coumadin, which she ran out of 3 days ago.

On the physical examination, the patient is profoundly diaphoretic and appears to be in severe respiratory distress. Although able to speak in full sentences with only brief pauses to catch her breath, she is visibly dyspneic and tachypneic. She is alert, oriented, and appears well-nourished. Vitals are as follows:

Pulse	Blood Pressure	Respirations	SpO_2	Temperature
96	130/84	28	93% on room air	97.7°F

The oropharynx is pink, moist, and nonerythematous. There is no JVD. Submandibular lymph nodes are tender, but not enlarged, on the right side. Auscultation of the lungs does not reveal any adventitious sounds, although breath sounds are decreased bilaterally. The thorax is symmetrical. No egophony or increased tactile fremitus is present. The patient consistently coughs when asked to take a deep inspiration. The heart has a regular rate and rhythm without any extra sounds. Abdominal examination fails to reveal any palpable organomegaly, masses, or tenderness; bowel sounds are present. There is no CVA tenderness. No palpable cords or TTP in the extremities bilaterally. The neurologic exam shows the patient to be tense but alert and cooperative. Pupils are brisk, equal in size, and reactive to light bilaterally, extraocular movements are intact, and there is no appreciable facial weakness. DTRs are 2/4 for L2-4, and C3-6 bilaterally. Strength is 5/5 throughout.

Laboratory Results and Studies

Labs were ordered with the following results:

ABGs: pH 7.39, P_{CO_2} 40, P_{O_2} 223, H_{CO_3} 23.7, S_{PO_2} 100%, base excess −1 (patient was on 9 L/min O_2 at time ABG was drawn; a repeat ABG on room air was normal).

CBCs: Noncontributory. No left shift. No leukocytosis. No evidence of polycythemia.

SMA-7: Within acceptable limits.

Coags: PT 12.4.

aPTT 20.4 (low).

INR 1.2 (nontherapeutic for warfarin therapy).

CXR: Moderate cardiomegaly. A right cavitary lesion is present in the right middle lobe. Infiltrates, present on a recent comparison study, appear to be resolved. Subpulmonary infiltrates are possibly present.

EKG: NSR at 90 bpm. Left atrial enlargement. Left ventricular hypertropy. T-wave inversions in V4-V6.

Cardiac Enzymes: CPK, LDH, CK-MB all within normal limits.

Spiral CT: Revealed a large right-sided pulmonary embolus.

Therapies Received to Date

Discussion and Presentation Summary

III. CLINICAL PEARLS

A. Pulmonary Embolism

1. Most DVTs are silent; most DVTs produce pulmonary embolism (PE).
2. Most PEs are asymptomatic.
3. Many DVTs and PEs are not detectable by current imaging techniques.
4. Many undetectable DVTs and PEs will progress to sudden death if not treated.

B. Brief Epidemiology of PEs

1. Most common preventable cause of death in hospitalized patients.
2. 50,000 deaths per year in the U.S. (third most common cause of death).
3. 650,000 cases annually in the U.S.

C. Brief Pathophysiology of PEs

1. All known clinical risk factors for DVT and PE have in common one or more predisposing factors from Virchow's triad: venostasis, vessel wall inflammation or endothelial injury, and hypercoagulability.
2. Hypercoagulable states are generally classified as inherited or acquired.

Inherited Hypercoagulable States	Acquired Hypercoagulable States
Antithrombin III deficiency	Pregnancy
Protein C, S deficiency	Chronic DIC (Trousseau's syndrome)
Protein C substrate deficiency	Oral birth control pills
Abnormal fibrinogens	Nephrotic syndrome
	Lupus anticoagulant and antiphospholipid antibodies

3. Thrombotic occlusion of large or medium-sized pulmonary artery is uncommon. Embolic in origin until proven otherwise.
4. 95% of all emboli arise in thrombi within the large deep veins of the lower legs.
5. Fate of emboli.
   a. Occlusion of main pulmonary artery.
   b. Saddle embolus formation (impact against the bifurcation of the pulmonary arteries).
   c. Passage into progressively branching pulmonary arteries.
6. Clinical consequences.
   a. 60% to 80% are silent because they are small.
   b. More than 60% of pulmonary vasculature must be obstructed for acute cor pulmonale or cardiovascular collapse to occur.
   c. Obstruction of small end arteries (10% to 15% of cases) causes centrally located pulmonary hemorrhage.
   d. Rarely, multiple small emboli lead to pulmonary hypertension and chronic right heart strain, causing progressively worsening dyspnea.
   e. If thromboembolus is allowed to organize, pulmonary vascular sclerosis may occur as an endothelium-covered fibrous mass develops.

D. PE Symptoms

1. Clinical diagnosis is unreliable.
2. Four most common: Dyspnea, tachypnea, pleuritic chest pain, apprehension.
3. Classic triad: Hemoptysis, dyspnea, chest pain (<20% of cases).
4. Young, active patients with pleuritic chest pain may be misdiagnosed with musculoskeletal pain or pleurisy.
5. Historical risk factors.
   a. History of previous DVT/PE.
   b. Recent surgery or pregnancy.
   c. History of immobilization.
   d. Underlying malignancy.

6. Differential diagnosis.
   a. Asthma (will not respond to beta-agonists).
   b. Pneumonia (fever and chills may overlap; most common discrepancy for pulmonary causes of death).

E. Diagnostic Evaluation

1. CBC, ESR, Chem-7 are normal in most patients.
2. D-dimer (degradation product of cross-linking fibrin).
   a. 90% negative predictive value.
   b. Only 30% that are positive have a positive angiogram.
3. Pulse oximetry is useful to monitor patients in need of O_2.
4. V-Q scan.
   a. A normal scan excludes PE 96% of the time.
   b. Classified into four categories: Normal, low, intermediate, high probability.
5. Angiography.
   a. "Gold standard" but small emboli can be missed.
   b. Extremely high negative predictive value.
6. Chest x-ray.
   a. Nonspecific and nonsensitive.
   b. Hampton's hump: Triangular infiltrate with apex toward hilum.
   c. Westermark's sign: Dilation of pulmonary vessels proximal to embolism.
7. Spiral (Helical) CT.
   a. Relatively noninvasive.
   b. Can miss peripheral emboli.

F. Treatment

1. Anticoagulation.
   a. Unfractionated versus fractionated heparin.
      (1) Reduces mortality to less than 10%.
      (2) Should be given as soon as diagnosis of PE is considered.
   b. Low-molecular-weight heparin.
      (1) May be safer and just as effective.
      (2) Doesn't require monitoring of coagulation tests.
      (3) Affects factor Xa more than IIa (heparin affects both equally).
2. Warfarin.
   a. Must give heparin first because warfarin will cause clot extension and early hypercoagulable state because protein C and factor VII have shorter half-lives than other vitamin K–dependent coagulation proteins.
   b. Continue heparin for first 5 to 7 days of warfarin therapy.
3. Thrombolytics indications.
   a. Severely hemodynamically unstable patients with PE.

   b. Patients with exhausted pulmonary reserves.
   c. Patients expected to have multiple recurrences of PE.
4. Other modalities.
   a. Embolectomy.
   b. Gradient compression stockings.
   c. Intermittent pneumatic compression.
   d. Greenfield filter (Vena cava filter).

6

DEATH CERTIFICATION

Stephen J. Cina, MD, and Thomas S. Neuhauser, MD

I. WHY COMPLETE A DEATH CERTIFICATE (DC)?

Despite the best efforts of the physician, some patients will die. When this occurs, a sequence of events is set into motion that affects the surviving family members and society in many ways. Prompt and accurate completion of a death certificate (DC) is essential to facilitate burial or cremation, to establish insurance benefits, to identify workmen's compensation issues, and to settle an estate. From a societal standpoint, accuracy in death certification allows for compilation of national epidemiologic data and statistics, identification of outbreaks of diseases, recognition of deaths related to adverse environmental conditions, monitoring of efficacy of therapy, and elucidation of various trends. Approximately 30% to 40% of death certificates are filled out incorrectly. Few medical students or residents are taught proper death certification. It requires some thought.

A. **Required by Law**: It is a legal document and should be completed accurately.

B. **Family Benefits**
1. Allows for collection of insurance.
2. Facilitates estate distribution.
3. Identifies inheritable diseases and risk factors.
4. Required before burial or cremation.

C. **Societal Benefits**
1. Accuracy of statistics.
2. Epidemiology.
3. Identification of infectious outbreaks/adverse environment.
4. Monitor efficacy of therapy.

II. WHAT DOES A DEATH CERTIFICATE LOOK LIKE?

A. **Design:** This varies somewhat by state, but a standardized national prototype is being designed.

B. **Top Half:** Demographic data.
1. Can be filled out by using the medical record or chart.
2. May be filled out by other hospital personnel.

C. **Bottom Half:** Cause of death, manner of death, and other conditions.
1. Requires medical expertise and judgment.
2. Should be filled out by primary caregiver (e.g., physician). Check hospital policy.
3. May be filled out by lay person (e.g. coroner) in some jurisdictions.

III. JURISDICTIONAL ISSUES

A. Legal: Certain deaths fall under the jurisdiction of the coroner, medical examiner, or Justice of the Peace.

1. Trauma deaths.
2. Deaths in hospital less than 24 hours after admission.
3. Overdose deaths.
4. Child/infant fatalities.
5. Other (check local statutes).
6. The authorities may defer cases to the medical staff for certification.
   a. Medical examiner/coroner may ask you to sign a DC on a patient who dies as an outpatient.
   b. You should sign the DC if you believe death is likely caused by a documented natural disease process.
   c. Broad causes of death may be used if necessary, but a specific cause of death is preferable.
   d. You are not obligated to sign a DC if you have no idea why the patient died.
   e. Most other in-hospital deaths will be certified by the primary caregiver.
   f. Example: A 75-year-old white male with chronic hypertension and a history of myocardial infarction is found dead in bed at home. It is likely that you may be asked to sign the death certificate. Although you cannot be sure whether this person suffered a cerebrovascular accident, myocardial infarct, an arrhythmia precipitated by cardiomegaly, or a ruptured abdominal aortic aneurysm, you can be comfortable that death was likely related to "hypertensive arteriosclerotic cardiovascular disease."

B. Physician Responsibility

1. Familiarize yourself with local jurisdiction and death reporting requirements.
2. If you are considering suicide, homicide, accident, or undetermined as the manner of death on a DC, this case likely falls under the jurisdiction of the coroner/medical examiner.

IV. THE CAUSE OF DEATH STATEMENT

A. Part I of Bottom of Form: Chain of events leading directly to death. (See Figure 6-1.)

B. Composition of Statement: Statement usually consists of three lines.

1. Top line is *immediate* cause of death.
2. Middle line is *intermediate* cause(s) of death.
3. Bottom line is *proximal* or *underlying* cause of death.

C. Definitions

1. Immediate cause of death.
   a. The specific event that led to the patient's death. Avoid cardiac arrest or cardiopulmonary arrest; it is nonspecific

ITEMS 24-28 MUST BE COMPLETED BY PERSON WHO PRONOUNCES OR CERTIFIES DEATH	24. DATE PRONOUNCED DEAD (Mo/Day/Yr)	25. TIME PRONOUNCED DEAD
26. SIGNATURE OF PERSON PRONOUNCING DEATH (Only when applicable)	27. LICENSE NUMBER	28. DATE SIGNED (Mo/Day/Yr)
29. ACTUAL OR PRESUMED DATE OF DEATH (Mo/Day/Yr) (Spell Month)	30. ACTUAL OR PRESUMED TIME OF DEATH	31. WAS MEDICAL EXAMINER OR CORONER CONTACTED? • Yes • No

CAUSE OF DEATH (See instructions and examples)

32. PART 1. Enter the chain of events-diseases, injuries, or complications—that directly caused the death. DO NOT enter terminal events such as cardiac arrest, respiratory arrest, or ventricular fibrillation without showing the etiology. DO NOT ABBREVIATE. Enter only one cause on a line. Add additional lines if necessary.

		Approximate interval: Onset to death
IMMEDIATE CAUSE (Final disease or condition - - - -> resulting in death)	a.______	______
	Due to (or as a consequence of):	
Sequentiaty list conditions, if any, leading to the cause listed on line a. Enter the UNDERLYING CAUSE (disease or injury that initiated the events resulting in death) LAST	b.______	______
	Due to (or as a consequence of):	
	c.______	______
	Due to (or as a consequence of):	
	d.______	______

Figure 6-1.

DEATH

To Be Completed By: MEDICAL CERTIFIER

PART II. Enter other significant conditions contributing to death but not resulting in the underlying cause given in PART I.

33. WAS AN AUTOPSY PERFORMED?
• Yes • No

34. WERE AUTOPSY FINDINGS AVAILABLE TO COMPLETE THE CAUSE OF DEATH? • Yes • No

35. DID TOBACCO USE CONTRIBUTE TO DEATH?
• Yes • Probably
• No • Unknown

36. IF FEMALE:
• Not pregnant within past year
• Pregnant at time of death
• Not pregnant, but pregnant within 42 days of death
• Not pregnant, but pregnant 43 days to 1 year before death
• Unknown if pregnant within the past year

37. MANNER OF DEATH
• Natural • Homicide
• Accident • Pending Investigation
• Suicide • Could not be determined

38. DATE OF INJURY (Mo/Day/Yr) (Spell Month)

39. TIME OF INJURY

40. PLACE OF INJURY (e.g., Decedent's home; construction site; restaurant; wooded area)

41. INJURY AT WORK?
• Yes • No

42. LOCATION OF INJURY: State: City or Town:
Street & Number: Apartment No: Zip Code:

43. DESCRIBE HOW INJURY OCCURRED:

44. IF TRANSPORTATION INJURY, SPECIFY:
• Driver/Operator
• Passenger
• Pedestrian
• Other (Specify)

45. CERTIFIER (Check only one):
• Certifying physician -To the best of my knowledge, death occurred due to the cause(s) and manner stated.
• Pronouncing & Certifying physician-To the best of my knowledge, death occurred at the time, date, and place, and due to the cause(s) and manner stated
• Medical Examiner/Coroner-On the basis of examination, and/or investigation, in my opinion, death occurred at the time, date, and place, and due to the cause(s) and manner stated.

Signature of certifier. ____________________

46. NAME, ADDRESS, AND ZIP CODE OF PERSON COMPLETING CAUSE OF DEATH (Item 32)

47. TITLE OF CERTIFIER

48. LICENSE NUMBER

49. DATE CERTIFIED (Mo/Day/Yr)

50. FOR REGISTRAR ONLY-DATE FILED (Mo/Day/Yr)

Figure 6-1. *cont'd*

and adds no information; everyone ultimately suffers cardiac arrest upon death.

b. If you must use a nonspecific mode of death, it must be further qualified in subsequent lines.

2. Intermediate cause of death: Any condition that gave rise to the immediate cause of death (e.g., myocardial infarction).

3. Underlying (proximal) cause of death. The underlying cause of death is the most important line on the DC. All effort must be made to maximize the accuracy of this determination.

a. The disease process or injury that initiated chain of events leading ultimately to death.

b. The underlying cause may occur years before the immediate cause of death.

D. Examples

1. A patient on the oncology service who has received chemotherapy and bone marrow transplant to treat acute myelogenous leukemia (AML) dies during the night. You may not know if death was caused by hemorrhage related to thrombocytopenia, sepsis resulting from immunosuppression, or a cytokine-mediated phenomenon. You can reasonably conclude, however, that if this patient never had AML, he would likely be alive. This allows for a cause of death of "Complications of AML." If you can ascertain a more specific chain of events (e.g., "Sepsis due to Staphylococcus bacteremia related to immunosuppression following bone marrow transplantation for AML"), it is preferable.

2. An elderly lady dies of a pulmonary thromboembolus caused by deep venous thrombosis following a hip fracture resulting from a fall at home. The manner of death in this case is "Accident," and this case must be reported to the proper authorities.

3. A one-line cause of death may be acceptable (e.g., hypertensive arteriosclerotic cardiovascular disease, diabetes mellitus, metastatic carcinoma of unknown primary).

E. Performance of Autopsy

1. Wait for the preliminary autopsy data if feasible rather than guessing at the cause of death.

2. If the DC must be issued before autopsy, you may use "Pending Autopsy" as the cause of death and then issue an amended DC.

F. Filling Out Part 1

1. To the right of each line on Part 1, estimate the interval between the presumed onset of each condition and the time of death.

2. Lines in Part I must be reasonably related to each other. Try to keep them in proper order.

V. OTHER SIGNIFICANT CONDITIONS

A. Pathologic Conditions: Conditions that contributed to death but did not enter the chain of direct causation (e.g., chronic alcoholism; diabetes in a person dying of acute myocardial infarction).

B. **Multiple Conditions:** If a person has two or more significant disease processes, choose the most likely cause of death for Part I and use Part II for the other (e.g., Part I: Congestive heart failure [CHF] resulting from ischemic cardiomyopathy caused by severe coronary artery disease [CAD], Part II: chronic obstructive pulmonary disease [COPD]).

VI. MANNER OF DEATH

The manner of death is usually determined by underlying cause of death (even if in remote past). It may be natural, suicide, accident, homicide, undetermined, or pending.

A. **Unnatural Deaths:** Anything other than natural death likely needs to be reported to authorities.

B. **Examples**

1. Cause of death: Aspiration pneumonia caused by paraplegia resulting from gunshot wound to the neck. If the wound was inflicted by someone else many years prior, the manner is homicide and the case is reportable. If the wound was self-inflicted, the manner would be suicide.
2. Death during medical/surgical treatment may be accident, homicide, natural, undetermined, or unclassifiable depending on the specifics of the case.
   a. A person who dies on the operating table while undergoing a triple coronary artery bypass graft (CABG) redo may be ruled as a natural cause of death because the procedure is high risk and was precipitated by severe coronary artery disease with few options left for survival. Cause of death: Complications of severe CAD, or death during bypass surgery for severe CAD.
   b. A death due to internal hemorrhage resulting from a lacerated spleen during placement of a chest tube may be an accident or unclassifiable death. Report the case to medical examiner (ME)/coroner and refer to local custom.

VII. MECHANISM OF DEATH

This is a pathologic process that culminates in death.

A. **Death Certificate:** In almost every case, the mechanism of death must be further qualified on the lower lines of Part 1 of the DC.

B. **Underlying Causes of Death:** Underlying causes may share a common mechanism of death (e.g., exsanguination due to a gunshot wound, multiple stab wounds, or gastrointestinal hemorrhage).

II

SPECIALTY HISTORY AND PHYSICAL EXAMINATION

7

ALLERGY AND IMMUNOLOGY

Jonathan W. Buttram, MD, Daniel R. More, MD, and James M. Quinn, MD

I. CHIEF COMPLAINT

A. Qualitative Aspects: Onset, duration, severity, diurnal or seasonal variations, triggers, exposures to dander or pollens, occupational or social exposures, symptoms with medication usage or ingestions, history of symptom relief with medication use.

B. Quantitative Aspects: Frequency of beta-agonist use (e.g., albuterol), frequency of nocturnal symptoms (e.g., wheezing, cough, dyspnea, chest tightness), and peak flow measurements.

C. Identifying Data: Name, age, sex, and race/ethnicity.

II. HISTORY OF PRESENT ILLNESS

Allergy and immunology symptoms may be system-specific (e.g., nasal or ocular symptoms in allergic rhinoconjunctivitis) or nonspecific (e.g., increased frequency of infections in primary immunodeficiency).

A. Characteristics of Symptoms, Conditions, or Syndromes

1. Chronology.
2. Quality.
3. Quantity.
4. Precipitators and exacerbators.
5. Alleviators.
6. Interventions.

B. Common Allergy and Immunology Conditions and Their Associated Symptoms (Table 7-1)

III. PAST MEDICAL AND SURGICAL HISTORY

A. Past Medical History

1. History of emergency room visits, hospitalizations, intubations, and need for oral steroids related to asthma or allergic disease.
2. Have you had any reactions to medications, latex, foods, or insect stings (e.g., anaphylaxis from eating peanuts or from being stung by a honey bee)?
3. Evaluate unrelated diseases that comprise syndromes (e.g., nasal polyposis, aspirin sensitivity, and asthma comprising Samter's syndrome).

B. Past Surgical History

1. Have you undergone sinus surgery for polypectomy, turbinectomy, or functional endoscopic sinus surgery (FESS) related to allergic disease or primary immunodeficiency?

Table 7-1. SYMPTOMS OF COMMON ALLERGY AND IMMUNOLOGY CONDITIONS.

Symptom	Conditions
Anaphylaxis or food, drug, insect, and latex allergy	Tachycardia, hypotension, presyncope, syncope; metallic taste in the mouth; itching, flushing, urticaria; itchy/watery eyes; nasal itching, congestion, rhinorrhea; difficulty swallowing and/or speaking; cough, wheezing, chest tightness; abdominal pain, cramping, nausea, vomiting, diarrhea; impending sense of doom
Allergic rhinoconjunctivitis	Itchy/watery eyes, conjunctival injection; nasal itching, congestion, rhinorrhea, sneezing, postnasal drip; itching of mouth and ears, ear fullness
Asthma	Fatigue, cough, wheeze, chest pain/ tightness, dyspnea, nocturnal cough or wheezing, cough or wheeze with exercise
Urticaria and angioedema	Flushing, itching, urticaria (single lesions lasting less than 24 hrs), angioedema
Immunodeficiency	Growth or developmental delay, fever, telangiectasias, purulent nasal discharge, nasal congestion, sinus pain, lymphadenopathy, cough, purulent sputum, wheeze, delayed separation of the umbilical cord, early satiety, abdominal fullness, abdominal pain, chronic diarrhea, malabsorption, skin infection, ataxia

2. Have you had a splenectomy as a result of trauma or hematologic disease? Such a procedure functionally results in an immunodeficiency.
3. Have you had a vasectomy (if a man)? Vasectomy places a patient at risk for sensitization to protamine because of the loss of antigenic isolation of sperm contents. Sensitization to protamine places patients at risk for anaphylaxis to NPH insulin and protamine, which is used for heparin reversal.

C. **Emergency and Trauma History (Hospitalizations, Transfusions, and Injuries)**

1. Have you had emergency visits, hospital admissions, ICU admissions, or intubations related to asthma or anaphylaxis?
2. Have you had a traumatic splenectomy (see immunizations)? This can necessitate additional immunizations to protect against encapsulated bacterial organisms (e.g., hemophilus influenza b vaccine [Hib], pneumococcal vaccine, and meningococcal meningitis vaccine).

D. **Childhood History**

1. Was your development and growth normal?
2. Did you experience recurrent sinopulmonary infection, which may indicate humoral immunodeficiency?
3. Have you had recurrent infections with intracellular pathogens, which may indicate cellular immunodeficiency?
4. Did you have delayed separation of the umbilical cord, gingivitis, or skin abscesses, all of which may indicate phagocytic immunodeficiency?
5. Have you had recurrent Neisserial infections, which are associated with complement (C5-9) deficiencies?

E. **Occupational History:** Any occupational exposures? These may be important triggers of allergic disease, especially asthma.

F. **Environmental History**

1. Do you have environmental exposure to such things as cockroach infestation at home? Is there water damage (leading to mold growth)? How much carpeting/draperies are in the home?
2. Do you employ environmental controls, such as house dust mite covers, frequent laundering of bedding, and presence of air filters/HEPA filters in the home?
3. As a child, did you live in an urban setting (which may increase the risk of allergic diseases, whereas rural life seems to protect against it)?

G. **Travel History:** Have you recently traveled? Within the United States? To foreign countries? Allergy symptoms may be influenced by changes in geographic location.

H. **Animals and Insects Exposure History**

1. Are you exposed to animals in your home?
2. Do you experience symptoms when exposed to animals?
3. Have you had previous envenomations? What were the resulting effects on your body?

IV. MEDICATIONS, ALLERGIES, AND ADVERSE REACTIONS

A. **Medications**

1. What prescription medications are you currently taking? Some medications may significantly alter the outcome of skin prick testing for allergens (e.g., H_1 and H_2 blockers). Other drugs impede the ability to treat anaphylaxis or other allergic reactions (e.g., beta-blockers, angiotensin-converting enzyme [ACE] inhibitors, and nonsteroidal anti-inflammatory drugs [NSAIDs]).
2. What over-the-counter (OTC) products are you taking?

3. Do you use herbal preparations or alternative medicine therapies?
4. Do you take supplements?

B. **Allergies to Medications and the Side Effects:** Have you had allergic reactions to medications? Individuals with a history of allergic reactions to medications may present a clue about their tendency toward atopic disease.

C. **Adverse Reactions to Medications**
1. What, specifically, was your reaction to the medication? The reaction often does not represent a true IgE-mediated allergy but rather intolerance (i.e., adverse reaction) to the medication (e.g., gastrointestinal upset with codeine).
2. Have you had a rash that lasted days to weeks, fever, arthralgias, and other constitutional symptoms? These features suggest a non-IgE-mediated etiology.

V. HEALTH MAINTENANCE

A. **Prevention**
1. Immunizations.
   a. Do you get annual influenza vaccination? Asthma patients should have annual influenza vaccinations performed regardless of age.
   b. Do you receive vaccinations against encapsulated bacterial organisms to prevent overwhelming sepsis? Splenectomy patients should have vaccinations against these organisms to prevent overwhelming sepsis (e.g., Hib, pneumococcal vaccination, meningococcal vaccination).

B. **Diet**
1. Do you avoid foods that cause allergic reactions?
2. Do you follow a special diet as a result of your allergic disease (e.g., gluten-free diet in patients with celiac sprue)?

C. **Exercise and Recreation:** Does your allergic disease limit your exercise or recreational activities?

D. **Sleep Patterns:** Do you experience poor sleep that is related to allergic disease (i.e., nocturnal cough related to asthma)?

E. **Social Habits:** Do you use tobacco? Tobacco use exacerbates asthma and places others at risk (e.g., maternal smoking increases the risk of asthma in newborns).

VI. FAMILY HISTORY

A. If patient is a child, what is the general health of the parents?

B. Do members of the family smoke, have poor dietary habits, or abuse substances?

C. How many siblings, if any, does the patient have? The number of siblings the patient has inversely correlates to the risk of developing allergic disease. What are the siblings' medical conditions?

D. **First-Degree Relative's Medical History:** Has there been any occurrence of atopic disease in first-degree relatives?

E. **Third-Generation Genogram:** Have any infant males suffered an early death? A history of early death in infant males may indicate X-linked primary immunodeficiency.

VII. PSYCHOSOCIAL HISTORY

A. **Personal and Social History:** Does the patient have access to health care and ability to obtain medications and other therapy (e.g., asthma education and immunotherapy)?

B. **Current Illness Effects on the Patient**

1. Has there been a decrease in your work or school performance because of allergy symptoms?
2. Has your exercise tolerance decreased because of asthma or allergy symptoms?

C. **Interpersonal and Sexual History**

1. Have you experienced gustatory rhinitis or nasal congestion with sexual activity?
2. Does contact with latex condoms produce irritation or anaphylactic symptoms?

D. **Family Aspects of Illness or Condition:** Have you had to make changes in your family, dwelling, or lifestyle because of this condition (e.g., pets, cover vents)? Are you able to afford medications for allergy treatment?

E. **Occupational Aspects of the Illness:** Are there any work-related issues (e.g., latex glove allergy) secondary to the condition?

VIII. REVIEW OF SYSTEMS (Tables 7-2 and 7-3)

Table 7-2. GENERAL ALLERGY AND IMMUNOLOGY SYMPTOMS BY SYSTEM.

System	Symptoms
General	Fatigue, height and weight percentiles
HEENT	Red, watery, itchy eyes; nasal congestion, rhinorrhea, itching, sneezing; ear fullness, itching; palatal itching, throat clearing; difficulty swallowing or speaking; hoarseness; sinus congestion, pain
Neck	Adenopathy
Cardiovascular	Tachycardia, hypotension
Chest	Cough, wheezing, chest pain or tightness, dyspnea, sputum production, nocturnal cough or wheezing
Gastrointestinal	Nausea, emesis, diarrhea, abdominal pain or cramping
Genitourinary	Itching, angioedema
Lymphatic	Adenopathy
Musculoskeletal	Arthralgias, myalgias, arthritis
Skin	Itching, urticaria, rash, pain, burning, hyperpigmentation, bruising, petechiae
Extremities	Angioedema

Table 7-3. NONSPECIFIC SYMPTOMS AND THEIR ALLERGIC AND IMMUNOLOGIC DISEASES.*

Symptom	Diseases
Abdominal pain	Anaphylaxis, angioedema, immunodeficiency
Anemia	Urticarial vasculitis
Anxiety	Anaphylaxis, asthma, vocal cord dysfunction, mastocytosis
Congestion	Allergic rhinitis, nonallergic rhinitis, nasal polyposis, sinusitis
Cough	Allergic rhinitis, nonallergic rhinitis, sinusitis, asthma, gastroesophageal reflux disorder (GERD), vascular ring, cystic fibrosis, primary ciliary dyskinesia, cardiac causes (see Chapter 9, Cardiology)
Diarrhea	Anaphylaxis, immunodeficiency
Fever	Primary or secondary immunodeficiency
Mood alteration	Mastocytosis
Sore throat	Allergic rhinitis, nonallergic rhinitis, sinusitis, GERD
Throat tightness	Anaphylaxis, vocal cord dysfunction, GERD
Urticaria	Acute or chronic urticaria, urticarial vasculitis, anaphylaxis, serum sickness, mastocytosis
Weakness and fatigue	Asthma, mastocytosis, primary or secondary immunodeficiency
Weight loss	Primary or secondary immunodeficiency
Wheezing	Asthma, vocal cord dysfunction, GERD, inhaled foreign body, vascular ring, cystic fibrosis, tracheobronchomalacia, primary ciliary dyskinesia, cardiac disease

*Best used to focus the HPI or when no obvious pattern emerges during the interview.

IX. PHYSICAL EXAMINATION (Table 7-4)

The list of allergic diseases is extensive, yet many present with similar symptoms (e.g., wheezing). This creates an enormous differential diagnostic list based on symptoms.

Table 7-4. ALLERGIC OR IMMUNOLOGIC DIAGNOSIS.

SYSTEM	PHYSICAL EXAMINATION FINDING	POSSIBLE DIAGNOSES
General	Difficulty speaking in complete sentences	Asthma
Vital Signs		
Temperature	Fever	Infection
Pulse	Tachycardia	Anaphylaxis, asthma
Blood pressure	Hypotension	Anaphylaxis, asthma
	Pulsus paradoxus	Asthma
Pulse oximetry	Hypoxemia	Asthma
Respiratory rate	Tachypnea	Anaphylaxis, asthma
HEENT		
Eyes	Conjunctival injections	Allergic rhinoconjunctivitis
	Allergic shiners	Allergic rhinoconjunctivitis
	Keratoconus	Allergic rhinoconjunctivitis
	Morning crusting	Allergic conjunctivitis
	Purulent discharge	Infection
	Telangiectasias	Primary immunodeficiency
Ears	Serous fluid collection	Allergic rhinoconjunctivitis
	Purulent fluid collection	Sinusitis, immunodeficiency
Nose	Edematous mucosa	Allergic rhinoconjunctivitis, nonallergic rhinitis
	Rhinorrhea	Allergic rhinoconjunctivitis, nonallergic rhinitis
	Purulent nasal discharge	Infection
	Mucosal erythema	Nonallergic rhinoconjunctivitis, rhinitis medicamentosa, infection
	Mucosal pallor	Allergic rhinoconjunctivitis
	Transnasal crease	Allergic rhinitis

Continued

Table 7-4. ALLERGIC OR IMMUNOLOGIC DIAGNOSIS—*cont'd*

SYSTEM	PHYSICAL EXAMINATION FINDING	POSSIBLE DIAGNOSES
	Nasal polyps	Nonallergic rhinitis, asthma, cystic fibrosis, allergic rhinitis
Mouth	Cobblestoning	Allergic rhinitis, nonallergic rhinitis, sinusitis
	Postnasal drip	Allergic rhinitis, nonallergic rhinitis, sinusitis
	Erythema	Allergic rhinitis, nonallergic rhinitis, infection
	Exudates	Infection
	Gingivitis	Immunodeficiency
Neck	Lymphadenopathy	Infection
	Stridor	Vocal cord dysfunction
Lung	Prolonged expiratory phase	Asthma
	Wheezing	Asthma, anaphylaxis, infection
	Rales	Infection
	Rhonchi	Infection
	Egophony	Infection
Chest	Supraclavicular or intercostal retractions	Asthma, anaphylaxis
Abdomen	Paradoxical movement	Asthma
	Organomegaly	Immunodeficiency
Skin	Urticaria	Anaphylaxis, acute and chronic urticaria/ angioedema, vasculitis, mastocytosis
	Angioedema	Chronic urticaria/ angioedema, hereditary angioedema
	Hyperpigmentation	Vasculitis, mastocytosis (urticaria pigmentosa)
	Petechiae/ecchymoses	Vasculitis
	Hypopigmentation	Atopic dermatitis
	Abscesses	Immunodeficiency
	Darier's sign	Mastocytosis

Table 7-4—cont'd

SYSTEM	PHYSICAL EXAMINATION FINDING	POSSIBLE DIAGNOSES
	Dermatographism	Urticaria/angioedema
Extremities	Clubbing	Asthma, immunodeficiency
	Cyanosis	Asthma, immunodeficiency, anaphylaxis
	Urticaria of palms and soles	Vasculitis
Neurologic	Ataxia	Immunodeficiency

A. Allergic Rhinoconjunctivitis Examination

1. When performing an ocular exam, look for the following:
   a. Eczema around the eyes involving the periorbital skin and cheeks.
   b. "Allergic shiners" or dark discolorations beneath the lower eyelids, resulting from venous stasis caused by mucosal edema of sinuses. Infraorbital creases (Dennie-Morgan lines) near the eyes are a result of chronic rubbing.
   c. Loss of the lateral eyebrow as a result of eye rubbing (de Hertoghe's sign).
   d. Evidence of conjunctival inflammation or injection.
2. Examination of the ears should include the appearance of the tympanic membrane (e.g., air bubbles or air-fluid level with serous otitis media is typical of allergic etiology).
3. When examining the nose, note the following:
   a. Transnasal crease caused by the frequent upward rubbing of the palm on the nose ("allergic salute").
   b. Color and quality of secretions (typically clear, serous, or watery discharge).
   c. Using an otoscope, examine the nasal passages and mucosa (pale, edematous boggy mucosa is often found in patients with allergic disease).
   d. Evidence of nasal septal deviation, which may provide a clue to a nonallergic etiology of disease.
   e. Presence of nasal polyps, which may be confused with edematous turbinates. Nasal polyps are smooth, pale, translucent structures that are insensitive and mobile to the touch.
4. Examination of the pharynx should focus on the following:
   a. Presence of high-arched palate, which may indicate allergic disease.
   b. Evidence of postnasal drainage on posterior aspect of pharynx.

c. "Cobblestoning" on pharyngeal mucosa often indicative of allergic disease.

B. Examination for Asthma

1. Because most patients with asthma are atopic, the examination for allergic rhinoconjunctivitis should also be performed, with special attention given to the possibility of nasal polyps.
2. Before the examination of the chest, note the patient's overall status.
   a. Determine the patient's vital signs, including the respiratory rate and pulse oximetry and presence or absence of cyanosis. An increase in the pulsus paradoxus may be present.
   b. Evaluate the patient's work of breathing and the ability, or inability, to speak in full sentences.
   c. Observe for any use of accessory muscles of respiration (e.g., scalenes, sternocleidomastoids), pursed lip breathing, flaring of the alae nasi. This may indicate a severe attack of asthma.
   d. Evidence of stridor, inspiratory wheezing heard over the larynx, may point to an alternative diagnosis, such as laryngospasm or vocal cord dysfunction.
3. Examination of the chest should include noting the following:
   a. Supraclavicular and intercostal muscle retractions, which also indicate increased work of breathing associated with a severe attack.
   b. Evidence of hyperinflation, which is manifested by increased anteroposterior diameter ("barrel chested") and hyperresonance to percussion.
   c. Auscultation of the chest, which may reveal inspiratory and expiratory crackles, rhonchi, and wheezes. Wheezing may diminish with decreased air movement ("silent chest syndrome"), which is an especially concerning finding and often associated with impending respiratory failure.

C. Urticaria/Angioedema Examination

1. Examination for urticaria/angioedema should also include looking for the presence of other atopic diseases, such as allergic rhinoconjunctivitis and asthma.
2. Examination of the skin should include the following:
   a. Note the location and morphology of the urticaria (size, erythema, blanchable) and well-demarcated swelling of the eyes, lips, hands, and feet (angioedema) that may give clues to the etiology.
   b. Evaluate for development of local hive after scratch on skin (dermatographism).
   c. Evaluate for urticaria pigmentosa (UP), which is seen in patients with systemic mastocytosis and is characterized by multiple small, tan to red-brown macules typically on the

trunk. Scratching one of these macular lesions results in a local wheal-and-flare reaction called Darier's sign.

d. Cholinergic urticaria often occurs during or shortly after exercise or exposure to heat. It is characterized by small, punctate papules without the occurrence of angioedema.

e. Various diagnostic tests can be performed as part of the physical examination if the urticaria is thought to be "physical" in nature. Types of physical urticaria include pressure, vibratory, solar, aquagenic, cold-induced, and heat-induced.

f. Hereditary angioedema occurs in the absence of urticaria.

g. Urticaria may occur as part of a rheumatologic or vasculitic disease process. Individual hives lasting longer than 24 hours, hives on the palms/soles, and scarring urticaria should raise suspicion of a vasculitic process.

h. Serpiginous bands of urticaria and erythema can be seen along the sides of the fingers, toes, hands, and feet in patients with serum sickness.

X. DIFFERENTIAL DIAGNOSIS (Table 7-5)

Many allergic diseases may present with similar symptoms and physical exam findings. The exam is best performed with a specific disease process in mind.

Table 7-5. DIFFERENTIAL DIAGNOSIS OF ALLERGY AND IMMUNOLOGY DISEASE.

SYMPTOM	POSSIBLE DIAGNOSES
Anaphylaxis	Shock (hemorrhagic, cardiogenic, septic), vasovagal reaction, carcinoid syndrome, systemic mastocytosis, pheochromocytoma, hereditary angioedema, panic disorder, vocal cord dysfunction, globus hystericus
Frequent infections	Primary immunodeficiency (B-cell, T-cell, phagocytic and complement defects), secondary immunodeficiency (human immunodeficiency virus [HIV], Epstein-Barr virus [EBV], malignancy), circulatory disorder (sickle-cell disease, diabetes mellitus), anatomic obstruction (cystic fibrosis, asthma, eustachian tube dysfunction), integument disruption (burns, atopic dermatitis), presence of foreign body (ventriculoperitoneal [VP] shunt, artificial heart valve), bacterial overgrowth, chronic bacterial carrier state, continuous recurrent infections

Continued

Table 7-5. DIFFERENTIAL DIAGNOSIS OF ALLERGY AND IMMUNOLOGY DISEASES—*cont'd*

SYMPTOM	POSSIBLE DIAGNOSES
Hives	Urticaria, insect stings/bites, urticarial vasculitis, serum sickness, Muckle-Wells syndrome, Schnitzler's syndrome, pruritus urticarial papules and plaques of pregnancy (PUPPP), infectious etiologies (Lyme disease, cat scratch disease), porphyria, mastocytosis
Red eye(s)	Infectious conjunctivitis, allergic conjunctivitis, blepharitis, subconjunctival hemorrhage, episcleritis, scleritis, uveitis, iridocyclitis, vernal conjunctivitis, atopic keratoconjunctivitis
Rhinitis	Allergic rhinitis, idiopathic nonallergic rhinitis (NARES, vasomotor rhinitis, gustatory rhinitis), infectious rhinitis, pregnancy, hypothyroidism, rhinitis medicamentosa, drug-induced (oral contraceptive pills [OCPs], alpha-blockers, beta-blockers, NSAIDs), granulomatous disease (Sarcoidosis, Wegener's, relapsing polychondritis), anatomic abnormality (septal deviation, choanal atresia) cerebrospinal fluid (CSF) rhinorrhea
Urticaria and angioedema	Acute urticaria (often IgE-mediated), chronic urticaria (often idiopathic), cholinergic urticaria (angioedema not present), physical urticaria (pressure, solar, vibratory, cold, heat, aquagenic), dermatographism, hereditary angioedema (urticaria not present), drugs (ACE inhibitors, NSAIDs). See also previous "hives" description
Wheezing	Asthma, upper airway disease (rhinitis, sinusitis), large/small airway obstruction, vocal cord dysfunction, vascular rings/ laryngeal webs, bronchiolitis, tracheomalacia, bronchopulmonary dysplasia, cystic fibrosis, cardiac causes, aspiration/GERD, chronic obstructive pulmonary disease (COPD), pulmonary embolism, masses obstructing the airway (lymph nodes, tonsillar abscess, tumor, retrosternal goiter)

XI. LABORATORY STUDIES AND DIAGNOSTIC EVALUATIONS

A. Procedures

1. Skin testing (epicutaneous and intradermal).
   - **a.** Sensitive and specific method of demonstrating *in vivo* specific IgE.
   - **b.** Useful in the diagnosis of allergic rhinoconjunctivitis, food allergy, venom allergy, latex allergy, and drug allergy.
   - **c.** Helpful in the determination of allergic triggers in extrinsic asthma.
   - **d.** Preferred method of diagnosing allergic diseases.
2. Pulmonary function testing: Useful in the diagnosis and management of chronic lung diseases, such as asthma.
3. Bronchoprovocation: Sensitive test for determining the presence of bronchial hyperreactivity and in the diagnosis of asthma.
4. Rhinoscopy.
   - **a.** Direct visualization of the nasal passages, sinus structures, and pharyngeal structures.
   - **b.** Useful in the differential diagnosis of chronic sinus diseases.

B. Blood and Serum Studies

1. Complete blood count (CBC).
   - **a.** Nonspecific test for quantification of white blood cell lineages.
   - **b.** Useful in the evaluation of primary immunodeficiency.
2. Radio-allergosorbent test (RAST).
   - **a.** *In vitro* method of demonstrating specific IgE.
   - **b.** Useful in the diagnosis of allergic rhinoconjunctivitis, food allergy, venom allergy, and latex allergy.
   - **c.** Helpful in the determination of allergic triggers in extrinsic asthma.
   - **d.** Alternative way to measure specific IgE when skin testing is not helpful or is unable to be performed.
3. Quantitative immunoglobulins.
   - **a.** Quantitative measurement of serum IgG, IgA, IgM, and IgE.
   - **b.** Useful in the evaluation of the humoral immune system and in the evaluation of primary immunodeficiency.

C. Radiographic Studies

1. Chest x-ray: Useful in the differential diagnosis of asthma and other chronic lung diseases.
2. Computed tomography of the sinuses: Useful in the diagnosis and management of chronic sinusitis and other sinus diseases.

D. Other Studies Available

1. Anergy panel.
   - **a.** Evaluation for the presence of delayed-type hypersensitivity; often to candida, mumps, and tetanus.
   - **b.** Useful in the evaluation of cell-mediated immunity and in the evaluation of primary immunodeficiency.

2. Nasal smear.
   a. Evaluation for the presence of nasal eosinophils.
   b. Useful in the differential diagnosis of allergic rhinitis.

XII. ACRONYMS AND ABBREVIATIONS (Table 7-6)

XIII. DEFINITIONS (Table 7-7)

XIV. SAMPLE H&P WRITE-UP

CC: "My nose is congested and runny in the morning and when I mow the grass."

HPI: The patient is a 24-year-old male with a history of many years of nasal congestion and clear rhinorrhea upon waking in the morning and on exposure to grasses. He also complains of increased symptoms when cleaning the house, especially while vacuuming. Has been treated with short-acting antihistamines in the past with some relief. Has never been treated with nasal steroids. There is no history of asthma symptoms. Has never been skin tested for allergies before.

Nasal symptoms: Congestion, rhinorrhea, sneezing, itching of nose, and frequent feeling of postnasal drip.

Eye symptoms: Watery, itching, injection.

Chest symptoms: Denies cough, wheezing. Wheezes zero times a week. Uses Albuterol metered-dose inhaler (MDI) zero times a week. No wheezing or coughing at night. No wheezing or coughing with exercise. Seasonal variation is perennial, with exacerbations during the summer.

Diurnal variation is evident, with nasal congestion noticeably worse in the morning.

Gastroesophageal reflux symptoms: Patient denies rising sensation of chest burning/dyspepsia.

Potential triggers include possibly dust and grasses. He denies allergic reactions to cigarette smoke, dog, cat, odors, perfumes, or temperature variations. He denies requiring emergency room visits, hospitalizations, intubations, or steroid bursts for this condition. The patient has carpets and drapes in the bedroom. He denies presence in any room of moisture or dampness, visible mold growth, cockroaches, wood-burning fireplace, heater, unvented stove, or heaters. He does not use HDM covers or HEPA filters for the air conditioner or vacuum. He does not have dogs, cats, birds, or other house pets. He has never smoked tobacco products.

Current occupation is a medical student. He denies occupational chemical exposures. No exacerbation of asthma symptoms at work. No exacerbation of allergic rhinitis and allergic conjunctivitis symptoms at work. He denies coughing, wheezing, shortness of breath, rhinorrhea, conjunctival irritation, or urticaria or angioedema after ingesting aspirin/nonsteroidals. He denies coughing, wheezing, or shortness of breath after eating shrimp, dried fruit, or processed potatoes or after drinking beer or wine. He denies allergic reactions after exposure to insects, eating foods, or latex exposure.

PMHx/PSHx: Noncontributory.

Table 7-6. ALLERGY AND IMMUNOLOGY ACRONYMS AND ABBREVIATIONS.

Acronym or Abbreviation	Definition	Acronym or Abbreviation	Definition
Ab	Antibody	**IT**	Immunotherapy
ABPA	Allergic bronchopulmonary aspergillosis	**NAR**	Nonallergic rhinitis
AFS	Allergic fungal sinusitis	**PAR**	Perennial allergic rhinitis
AIT	Aeroallergen immunotherapy	**PF**	Peak flow
AKC	Allergic keratoconjunctivitis	**PND**	Postnasal drip
AR	Allergic rhinitis	**PST**	Prick skin testing
BHR	Bronchial hyperresponsiveness	**RIT**	Rush immunotherapy
CGD	Chronic granulomatous disease	**SAR**	Seasonal allergic rhinitis
CVID	Combined variable immunodeficiency	**SCID**	Severe combined immunodeficiency
EIA	Exercise-induced anaphylaxis	**T/A**	Tonsillectomy and adenoidectomy
EIB	Exercise-induced bronchospasm	**TM**	Tympanic membrane
GERD	Gastroesophageal reflux disease	**VCD**	Vocal cord dysfunction
ID	Intradermal skin test or Immunodeficiency	**VIT**	Venom immunotherapy
Ig	Immunoglobulin	**VKC**	Vernal keratoconjunctivitis

Table 7-7. ALLERGY AND IMMUNOLOGY DEFINITIONS.

TERM	DEFINITION
Anaphylaxis	Immediate, transient immunologic reaction characterized by smooth muscle contraction and capillary dilation caused by release of mast cell mediators, classically initiated by cross-linking of mast cell–fixed IgE by an antigen
Angioedema	Well-demarcated swelling in the dermis
Darier's sign	Wheal-and-flare reaction as a result of scratching the macular lesion seen in patients with urticaria pigmentosa
Gustatory rhinitis	Watery nasal discharge associated with stimulation of the sense of taste
Keratoconus	Conical protrusion of the cornea caused by thinning of the stroma; may be caused by repeated rubbing of the eyes
Mastocytosis	Abnormal proliferation of mast cells; may be systemic, involving a variety of organs, or cutaneous only (urticaria pigmentosa)
Muckle-Wells syndrome	Familial amyloidosis, progressive neural hearing loss, and periodic febrile urticaria associated with joint and muscle pain
NARES	Nonallergic rhinitis with eosinophilia syndrome
NBT test	Nitroblue tetrazolium test; a test to detect the phagocytic ability of polymorphonuclear leukocytes (neutrophils) by measuring the capacity of the oxygen-dependent leukocytic bactericidal system
PUPPP	Pruitic urticarial papules and plaques of pregnancy; intensely pruritic, occasionally vesicular eruption of the trunk and arms, appearing in the third trimester; spontaneous involution occurs within 10 days of term
Rebuck skin window	*In vivo* test of the inflammatory response in which the skin is abraded and a glass slide is then placed over the abraded area. Leukocytes adhere to the slide and thus permit subsequent visualization of leukocyte mobilization
Rhinitis medicamentosa	Rhinitis secondary to improper or excessive use of topical decongestants

Table 7-7—cont'd

TERM	DEFINITION
Samter's syndrome	Nasal polyposis, aspirin sensitivity, and asthma (a.k.a. triad asthma)
Schnitzler's syndrome	Urticaria, fever, bone pain with osteocondensation, and IgM gammopathy
Urticaria	Eruption of pruritic wheals resulting from hypersensitivity, foci of infection, physical stimuli, or psychic stimuli
Urticaria pigmentosa	Characterized by multiple small, tan to red-brown macules typically on the trunk. Scratching one of these macular lesions results in a local wheal-and-flare reaction called Darier's sign. See also mastocytosis
Vocal cord dysfunction	Paradoxical adduction of the vocal cords on inspiration, which may cause dyspnea and stridor, often mimicking asthma (typically during emotional or physical stress)
Wheal	Circumscribed, evanescent papule or irregular plaque of edema of the skin, slightly reddened, often changing in size and shape, and accompanied by intense itching

Medications: Benadryl prn and no known drug allergies (NKDA).

Family HX: Positive for hay fever.

Physical Exam: General: Well-developed, well-nourished male in no acute distress; mouth breathing with "allergic shiners."

HEENT: Conjunctiva: Clear without significant chemosis or injection. Tympanic membranes: Clear without evidence of retraction, fluid, erythema, or sclerosis. Nares: Nasal mucous pale grey with bogginess and moderate edema, scant clear discharge, no crusting, bleeding, or polyps visualized, no transverse nasal crease. Oropharynx: Clear PND and cobblestoning. Neck: Supple without adenopathy.

Lungs: Clear with good air movement, no evidence of wheezing, rhonchi, rales, or prolonged expiratory phase.

Heart: Regular rate and rhythm without murmurs or gallops.

Extremities: No evidence of clubbing or cyanosis.

Skin: No observed eczema or urticaria.

8

ANESTHESIA

Dorene A. O'Hara, MD, MSE

I. CHIEF COMPLAINT

A. Anesthesiology Evaluation Goals

Because anesthetics interact with medications and alter physiology, the patient undergoing anesthesia requires thorough medical and surgical evaluation. The goals for this evaluation are to;

1. Assess the current state of the surgical problem and any concomitant disease.
2. Plan for the anesthesia, fluid, electrolyte, blood or coagulation management, and postoperative (postop) recovery period.
3. Identify disease processes, which can increase patient risk. This will aid in the surgeon's decision-making process whether to manage acutely or to postpone the procedure (e.g., new diseases are often diagnosed before [in preoperative work-up] or during the surgery, especially in a patient who has not had regular medical care).
4. Relieve the patient's pain, suffering, and anxiety.

B. Identifying Data: Name, age, gender, race/ethnicity, and location of admission/evaluation.

II. HISTORY OF PRESENT ILLNESS

This chapter focuses primarily on the evaluation of a patient requiring anesthesia for a procedure.

A. Preoperative Evaluation (The Procedure).

1. What is the nature of the procedure? Does it require general or regional anesthesia, with or without sedation?
2. Is there likely to be blood loss during the procedure? Large fluid shifts? Major organs involved?
3. What kind of intravenous or arterial access is needed (e.g., central line, arterial line)?

B. Preexisting Medical Conditions (see Table 8-1)

1. What is the severity of, and control over, all concurrent disease?
2. What does a detailed evaluation of the patient's cardiac and respiratory systems reveal?
3. Has the patient had recent oral intake: What type of fluid or food, how much, and when (a full stomach increases risks of regurgitation/aspiration and death)?
4. Does the patient have a current infection unrelated to the surgery? Even if currently treated, discuss with surgeon whether surgery should be delayed.

C. **For Emergencies Without Time for Full Evaluation:** Obtain the following minimum of information, as time permits: Allergies, nil per os (NPO) status, medications, acute cardiac disease, possibility of pregnancy, and information from family.

III. PAST MEDICAL AND SURGICAL HISTORY

A. Past Medical History

1. Has the patient received regular medical care? Assess previous level of health care. In some populations, patients have no regular care.
2. What is the patient's medical history? Be aware that history may be unreliable.
3. Are any advanced and untreated diseases present (typically infectious disease, such as tuberculosis or hepatitis, or other chronic conditions like diabetes, asthma, hypertension, or other cardiac disease)?

B. Past Surgical and Anesthetic History

1. Has the patient had previous operations, when and where, and any adverse events?
2. Is there a history of prolonged anesthesia, unanticipated postoperative ICU stay, ventilation, or cardiac arrest?
3. Do any family members have anesthesia problems, been screened for muscle disease, pseudocholinesterase deficiency, or malignant hyperthermia?

C. Emergency and Trauma History

1. History and physical are often abbreviated in format, presented together, with treatment, diagnosis, and transport information. Resuscitation measures—airway, breathing, and circulation—and evaluation of life-threatening injuries and bleeding always come first.
2. What are the patient's previous hospitalizations, transfusions, and injuries?

D. Childhood History

1. Does the patient have any congenital conditions that increase anesthetic risk?
2. Does the patient have congenital cardiac disease?
3. Does the patient have any diseases or congenital conditions that affect facial structures or the airway?

IV. MEDICATIONS, ALLERGIES, AND ADVERSE REACTIONS

A. Medications

1. Is the patient currently taking prescription and over-the-counter (OTC) medications? Most important to consider are insulin, steroids, psychiatric drugs (especially monoamine oxidase [MAO] inhibitors due to anesthesia and narcotic interactions), nitroglycerin and cardiac medications, asthma inhalers, aspirin/NSAIDs (some bleeding risk), chemotherapy, thyroid medications, chronic pain treatments, anxiety medica-

tions, muscle relaxants, and diuretics. Medication lists often provide clues to disease processes present in the patient.

2. Is the patient using herbals, supplements, or diet pills? Some contain ma huang/ephedra (risk of severe hypertension). Many herbals and vitamins increase risk of bleeding (e.g., ginger, gingko, vitamin E, garlic). Herbals for anxiety, depression, or sleep may interact with anesthetics (e.g., valerian, St. John's wort, kava).

B. Allergies and Adverse Reactions

1. Is the patient allergic to drugs? What are the symptoms and severity? Differentiate nasal allergies from new upper respiratory infections.
2. Does patient have a latex allergy (must inform the operating room [OR] personnel)?
3. Has patient had an allergic reaction to local anesthetics or while under anesthesia?
4. Is patient allergic to narcotics? Is it a true allergy or was any reaction a side effect (e.g., nausea)?
5. Is patient allergic to soy or eggs (e.g., concern about using Diprivan) or barbiturates? This information is very important for the anesthesiologist.

V. HEALTH MAINTENANCE

A. Diet: What is the patient's diet? Does the patient take diet aids (see previous section)? Has the patient experienced recent weight gain or loss (signs of possible undiagnosed disease)?

B. Exercise: Is the patient able to walk or use stairs? If so, how far or long can they go? What are the patient's daily activities, including carrying groceries and working around the house? Exercise tolerance is one of the best measures of cardiopulmonary function.

C. Sleep Patterns: Does the patient have a history of severe snoring or apnea?

D. Social Habits

1. Does the patient smoke? If yes, what type of tobacco (or marijuana), how much, and for how long?
2. Does the patient use alcohol?
   a. Amount, type, and frequency? Does patient become acutely intoxicated?
   b. Is there a history of liver involvement?
   c. What is the risk of acute withdrawal postprocedure?
3. Does patient abuse IV or inhaled drugs?
   a. Which drugs and how recently used? Has the patient shared needles? Assess for infection and hepatitis issues.
   b. Is the patient at risk for HIV/AIDS?
   c. Does the patient have risks of systemic effects (e.g., heart murmur and drug-related endocarditis)?

VI. FAMILY HISTORY

Is there any history of anesthesia or anesthetic complications, heart disease, or muscle disease in patient's first-degree relatives?

VII. PSYCHOSOCIAL HISTORY

A. Personal and Social History

1. In what city and country was the patient born?
2. What is the patient's religious and ethnic background?

B. Current Illness Effects on the Patient

1. Does the patient have an accurate and appropriate perception of the severity of the illness?
2. Has the patient addressed death and dying issues, as applicable (e.g., Do Not Resuscitate [DNR] orders)?
3. Has the patient put any advanced directives in place (e.g., Living Will, Durable Power of Attorney for Health Care [DPAHC])?

C. Family Support

1. Will the patient have family members, friends, and other sources of support present during the emergency or elective procedure?
2. Are family members available for support? Have important phone numbers been obtained (helpful when information is needed or if information must be relayed to family)?

VIII. REVIEW OF SYSTEMS (Tables 8-1 and 8-2)

Text continued on p. 78.

Table 8-1. ANESTHESIOLOGY-FOCUSED REVIEW OF SYMPTOMS BY SYSTEM.

System	Symptoms
General	Fatigue, appetite, sleep patterns, and sleep apnea (sleep apnea risk postop)
HEENT	Oral opening, teeth/dentures, airway classification for intubation (is posterior pharynx visible?), facial abnormalities, loose teeth, caps
Neck	Short/long, measure chin (three fingerbreadths sign for intubation), mobility, stability (especially in trauma patients with neck collar on)
Cardiovascular	Myocardial infarction (within 6 months is a high risk), chest pain, angina, congestive heart failure (serious risk), valvular disease, hypertension, syncope, arrhythmias/ palpitations, positional or exercise-related shortness of breath, hypertension, exercise tolerance

Continued

Table 8-1. ANESTHESIOLOGY-FOCUSED REVIEW OF SYMPTOMS BY SYSTEM—*cont'd*

System	Symptoms
Chest/pulmonary	Acute bronchitis/pneumonia (high risk), shortness of breath, asthma (severity, inhalers used, emergency department treatment history), smoking and chronic obstructive pulmonary disease (COPD), cough, airway/pulmonary surgery, recent upper respiratory tract infection (URI, increased risk)
Gastrointestinal	Ulcer, GERD (check if food or acid refluxes), gastrointestinal (GI) bleeding, "heartburn" as undiagnosed cardiac disease, abdominal pain (evaluate for source), nil per os (NPO) or nothing by mouth status, problem swallowing (possible obstruction or mass)
Neurologic	Neurologic deficits, stroke, multiple sclerosis (can worsen with surgery), spinal surgery or injury, dizziness (requires evaluation), back or neck injury (positioning issues), seizures and degree of control, increased intracranial pressure risk (e.g., bleed, tumor, or trauma), preoperative confusion, Alzheimer's
Psychiatric	History, medications, informed consent issues
Obstetrics/ gynecologic	Pregnancy risk (many centers require test before surgery); surgery on pregnant patient has special risks
Hematologic/ cancer	Anemia (source, severity, acute versus chronic), coagulation defects, easy bruising, bleeding with dental work, platelets (number and function), von Willebrand's, hemophilia, consumption coagulopathy (severe risks), sickle cell disease (special anesthesia technique), systemic/metastatic cancer and chemo used (interactions with anesthesia), radiation (especially to chest or neck), cancer pain control (need even more pain meds postop), IV access issues (may need cut down or implanted line)

Table 8-1—cont'd

SYSTEM	SYMPTOMS
Musculoskeletal	Myasthenia gravis (high risk, plan for postoperative ventilation), muscle-wasting diseases (increases risk of potassium release and cardiac arrest), myoglobinemia (risk of acute renal failure), patient or family history of malignant hyperthermia (must see anesthesiologist preop), positioning issues (e.g., contractures), arthritis and pain (limitations of movement, especially the cervical spine), recent trauma
Skin	Open wounds, bedsores, rashes over IV or regional sites, burns (full- or partial- thickness burns cause fluid and heat losses, special techniques used, also severe pain), color (pallor or cyanosis)
Hepatic	Acute hepatitis (contraindication for surgery), risk of fulminate hepatic failure, chronic hepatitis (metabolism altered, bleeding effects, needle-stick risks), IV access problems, biliary disease, ethanol use
Renal/urologic	Hydration status, renal function (acute versus chronic failure), electrolytes (risks under anesthesia), dialysis (type, whether recent, new electrolyte levels, and state of hypovolemia), unrecognized urinary tract infection is common
Endocrine	Diabetes mellitus (diagnosed or new symptoms, must be under control, insulin-dependent or adult-onset, controlled by diet or oral medication, glucose level), thyroid or parathyroid (enlargement, possible airway obstruction), new endocrine-related symptoms need full evaluation (thyroid storm, calcium abnormalities risk of death under anesthesia), corticosteroid dependence (need coverage for surgery), unexplained general symptoms such as fatigue need work-up

Continued

Table 8-1. ANESTHESIOLOGY-FOCUSED REVIEW OF SYMPTOMS BY SYSTEM—cont'd

System	Symptoms
Infectious disease	Type and source of infection, treated or partially treated, risks of resistant superinfection in hospital, urinary tract infection (frequency, burning, urgency), upper respiratory (cough, sputum characteristics, fever, sore throat, ear pain, wheezing), chronic infections, including AIDS (counts, contact precautions, needle-stick risks), sepsis (cardiovascular effects, severity, need for invasive monitoring)
AGE-RELATED CONCERNS	
Pediatric	Normal gestation/delivery? Congenital abnormalities, especially cardiac or facial/airway deformities, current infections, patient/parental anxiety and preop preparation, NPO requirements are different in children and infants, airway, mouth opening, size of tongue
Adolescent/emancipated minor	Consent issues, discussion with patient and parent/guardian, private discussions regarding smoking, drugs, alcohol, sexual activity and pregnancy, postop pain control, anxiety, desire for autonomy
Females of childbearing potential	Any risk of pregnancy? Must obtain pregnancy test, history of previous pregnancies, complications, anesthesia issues
Elderly	Polypharmacy and drug interactions, increased risks with underlying systemic diseases, neurologic function, depression and increased risk of postoperative memory loss or confusion, decreased metabolism, increased drug effects, home care issues

Table 8-2. ANESTHETIC IMPLICATIONS OF COMMON DISEASES/CONDITIONS.

Disease/Condition	Implications for Anesthesia
Alcohol/drug use	Acute intoxication (delay surgery), withdrawal, concurrent hepatitis or other infection, needle-stick risk, undiagnosed disease
Anemia	Concern for more blood loss, inadequate oxygen-carrying capacity for surgery, transfusion risks, source, whether ongoing, coagulation status
Arthritis	Pain limiting motion, positioning, neck mobility and intubation difficulty, use of NSAIDs and clotting, use of steroids
Asthma	Current wheezing: risk of death in operating room, concurrent infection, current medications: adequate? Use of steroids, history of exacerbations and emergency department visits, intubations
Cancer	Spread to key organs, pain, radiation history (lung or airway?), chemotherapy affecting heart or lung, hepatic function
Coronary artery disease	Status of current angina and how controlled, triggers, recent myocardial infarction (MI, <6 months increases risk of death), medications used (possible interactions with anesthesia, e.g., diuretics cause relative hypovolemia), plans for angioplasty, stents or surgery, valvular disease, carotid insufficiency (risk of stroke)
Diabetes mellitus	Glucose preop, taking medications on day of surgery?, degree of control, associated end-organ effects, risk of intraoperative hypoglycemia
Ear infection	Treatment for how long? Other upper respiratory symptoms, signs of meningitis
Hepatitis	Acute or chronic, signs of adequate hepatic function (bleeding, ascites, jaundice), type of hepatitis and source, contact precautions
HIV infection/AIDS	Is patient just exposed (HIV) or ill (AIDS)? Cell counts (e.g., CD4 count), current opportunistic infections, contact precautions

Continued

Table 8-2. ANESTHETIC IMPLICATIONS OF COMMON DISEASES/CONDITIONS—*cont'd*

Disease/Condition	Implications for Anesthesia
Hypertension	How high, medication(s)? Taken on surgical day? Other end-organ effects, especially cardiac, vascular, and renal
Hypothyroidism	Medication for thyroid treatment? Currently symptomatic? (if so, need better control before surgery)
Hyperthyroidism	If uncontrolled, this is a serious operative risk, which requires full evaluation and treatment before surgery if possible
Pain	What is the source? Is the surgical lesion the cause? Treat if possible in consultation with surgeon, limit unnecessary patient movement, limit multiple attempts to elicit pain once diagnosis is made. If unrelated, is there other pathology? What medications taken?
Pneumonia	Should be fully treated and recovered before surgery
Psychiatric illness	Some medications interact with anesthetics (especially tricyclics and MAO inhibitors), anxiety may be severe, consent issues
Renal insufficiency	Severity, if dialysis, type and frequency, volume and electrolyte status
Stroke	Should be >6 months prior, assess and document deficits, risk of intracranial hypertension with recent bleeds, check blood pressure
Upper respiratory infection (URI)	Severity, lung involvement, normal cold, or flu onset? With pediatric patients, evaluate with parents, consider postponing if new infection
Urinary tract infection (UTI)	Often asymptomatic, check urinalysis, may need antibiotic coverage preoperative or for hardware insertion, may postpone

IX. PHYSICAL EXAMINATION (Table 8-3)

A. Anesthesia History and Physical Exam General Considerations: This is focused on airway (head and neck), heart and lungs, spine (if spinal, epidural or caudal are planned), and overall neurologic and muscular function. The basic exam should be documented in the anesthesia record.

Text continued on p. 83.

Table 8-3. FINDINGS OF ANESTHESIOLOGY-FOCUSED PHYSICAL EXAMINATION AND POSSIBLE DIAGNOSES.

Systems	Physical Exam Finding	Possible Diagnoses
Pulse	Bradycardia	Drug effects, cardiac disease versus athletic heart, hypothyroidism
	Tachycardia	Hypovolemia, anxiety, pain, primary arrhythmia, anemia, bleeding, thyrotoxicosis
Blood pressure	Hypertension	Anxiety, pain, full bladder, poorly controlled hypertensive disease, fluid overload/renal disease
	Hypotension	Hypovolemia, bleeding, major trauma
Respiratory rate	High (e.g., >15-18 in adult)	Hypoxia, anxiety, pain, asthma or COPD, airway obstruction, cardiac, abdominal, or neurologic event
	Low (e.g., <10 in adult)	Drug effects, acute neurologic event
Weight	>100 lbs overweight, or two times ideal weight	Morbid obesity: multiple anesthetic considerations (e.g., airway, cardiac reserve, pulmonary reserve, full stomach)
	Cachexia	Poor surgical candidate: anticipate difficulty, increased sensitivity to anesthesia, poor wound healing
HEENT		
Head	Facial deformities, short neck, poor neck mobility	Anticipate difficult intubation
Eyes	Abnormal eye movements	Evaluate for new neurologic event
	Contact lenses	Remove for surgery
	Glaucoma or other	Some drug interactions possible

Continued

Table 8-3. FINDINGS OF ANESTHESIOLOGY-FOCUSED PHYSICAL EXAMINATION AND POSSIBLE DIAGNOSES—*cont'd*

SYSTEMS	PHYSICAL EXAM FINDING	POSSIBLE DIAGNOSES
Mouth	See uvula, soft palate, tonsils	Mallampati Class I: No special difficulty
(Full mouth opening and protrude tongue)	See base of uvula, tonsillar pillars obscured by tongue	Mallampati Class II: No special difficulty
	See only soft palate, no uvula	Mallampati Class III: Expect difficult intubation
	Soft palate not visible	Mallampati Class IV: Expect significant difficulty with intubation. Plan for fiber-optic and possibly other techniques
Teeth	Missing, cracked or poor dentition (brown, loose)	Aspiration risks (e.g., lost tooth intraoperatively), consider dental consult, especially for hardware, cardiac surgery
	Dentures	Remove for general anesthesia
Oral cavity	Masses, infection	New infection? Intubation risks, possible problems postoperative
NECK		
	Mass	Possible obstruction: need ENT evaluation, pulmonary flow-volume loops
Thyroid	Enlarged	Rule out mass: possible neck obstruction; tracheal deviation, check thyroid functioning tests (TFTs)
Carotids	Bruits	Evaluate dizziness, especially with neck extension; risk of stroke, check murmurs
Jugular veins	Distention	CHF, possible cardiac tamponade

Neck mobility	Decreased forward or back (<35%) range of motion	Possible difficult intubation, risk of injury with head positioning
Thyromental distance	<3 fingerbreadths under chin to thyroid cartilage	Possible difficult intubation
Neck trauma	Neck not "cleared" with x-ray and trauma/neuro evaluation	Must intubate and position with collar; one person assigned to hold head neutral
Lungs	Wheezing	Asthma versus pneumonia versus foreign body
	Rales	CHF, must evaluate and treat
	Decreased breath sounds	Pneumonia versus traumatic or spontaneous pneumothorax
Chest	Using accessory muscles to breathe	Respiratory distress; evaluate cause
Cardiovascular	Murmur	Valvular disease versus mitral valve prolapse versus functional; check symptoms, evaluation completed, and patient stable? Need for antibiotics/subacute bacterial endocarditis (SBE) prophylaxis?
	Irregular heart sounds	Atrial fibrillation, PVCs, APCs, SVT; assess if rhythm stable or unstable and symptoms, rate of pulse at wrist or groin
Abdomen	Tenderness	Surgical diagnosis: how acute (i.e., how much time to surgery to prepare patient)?
	Distention	Ascites, bowel obstruction or perforation, obesity
Skin	Rashes	New infectious process versus chronic
	Pallor	Rule out chronic anemia, new bleeding

Continued

Table 8-3. FINDINGS OF ANESTHESIOLOGY-FOCUSED PHYSICAL EXAMINATION AND POSSIBLE DIAGNOSES—*cont'd*

Systems	Physical Exam Finding	Possible Diagnoses
	Jaundice	Evaluate hepatic or biliary source
	Cyanosis	Hypoxia or circulation defect
	Burns	Depends on percentage of body involved. Special burn care, pain relief, temperature control, fluids
	Tracks/pin marks on forearms	IV drug use, multiple sticks for other purposes (e.g., chemotherapy, transfusions, renal)
Spine	Curvature, scoliosis	Possible difficult spinal, epidural, or intubation
	Back surgery history	Evaluate for neurologic deficits; spinal or epidural may be difficult
Extremities	IV sites	Evaluate for size of IV needed, possible need for cut down, central line
	Pulses	Rate and strength, assess if adequate circulation, especially for arterial line
	Edema	Consider CHF, lymphatic obstruction
	Contractures	Muscle and neurologic disease; positioning problems
Neurologic	Confused, obtunded	Rule out new neurologic event, possible drug effects, consent issues
	Paralysis	Stroke versus nerve injury
	Paraplegia	Multiple anesthetic issues, especially autonomic hyperreflexia

1. The anesthesiologist evaluates the airway to assess ease of ventilation (neck mobility, size of tongue, shape of face and chin) and intubation (neck mobility, jaw size and mobility, teeth, caps and dentures, neck size and length).
2. Heart and lungs are assessed to determine risk under anesthesia because general and regional anesthetics can alter blood pressure, blood flow to vital organs, cardiac work, and respiratory mechanics. Major physiologic abnormalities in either the heart or lungs may require treatment before surgery.
3. The neurologic and musculoskeletal exams assess the level of consciousness, any chronic or acute neurologic changes that might indicate risk of further injury with anesthesia, positioning issues (under anesthesia the patient cannot protect him or herself), and special anesthetic drug interactions known to occur with neurologic and muscular diseases.
4. Finally, overall, the anesthesiologist assesses the severity of illness and patient compensation for chronic conditions (maximized given good medical care) before surgery.

B. **Special Anesthesia Concern: IV Access Issues**

1. Peripheral veins (location and size) and broken skin.
2. Evidence of multiple IV sticks, damage caused by chemotherapy or long-term IV access, and evidence of IV drug abuse.
3. For central access, assess neck anatomy, visualize external jugular veins, and assess upper chest anatomy.
4. Refer pediatric IV placement to anesthesia and surgery unless absolutely necessary for current treatment.
5. Even though internist and surgeon may have completed a physical examination, a brief exam must also be done and documented by anesthesia.

X. **DIFFERENTIAL DIAGNOSIS (Table 8-4)**

Table 8-4. DIFFERENTIAL DIAGNOSIS OF COMMON CONDITIONS SEEN IN ANESTHESIOLOGY.

Condition	Possible Diagnoses
Shortness of breath	Asthma, airway disease, airway obstruction, CHF acute arrhythmia or MI, severe valvular disease, hypoxia, mild URI versus pneumonia, COPD, anxiety, anemia, hemoglobin abnormalities, pulmonary embolus, overdose of skeletal muscle relaxants
Chest discomfort	Acute MI, heartburn, GERD, surgery-related anxiety, hypoxia, costochondritis, chest trauma, pneumonia, herpes zoster (shingles), pulmonary embolism

Continued

Table 8-4. DIFFERENTIAL DIAGNOSIS OF COMMON CONDITIONS SEEN IN ANESTHESIOLOGY—*cont'd*

CONDITION	POSSIBLE DIAGNOSES
Anemia	Preoperative blood loss, surgical blood loss, undiagnosed trauma, hemolysis, overhydration, autologous blood donation, pregnancy-related, sickle cell, thalassemia, intrinsic coagulation defect, high-dose Coumadin or heparin, drug effects
Hypotension	Hypovolemia, blood loss, NPO status, GI losses, acute cardiac event, status post dialysis for surgery, undiagnosed trauma, vasovagal reaction, pulmonary embolus
Hypertension	Inadequate blood pressure (BP) medication, pain, anxiety, endocrine abnormality, renal disease, fluid overload, CHF, intracranial pathology
Pain	Recent injury, chronic systemic illness, normal postsurgical pain versus new event, inadequate pain medication ordered (dose too low, interval too long), ischemia or obstruction of internal organ(s)
Arrhythmia	Electrolyte imbalance, intrinsic cardiac rhythm disturbance, acute cardiac event, hypoxia, hypercarbia (respiratory failure), high digitalis level, other drug effects, thyrotoxicosis, anemia, anxiety, hypoglycemia, pheochromocytoma, high caffeine intake, effects of anesthetics
Confusion	Effect of anesthetics, other drug effects, hypoxia, hypercarbia, anxiety with hyperventilation, older patient in different environment, electrolyte imbalance, stroke, seizure, hypoglycemia, new head injury, cardiac abnormalities, carotid artery disease, psychiatric illness
Somnolence	Normal anesthetic/analgesic effect, anesthetic overdose, electrolyte imbalance, stroke, COPD with hypercarbia, new head injury, seizures, hypoglycemia

XI. LABORATORY STUDIES AND DIAGNOSTIC EVALUATIONS

Required tests for surgery are based primarily on preexisting medical conditions, a history of smoking, ethanol and/or drug use. Age and the type of procedure are also important. The minimal recommended tests are requested after an adequate history and physical exam, which is the best screen for disease. Some patient populations have a high incidence of poorly treated or undiagnosed conditions. Lab normal ranges for anesthesia are equivalent to those of medical/surgical services.

A. **Tests:** General recommendations (best information at time of publication; recommendations continue to be revised):
   1. **Electrocardiogram (ECG):** Recommended for patients age 40 years or older, history of hypertension, diabetes, other coronary risk factors. (Note, in some centers, women require an ECG if 50 to 55 years or older, not 40. This recommendation may change in the future in all centers because of the prevalence of undiagnosed cardiac disease in women).
   2. **Hemoglobin/hematocrit:** Recommended if blood loss is expected, there are symptoms suggestive of anemia, a history of bleeding problems, a history of chronic medical conditions associated with changes in red cell type or number, and, generally, if the patient is 40 years of age or older.
   3. **Chest x-ray (CXR):** Recommended if a history of smoking, if the patient is age 60 years or older, there is a history or symptoms of chronic cardiac or pulmonary disease, symptoms of acute pulmonary disease or asthma, or major general, pulmonary, or cardiac surgery is planned.
   4. **Urinalysis:** Useful if there are urinary or renal symptoms, history of diabetes, fever without known source, or back or flank pain.
   5. **Pregnancy test:** Obtained in females of childbearing potential. Rapid urine pregnancy screening tests should be available on wards and in preoperative areas.
   6. **Chemistries:** Medications (such as diuretics) or diseases known to alter electrolytes, renal or liver function; diabetes, history of renal, pancreatic, or liver disease, endocrine disease, history of ethanol or drug abuse, and generally, if the patient is 40 years of age or older.
   7. **Coagulation tests:** Recommended if a history of abnormal bleeding or bruising, planned vascular surgery, known hematologic diseases, and sometimes by surgical preference.
   8. **White count with differential:** Recommended for signs of infection or cancer, exposure to parasitic or other infections resulting from travel, occupation, or contacts; HIV patient requires additional testing (e.g., CD4 counts).
   9. Therapeutic drug levels (e.g., digoxin, theophylline, or Dilantin).
   10. More advanced tests to evaluate disease may be required, depending on the patient's disease and planned surgery. These include pulmonary function tests (PFTs), arterial blood gases (ABGs), pulmonary flow loops, electroencephalograms (EEGs), Holter monitor, and echocardiogram.

B. **Classification of Risk**
   1. American Society of Anesthesiologists (ASA) Classification (Table 8-5).

Table 8-5. AMERICAN SOCIETY OF ANESTHESIOLOGISTS (ASA) CLASSIFICATION OF RISK.

ASA CLASSIFICATION	DESCRIPTION
ASA I	Healthy patient with only the surgical problem
ASA II	A patient with mild systemic disease, such as early, orally controlled diabetes, or mild hypertension on medication
ASA III	A patient with moderate to severe systemic disease that is limiting but not incapacitating, such as controlled hypertension and stable angina, insulin-dependent diabetes, cancer well-controlled with chemotherapy or radiation, asthma maintained with systemic steroids and inhalers
ASA IV	A patient with severe systemic disease that is a constant threat to life, such as sepsis, widely metastatic cancer with cachexia, acute stroke, or escalating angina
ASA V	A patient not expected to survive 24 hours, with or without surgery (e.g., a patient with extensive necrotic bowel)
ASA VI	Sometimes this score is used to indicate that the patient is declared brain dead, scheduled for organ harvest, and maintained on life support to preserve organs
Add the letter "E"	This is added to VI when the surgical procedure is an emergency

2. Other scoring systems.
   a. Goldman cardiac risk classification: High scores are associated with severe risk, especially with signs of congestive heart failure (CHF).
   b. Charlton scale: Evaluates comorbidity and prognostic risk.
   c. Acute Physiology and Chronic Health Evaluation (APACHE II): A severity of disease classification; predicts in-hospital mortality.
   d. New York Heart Association: Cardiac risk.

C. **Evaluation for Sedation or Local Anesthesia with Monitoring**

1. The general principles for evaluation are the same for any procedure requiring sedation and even possibly requiring a

conversion to general anesthesia (e.g., if the patient becomes uncooperative during the procedure, the local block fails, or the surgery becomes more invasive).

2. Risks of anesthesia occur even with "minor" procedures.
3. Deep invasive or diagnostic procedures are often painful and stressful on the cardiovascular and pulmonary systems.

D. **Anesthesia for the Pregnant Patient**

1. Elective surgery should be avoided in pregnant patients. History and lab tests for pregnancy are listed in the previous section.
2. Pregnant patients who require anesthesia should be jointly evaluated and managed by anesthesia and the obstetrician.
3. For nonobstetric surgery during pregnancy, minimum evaluations include fetal heart monitoring preop, and sometimes, intraoperatively.
4. Known teratogens and newer, untested drugs are avoided.

E. **Acute and Chronic Pain Evaluation**

1. The anesthesia evaluation includes preparation for treatment of pain postoperatively and discussion with the patient and surgeon.
2. Local anesthesia, regional blocks, epidural catheters, and patient-controlled analgesia are options for pain therapy. History, physical exam, and lab tests may be helpful in planning phases.
3. Patients with a history of chronic pain usually require higher doses of postoperative pain medications.
4. Patients with narcotic addiction on maintenance (such as methadone) require additional medications for superimposed acute pain. Continue current pain medications as much as possible.

XII. ACRONYMS AND ABBREVIATIONS (Table 8-6)

XIII. DEFINITIONS (Table 8-7)

XIII. SAMPLE H&P WRITE-UP

CC: The patient is a 63-year-old male admitted for laparoscopic, possible open cholecystectomy.

HPI: The patient admits to a history of waxing and waning abdominal pain for many years. The pain was worse following consumption of fatty foods. Work-up revealed the presence of gallstones within the gallbladder and common bile duct. Surgery was scheduled by general surgery.

PMHx:

Cardiac: The patient has a history of angina, status post angioplasty 2 years ago. He experiences mild shortness of breath climbing one flight of stairs and does no regular exercise. The angina is sporadic.

Pulmonary: The patient smokes one pack per day (ppd) of cigarettes. He has a chronic, nonproductive cough.

Text continued on p. 95.

ANESTH

Table 8-6. ANESTHESIOLOGY-FOCUSED ACRONYMS AND ABBREVIATIONS.

Acronym or Abbreviation	Definition	Acronym or Abbreviation	Definition
ABG	Arterial blood gas	**LV**	Left ventricle
ABO	Major compatibility system for blood	**LVEDP**	Left ventricular end-diastolic pressure
ACE	Angiotensin-converting enzyme	**MAC**	Monitored anesthesia care
Ach	Acetylcholine	**MAC**	Minimum alveolar concentration (of gas)
ACT	Activated clotting time	**MAOI**	Monoamine oxidase inhibitor (antidepressant)
ACLS	Advanced cardiac life support	**MAP**	Mean arterial pressure
AF	Atrial fibrillation	**MAST**	Military anti-shock trousers
Alpha	Receptor subtype	**MH**	Malignant hyperthermia (anesthetic emergency)
Ambu	Brand name of bag-valve-mask device	**MI**	Myocardial infarction
ANS	Autonomic nervous system	**mmHg**	Millimeters of mercury (pressure)
AR	Aortic regurgitation	**Modified V5 lead**	ECG lead used to monitor for ischemia
ARDS	Adult respiratory distress syndrome	**MR**	Mitral regurgitation
AS	Aortic stenosis	**MRI**	Magnetic resonance imaging
ASA	Aspirin (acetyl salicylic acid)	**MS**	Mitral stenosis
ASA	American Society of Anesthesiologists	**MS**	Multiple sclerosis
ATLS	Advanced trauma life support	**MSO_4**	Morphine sulfate
ATN	Acute tubular necrosis	**Mu receptor**	Morphine receptor in brain and spinal cord

AV	Aortic valve	**MV**	Mechanical ventilation
Beta	Receptor subtype, autonomic nervous system	**MVP**	Mitral valve prolapse
BE	Base excess	**Neo**	Neosynephrine, or phenylephrine (vasopressor)
Bier block	Nerve block of the arm using IV local anesthetic	**NG**	Nasogastric (tube)
BLS	Basic life support	**NIDDM**	Non-insulin-dependent diabetes mellitus
BP	Blood pressure	**NMDA**	N-methyl-D-aspartate (receptor)
CABG	Coronary artery bypass graft	**NMJ**	Neuromuscular junction
CAD	Coronary artery disease	**Norepi**	Norepinephrine (Levophed)
CBF	Cerebral blood flow (or coronary blood flow)	**NO**	Nitric oxide
CHF	Congestive heart failure	**N_2O**	Nitrous oxide (anesthetic)
$CMRO_2$	Cerebral metabolic rate of oxygen consumption	**NPO**	Nil per os (nothing by mouth)
CNS	Central nervous system	**NSAID**	Nonsteroidal anti-inflammatory drug
CO	Cardiac output	**NTP**	Sodium nitroprusside
COPD	Chronic obstructive pulmonary disease	**O_2**	Oxygen
COX-2	Cyclo-oxygenase subtype 2 receptor (analgesia)	**OR**	Operating room
CPAP	Continuous positive airway pressure	**PAC**	Premature atrial contractions
CPB	Cardiopulmonary bypass	**PACU**	Postanesthesia care unit (or recovery room)

Continued

Table 8-6. ANESTHESIOLOGY-FOCUSED ACRONYMS AND ABBREVIATIONS—*cont'd*

Acronym or Abbreviation	Definition	Acronym or Abbreviation	Definition
CPR	Cardiopulmonary resuscitation	**PCA**	Patient-controlled analgesia
CRF	Chronic renal failure	**PCO_2**	Partial pressure of carbon dioxide
CSF	Cerebrospinal fluid	**PCWP**	Pulmonary capillary wedge pressure
CVP	Central venous pressure	**PDPH**	Post dural puncture headache
CXR	Chest x-ray	**PEEP**	Positive end-expiratory pressure
DIC	Disseminated intravascular coagulation	**PFTs**	Pulmonary function tests
DNR	Do Not Resuscitate	**PGE1**	Prostaglandin E1
DTC	d-Tubocurarine	**pH**	Power of hydrogen
E cylinder	Standard-size cylinder for oxygen, anesthesia gases	**PHN**	Postherpetic neuralgia
ECG	Electrocardiogram	**Pk/Pd**	Pharmacokinetic/pharmacodynamic
ECMO	Extracorporeal membrane oxygenation (used in infants)	**PLT**	Platelets
ECT	Electroconvulsive therapy	**Po_2**	Partial pressure of oxygen
EEG	Electroencephalogram	**PONV**	Postoperative nausea and vomiting
EF	Ejection fraction	**ppm**	Parts per million
EJ	External jugular vein	**PRBCs**	Packed red blood cells

EMLA	Eutectic mixture of local anesthetics (topical agent)	**PSI**	Pounds per square inch
Epi	Epinephrine	**PTF**	Post-tetanic fade
$ETCO_2$	End-tidal carbon dioxide	**PT**	Prothrombin time
ETT	Endotracheal tube	**PTT**	Partial thromboplastin time
Fa/Fi	Fraction of alveolar to fraction inspired gas ratio	**PVCs**	Premature ventricular contractions
FFP	Fresh frozen plasma	**PVR**	Pulmonary vascular resistance
FIO_2	Fraction of inspired oxygen	**RA**	Right atrium
FROM	Full range of motion	**RR**	Respiratory rate
FRC	Functional residual capacity	**RSD**	Reflex sympathetic dystrophy
GA	General anesthesia	**RV**	Right ventricle
GABA	Gaba-amino benzoic acid	**SB**	Sinus bradycardia
HCT	Hematocrit	**SpO_2**	Oxygen saturation
Hespan	Brand name for hetastarch plasma expander	**SSEP**	Somatosensory evoked potential(s)
Hgb	Hemoglobin	**ST**	Sinus tachycardia
HR	Heart rate	**Sux**	Succinylcholine
HTN	Hypertension	**SVR**	Systemic vascular resistance
IABP	Intra-aortic balloon pump	**SVT**	Supraventricular tachycardia
ICP	Intracranial pressure	**T**	Temperature
ICU	Intensive care unit	**T10**	10th thoracic dermatome level
IDDM	Insulin-dependent diabetes mellitus	**T-piece**	Breathing circuit used sometimes in pediatrics

Continued

Table 8-6. ANESTHESIOLOGY-FOCUSED ACRONYMS AND ABBREVIATIONS—*cont'd*

Acronym or Abbreviation	Definition	Acronym or Abbreviation	Definition
IJ	Internal jugular (vein)	**3-in-1 block**	Block of femoral, lateral femoral,cutaneous, and obturator
IM	Intramuscular	**TIVA**	Total intravenous anesthesia
IMV	Intermittent mandatory ventilation	**TLC**	Total lung capacity
IV	Intravenous	**TOF**	Train of four (muscle relaxation)
K	Potassium	**TR**	Tricuspid regurgitation
LA	Left atrium	**UE**	Upper extremity
LE	Lower extremity	**V/Q**	Ventilation/perfusion
L3-4	Lumbar 3 to 4 vertebrae	**VF**	Ventricular fibrillation
Lead II	Second lead of ECG, monitored for rhythm	**VT**	Ventricular tachycardia
LMA	Laryngeal mask airway	**WPW**	Wolff-Parkinson White syndrome

Table 8-7. ANESTHESIOLOGY-SPECIFIC DEFINITIONS.

Term	Definition
Airway/airway algorithm	Adequate anatomic or assisted pathway for respiration, scheme for establishing airway under anesthesia or with emergency respiratory failure or obstruction
Increased anesthetic risk	Condition or procedure increases risk over normal anesthetic mortality of <1/250,000 (e.g., uncontrolled disease, emergency, extremes of age, prolonged of >4 hours surgery)
General anesthesia	Provision of loss of consciousness, loss of normal reflexes, amnesia and analgesia
Local/regional	Infiltration of local anesthetic, nerve block, field block, spinal, or epidural. May also include some sedation
Conscious sedation	Patient maintains reflexes, respiration, responds to commands, but is comfortable. Does not replace adequate local for procedure
"Deep" sedation	State in which some reflexes are depressed and loss of consciousness may occur, with similar risks of general anesthesia. May only be provided by anesthesia-trained, licensed personnel
IV access	Assessment by anesthesia of IV sites based on surgical requirements, state of patient, intact skin areas. Secure IV access is critical to provision of safe anesthesia
True surgical emergency	Surgery should proceed immediately, with or without time for lab evaluation and possibly even full history and physical so as to save life (e.g., massive trauma with abdominal or chest bleeding)
True obstetrical emergency	Delivery or cesarean section should proceed immediately, generally without time for regional anesthesia or full history and physical or lab tests so as to save mother or baby
"Cleared" for surgery	Term not used by anesthesiologists, but implies patient is in the best possible medical condition to undergo the procedure such that no undue risk of mortality or morbidity. Implies that a full and careful medical evaluation has been completed

Continued

Table 8-7. ANESTHESIOLOGY-SPECIFIC DEFINITIONS—*cont'd*

Term	Definition
Full stomach	Any adult patient who has ingested food (within 6 hours) or liquids (within 4 hours) of surgery is considered to be at risk for aspiration of stomach contents under anesthesia. Pregnancy, major trauma slow gastric emptying (always consider full stomach); infants on breast milk have shorter interval (2 hours)
Intubation	Place endotracheal tube (ET) by variety of techniques. Standard is direct view with laryngoscope, place tube between vocal cords
Extubation	Removal of ET tube under controlled conditions
Fiber-optic intubation	Controlled intubation method, awake or asleep, sedated or not, usually with some topical anesthesia method, direct view of cords and trachea
Laryngeal mask airway (LMA)	Important device, blind technique, tiny mask goes over trachea inside pharynx. Does not protect against aspiration; can then use to guide small endotracheal tube
Mask ventilation	Most important technique to learn in airway resuscitation. Apply mask with good fit, maintain respiration by bag-valve-mask device or anesthesia circuit. Requires skill and practice for correct "feel"; critical skill in ACLS algorithms
"Wean" from ventilation	Usually postoperative, assess patient's spontaneous respiration/airway control, cut down on ventilator rate before extubation
Desaturation/ hypoxia	Drop in blood oxygen level, measured by pulse oximeter (saturation) or blood gas (saturation and Po_2), in normal patients below 90% is definite cause for concern, or rapidly dropping
Respiratory distress	Difficulty in breathing may show in rate, type of breathing, and whether labored or not
Monitoring requirements	Vital sign monitoring requirements to safely perform procedure with anesthesia or sedation. Many states have requirements in law. Minimums include BP, O_2 saturation, pulse, and ECG. Need for O_2 monitor on delivery device and end-tidal CO_2 varies

Hepatic: The patient had a recent bout of abdominal pain and a positive ultrasound for gallstones. He denies history of hepatitis or jaundice. **Renal:** One episode of kidney stone in the past and benign prostatic hyperplasia (BPH). **GI:** History of gastroesophageal reflux disease (GERD). He was treated with Prevacid for 4 years. **Neuro:** Negative history of stroke, falls, motor or neurologic weakness.

PSHx: Tonsils and adenoids at age 7, right inguinal hernia 5 years ago with spinal anesthesia, two colonoscopies for screening with polyp removal under sedation. No history of anesthesia problems.

Emergency and Trauma History: Hospitalizations as above.

Medications: Zocor, Metoprolol, Prevacid, rarely takes nitroglycerin (NTG) for angina. Also vitamins C, E, saw palmetto, ginkgo.

Allergies: Penicillin.

Dental History: Patient has partial upper plate, no loose teeth or caps.

Health Maintenance: Smokes 1 ppd as noted above, 1 glass of beer per day.

Social History: Lutheran religious preference. No restrictions on medical care, living will in place. Patient is not in do-not-resuscitate (DNR) status.

Review of Systems: Otherwise negative.

PHYSICAL EXAM (Table 8-8)

Vital signs: BP 150/95, HR 72, RR 18, Temp 99.0°F, Weight 190, Height 5′9″.

Moderately obese male in nonacute distress (NAD).

HEENT: Full jaw opening, dental work intact. Mallampati class II airway. Three fingerbreadth distance under jaw, full range of motion (ROM) of head and neck. Carotid bruit noted on the left side.

Lungs: Wheezing right side, cleared with cough. No rales.

Cardiovascular: Normal S1, S2, without murmur.

Extremities: No cyanosis, clubbing, or edema.

Lab Evaluation and Plan: Preoperative labs to include CBC, U/A, CXR, and ECG, electrolytes (required for cardiac and smoking history as well as age). Patient instructed to stop Vitamin E and ginkgo for 2 weeks (risk of bleeding) and to take his metoprolol on day of surgery with a sip of water.

Further questioning regarding bruit reveals that the patient is asymptomatic, but the finding has not been evaluated; however, the patient's exercise tolerance is poor. A carotid ultrasound is recommended by the patient's primary doctor. Review of the ECG also shows new nonspecific ST changes, and patient also undergoes repeat cardiac catheterization and angioplasty. The carotid artery is less than 50% occluded on the left, so no treatment except addition of Plavix recommended (stopped 1 week for surgery). The patient returns 1 month later for procedure.

Table 8-8. BRIEF SAMPLE WRITE-UP FOR A NORMAL ADULT ANESTHESIOLOGY-DIRECTED PHYSICAL EXAMINATION.

System	Sample Findings
Vital Signs	Awake, alert, oriented. HR 60-90, RR 10-15, unlabored, BP 90/60-140/90, O_2 sat 95-100%. Weight within 50% +/-ideal body weight, assuming no recent unexpected weight changes
Head and neck, airway	Full mouth opening, Mallampati I, tongue midline, no oral masses, no decayed/loose teeth, ROM neck ≥35 degrees forward and back, thyromental distance ≥3 fingerbreadths under jaw. Also dentures, contact lenses, earrings, tongue jewelry, hearing aids need to be removed
Chest	Lungs clear bilaterally, no wheezes, good air movement, no kyphoscoliosis or chest wall abnormalities
Cardiac	Normal heart sounds, no murmurs, no carotid bruits, rate regular with pulses conducted to extremities. Sinus arrhythmia and occasional premature beats are considered within normal limits
Back	No scoliosis, spine normal, no skin abnormalities over lumbar area for spinal or epidural
Extremities	Good capillary flow, normal color, normal pulses, veins observable for IV start, no contractures. Also, watches and rings are usually removed

Note: It is very common for uncontrolled or previously unknown disease to present at the time of surgery and for screening tests to reveal new pertinent findings. Vitamins and herbal supplements must be included in medication history.

9

CARDIOLOGY

Carey L. O'Bryan IV, MD

I. CHIEF COMPLAINT

Chronology of events (e.g., chest pain following mowing the grass) is very important with cardiology patients, and this information is often recorded within the chief complaint.

II. HISTORY OF PRESENT ILLNESS

A. Five Most Common Complaints Leading to a Cardiovascular Evaluation

1. Do you have **chest pain**?
2. Have you experienced **shortness of breath**?
3. Has there been any **swelling in your lower extremities**?
4. Do you have **palpitations**?
5. Have you experienced **loss of consciousness (syncope)**?

B. Chief Complaint Characteristics

For each symptom described previously, the following information must be obtained:

1. What is the **quality (character)** of your symptom (e.g., is the chest pain sharp, dull, squeezing, burning)?
2. When did the symptom begin **(onset)** and how long have you been experiencing the symptom **(duration)**?
3. How often does the symptom occur **(frequency)**?
4. How long does the symptom last when it is present **(length)**?
5. If the symptom is chest pain, does the pain travel to the neck, jaw, arm, back, or other parts of the chest **(radiation)**?
6. What type of activity causes the symptom to occur **(precipitators)**?
7. What type of activity makes the symptom worse **(exacerbators)**?
8. What type of activity, or cessation of activity, makes the symptom better **(relievers)**?
9. What additional symptoms **(associations)** occur with the primary symptom?

C. Angina Versus Nonanginal Chest Pain

Historical characteristics help distinguish pain caused by angina pectoris from other causes of chest pain. It should be noted, however, that some patients with myocardial ischemia experience symptoms not considered typical of angina (Table 9-1).

Table 9-1. PAIN CHARACTERISTICS TYPICAL OF ANGINA AND NOT TYPICAL OF ANGINA.

Feature	Typical of Angina	Not Typical of Angina
Location	Substernal, diffuse, left-sided	Focal, extrathoracic, right-sided
Character	Pressure, squeezing or burning	Sharp, "knifelike," electric, pleuritic
Radiation	Inner left arm, jaw	Right arm, midepigastrium, back, leg(s)
Onset and resolution	Gradual	Sudden
Length	Minutes (one or more hours in infarction)	Fleeting (seconds) or protracted (days to weeks)
Precipitators	Physical exertion, emotional distress, postprandial, cold weather	A specific body motion, occurring after exercise
Relievers	Rest, nitroglycerin	Exercise, massage, belching, antacids, changing positions, bronchodilators
Associations	Nausea, diaphoresis, dyspnea, light headedness	—

III. PAST MEDICAL AND SURGICAL HISTORY

A. Past Medical History: Cardiac Disease Risk

The following questions concern factors that may influence the risk for cardiac disease and that should be inquired about for every patient:

1. Have you been diagnosed as hypertensive?
2. Do you have diabetes mellitus?
3. Do you have hyperlipoproteinemia?
4. Have you been diagnosed with peripheral vascular disease, including carotid, aortic, and lower extremity disease?
5. Do you have a thyroid disease?
6. Have you had rheumatic fever?
7. Have you recently been, or are you currently, pregnant?
8. Do you have a history of malignancy or treatment with chemotherapy or radiation?
9. Have you been diagnosed with a rheumatologic condition, including rheumatoid arthritis, systemic sclerosis, systemic lupus erythematosus (SLE), and vasculitides?

10. What medications are you currently taking? What medications have you taken in the past?

B. **Past Surgical History**

1. Have you undergone coronary artery bypass surgery?
2. Have you had heart valve surgery?
3. Have you undergone aortic surgery?
4. Has surgery for congenital heart disease been performed?

C. **Emergency and Trauma History**

1. Have you previously presented to a hospital for a cardiac symptom or condition? When and at which hospital?
2. Do you have a history of cardiac trauma?

D. **Childhood History**

1. Did you have rheumatic fever as a child?
2. Do you have a history of congenital heart disease, either repaired or unrepaired?

E. **Occupational History:** Are you currently exposed, or have you been exposed, to substances that could contribute to heart disease (e.g., second-hand smoke, radiation exposure to the chest, or professional work with microbes).

F. **Travel History:** Have you traveled to areas where infectious diseases that are associated with specific cardiac complications are endemic, such as South America (Chagas disease) and the northeastern United States (Lyme disease)?

G. **Animals and Insects Exposure History**

1. Have you traveled to areas where livestock is raised? There are few zoonoses in cardiology. Occasionally, hydatid cysts from echinococcal infection can be seen in the myocardium.
2. Have you received an insect bite that produced a rash? Diseases such as Lyme and Chagas are transmitted by insect bites and may be associated with rashes.

IV. **MEDICATIONS, ALLERGIES, AND ADVERSE REACTIONS**

A. **Medications**

1. Are you currently taking any prescription medications, especially antihypertensive agents, cardiac agents (e.g., digoxin), anticoagulants, and nitrogen-based compounds?
2. Are you taking any over-the-counter (OTC) medications?
3. Do you take herbal preparations?
4. Are you taking supplements?

B. **Allergies to Medications and Side Effects**

1. It is critical to note all true drug allergies.
2. True allergies to aspirin or clopidogrel are of particular importance given their widespread use in treating coronary artery disease (CAD).
3. It is important to ask about allergic reactions to anticholinesterase (ACE) inhibitors that have caused swelling or dyspnea.

C. Adverse Reactions to Medications

1. Many people will have adverse reactions to both aspirin and ACE inhibitors that are not true allergies (such as GI bleeding with aspirin or renal insufficiency with ACE inhibitors). These should be determined.
2. Any adverse reaction to an anticoagulant (such as coumadin or heparin) should be noted.

V. HEALTH MAINTENANCE

A. Prevention

1. What were the results of your last cholesterol profile?
2. How often do you have your blood pressure checked? Was the most recent measurement high?

B. Diet

1. How much animal fat and cholesterol is contained in your regular diet? These substances can increase the risk of atherosclerosis.
2. Does your diet contain potassium or selenium? Inadequate intake of substances such as selenium can lead to heart complications. Both hypo- and hyperkalemia can lead to arrhythmias.

C. Exercise and Activities

1. Do you regularly partake in exertional activities?
2. Do you exercise regularly? If so, what specific exercises do you do and for what length of time? If you do not exercise, what do you do (e.g., housework, golf, shopping, climb stairs, lift heavy objects)? The goal is to determine the following:
   a. Aerobic Functional Status: This is often expressed in terms of metabolic equivalents (METs).
      (1) 1 MET = 3.5 mL of oxygen uptake per kilogram of body weight and reflects the metabolic cost of sitting at rest for a 70-kg male.
      (2) 3-5 METs = raking leaves, light carpentry, walking 3 to 4 miles per hour.
      (3) 5-7 METs = singles tennis, light backpacking.
      (4) >9 METs = heavy manual labor, running 6 miles per hour.
   b. Inability to achieve 5 METs is considered significant impairment. If the impairment results from neurologic, pulmonary, or musculoskeletal causes, significant cardiac disease may be present but symptoms masked by the patient's relative inactivity.

D. Sleep Patterns

1. Is your sleep disrupted from needing to sleep in a sitting position? Sleep may be disrupted from needing to sleep sitting up when in heart failure.
2. Are you experiencing alterations in your sleep patterns? Have you been feeling fatigue or drowsiness as a result? Chronic

heart failure can result in altered sleep patterns that may produce fatigue or drowsiness.

3. Have you experienced sleep apnea? Sleep apnea is associated with a variety of arrhythmias, most commonly bradyarrhythmias.

E. Social Habits

1. Do you drink alcohol? If so, what type, how much (quantify amount by day, week, or month), and for how long? Have you experienced complications from excessive alcohol ingestion?
2. Do you smoke? If so, what type of tobacco and for how long (e.g., how many pack-years)? Any complications?
3. Do you use intravenous or illicit drugs? If so, what type and how long? Have you experienced any complications from this drug use?

VI. FAMILY HISTORY

First-Degree Relative's Medical History and Three-Generation Genogram.

1. Do any family members have coronary artery diseases?
2. Do any blood relatives have heart failure or arrhythmias. If so, how old were they at diagnosis?
3. Have any blood relatives died suddenly? If so, at what age?

VII. PSYCHOSOCIAL HISTORY

A. Personal and Social History

1. What is your ethnic background? Ethnicity/race may identify increased risk of disease or variable responses to therapy (e.g., diabetes in Hispanics and sodium-avid hypertension in African Americans).
2. Are you able to afford medications and therapies that may be required to treat your condition?
3. What is the highest level of formal education you have attained? The ability of a patient to understand his or her own disease(s) and make lifestyle adjustments correlates with level of education.

B. Current Illness Effects on the Patient

1. How has this illness affected you? Do you feel that you are able to cope well with it? Do you have friends and family who might support you throughout this illness?
2. Is the patient's expectations of his or her illness and therapy realistic?
3. Are there signs/symptoms of depression?
4. Inquire about living wills and advanced directives.

C. Interpersonal and Sexual History: Are you concerned that some medications used to treat your condition (e.g., some hypertensive agents) may adversely affect your ability to achieve erection or may decrease your sexual appetite (i.e., libido)? How do you feel about these possibilities? How will such side effects affect your life?

D. Family Support and Risk

1. Are any family members in need of tutoring on cardiac emergencies and basic life support (BLS)?
2. Are any family members at risk for cardiovascular disease?

E. Occupational Aspects of the Illness

1. Does your work require you to be physically active? The patient may require restriction of physical activity at work.
2. Does your occupation require you to perform risky tasks (such as piloting a plane or driving a bus)? If the patient has an occupation that would make the occurrence of a cardiac event at work particularly risky, he or she may need to be restricted from performing his or her usual job.

VIII. REVIEW OF SYSTEMS

The primary purpose of the review of systems is to uncover any evidence of the diseases or conditions mentioned previously that can influence a patient's risk for cardiac disease (Tables 9-2, 9-3, and 9-4).

Table 9-2. GENERAL CARDIOVASCULAR SYMPTOMS BY SYSTEM.

SYSTEM	SYMPTOMS
General	Fever, night sweats, weight loss or gain, general energy level
Neurologic	Loss of consciousness, headache, transient speech problems, numbness, weakness
Respiratory	Shortness of breath, cough (productive or not), hemoptysis, wheezing
Cardiovascular	Chest pain, palpitations, orthopnea, nocturnal dyspnea, exertional leg (buttock, thigh,or calf) or arm pain, cold extremities, changes in skin color in extremities, leg swelling
Gastrointestinal	Abdominal pain or swelling, nausea, change in bowel habits, GI bleeding, reflux symptoms
Genitourinary	Urinary retention, frequent or reduction in urination, frothy urine
Obstetric/ gynecologic	First day of last normal menstrual period (LNMP)
Musculoskeletal	Back pain, leg pain or swelling
Rheumatologic	Joint pain or swelling, rashes, mouth ulcers, skin changes
Endocrinologic	Cold or heat intolerance, hunger, thirst

Table 9-3. NONSPECIFIC SYMPTOMS AND THEIR CARDIOVASCULAR DISEASES.

SYMPTOM	DISEASES
Chest pain	Myocardial ischemia, aortic dissection, aortic stenosis, pericarditis
Shortness of breath	Heart failure (systolic or diastolic), myocardial ischemia, disease of any valve, chronotropic incompetence, tachyarrythmias, tamponade, constrictive pericarditis
Lower extremity swelling	Heart failure from any cause (e.g., myocardial, valvular, pericardial), deep venous thrombosis (DVT)
Palpitations	Premature atrial contractions (PACs), premature ventricular contractions (PVCs), atrial or ventricular arrhythmias, sinus pauses
Loss of consciousness	Ventricular arrhythmias, bradyarrhythmias, neurocardiogenic, severe stenotic valvular disease, severe ventricular dysfunction, cardiac tamponade, aortic dissection
Fatigue	Left ventricular dysfunction, chronotropic incompetence, valvular disease, CAD

Table 9-4. COMMON CARDIOVASCULAR DISEASES AND THEIR SYMPTOMS.

DISEASE	SYMPTOMS
Angina pectoris	Substernal chest pain, pressure or burning, often with radiation to jaw or arm; symptoms brought on with exertion and relieved with rest
Aortic regurgitation	Dyspnea, exertional fatigue
Aortic stenosis	Angina, syncope, dyspnea, exertional fatigue
Heart failure, left	Dyspnea, orthopnea, paroxysmal nocturnal dyspnea (PND), exertional fatigue
Heart failure, right	Dyspnea, lower extremity edema, ascites
Mitral regurgitation	Dyspnea, exertional fatigue, palpitations
Mitral stenosis	Dyspnea, exertional fatigue, palpitations
Arrhythmia	Palpitations, syncope, light-headedness, dyspnea, chest pain/pressure
Myocardial infarction	Anginal chest pain at rest, dyspnea, diaphoresis, nausea

IX. PHYSICAL EXAMINATION

The three primary modalities for the cardiovascular examination are inspection, palpation, and auscultation.

A. **General Inspection:** Observe the following:
   1. Distress: Is the patient in obvious discomfort from chest pain or dyspnea?
   2. Body habitus: Observe for stigmata of syndromes with cardiac associations such as Marfan's, Turner's, Down's, or Holt-Oram.
   3. Head: Conjunctival injection (endocarditis), arcus senilis (hyperlipoproteinemia), bilateral diagonal earlobe creases (associated with coronary artery disease).
   4. Fundi: Copper or silver wiring changes of arterioles, cotton wool spots, papilledema (all associated with systemic hypertension), Hollenhorst plaques (cholesterol emboli), Roth spots (endocarditis).
   5. Neck: Jugular venous pulses (see following section).
   6. Extremities: Cyanosis (Eisenmenger's syndrome, severe heart failure), clubbing (Eisenmenger's syndrome), swelling, signs of endocarditis (e.g., Osler's nodes [painful, nonblanching papules on palms or soles], Janeway lesions [painless, nonblanching macules on palms or soles], splinter hemorrhages [red, linear streaks at base of nails]).

B. **Jugular Venous Pulses**
   1. The jugular venous pulse (JVP) is best observed with the head turned slightly leftward. The head of the bed should be elevated to whatever degree necessary to locate the top of the pulsating venous fluid column. Usually this can be accomplished with the patient at a 45-degree angle.
   2. The jugular vein is deep to the skin and medial head of the sternocleidomastoid muscle, so its pulsations are not directly observed. Observe for the skin flickering, which represents transmitted JVPs.
   3. The A wave reflects atrial contraction, the X descent occurs with right atrial relaxation, the C wave coincides with the carotid pulse, the V wave reflects passive right atrial filling behind a closed tricuspid valve (TV), and the Y descent reflects sudden opening of the TV.
   4. One can distinguish JVPs from carotid pulsations by noting or performing the following:
      a. The carotid pulsation is medial to the JVP.
      b. The A wave of the JVP occurs slightly before the carotid pulsation.
      c. Moderate compression at the root of the neck often obliterates venous pulsations but should not alter carotid pulsations.
      d. The A wave of the JVP occurs nearly simultaneously with S1.

5. Utility of estimating jugular venous pressure:
   a. Because the jugular vein is in direct communication with the right atrium, it can be used as a measurement of right atrial pressure.
   b. In the absence of obstruction at the level of the tricuspid valve, mean right atrial pressure should equal right ventricular diastolic pressure.
   c. Right ventricular diastolic pressure is most commonly elevated because of left ventricular dysfunction. Consequently, an elevation of jugular venous pressure usually implies some degree of heart failure. Other causes of elevated right ventricular diastolic pressure include tricuspid regurgitation, pulmonic stenosis or regurgitation, pulmonary hypertension, volume-overloaded states, and pericardial disease.
6. Estimating the JVP:
   a. Position the patient as described previously.
   b. Determine the height of the JVP (pointing a penlight tangential to the neck will help make the pulsations visible).
   c. Measure in centimeters how far this extends above the sternal angle.
   d. Any value greater than 4 cm is elevated.
   e. *Note:* The right atrium is approximately 5 cm below the sternal angle. To estimate the actual jugular venous pressure (in centimeters of water), simply add 5 to the number of centimeters the JVP rises above the sternal angle. For example, if you measured the JVP to be 7 cm above the sternal angle, then the actual jugular venous, and therefore right atrial, pressure would be approximately 12 cm H_2O. Normal is approximately 5 to 9.

C. Palpation

1. Pulses.
   a. The following pulses should be palpated: Carotid, brachial, radial, femoral, popliteal, posterior tibial, and dorsalis pedis. A cautious attempt to palpate the abdominal aorta should also be made (Table 9-5).
   b. Notation should be made of pulse fullness, symmetry, regularity of cardiac rhythm, and heart rate.
   c. When assessing for the specific pulse abnormalities described as follows, it is best to palpate the carotid pulse (unless otherwise noted).
2. Precordium.
   a. Open hand.
      (1) Examine the patient in both the supine and left lateral decubitus positions. Place the right hand on the sternum such that the heel of the hand is at the inferior sternal border with the fingers extended and overlying the right sternal border. Move the hand through

Table 9-5. ABNORMAL PULSES AND ASSOCIATED CONDITIONS.

Abnormal Pulse	Description	Associated Condition(s)
Pulsus parvus	Small pulse amplitude	Any severe stenotic valvular lesion, heart failure, pericardial disease
Pulsus magnus	Increased pulse amplitude	Anxiety, anemia, thyrotoxicosis, hypertension
Water-hammer (Corrigan) pulse	Extremely rapid rise and collapse caused by elevated systolic pressure, low diastolic pressure, and large stroke volume	Aortic regurgitation
Pulsus alternans	Alternating large and small pulse waves	Severe heart failure
Pulsus paradoxus	Decrease in pulse amplitude (systolic blood pressure) by more than 10 mmHg with inspiration	Cardiac tamponade, severe airways obstruction
Pulsus parvus et tardus	Small amplitude pulse that has a delayed peak*	Severe aortic stenosis (AS)
Pulsus bisferiens (bifid pulse)	Pulse wave has two narrowly separated peak impulses	AS with atrial regurgitation (AR), AR alone, or hypertrophic obstructive cardiomyopathy (HOCM)
Arm-Leg Pulse Discrepancy	The pulses in the leg are diminished and delayed compared to the pulses in the arms	Coarctation of the aorta; always check this in a young patient with hypertension

*To determine if the pulse is delayed, simultaneously palpate the apical impulse and the carotid pulse. Both pulsations should be felt at the exact same time. If the carotid lags the apical pulse even slightly, delay is present. If the apical impulse cannot be palpated, S1 may be used as a surrogate. In elderly patients with severe AS and stiff arteries, a pulsus parvus et tardus may not be present because of pseudonormalization.

and arc to the patient's left until the hand is 90 degrees to the sternum.

(2) Palpate for exaggerated motion of the entire parasternal area, which implies hyperdynamic right ventricle (RV) from volume overload (e.g., CHF, ASD, or severe TR) or left parasternal lift (systolic anterior motion of the left parasternal region), which implies right ventricular enlargement or hypertrophy or left ventricular aneurysm.

b. Finger tips and point of maximum impulse (PMI): Once the hand has rotated 90 degrees to the patient's left, palpate for the PMI with the distal third of the fingers.

(1) The PMI is located in the 4th or 5th intercostal space (ICS) in the midclavicular line and is most readily found with the patient in the left lateral decubitus position. If not readily palpable, ask the patient to exhale completely and hold his or her breath out. This will bring the heart closer to the chest wall.

(2) The normal PMI is no more than 2 cm (a quarter) in size and produces a light tapping sensation.

(a) Sustained PMI: A PMI that is palpable for two thirds or more of systole (must auscultate and palpate simultaneously). Implies chronic pressure overload from conditions such as hypertension or aortic stenosis (AS).

(b) Displaced PMI: Chronic volume overload or left ventricular enlargement from systolic dysfunction will typically displace the PMI inferiorly and laterally. The PMI is often diffuse (>2 cm) in this setting.

(c) S3 and S4: Occasionally these sounds will be palpable at the PMI.

(d) Triple ripple: Felt in hypertrophic obstructive cardiomyopathy (HOCM) and consists of a palpable S4, sustained PMI, and an end-systolic bulge caused by obstruction occurring when the heart is nearly empty.

(e) Thrills: A thrill is a palpable vibration caused by a heart murmur. These are best palpated in the ICS, where the respective murmur is best heard (see following section on murmurs). The presence of a thrill implies a murmur of grade 4/6 or higher.

(f) Pulmonary artery: If enlarged (as seen in conditions such as pulmonary hypertension or increased pulmonary blood flow) may palpate systolic pulsations in the second left ICS. Often associated with evidence of RV enlargement or hypertrophy.

(g) Aorta: Enlargement or aneurysm of the ascending aorta or the arch may be palpable in the suprasternal notch.

D. Auscultation

1. General approach.
   - **a.** Do not attempt to auscultate through clothing.
   - **b.** All heart sounds can be described in terms of frequency (pitch), amplitude (loudness), and duration.
   - **c.** The diaphragm of the stethoscope is best for hearing medium- to high-frequency sounds, whereas the bell is best for hearing low-frequency sounds.
   - **d.** Auscultate with the patient upright and in the left lateral decubitus position.
   - **e.** Auscultate S1, systole, S2, and diastole with both the diaphragm and the bell in each of the four major listening areas.

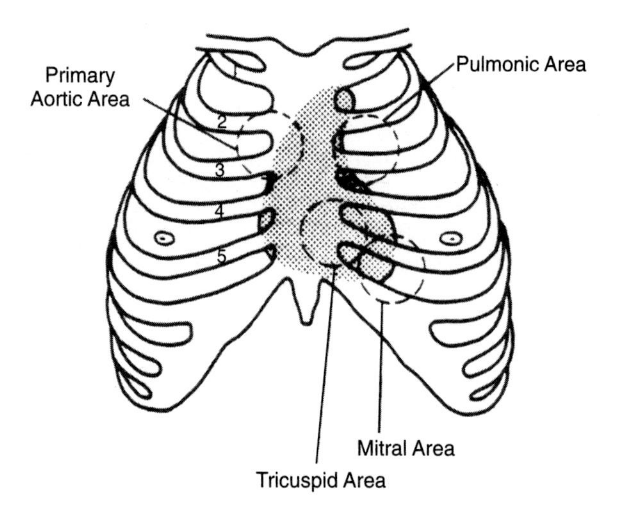

2. First heart sound (S1).
   - **a.** Caused by the closure of the mitral (M1) and tricuspid (T1) valves in that order.
   - **b.** Best heard (loudest) at the mitral and tricuspid areas.
   - **c.** M1 is louder than T1 in normals.
   - **d.** S1 is usually a single sound, but when listening at the tricuspid area, splitting may be heard because of optimal transmission of the sound of T1 at this site. In this case, the frequency of the sounds will be similar, but the amplitude (volume) of T1 will still be smaller than M1.

e. S1 is louder than S2 at the mitral and tricuspid area, whereas S2 is louder than S1 at the base.
f. Amplitude of S1: A loud S1 is defined as an S1 that is louder than S2 at the base. The major causes include:
   (1) Hyperdynamic heart (with anemia, thyrotoxicosis, anxiety, and exercise).
   (2) Mitral stenosis.
   (3) Short PR interval (caused by wide-open position of valves at the onset of ventricular contraction).
g. A soft S1 is defined as an S1 that is quieter than S2 at the mitral and tricuspid areas. The major causes include:
   (1) Long PR interval (atrioventricular valves have moved closer together by the time of ventricular systole resulting in reduced force of closure).
   (2) Poorly contracting ventricle (reduced force of closure caused by shock or severe systolic dysfunction).
   (3) Masking of S1 by a loud mitral regurgitation murmur.
h. Variable S1 will be seen in conditions of variable preload, such as:
   (1) Atrial fibrillation.
   (2) Ventricular tachycardia (VT) (preload varies because of atrioventricular [AV] dissociation; this finding can help distinguish VT from supraventricular tachycardia [SVT] with aberrancy because S1 intensity should be constant in the latter).

3. Second heart sound (S2).
   a. Caused by the closure of the aortic (A2) and pulmonic (P2) valves in that order.
   b. Best heard (loudest) at the base of the heart (aortic and pulmonic areas).
   c. A2 is louder than P2 in normals.
   d. Amplitude of S2:
      (1) A loud S2 is defined as an S2 that is louder than S1 at the tricuspid or mitral areas.
      (2) It will be caused by anything that increases the intensity of A2 or P2, such as arterial or pulmonary hypertension, respectively.
      (3) A loud P2 is established if P2 is louder than A2 at the base; a loud P2 is suggested if P2 can be heard at the apex.
      (4) A quiet S2 can be heard in the setting of arterial or pulmonary hypotension, AS, or pulmonic stenosis (PS).
   e. Normally the S2 demonstrates splitting.
4. Normal (physiologic) splitting.
   a. S2 splits (separates) on inspiration, and is single on expiration.

CARD

b. On inspiration venous return to the RV is increased resulting in prolonged ejection of blood. This delays the closure of the pulmonic valve (PV) and results in splitting.
c. On expiration, venous return to the RV decreases, as does the ejection time, causing P2 to move closer to A2.
d. Exaggerated splitting: Seen in conditions that cause either delay in PV closure (e.g., right bundle branch block [RBBB] or pulmonic stenosis) or early aortic valve closure (e.g., MR or ventriculoseptal defect [VSD]).
e. Paradoxical splitting: S2 splits on expiration and is single on inspiration.
   (1) Seen in conditions that cause delayed closure of the AV.
   (2) With delayed AV closure, P2 occurs before A2 on expiration.
   (3) On inspiration, with increased venous return to the RV and prolonged RV ejection, P2 occurs later, which places it simultaneous with A2.
   (4) Causes include left bundle branch block (LBBB) and severe AS.
f. Fixed splitting.
   (1) This is the hallmark of hemodynamically significant left-to-right shunting through an ASD.
   (2) Mechanism:
      (a) The left-to-right shunt is so large that the right ventricle becomes volume overloaded, leading to a prolonged ejection time.
      (b) This results in P2 occurring after A2 with both inspiration and expiration.
      (c) Although there may be some movement of P2 closer to A2 during the respiratory cycle, the sounds will never become one (i.e., there will always be some fixed splitting present).

3. Third heart sound (S3).
   a. A low-pitched sound heard after S2.
   b. Through the third decade, can be a normal finding.
   c. In most patients it is a reliable sign of heart failure.
   d. Best heard with the patient in the left lateral decubitus position with the bell placed lightly over the PMI.
   e. Can distinguish an S3 from a split S2 by noting that an S3 can be made quieter or possibly made to disappear by applying firm pressure with the bell.
4. Fourth heart sound (S4).
   a. A low-pitched sound heard just before S1.
   b. Caused by atrial contraction into a stiff ventricle.
   c. Always signifies an abnormal ventricle.
   d. Best heard with the patient in the left lateral decubitus position with the bell placed lightly over the PMI.

e. Can distinguish an S4 from a split S1 by using the same criteria described previously for distinguishing an S3 from an S2.

5. Summation Gallop.

a. A four-component sound consisting of an S4, S1, S2, and S3.

b. Has the rhythm of a galloping horse.

6. Additional heart sounds are described in Table 9-6.

7. Murmurs (general).

a. Murmurs are prolonged auditory vibrations caused by blood flowing through the heart.

b. These may be innocent, in which case the murmur is caused by blood flowing out of the left or right ventricle, usually in the setting of a healthy, vigorously contracting heart.

c. Murmurs are often pathologic, implying disease in a heart valve or some other structure (e.g., patent ductus arteriosus [PDA], ventricular septal defect [VSD]).

d. By convention, murmurs are graded on a scale of 1–6.

HEART MURMUR SCALE.

1. A grade 1 murmur requires special effort to hear.
2. A grade 2 murmur is soft but readily heard.
3. A grade 3 murmur is loud but not associated with a thrill.
4. A grade 4 murmur is loud and is associated with a thrill.
5. A grade 5 murmur is very loud and associated with an easily palpable thrill.
6. A grade 6 murmur can be heard at a distance from the chest wall and is associated with an easily palpable thrill.

e. The following should be determined when auscultating a murmur:

(1) Location best heard.

(2) Timing within the cardiac cycle (systole or diastole).

(3) Grade.

(4) Pitch (high or low).

(5) Character (e.g., crescendo, decrescendo, crescendo-decrescendo, early systolic, holosystolic).

(6) Radiation (i.e., where else can the murmur be heard besides its site of maximal intensity?).

Table 9-6. ADDITIONAL HEART SOUNDS.

SOUND	MECHANISM	FEATURES	CAUSE
Ejection sound	Blood flowing through an abnormal PV or AV and snapping it tight	Occurs shortly after S1 and is best heard at base	Most common cause is bicuspid AV
Systolic clicks	Likely from chordae tendonae being pulled tight	High-pitched sound in midsystole; more than one click may be present; often followed by systolic murmur of MVP	MVP
Opening snap	Caused by the opening of a stenotic but mobile MV or TV	High-pitched sound closely following S2 heard best at apex; may be mistaken for split S2	MS >> TS
Pericardial knock	Sudden cessation of ventricular expansion	Low- to medium-pitched sound in diastole, which may be mistaken for S3	Constrictive pericarditis
Tumor plop	Atrial myxoma prolapsing across MV or TV during diastole	Low-pitched early diastolic sound, which may be mistaken for an S3	Atrial myxoma

8. Systolic murmurs.
   a. Systolic ejection murmurs (SEM, also known as midsystolic murmurs): Caused by ejection of blood into one of the great vessels (aorta or pulmonary artery).
   b. Holosystolic murmurs (HS, also known as early systolic murmurs): Caused by regurgitation of blood across an AV or across a VSD; these murmurs typically obscure S1 and often occupy all of systole.
   c. Some of the more common murmurs are described in Table 9-7.
9. Diastolic murmurs (Table 9-8).
   a. Early diastolic murmurs: Decrescendo pattern, often "blowing" in quality.
   b. Middiastolic murmurs: Lower frequency, "rumbling" in quality, and often preceded by an opening snap.
10. Continuous murmurs, heard in both systole and diastole.
   a. PDA.
   b. Aortovenous fistula (e.g., ruptured sinus of Valsalva).
   c. Cervical venous hum.
   d. Mammary soufflé.

E. Dynamic Auscultation

1. It is often impossible to accurately diagnose a murmur by simply auscultating the patient at rest.
2. Most murmurs behave in predictable ways with certain maneuvers, and performing such maneuvers can help confirm a specific diagnosis.
3. The examiner listens for a change in amplitude (loudness) of the murmur with the standard maneuvers presented in Table 9-9.
4. The following associations between maneuvers and murmurs are well described (Table 9-10).
5. The click and murmur of mitral valve prolapse (MVP) also change with maneuvers (Table 9-11).

X. DIFFERENTIAL DIAGNOSIS (Table 9-12)

XI. LABORATORY STUDIES AND DIAGNOSTIC EVALUATIONS

A. Cardiac Enzymes

1. Myoglobin: A nonspecific marker of myocyte injury.
2. Creatine kinase (CK): A nonspecific marker of myocyte injury.
3. CK-MB: An isoenzyme of CK that is relatively specific for cardiac myocyte injury.
4. Troponin (Tn).
   a. Two forms are in clinical use: Tn T and Tn I.
   b. The most specific markers of cardiac myocyte injury currently available.
   c. Rises as quickly as CK, but stays elevated longer.

B. C-reactive protein (CRP): An inflammatory marker that, when elevated, has been associated with increased risk for cardiac events in certain patient populations.

CARD

Table 9-7. COMMON SYSTOLIC MURMURS.

Murmur	Type	Location	Quality	Radiation	Comments
Flow murmur	SEM	Usually LUSB	Low-amplitude, early or midsystolic murmur	No radiation	Heard more often in younger patients with thinner chests and vigorous contractility
AS	SEM	RUSB	Harsh, crescendo-decrescendo	Neck	Infrequently can radiate to apex/axilla
PS	SEM	LUSB	Harsh, crescendo-decrescendo	—	Quieter than AS murmur
ASD	SEM	LUSB	Quiet midsystolic murmur	—	Caused by increased flow across PV, not the ASD itself; should also hear an S2 with fixed splitting
HOCM	SEM	LLSB	Harsh	May radiate to apex	—
MR	HS	LLSB	Medium to high pitch	Apex, axilla, back	Can radiate to base if MR occurs through an incompetent posterior leaflet; the murmur of acute MR may be an early systolic, decrescendo murmur
TR	HS	Tricuspid area	Similar in quality to MR but often quieter	—	If severe may see pulsatile liver or "no, no" sign (head tilting left and right)
VSD	HS	LLSB	Medium pitch; often musical	Across precordium but not axilla	—

SB = Sterna border.

Table 9-8. DIASTOLIC MURMURS.

Murmur	Type	Location	Quality	Radiation	Comments
AR	Early diastolic	Aortic area	High pitched	Apex	May hear Austin Flint murmur (see Table 9-13)
PR	Early diastolic	Pulmonic area	High pitched	—	Most commonly caused by pulmonary hypertension; may also hear loud P2
MS	Early diastolic	Apex	Low pitched	—	Often follows an opening snap; S1 usually loud
TS	Middiastolic	Tricuspid	Low pitched	—	Rare

Table 9-9. DYNAMIC AUSCULTATION MANEUVERS.

MANEUVER	DESCRIPTION	PHYSIOLOGIC EFFECT
Inspiration	The patient takes a slow deep breath in	Venous return increases to the right side of the heart and decreases to the left
Valsalva	The patient strains abdominal muscles and expires against a closed glottis for several seconds and then releases. The examiner listens during both the strain and release phases	Venous return to the right side of the heart is decreased with strain and restored with release
Squatting	The patient stands upright while the examiner sits with the stethoscope positioned on the chest in the position where the murmur is best heard. The patient then squats down and stays squatting while the examiner listens	Squatting simultaneously increases venous return (preload) and afterload
Standing	From the squatting or sitting position, the patient stands while the examiner listens	Venous return and afterload decrease
Handgrip	The patient extends arms and clenches fists tightly for several seconds	Afterload is increased
Leg elevation	While supine the patient's legs are elevated to 30 degrees	Venous return is increased

C. Cardiac Catheterization

1. Invasive test, which involves inserting catheters into the aorta, cardiac chambers, coronary arteries, and pulmonary vessels.
2. Images are obtained using the injection of contrast and x-ray imaging.
3. Coronary interventions (angioplasty, stents) and valvuloplasties can be performed in the catheterization lab.
4. Pulmonary, intracardiac, venous. and arterial pressures can be measured by connecting the catheters to a pressure transduction system.

Table 9-10. ASSOCIATIONS BETWEEN MANEUVERS, MURMURS, AND MURMUR AMPLITUDE.

MANEUVER	MURMUR	EFFECT ON MURMUR AMPLITUDE
Inspiration	All right-sided murmurs	Increases
Valsalva	HOCM	Increases with strain, decreases with release
	AS	Decreases with strain, increases with release
Squatting	AS, MR, AR	Increases
	HOCM	Decreases
Standing	HOCM	Increases
Handgrip	MR, VSD, AR, MS	Increases
	PDA	Increases diastolic component
	HOCM	Decreases
	AS	Decreases
Leg elevation	AS, TR, TS	Increases

Table 9-11. MANEUVER EFFECTS ON MVP.

MANEUVERS	EFFECT
Standing, Valsalva strain	Click moves closer to S1 and murmur starts earlier
Squatting, leg elevation	Click moves closer to S2 and murmur starts later

D. Echocardiography

1. Noninvasive, ultrasound study, which provides images of the heart chambers, valves, pericardium, and often portions of the aorta and inferior vena cava (IVC).
2. Varieties include transthoracic echo (TTE), which is the standard and can be done at the bedside; transesophageal echo (TEE), which is more invasive but gives better-quality images, improved spatial resolution, and can also be done at the bedside; and stress echo, which indirectly tests for ischemia based on identifying ventricular wall motion abnormalities at stress (either exercise or chemical stress).

E. Nuclear Cardiology

1. Tests that involve administering a radioactive tracer that is deposited (relatively) selectively in the heart.

Table 9-12. DIFFERENTIAL DIAGNOSIS OF CARDIOVASCULAR DISEASE.

Symptom	Cardiovascular Diagnoses	Noncardiac Causes
Chest pain	Myocardial ischemia, aortic dissection, aortic stenosis, pericarditis	Pulmonary embolus (PE), pneumothorax, pleural disease, pulmonary hypertension, esophageal, gastric or liver/gallbladder disease, disorders of the chest wall, diseases of the skin, disorders of peripheral nerves
Shortness of breath	Heart failure (systolic or diastolic), myocardial ischemia, disease of any valve, chronotropic incompetence, tachyarrythmias, tamponade, constrictive pericarditis	Lung disease, anemia, disorders resulting in impaired venous return, deconditioning, neuromuscular disorders
Lower extremity swelling	Heart failure from any cause (myocardial, valvular, pericardial), DVT	Venous insufficiency, lymphatic obstruction, liver disease, renal disease, trauma, infection, ruptured Baker's cyst
Palpitations	PACs, PVCs, atrial arrhythmias, ventricular arrhythmias, sinus pauses	Sinus tachycardia secondary to PE, pericardial disease, thyrotoxicosis, shunts, hypovolemia, hyperadrenergic states
Loss of consciousness	Ventricular arrhythmias, heart block, sinus arrest, neurocardiogenic, severe stenotic valvular disease, severe ventricular dysfunction, tamponade, aortic dissection	PE, severe pulmonary hypertension, severe hypoxemia, CVA/TIA, seizure, hypovolemia, disorders of autonomic nervous system

2. Cameras detect this activity, and images are generated based on the degree to which the tracer is taken up by various parts of the myocardium.
3. Stress perfusion tests are most common and detect obstructive coronary artery disease based on a reduction in tracer activity in areas of the heart that have a reduced blood supply at stress (either exercise or chemical).
4. Nuclear studies can also give information on ejection fraction and viability of ischemic myocardium.

F. **Computed Tomography (CT)**
1. Certain techniques (electron beam CT [EBCT] or newer multi-slice CT) can detect and quantify coronary calcium, which is used as a surrogate marker of atherosclerosis. Higher calcium scores generally correspond to higher risk for coronary events.
2. Useful for evaluating for pericardial calcium and thickening, which are often seen in constrictive pericarditis.
3. May be able to perform diagnostic-quality, noninvasive coronary angiograms in the near future.

G. **Magnetic Resonance Imaging (MRI)**
1. Established uses for MRI include diagnosing congenital heart disease, anomalous coronary arteries, cardiac masses, diseases of the right ventricle, and pericardial and aortic disease.
2. State-of-the-art centers can also use MRI to evaluate myocardial perfusion, viability, and valvular disease, and to perform limited coronary angiograms.

XII. **EPONYMS, ACRONYMS, AND ABBREVIATIONS (Table 9-13, 9-14, and 9-15)**

Table 9-13. EPONYMS ASSOCIATED WITH CARDIAC DISORDERS.

Name	Description	Cause
Austin Flint murmur	Mid- to late-diastolic murmur heard best at mitral area	Severe AR caused by rapid blood flow across a mitral valve whose orifice is quickly diminishing; to be distinguished from the early diastolic murmur of AR per se

Continued

CARD

Table 9-13. EPONYMS ASSOCIATED WITH CARDIAC DISORDERS—*cont'd*

Name	Description	Cause
Carey-Coombs	Early diastolic murmur head best at mitral area	Active mitral valvulitis from acute rheumatic fever
Caravhallo's sign	Holosystolic murmur that increases with inspiration	Seen in association with severe TR
Gallavardin phenomenon	High-frequency, musical systolic murmur radiating to the apex	Vibrations of the fibrocalcific cusps of the aortic valve in the setting of severe AS
Graham Steel murmur	Early diastolic murmur heard best at pulmonic area	PR from pulmonary hypertension
Hollenhorst plaques	Atheromatous emboli containing cholesterol crystals noted in retinal arterioles on fundoscopic exam	Seen in severe atherosclerosis
Janeway lesions	Painless, nonblanching macules on palms or soles	Infective endocarditis
Means-Lerman murmur	Scratchy, midsystolic sound, which can be confused with a rub	Seen with thyrotoxicosis
Osler's nodes	Painful, nonblanching papules on palms or soles	Infective endocarditis
Roth's spots	Round/oval white spots in retina	Coagulated fibrin resulting from vascular insult/hemorrhage followed by healing; seen in infective endocarditis
Still's murmur	Short, midsystolic murmur	Innocent flow murmur in children

Table 9-14. EPONYMS ASSOCIATED WITH SEVERE ATRIAL REGURGITATION.

NAME	DESCRIPTION	CAUSE
Austin Flint murmur	Mid- to late-diastolic murmur heard best at mitral area	Rapid blood flow across a mitral valve whose orifice is quickly diminishing due to AR
Corrigan's pulse	Rapid rise and collapse of the systemic pulse	Widened pulse pressure
De Musset's sign	Movement of the head up and down	Widened pulse pressure
Duroziez's sign	Murmurs over femoral arteries	Widened pulse pressure
Hill's sign	BP in legs exceeds arm pressures by more than 60 mmHg	Widened pulse pressure
Muller's sign	Bobbing uvula	Widened pulse pressure
Oliver's sign	Tracheal tug	Widened pulse pressure
Quincke's pulses	Systolic flushing of the nailbeds	Widened pulse pressure
Traube's sign	Cracking sounds over the femoral vessels ("pistol shot femorals")	Widened pulse pressure

XIII. DEFINITIONS (Table 9-16)

XIV. SAMPLE H&P WRITE-UP

CC: "I've had chest pain for three hours."

HPI: J.R. is a 45-year-old married white male who presented to the Emergency Department with complaints of chest pain. He describes the pain as substernal pressure that radiates to the left arm. The pain began at rest and has been associated with mild nausea and shortness of breath. The pain was not relieved with positional changes or antacids but improved with nitroglycerin administered in the emergency department. It was made worse with ambulation but not with respiration. The pain did not radiate to his back and was not associated with a sour taste in his mouth. The chest pain was new for the patient; however, he had experienced three episodes of pain that were similar in quality but much less severe in intensity over the prior week. These episodes always resolved spontaneously within five minutes. The patient denied palpitations or loss of consciousness. He has no prior history of cardiac illness.

Text continued on p. 126.

Table 9-15. CARDIOLOGY ACRONYMS AND ABBREVIATIONS.

Acronym or Abbreviation	Term	Description
AF	Atrial fibrillation	Chaotic atrial electrical activity resulting in irregularly irregular tachycardia
AFL	Atrial flutter	Atrial arrhythmia resulting in an often regularly irregular tachycardia
AR	Aortic regurgitation	Abnormal flow of blood from aorta through the aortic valve into the left ventricle during diastole
AS	Aortic stenosis	Disease resulting in narrowing of the aortic valve
ASD	Atrial septal defect	Defect in the interatrial septum leading to abnormal communication between atria
CABG	Coronary artery bypass grafting	Surgical procedure performed on patients with severe coronary artery disease
CAD	Coronary artery disease	A disease of the arterial wall resulting in inflammation, lipid deposition, calcification, and obstruction of the coronary lumen
CHF	Congestive heart failure	The pathologic state in which the heart cannot eject blood sufficient to meet the body's metabolic needs, or does so at elevated filling pressures
CK	Creatine kinase	Serum protein; nonspecific marker of myocyte injury; used in diagnosing and quantifying myocardial infarctions
CRP	C-reactive protein	Serum protein; an inflammatory marker that, when elevated, has been associated with increased risk for cardiac events in certain patient populations
EF	Ejection fraction	The fraction of blood ejected with each contraction; usually refers to the left ventricle unless specified

HCM	Hypertrophic cardiomyopathy	Genetic disorder leading to abnormal thickening of the left ventricle and usually conferring an increased risk of sudden death
HOCM	Hypertrophic obstructive cardiomyopathy	A variant of HCM in which there is obstruction to outflow of blood at the left ventricular outflow track; the risk of CHF is higher than in those with non-obstructive HCM
HS	Holosystolic murmur	Also known as early systolic murmurs, caused by regurgitation of blood across an atrioventricular valve or a VSD
ICD	Internal cardiac defibrillator	Device surgically implanted, which automatically detects ventricular arrhythmias and treats them with either rapid pacing or a shock
ICS	Intercostal space	Spaces between ribs
JVD	Jugular venous distention	Abnormal fullness of the jugular veins caused by elevated right heart pressures
JVP	Jugular venous pressure	An estimate of right atrial pressure made by measuring the height of the fluid column in the internal jugular vein
LBBB	Left bundle branch block	Abnormality noted on ECG resulting from the inability of the left branch of the ventricular conduction system to conduct electrical impulses
LV	Left ventricle	Main cardiac pumping chamber
MET	Metabolic equivalent	Used to quantify functional status or physical performance
MI	Myocardial infarction	Focus or foci of myocyte death caused by prolonged ischemia
MR	Mitral regurgitation	Abnormal flow of blood from left ventricle into left atrium during ventricular contraction
MS	Mitral stenosis	Narrowing of the mitral valve resulting in obstruction of blood flow from the left atrium to the left ventricle

Continued

Table 9-15. CARDIOLOGY ACRONYMS AND ABBREVIATIONS—*cont'd*

Acronym or Abbreviation	Term	Description
MUGA	Multiple gated acquisition	Nuclear medicine test to determine left or right ventricular ejection fraction
MV	Mitral valve	Left-sided heart valve between left ventricle and left atrium
MVP	Mitral valve prolapse	Prolapse of histologically abnormal mitral valve leaflet(s) into left atrium during ventricular contraction
PDA	Patent ductus arteriosus	Persistent, abnormal connection between the pulmonary artery and aorta
PMI	Point of maximum impulse	Point at which ventricular contraction is most strongly palpated on chest well
PND	Paroxysmal nocturnal dyspnea	Dyspnea occurring during sleep requiring sitting upright or standing for several minutes to relieve
PR	Pulmonic regurgitation	Leaking of blood from the pulmonary artery through the pulmonic valve into the right ventricle during diastole
PS	Pulmonic stenosis	Narrowing of the pulmonic valve resulting in obstruction to blood flow to the pulmonary artery
PTCA	Percutaneous transluminal coronary angioplasty	Procedure in which a balloon is inflated in a coronary artery to relieve an atherosclerotic obstruction
PV	Pulmonic valve	Heart valve separating right ventricle from the pulmonary artery
RBBB	Right bundle branch block	Abnormality noted on ECG resulting from the inability of the right branch of the ventricular conduction system to conduct electrical impulses
RV	Right ventricle	Heart chamber that pumps blood to lungs

SEM	Systolic ejection murmur	Also known as midsystolic murmurs, caused by ejection of blood into one of the great vessels (aorta or pulmonary artery)
SVT	Supraventricular tachycardia	Abnormally fast heart rate caused by atrial arrhythmias, abnormal conduction through the AV node, or the presence of an accessory pathway connecting the atrium to the ventricle
TEE	Transesophageal echocardiogram	Ultrasound study performed with probe in the esophagus; provides better resolution than TTE
TTE	Transthoracic echocardiogram	Ultrasound study of the heart performed with the probe on the chest wall; also known as an "echo"
Tn	Troponin	Serum protein; most specific marker of cardiac myocyte injury currently available
TR	Tricuspid regurgitation	Abnormal blood flow from right ventricle to right atrium
TS	Tricuspid stenosis	Narrowing of the tricuspid valve resulting in obstruction of blood flow from right atrium to right ventricle
TV	Tricuspid valve	Right-sided heart valve between right atrium and right ventricle
TVP	Transvenous pacemaker	A system for pacing the heart that involves placing pacing leads through the venous system and into the right ventricle; can be temporary or permanent
VSD	Ventricular septal defect	Defect in the interventricular septum resulting in abnormal communication of blood between the ventricles
VT	Ventricular tachycardia	Fast heart rate caused by a focus/foci of abnormal electrical activity in one of the ventricles; usually an unstable rhythm

Table 9-16. DEFINITIONS OF CARDIOLOGY TERMS.

TERM	DESCRIPTION
Angina	Substernal chest pain, pressure or burning brought on with exertion and relieved with rest, often radiating to jaw or arm
Atrial gallop	The S4; the sound associated with atrial contraction into a stiff ventricle; always signifies an abnormal ventricle
Atypical chest pain	Chest pain without obvious alternative cause that suggests ischemia but doesn't meet the criteria for angina
Cotton wool spot	Whitish discoloration on retina associated with systemic hypertension
Dyspnea	Shortness of breath
Edema	Swelling in dependent areas, usually the legs
Functional status	The ability or inability of a patient to perform aerobic activities; expressed in terms of METs
Orthopnea	Shortness of breath when recumbent
Palpitations	Fluttering, racing, or skipping sensation in chest often caused by irregular heart rhythm
Stent	A device usually made of stainless steel placed into a coronary (or other) artery to relieve a stenosis
Stress test	A test used to assess myocardial perfusion; usually done with exercise on a treadmill but can also be done using medications such as adenosine or dobutamine
Syncope	Loss of consciousness resulting from cerebral hypoperfusion
Ventricular gallop	The S3; may be normal in young patients, but in most patients it is a reliable sign of heart failure

PMHx: The patient has a 10-year history of hypertension. He has no history of hyperlipoproteinemia, diabetes mellitus, prior thromboembolic disease, peripheral arterial disease, hypercoagulable syndromes, rheumatic fever, connective tissue or autoimmune diseases. No history of psychiatric disorders.

PSHx: No prior surgeries and no history of trauma.

Occupational History: The patient has a college degree and works as an accountant.

Medications: Hydrochlorothiazide 25 mg po qd.

Allergies: No known allergies to medications.

HEALTH MAINTENANCE

Prevention: The patient has not had a lipid panel in more than 10 years.

Diet: Regular diet with no restrictions.

Exercise: The patient coaches his 8-year-old son's soccer team but does not engage in regular exercise otherwise.

Social Habits: The patient is an active smoker with a 30 pack-year history. He consumes six beers per week and denies illicit drug use.

FAMILY HISTORY

First-Degree Relatives' Medical History: The patient's father has hypertension and adult-onset diabetes mellitus but no history of coronary disease. The patient's mother and 42-year-old sister are healthy. No history in the extended family of sudden death or cardiac diseases.

PSYCHOSOCIAL HISTORY

Personal and Social History: The patient is married with two children. He reports no undue emotional stress associated with either his domestic or professional environments.

REVIEW OF SYSTEMS

General: No recent weight gain or loss. No fevers. No change in baseline energy level.

HEENT: No epistaxis.

Respiratory: No cough, hemoptysis, shortness of breath, or pleuritic chest pain.

Cardiovascular: As discussed in the HPI.

Gastrointestinal: No right upper quadrant (RUQ) or epigastric pain, no diarrhea. No hematemesis, hematochezia, or black stools.

Genitourinary: No erectile dysfunction. No dysuria, urinary urgency, or increase in urinary frequency.

Hematologic/lymphatic: No easy bruising or bleeding tendencies.

Skin: No rashes.

Neurological: No history of weakness, dysarthria, paresthesias, numbness, headaches, or visual changes.

Musculoskeletal: No back pain.

Extremities: No arthralgias or joint swelling. No arm or leg swelling. No leg or buttock pain with ambulation.

PHYSICAL EXAM

Vitals: T 98.8°F P 95 BP 158/94 RR 18 Weight 180 lbs

HEENT: Positive diagonal skin creases on both earlobes.

Neck: JVP of approximately 8 cm of water. Carotid pulses were full with brisk upstrokes bilaterally. No carotid bruits.

Lungs: Clear to auscultation and percussion (CTAP) bilaterally.

Chest: No tenderness to palpation of the sternal area or costochondral junction.

Cardiac: The PMI was normal in size, duration, and location. There were no lifts. The rhythm was regular. S1 was normal in intensity. There was physiologic splitting of S2 with normal intensity of both components. An S4 was present. There was no S3. There was a II/VI holosystolic murmur heard best at the left lower sternal border, which radiated into the axilla and increased with handgrip.

Abdomen: Soft, nontender, and nondistended. There were no pulsatile masses and no bruits.

Genitourinary: No CVA tenderness. Prostate was normal in size and without masses or tenderness. Bedside study for occult blood in the stool was negative.

Skin: No rashes.

Extremities: The extremities were warm and demonstrated normal color. The brachial, radial, femoral popliteal, dorsalis pedis, and posterior tibial pulses were normal bilaterally. The capillary refill time at the toes and fingers was less than 3 seconds. There was no lower extremity edema. There were no femoral artery bruits.

Neurologic: There were no motor or sensory deficits. Reflexes were 2+ and symmetric bilaterally. Mental status was normal.

10

DERMATOLOGY

Todd Kobayashi, MD, Eric H. Hanson, MD, MPH,
and Richard Bernert, MD

I. CHIEF COMPLAINT

A. Chief Complaint: In the patient's own words, why he or she sought attention for this problem.

B. Identifying Data: Age, gender, race/ethnicity, geographic location, and occupation.

II. HISTORY OF PRESENT ILLNESS

A. History of Lesion/Eruption

1. When and how did the lesion or eruption start (chronology)? For what length of time (duration)?
2. Is the lesion or eruption pruritic, painful, burning, or anesthetic?
3. Did it spread? If so, describe the pattern.
4. Did individual lesions evolve in a pattern?
5. Were you exposed to any provocative factors, such as stress, sunlight, heat, cold, pressure, vibration, water, or irritating chemicals? Did you engage in a form of exercise that might have been provocative?
6. Have you noticed any factors that have had an alleviative effect?
7. Has the lesion or eruption been constant, progressive, intermittent, or waxing and waning in nature?
8. Have you received previous treatments for the condition? What therapy was used and how effective was it?

B. Focused History as Indicated

1. Before the lesion or eruption, did you experience prodromal symptoms, such as headache, nausea, vomiting, diarrhea, myalgia, arthralgia, fevers, or chills?
2. Have you had any chronic symptoms (e.g., fevers, night sweats, generalized pruritus, weight loss, or fatigue)?
3. Any other associated symptoms, including neurologic, gastrointestinal, cardiopulmonary, musculoskeletal, genitourinary, or ocular symptoms?
4. Are you currently taking any prescribed or OTC medications? Which ones? What medications have you taken in the past? Are you currently using herbal supplements, aspirin, oral contraceptive pills, laxatives, or vitamins?
5. Have you used topical agents; chemical contactants, at home or at work; eye, ear, or nose drops; vaginal or rectal suppositories; bath oils; aromatherapy substances; or tattoo ink? Have you worn any jewelry recently?

6. Have you had any infectious contacts?
7. Any plant or animal contacts?
8. Have you recently been traveling, hiking, swimming, or bathing?
9. Did you recently undergo surgery or cardiac catheterization?
10. Do you, or does anyone in your family, have a history of skin cancer (e.g., melanoma, basal cell carcinoma, or squamous cell carcinoma), diabetes mellitus, systemic lupus or other autoimmune diseases, psoriasis, neurofibromatosis, or atopy (i.e., asthma, eczema, allergic rhinitis, or conjunctivitis)? Are there any genetic or familial diseases?
11. Have you had any previous skin disorders?
12. Are you pregnant or breast-feeding?

III. PAST MEDICAL AND SURGICAL HISTORY

A. Past Medical History

1. Have you had skin cancer (i.e., basal cell carcinoma, squamous cell carcinoma, malignant melanoma)? When did it occur, where, how deep was it, and how was it treated?
2. Have you had any other malignancies (e.g., breast, ovarian, renal, lung, or gastrointestinal)?
3. Have you had asthma, allergic rhinitis, allergic conjunctivitis, eczema, or atopic dermatitis?
4. Have you experienced allergic contact dermatitis (e.g., nickel, other metals, Neosporin, Bacitracin)?
5. Have you been diagnosed previously with other chronic or recurrent conditions that required treatment?

B. Past Surgical History

1. Have you undergone Mohs' micrographic surgery, simple excision (what margins were taken), electrodesiccation and curettage, or laser oblation?
2. Was any dental work performed recently? Was an amalgam used? What type?
3. Have you undergone surgery for artificial or replaced heart valves or joints, which requires antibiotic prophylaxis before surgery?
4. Do you have a pacemaker? What type is it and when was it placed? (Electrocautery cannot be used near the device.)

C. Emergency and Trauma History

1. Have you experienced anaphylaxis in response to medications, latex, nuts, shellfish, bees, or other substances?
2. Has a foreign body or infectious agent been introduced percutaneously through trauma?

D. Childhood History

1. Did you experience eczema or atopic dermatitis, asthma, or hay fever?
2. Did you have frequent sunburns? How many?
3. Did you ever have pigmented skin lesions?
4. Did you have any other skin conditions?

E. **Occupational History**

1. At work, are you exposed to chemicals (e.g., inhaled, percutaneously absorbed, accidental ingestion) or have infectious contacts? Do you have contact with plants, water, or animals?
2. Are you exposed to solar or other radiation?
3. What, if any, personal protective equipment (PPE) do you use?

F. **Travel History**

1. Do you travel within the United States? Do you travel to foreign countries?
2. Have you recently been on a camping trip or an excursion?

G. **Animals and Insects Exposure History**

1. What exposure to animals and insects do you have at home?
2. Do you have any exposure to animals or insects at work?
3. Have you had any incidental or accidental exposure to an animal or insect?

IV. MEDICATIONS, ALLERGIES, AND ADVERSE REACTIONS

A. **Medications**

1. Which prescription medications are you currently taking?
2. Which OTC medications are you taking? Aspirin (acetylsalicylic acid [ASA]); nonsteroidal anti-inflammatory drugs (NSAIDs); cold medicines; decongestants; eye, nose, or ear drops; vaginal or rectal suppositories; or laxatives?
3. Are you taking any herbal preparations (e.g., ginkgo biloba, garlic, Vitamin E, St John's Wort)?
4. Are you taking any supplements (e.g., vitamins or weight loss preparations)?

B. **Allergies to Medications and the Side Effects**

1. What type of reaction, if any, have you had to medications? Morbilliform, erythema multiforme, Stevens-Johnson syndrome, and toxic epidermal necrolysis (SJS and TEN; often caused by sulfa and anticonvulsants), urticarial, anaphylaxis, fixed drug eruption, granulomatous, lichenoid, pityriasis rosea-like, bullous, or pseudo-porphyria cutanea tarda (pseudo-PCT, e.g., naproxen)?
2. Have you experienced drug-induced lupus, hypersensitivity syndrome, or hepatitis (e.g., minocycline and others)?
3. Have you had a photoallergic reaction (e.g., HCTZ, gold), phototoxic reaction (doxycycline), or photoreactivation (methotrexate) reaction?
4. Have you ever been diagnosed with drug-induced immunobullous disease (e.g., Vancomycin and linear IgA bullous dermatosis)?

C. **Adverse Reactions to Medications**

1. Have you had an adverse reaction to medication (e.g., antibiotics or pain relief medication) that consisted of gastrointestinal upset or an ulcer?
2. Have you had a reaction of headache or pseudotumor cerebri (e.g., tetracyclines, isotretinoin)?

3. Have you reacted to medication with depression, dry mucous membranes, myalgias, arthralgias, elevated lipid levels, elevated liver enzymes, or photosensitivity (isotretinoin)?

V. HEALTH MAINTENANCE

A. Prevention

1. What type of preventive measures against sun exposure do you take? Photoprotection: sun block (both UVB and UVA), proper clothing, limit activity outdoors between 10 a.m. and 2 p.m. Avoid burning at all times.
2. Do you use emollients or moisturizers and avoid irritants and allergens to protect sensitive skin? These measures also guard against allergic contact dermatitis.

B. Diet

1. Do you include antioxidants in your diet? Do you take them as supplements? Antioxidants may help prevent skin cancer and reduce inflammatory skin conditions.
2. Are you now, or have you ever been, on an elimination diet? Some patients with urticaria or atopic dermatitis respond to elimination diets.

C. Exercise

1. Do you partake in outdoor exercise activities? If so, what type and for what period of time? Outdoor activities greatly increase the risk for sunburn and skin cancer/aging if not protected.
2. Do you exercise regularly? Regular exercise can help prevent cholinergic urticaria.

D. Sleep Patterns: Have you experienced any loss of sleep or developed unusual sleep patterns? Inadequate sleep, as well as stress and depression, exaggerates many common dermatoses (e.g., acne, neurotic excoriations, urticaria, rosacea).

E. Social Habits

1. Do you smoke, chew tobacco, or drink alcohol? If so, how much and for how long? Smoking, chewing tobacco, and alcohol use greatly increase the risk of oral and esophageal cancer. Smoking increases the rate of skin aging/wrinkling and decreases the effectiveness of hydroxychloroquine in the treatment of cutaneous lupus. Alcohol can exacerbate psoriasis.
2. Do you sunbathe or use artificial tanning booths? Sunbathing and artificial tanning greatly increase the risk of skin cancer.

VI. FAMILY HISTORY

First-Degree Relative's Medical History and Third-Degree Relative's Genogram: Do any first-degree relatives have a history of atopic dermatitis, asthma, or hay fever? Genetic syndromes or other heritable conditions?

VII. PSYCHOSOCIAL HISTORY

A. Personal and Social History: Occupation, hobbies, exposure, travel.

B. Current Illness Effects on the Patient

1. Have you experienced anxiety, depression, or loss of self-esteem as a result of your condition? Dermatologic diseases

often carry with them significant psychological morbidity (e.g., acne, psoriasis, atopic dermatitis; they are associated with anxiety, depression, and loss of self-esteem).

2. Have you had any loss of sleep, depressive symptoms, or social isolation? Intractable pruritus can cause loss of sleep, excoriations, depression, and social isolation.

C. Interpersonal and Sexual History

1. Have you had a sexually transmitted disease? Syphilis, gonorrhea, chlamydia, chancroid, lymphogranuloma venereum (LGV), granuloma inguinale, trichomoniasis, condyloma accuminata, human immunodeficiency virus (HIV), hepatitis B, hepatitis C, herpes simplex virus (HSV), or candidiasis?
2. Have you had vaginal or penile discharge, dysuria, erosions, ulcerations, warts, enlarged inguinal lymph nodes, or other lesions of the genitals?

D. Family Support

1. Are family members or other support persons available to care for biopsy or surgery sites?
2. Are family members or other support persons available to drive you home or to work after surgery, especially if eye is covered with bandage or unable to wear glasses?
3. Will income for family be adversely affected while you are in the hospital or clinic?
4. Do you have sources for psychological support and encouragement?

E. Occupational Aspects of Illness

1. Will you be able to cross-train or switch jobs if your skin condition is caused by your occupation?
2. Will you be able to be absent from work to make frequent follow-up appointments for difficult skin condition?
3. If necessary, can you wear protective gear to prevent exposure?

VIII. REVIEW OF SYSTEMS (Tables 10-1 to 10-4)

IX. PHYSICAL EXAMINATION

A. Anatomy

The cutaneous exam includes the skin, hair, nails, mucosal surfaces, genitals, and conjunctiva.

B. Describing a Lesion

1. Identify the primary lesion (e.g., macule, papule).
2. Add the appropriate adjectives on morphology (i.e., size, color, consistency, configuration, margination, and surface characteristics).
3. Note the distribution (scalp, nails, mucous membranes, palms, and soles): Localized, generalized, symmetric, photodistributed, follicular or perifollicular, periungual, exposed areas, protected areas, sites of pressure, intertriginous, flexural, extensor, glabrous, central, peripheral, palmar or plantar, trunk, upper or lower extremity, head and neck, girdle, mucosal, genital, sebaceous areas, or name specific locations.

Text continued on p. 144.

DERM

Table 10-1. DISEASES WITH DERMATOLOGIC SIGNS AND SYMPTOMS BY SYSTEM.

System	Signs and Symptoms	Diseases
Cardiopulmonary	Chest pain on exertion, claudication, digital infarcts	Atherosclerosis
	Cyanosis	Congenital heart defects, methemoglobinemia from Dapsone
	Shortness of breath, wheezing, urticaria	Allergic reaction/anaphylaxis
	Stasis dermatitis	Congestive heart failure
	Pulmonary arteriovenous malformations, telangiectases of skin and mucosa	Hereditary hemorrhagic telangiectasia (Osler-Weber-Rendu)
	Clubbing of nails	Congenital heart defects, congestive heart failure, COPD, left to right shunts
Gastrointestinal	Enlarged male breasts (i.e., gynecomastia), palmer erythema, telangiectases, jaundice eyes, mucosa, or skin	Liver disease
	Malabsorption, pruritic vesicles on elbows and knees	Dermatitis herpetiformis
	Constipation, diarrhea, abdominal pain, bloating, GI bleeding, acanthosis nigricans, eruptive seborrheic keratoses, Bazex syndrome (acrokeratosis paraneoplastica)	Gastrointestinal carcinoma or upper aeroesophageal carcinoma

	Sebaceous neoplasms and colon cancer	Muir-Torre syndrome
	Cutaneous cysts and GI cancer	Gardner's syndrome
	Pyoderma gangrenosum, cutaneous Crohn's	Inflammatory bowel disease
	Morbilliform or maculopapular eruption/exanthem	Viral gastroenteritis
	Hematochezia or dark, tarry stools, gastrointestinal bleeding, telangiectases, venous malformations, multiple cutaneous hemangiomas	Hereditary hemorrhagic telangiectasia, blue rubber bleb nevus syndrome, disseminated hemangiomatosis
	Bowel perforations and "plucked chicken" skin of neck and axilla	Pseudoxanthoma elasticum
	Periodic abdominal pain with swelling of tongue, throat, lips, genitals, skin	Hereditary or acquired angioedema
	Abdominal pain, gastrointestinal bleeding, cutaneous infarcts	Polyarteritis nodosa, Henoch-Schönlein purpura, leukocytoclastic vasculitis, Degos' malignant atrophic papulosis
	Pigmented macules of lips, oral mucosa, genitals, or hands and gastrointestinal tumors	Peutz-Jeghers, Cronkhite-Canada
	Facial flushing	Carcinoid
Musculoskeletal	Absent or hypoplastic patella, posterior iliac horns, radial head subluxation, glomerulonephropathy, Lester iris, triangular lunula, nail defects	Nail-patella syndrome
	Stippled cartilage, shortened limbs and dwarfism, linear ichthyosis, hyperkeratosis, and follicular atrophoderma	Conradi-Hünermann (chondrodysplasia punctata)

Continued

Table 10-1. DISEASES WITH DERMATOLOGIC SIGNS AND SYMPTOMS BY SYSTEM—*cont'd*

System	Signs and Symptoms	Diseases
	Congenital hemidysplasia, ichthyosiform erythroderma, limb defects	CHILD syndrome
	Osteolytic bone lesions	Langerhans cell histiocytosis (Hand-Schüller-Christian disease, Letterer-Siwe disease, or eosinophilic granuloma)
	Port-wine stain with associated limb and soft tissue hypertrophy	Klippel-Trenaunay-Weber syndrome, Parkes-Weber syndrome
Rheumatologic	Stiff skin, arthralgias, myalgias, weakness, intolerance of fingers to cold	Limited or progressive systemic sclerosis
	Photosensitivity, renal disease, arthritis, serositis, cytopenias, fatigue, oral aphthae, cognitive dysfunction, malar rash, scarring alopecia, discoid lesions	Systemic lupus erythematosus (SLE)
	Dry eyes, dry mouth, annular erythema	Sjögren's syndrome
	Pruritus, heliotrope rash, Gottron's papules, Gottron's sign, shawl sign, ragged cuticles, proximal muscle weakness, myalgias, photosensitivity	Dermatomyositis
	Difficulty swallowing, sclerodactyly, telangiectases, Raynaud's phenomenon, tight, bound-down skin, circumoral rhagades, calcinosis cutis	Systemic sclerosis

Neurologic	Paresthesias, numbness, hyperhidrosis, hypohidrosis	Hansen's disease, reflex sympathetic dystrophy, zoster, focal hyperhidrosis, diabetes
	Cognitive dysfunction or focal defects, cutaneous vasculitis	Acute SLE or other vasculitis
	Seizures, angiofibromas of face, Koenen's tumors, ash leaf macules, Shagreen patch	Tuberous sclerosis
	Seizures, port-wine stain of face	Sturge-Weber syndrome
	Headaches, diplopia, focal defects, cutaneous nodules	Metastatic disease
	Cutaneous tumors, café-au-lait macules, axillary freckling, Lisch nodules of iris, central nervous system (CNS) tumors, pheochromocytoma	Neurofibromatosis
	Medulloblastoma, basal cell carcinomas	Nevoid basal cell carcinoma syndrome
	Photosensitivity with blisters, acute neuropsychiatric changes, abdominal pain	Variegate porphyria
	Epidermal nevus, neurologic defects, other internal organ defects	Schimmelpenning's syndrome or epidermal nevus syndrome
	Giant melanocytic nevus with associated leptomeningeal melanocytosis and high risk of melanoma	Neurocutaneous melanosis
Hematologic	Pruritus, fatigue, opportunistic infection, anemia, weight loss, anorexia, cachexia	Lymphoma, leukemia

Continued

Table 10-1. DISEASES WITH DERMATOLOGIC SIGNS AND SYMPTOMS BY SYSTEM—*cont'd*

System	Signs and Symptoms	Diseases
	Pruritus, bone pain or fracture, urticaria, diarrhea, headache, flushing or sweating, pigmented macules or patches on skin	Mastocytosis
	Pallor	Anemia
	Spooning of nails	Iron deficiency
	Plethora, pruritus in shower/water, thrombosis	Polycythemia
	Red, scaly patches, plaques, or tumors +/– adenopathy, fatigue, opportunistic infections	Mycosis fungoides
	Infiltrative skin tumors	Cutaneous metastases
Endocrine	Brittle or coarse hair, lethargy, cold intolerance, constipation, poor cognition, weight gain, fluid retention	Hypothyroidism
	Hair thinning, heat intolerance, sweating, diarrhea, fatigue, pretibial myxedema, proptosis	Hyperthyroidism
	Excess hair growth, deepening voice, hair thinning, worsening or new-onset acne, increased muscle mass, enlarged clitoris	Androgen-secreting tumor, familial, 21-hydroxylase deficiency, 17-B-hydroxylase deficiency
	Enlarged tongue and hands, thickening of skin, headaches	Growth hormone-secreting tumor of pituitary

	Palpitations, sweating, hypertension, flushing	Pheochromocytoma
	Dermatitis of periorificial skin, acral skin, perineal skin	Glucagonoma, zinc deficiency, essential fatty acid deficiency, amino acid deficiency
	Increased pigmentation of skin, mucous membranes, and nevi	Addison's disease, ACTH-secreting tumor
	Striae, plethora, buffalo hump, moon facies	Cushing's syndrome
Infectious	Palpable purpura, fever, chills, multi-organ failure	Sepsis
	Splinter hemorrhages, Janeway lesions, fever, heart murmur	Bacterial endocarditis
	Opportunistic infections, Kaposi's sarcoma, bacillary angiomatosis	HIV, AIDS
	Painless chancre, copper-colored papules and plaques on palms, soles, trunk	Syphilis
	Red, "slapped" cheek appearance, reticulate erythema, feels well	Parvovirus B19
	Erythema migrans, arthritis, focal neurologic defects	Lyme disease
	Pustules over joints, arthritis, penile or vaginal discharge	Gonorrhea
	Anesthetic, annular or circular patch	Hansen's disease (leprosy)
	Painful ulcers mucosa or genitals, recurrent nature, and erythema multiforme	Herpes simplex virus (HSV)

Continued

Table 10-1. DISEASES WITH DERMATOLOGIC SIGNS AND SYMPTOMS BY SYSTEM—*cont'd*

System	Signs and Symptoms	Diseases
	Fever, headache, myalgias, arthralgias, centripetal spreading red spots: from wrists and ankles to trunk	Rocky mountain spotted fever
	Fever, headache, myalgias, arthralgias, centrifugal spreading rash: from trunk to extremities	Typhus
	Red papules of genitals, nipples, periumbilical skin with associated interdigital web space burrows and tracks	Scabies
	Red tongue, peeling palmoplantar and genital skin, edema of hands and feet, conjunctivitis, fever, adenopathy	Kawasaki's syndrome
	Sandpaperlike rash, red tongue, circumoral pallor, fever, sore throat, adenopathy	Scarlet fever/streptococcal infection

DERM

Table 10-2. DERMATOLOGIC DISEASES AND THEIR CUTANEOUS FINDINGS.

Disease	Findings
Tuberous sclerosis	Acnelike red papules of perinasal and cheek areas, ash leaf hypopigmented macules, Shagreen patches, angiofibromas of nail folds
Cirrhosis of the liver	Angiomas, spider (face and chest), palmar erythema, diminished secondary sexual hair
Porphyria cutanea tarda	Vesicles, bullae, and milia on dorsum of hands, sclerodermalike changes of face, hypertrichosis
Neurofibromatosis type I	Café-au-lait macules, neurofibromas, Lisch nodules of iris, axillary freckling
Pseudoxanthoma elasticum	Yellow, "plucked chicken" like skin of neck, axilla, groin
Gardner's syndrome	Multiple cutaneous cysts (with pilomatrical differentiation)
Acanthosis nigricans	Velvety, dirty-appearing skin of neck, axilla, groin, flexures
Hypothyroidism (myxedema)	Generalized edema, dry, rough skin, loss of lateral brows, coarse and brittle hair
Acrodermatitis enteropathica (zinc deficiency, also seen with essential fatty acid and amino acid deficiencies)	Erosions and dermatitis of periorificial skin, acral and perineal skin, alopecia, diarrhea
Dermatomyositis	Erythematous papules over knuckles, cuticular damage with dilated capillary loops, periorbital edema with heliotrope rash, shawl sign, calcinosis cutis, proximal muscle weakness
Hereditary hemorrhagic telangiectasia (Osler-Weber-Rendu disease)	Multiple to numerous spiderlike telangiectases on tongue, mucous membranes, lips, fingers, palms and soles, face and trunk (epistaxis, GI bleeding, CNS bleeding)
Addison's disease	Hyperpigmentation of palmar creases, knuckles, scars, buccal mucosa, scrotum, linea alba, nevi
Pretibial myxedema (hyperthyroidism, Graves' disease)	Nodular, waxy violaceous plaques on pretibial skin

Continued

Table 10-2. DERMATOLOGIC DISEASES AND THEIR CUTANEOUS FINDINGS—*cont'd*

Disease	Findings
Sarcoidosis	Skin colored to erythematous papules on face, perinasal skin, angle of mouth (split papule) with apple jelly color by diascopy
Necrobiosis lipoidica (diabeticorum)	Atrophic, erythematous pretibial plaques with central yellowish coloration and telangiectases
Ehlers-Danlos	Easily stretchable skin with good recoil (hyperextensible joints)
Cutis laxa	Stretchable skin with poor recoil in axilla, groin, face
Systemic sclerosis (limited or progressive)	Sclerodactyly with tight, bound-down skin, telangiectases of face and fingers/palms, Raynaud's phenomenon, calcinosis cutis
Pyoderma gangrenosum	Widely undermined ulcers with purple/red border and characterized by pathergy (often associated with inflammatory bowel disease)
Herpes simplex or zoster	Grouped vesicles on an erythematous base
Vitiligo (associated with pernicious anemia, Hashimoto's thyroiditis, Addison's disease, Type I diabetes mellitus)	Depigmented patches of acral skin, periorbital, periorificial, nipples, genitals
Xanthoma (hypercholesterolemia)	Yellow, lobulated papules of upper or lower eyelids, nodules of tendons, or elbows and knees
Eruptive xanthomas (hypertriglyceridemia)	Eruptive erythematous to yellowish papules over buttocks, arms, thighs
Primary systemic amyloidosis (multiple myeloma)	Pinch purpura, petechiae of eyelids, easy bruising
Systemic lupus erythematosus	Malar rash, photosensitivity, scarring discoid lesions (face, scalp, ears), conchal bowl follicular plugging, oral aphthae
Kaposi's sarcoma (HIV)	Purplish plaques of face, oral mucosa, legs

Table 10-3. NONSPECIFIC CUTANEOUS FINDINGS AND THEIR ASSOCIATED DERMATOLOGIC DISEASE PROCESSES.

Findings	Diseases
Pruritus	Lymphoma, leukemia, urticaria, atopic dermatitis, contact dermatitis, neuropathy, drug eruption, xerosis, renal disease, liver disease
Palpable purpura	Leukocytoclastic vasculitis from sepsis/infection, lupus, rheumatoid arthritis, Sjogren's, mixed cryoglobulinemia, polyarteritis nodosa, microscopic polyarteritis, Henoch-Schönlein purpura, Wegener's, Churg-Strauss, antiphospholipid syndrome, drug reaction, erythema elevatum diutinum, granuloma faciale, nodular vasculitis
Eczema	Atopic dermatitis, allergic contact dermatitis, irritant contact dermatitis, nummular dermatitis, dyshidrotic eczema, id reaction
Morbilliform rash	Drug or viral most common (numerous causes)
Urticaria	Drug, food, viral, chronic idiopathic, autoimmune, vasculitic, thyroid induced, stress, contact urticaria, lymphoma, mastocytosis
Blisters, bullae, and sloughing	Bullous impetigo, immunobullous diseases, lupus, bullous lichen planus, arthropod, epidermolysis bullosa, Stevens-Johnson syndrome, toxic epidermal necrolysis, grade IV graft versus host disease, friction blister, porphyria, drug effect
Alopecia	Androgenetic (male or female pattern), thyroid disorder, iron deficiency, telogen effluvium, anagen effluvium, trichotillomania, alopecia areata, hair shaft abnormalities, traction, lupus, lichen planopilaris, folliculitis decalvans, tinea capitis, pseudopelade, acne keloidalis nuchae
Genital ulcer	HSV 1 and 2, syphilis, chancroid, chlamydia, lymphogranuloma venereum, granuloma inguinale, Behçet's, aphthae, cutaneous Crohn's, amebiasis, erosive lichen planus, lichen sclerosus, erosive candidiasis
Palmoplantar keratoderma	Hereditary (numerous types), pityriasis rubra pilaris, paraneoplastic, pachyonychia congenita, Richner-Hanhart, hidrotic ectodermal dysplasia

Continued

Table 10-3. NONSPECIFIC CUTANEOUS FINDINGS AND THEIR ASSOCIATED DERMATOLOGIC DISEASE PROCESSES—*cont'd*	
FINDINGS	DISEASES
Nail dystrophy	Trauma, stasis, ill-fitting shoes, onychomycosis, lichen planus, psoriasis, Reiter's, pseudomonas, pachyonychia congenita, habitic deformity, chronic paronychia, yellow nail syndrome, dyskeratosis congenita
Red, scaly, plaque	Tinea, psoriasis, eczematous dermatitis (contact, nummular, id), mycosis fungoides, erythema annulare centrifugum, pityriasis rosea, seborrheic dermatitis, Bowen's disease

C. Primary, Secondary, and Special Lesions

1. PRIMARY LESIONS	
LESION	DESCRIPTION
Macule	Circumscribed flat (nonpalpable) discoloration <1 cm; smooth surface, occasionally fine scale (e.g., tinea versicolor); an atrophic macule is depressed below the surface
Patch	Similar to a macule but >1 cm in diameter (e.g., melasma, tinea versicolor)
Papule	Small, palpable, usually raised lesions <1 cm; any color; smooth or rough surface; variety of shapes; sessile, pedunculated, filiform, verrucous (e.g., insect bite, wart)
Plaque	Similar to a papule but larger in surface area >1 cm (e.g., psoriasis, seborrheic keratoses) and usually elevated. Some lesions are indurated, thickened, or atrophic (e.g., morphea, lichen sclerosus)
Wheal	Edematous papule or plaque (e.g., hive)
Nodule	Similar to a papule but with some depth and >1 cm; solid, semi-solid, or liquid (e.g., epidermal cyst)
Tumor	Similar to a nodule but >2 cm in diameter (e.g., giant hairy nevus, large basal cell carcinoma, melanoma and dermatofibrosarcoma protuberans)
Vesicle	Clear, fluid-filled blister <1 cm; fluid may become cloudy with time (e.g., herpes simplex virus)
Bulla	Vesiclelike >1 cm (e.g., bullous impetigo)
Pustule	Blisterlike but filled with white or yellow-white fluid (e.g., acne)
Rash	Describes all of the lesions as a whole; synonymous with eruption

Table 10-4. DERMATOLOGIC DISEASES, PATHOGENESIS, AND FINDINGS.

Disease	Pathogenesis	Findings
Acne	Follicular plugging, sebum production and retention, bacterial inflammation	Comedones, papules, pustules, nodules, and cysts of face and trunk
Actinic keratosis	UV damage, p53 gene defect and others	Rough, keratotic, gritty or sandpaperlike papules or macules on sun-exposed skin (face, ears, forearms, dorsal hands)
Allergic contact dermatitis	Type IV delayed-type hypersensitivity response to contact allergen	Patterned erythema, vesicles, scale, crust (acute) or lichenification (chronic)
Alopecia areata	Autoimmune destruction of hair matrix	Nonscarring episodes of sudden hair loss, usually in circular patches, which commonly regrows and then repeats the cycle in different location
Androgenetic alopecia	Dihydrotestosterone-mediated miniaturization of hair follicles on scalp, controlled by 5α-reductase enzyme	Patterned loss and miniaturization of scalp hair, usually frontal, bitemporal, and vertex; females have Christmas tree-like pattern of thinning
Angioedema	C1 inhibitor deficiency (hereditary) or lymphoma (acquired)	Subcutaneous swelling without significant pruritus of lips, tongue, throat, face, hands, and sometimes feet
Atopic dermatitis	Hypersensitive cutaneous immune response	Pruritus, erythema, scale, cracks, fissures, and lichenification of antecubital fossa, popliteal fossa (adults); face and extensor surfaces of extremities (toddlers)
Basal cell carcinoma	UV damage, PTCH gene defect	Pearly white papule with telangiectases or pink papule with translucent quality and rolled edges

Continued

Table 10-4. DERMATOLOGIC DISEASES, PATHOGENESIS, AND FINDINGS—*cont'd*

Disease	Pathogenesis	Findings
Condyloma accuminata	HPV types 6, 11, etc.	Rough-surfaced, verruciform, skin-colored to hyperpigmented papules on genital skin
Condyloma lata	Treponema pallidum	Fleshy, taglike papule of genital or perineal skin
Dyshidrotic eczema	Unknown	Pruritic, tapioca pudding-like, deep-seated vesicles along sides of fingers, palms, and soles
Herpes simplex	HSV 1 and 2	Grouped vesicles on an erythematous base (Tzanck positive)
Impetigo	Staphylococcus aureus	Honey-crusted erosions, vesicles, and bullae
Lichen planus	Unknown	Pruritic, purple, planar, polygonal papules on the volar wrists, dorsal ankles, extremities, and trunk
Melanocytic nevi	Collection of pigmented melanocytes in skin	Brown, homogenously pigmented, flat or dome-shaped, well-demarcated papules or macules
Melanoma	UV damage, p16 gene defect and others	A, B, C, D criteria: *A*symmetry, *b*order irregularity, *c*olor variation, *d*iameter greater than 6 mm
Molluscum contagiosum	DNA pox virus	Skin-colored to pink, umbilicated papules on face, trunk, extremities, genitals
Nummular dermatitis	Unknown, but exacerbated by dry, cold, climates	Coin-shaped erythematous, scaly plaques of lower extremities, upper extremities, and trunk
Onychomycosis	Trichophyton rubrum, Trichophyton mentagrophytes, others	Distal onycholysis with subungual debris, dystrophic appearance, discoloration, pain
Pityriasis rosea	Possible viral etiology	Herald patch followed by numerous smaller similar lesions: Oval plaques with central collarette of scale in "Christmas tree" pattern on trunk

Psoriasis	Possible autoimmune T-cell phenomenon in susceptible host	Erythematous, circular plaques with thick silvery scale over elbows, knees, scalp most commonly, but also intertriginous, extremities, trunk, palmoplantar skin, nails, and gluteal cleft
Rosacea	Unknown pathogenesis: vascular flushing, perifollicular inflammation	Flushing, erythema of central face convexities, papules, pustules, phymatous changes of nose, telangiectases
Seborrheic dermatitis	Unknown, possible hypersensitivity response to pityrosporum yeast	Erythema and waxy or fluffy scale of nasolabial folds, brows, scalp, retroauricular, auditory canals, chest, axilla, pubic and genital skin
Seborrheic keratosis	Unknown	Warty, rough-surfaced, scaly or waxy-appearing yellow, brown "stuck-on" appearing papules and plaques on face, trunk, and extremities
Squamous cell carcinoma	p53 gene defect and others, UV damage	Indurated (thickened at base) hyperkeratotic papule or nodule
Tinea corporis, cruris, pedis, manum, unguium	Trichophyton rubrum most common	Erythematous, scaly, annular plaques, sometimes with central clearing (KOH positive)
Tinea capitis	Trichophyton tonsurans (in United States) most common	"Black dot tinea capitis" with broken hair shafts at level of scalp; may also be red, boggy kerion or follicular pustules or scale
Tinea (pityriasis) versicolor	Malassezia furfur	Hypo- or hyperpigmented, finely scaly, circular macules of upper back, chest, neck, shoulders
Urticaria	Numerous causes (See Table 10-3.)	Evanescent, pink papules and plaques lasting less than 24 hours, sometimes in arcuate patterns

2. SECONDARY LESIONS

Lesion	Description
Scale	Desiccated plates of normal or abnormal keratosis or exfoliations (e.g., psoriasis, ichthyosis)
Lichenification	Accentuated skin lines and thickening of the skin (e.g., lichen simplex chronicus)
Crust	Dried serum, pus, or blood mixed with epithelial and bacterial debris (e.g., impetigo, scabs)
Eschar	Necrotic crust
Fissure	Linear break in the skin down to the dermis, causing cracks or clefts (e.g., cheilitis)
Erosion	Epidermis is partially missing; slightly depressed lesion that usually does not scar (e.g., aphthae, ruptured vesicles)
Ulceration	Total loss of the epidermis and some dermis—significantly depressed lesion that usually scars (e.g., bedsore)
Atrophy	Loss of skin substance, resulting in depression of the skin that can involve epidermal, dermal, and subcutaneous layers (e.g., lipoatrophy)
Scar	Fibrous replacement of lost substance in the dermis or subcutis (e.g., keloid, cicatrices)
Pigmentary change	Macular changes in skin color; hypo- or hyperpigmented (e.g., melasma)
Excoriation	Oval or linear crusts (e.g., abrasions, scratch marks)
Induration	Thickening of the skin without accentuation of the skin lines

3. SPECIAL LESIONS

Lesion	Description
Burrow	Tiny, superficial, subcorneal, serpiginous tunnels approximately 5 mm long, but may be longer (e.g., scabies)
Comedo/comedones	Plug of keratinous debris lodged in hair follicle opening (e.g., acne)
Milium/milia	Small superficial cyst without an opening
Telangiectasia	Tiny, dilated superficial blood vessels (e.g., rosacea)
Ecchymosis	Circumscribed deposit of extravasated blood into the skin; petechiae are less than 0.5 cm diameter, purpura are more than 0.5 cm diameter

4. SHAPE OF LESIONS.

Lesion	Description
Round	Tinea, mycosis fungoides, nummular eczema
Oval	Pityriasis rosea; hand, foot, and mouth disease
Asymmetric	Malignant melanoma
Annular (ring-like)	Granuloma annulare, mycosis fungoides, erythema migrans, tinea, subacute cutaneous lupus
Serpiginous	Urticaria, subacute cutaneous lupus
Arciform (partial ring)	Urticaria, subacute cutaneous lupus
Umbilicated	Central dell on top of papule (e.g., molluscum contagiosum, small pox)
Indistinct	Not easily detectable or obvious
Atrophic	Flat or depressed with fine wrinkling of epidermis (e.g., lichen sclerosus, atrophie blanche, Ehlers-Danlos [EDS] scars)
Dome-shaped	Intradermal nevi, neurofibromas
Pedunculated	Skin tags, condylomata, intradermal nevi
Verruciform (wart-like)	Verruca, seborrheic keratosis, tricholemmoma
Filiform	Warts, tongue papillae, skin tags
Flat topped	Lichen planus, certain seborrheic keratoses

5. ARRANGEMENT OF LESIONS.

Lesion	Description
Isolated	Single lesion (e.g., tumor)
Scattered	Sparsely arranged without particular pattern (e.g., arthropod bites)
Confluent	Macules merging together to form patches, or papules merging together to form plaques (e.g., morbilliform eruptions, granuloma annulare, PRP)
Grouped	Smaller lesions grouped together (e.g., herpes: grouped vesicles)
Herpetiform	Grouped as in herpes (e.g., dermatitis herpetiformis, pemphigoid gestationis)
Zosteriform	Dermatomal distribution
Linear	In a line (e.g., linear epidermal nevus, lichen striatus, linear morphea)
Reticulate	Netlike (e.g., livedo reticularis)
Skin cleavage lines	Christmas tree-like pattern on back (e.g., pityriasis rosea), following wrinkles
Blaschkoid	Along lines of embryonic epidermal migration (e.g., incontinentia pigmenti, hypomelanosis of Ito, focal dermal hypoplasia)
Circumferential	Encircling completely (e.g., rope burns from tying down or handcuffing)

6. Other descriptors: Temperature, color (red, blue, gray, brown, black, yellow, pink, salmon, copper, orange, violaceous, purple, white, porcelain, erythematous), blanching, nonblanching, petechial, purpuric, palpable, tender, scaly, keratotic, rough surfaced, smooth, glossy, lichenified, indurated, papulosquamous, atrophic, ulcerated, eroded, excoriated, crusted, pustular, edematous, juicy, weepy, soft, fleshy, firm, doughy, scarring, sclerosing, evanescent, morbilliform, maculopapular, transient, persistent, gangrenous, necrotic, cyanotic, eczematous, anesthetic, hyperesthetic, cracked, fissured, epidermal, dermal, subcutaneous, fixed, firm, mobile, calcified.

7. LOCATION OF THE LESIONS.

Lesion	Description
Exposed surfaces	Face, ears, neck, arms, hands, eyelids; spares creases (airborne contact)
Photodistributed	Dorsal hands, extensor forearms, face, ears, anterior chest, posterior and lateral neck; spares submental, mid upper lip, eyelids, and covered areas (e.g., photoallergic, phototoxic, recall phenomenon)
Acral or distal	Hands, feet and distal extremities (e.g., acrodermatitis enteropathica, acrokeratosis paraneoplastica, Raynaud's syndrome)
Intertriginous	Neck, axillae, groin, toe webs and gluteal fold (e.g., candidiasis, erythrasma, fungal infections, psoriasis, Hailey-Hailey)
Bony prominences	Shoulders, knees, elbows, ankles and wrist (e.g., psoriasis, dermatitis herpetiformis)
Mucous membranes	Oropharynx, conjunctiva, genitalia and perianal (e.g., herpes simplex virus, syphilis, wart, mucous membrane pemphigoid, Behçet's, lichen planus)
Glabrous	Nonterminal hair bearing skin (e.g., parts of face, palms, soles)
Sebaceous areas	Face, chest, upper back (e.g., Darier's, seborrheic dermatitis)
Cephalic	Head and neck (e.g., cephalic histiocytosis, variants of pityriasis rosea)
Pressure areas	Plantar, buttock, elbows, knees, forearms, hands

D. **General Physical Exam as Indicated:** Vitals, HEENT, neck, heart, lungs, chest, abdomen, pelvis, genitourinary, neurologic, lymphatic, cardiovascular, skeletal, muscular, endocrine, ophthalmologic.

X. LABORATORY STUDIES AND DIAGNOSTIC EVALUATIONS

A. Studies and Tests Performed in Clinic

1. KOH (fungal), Gram stain (bacterial), Tzanck smear (viral), darkfield microscopy (spirochetes), scabies prep.
2. Cultures: Viral, bacterial, or fungal.
3. Wood's lamp exam (melanocytic lesions).
4. Patch testing (allergic disease).
5. Biopsy (shave, punch, excisional, incisional): Hematoxylin and eosin (H&E; standard general stain), periodic acid schiff (PAS; fungal organisms, glycogen), immunofluorescence (immunoglobulins, complement), electron microscopy (study ultrastructure, e.g., melanosomes), Warthin-Starry (specific bacterial organisms).

B. Possible Useful Laboratory Studies: Complete blood count (CBC), specific chemistry studies, urinalysis, serologic tests (e.g., RPR, ANA), stool analysis.

C. Possible Useful Radiology Studies: Chest x-ray (CXR), computed tomography (CT), magnetic resonance imaging (MRI), ultrasound (US), lymphoscintigraphy.

XI. EPONYMS, ACRONYMS, AND ABBREVIATIONS (Table 10-5)

TABLE 10-5. DERMATOLOGY EPONYMS, ACRONYMS, AND ABBREVIATIONS.

AA	Alopecia areata	**LP**	Lichen planus
AK	Actinic keratosis	**LPP**	Lichen planopilaris
AN	Acanthosis nigricans	**LS(A)**	Lichen sclerosis (et atrophicus)
BCC	Basal cell carcinoma	**MF**	Mycosis fungoides
BP	Bullous pemphigoid	**MIS**	Melanoma in situ
CCLE	Chronic cutaneous lupus erythematosus	**MM**	Malignant melanoma
CNCH	Chondrodermatitis nodularis chronica helicis	**NF**	Neurofibroma
DEB	Dystrophic (dermolytic) epidermolysis bullosa	**NL(D)**	Necrobiosis lipoidica (diabeticorum)
DF	Dermatofibroma	**PAN**	Polyarteritis nodosa
DFSP	Dermatofibrosarcoma protuberans	**PCT**	Porphyria cutanea tarda
DH	Dermatitis herpetiformis	**PFB**	Pseudofolliculitis barbae
DLE	Discoid lupus erythematosus	**PF**	Pemphigus foliaceus

Continued

TABLE 10-5. DERMATOLOGY EPONYMS, ACRONYMS, AND ABBREVIATIONS—*cont'd*			
EAC	Erythema annulare centrifugum	**PG**	Pyogenic granuloma, pyoderma gangrenosum
EBA	Epidermolysis bullosa acquisita	**PSS**	Progressive systemic sclerosis
EB(S)	Epidermolysis bullosa (simplex)	**PV**	Pemphigus vulgaris
ECM	Erythema chronicum migrans	**PWS**	Port wine stain
EDS	Ehlers-Danlos syndrome	**RA**	Rheumatoid arthritis
EHK	Epidermolytic hyperkeratosis	**SCC**	Squamous cell carcinoma
EM	Erythema multiforme	**SCLE**	Subacute cutaneous lupus erythematosus
GA	Granuloma annulare	**SK**	Seborrheic keratosis
HHT	Hereditary hemorrhagic telangiectasia	**SJS**	Stevens-Johnson syndrome
HSP	Henoch-Schönlein purpura	**SLE**	Systemic lupus erythematosus
IP	Incontinentia pigmenti	**TEN**	Toxic epidermal necrolysis
JEB	Junctional epidermolysis bullosa	**TMEP**	Telangiectasia macularis eruptiva perstans
KP	Keratosis pilaris	**TS**	Tuberous sclerosis
KS	Kaposi's sarcoma	**UP**	Urticaria pigmentosa
LCV	Leukocytoclastic vasculitis	**XP**	Xeroderma pigmentosum

XII. DEFINITIONS (Table 10-6)

XIII. SAMPLE H&P WRITE-UP

CC: "I have itchy bumps on my wrists."

HPI: Healthy-appearing, 43-year-old white female presents with a 2-week history of pruritic lesions on her wrists and ankles. The lesions initially started on the volar wrists and dorsal ankles and have started progressing proximally. There are no alleviating or exacerbating factors. No prior similar eruptions in past. No new medications, OTC medications, herbal supplements, but does occasionally drink a "gold"-containing drink. Current medications include only oral contraceptive pills and occasional ibuprofen. Patient has been using 1% hydrocortisone cream twice daily for 2 weeks without benefit.

Text continued on p. 161.

TABLE 10-6. DERMATOLOGY TERMS AND DEFINITIONS.

TERM	DEFINITION	EXAMPLES
Abscess	Pus (neutrophil/granulocyte)-filled cystic cavity, may or may not be encapsulated	Acne, furunculosis, dissecting cellulitis, infection, hidradenitis suppurativa
Actinic	Caused by or related to solar radiation	Actinic keratosis, actinic purpura
Alopecia	Hair loss	Alopecia areata, telogen effluvium, androgenetic alopecia, alopecia mucinosis, scarring alopecias (lupus, lichen planopilaris, folliculitis decalvans, pseudopelade)
Angioedema	Deep, edematous urticarial reaction that occurs in the deep, loose reticular dermis or subcutis, usually on mucosal surfaces, eyelids, or genital skin, but may occur anywhere	Hereditary angioedema, acquired angioedema (lymphoma), chronic urticaria, anaphylaxis, drug reaction, urticarial vasculitis
Annular	Round with central clearing	Tinea corporis, granuloma annulare, subacute cutaneous lupus erythematosus
Asbo-Hansen sign	Lateral spread of blister with gentle pressure over top	Pemphigus vulgaris, pemphigus foliaceus, toxic epidermal necrolysis, Stevens-Johnson syndrome, bullous impetigo
Atopic	Predisposition to develop eczema, asthma, allergic rhinitis, and other hypersensitivity reactions	Atopic dermatitis, Job's syndrome, hyper IgE syndrome, Netherton's syndrome
Atrophic	Diminution of size of a cell, tissue, organ, or part of the body. Epidermal atrophy: Thin, translucent, with cigarette paper-like quality. Dermal atrophy: Depression, outpouching, or sclerotic variants	Lichen sclerosus et atrophicus, atrophoderma, morphea, steroid atrophy, focal dermal hypoplasia, anetoderma, Ehlers-Danlos' scars, atrophie blanche, aplasia cutis congenita

Continued

TABLE 10-6. DERMATOLOGY TERMS AND DEFINITIONS—*cont'd*

TERM	DEFINITION	EXAMPLES
Auspitz's sign	Appearance of pinpoint dots of blood at the tops of ruptured capillaries when scale is removed from psoriatic plaques	Psoriasis
Blaschko's lines	Lines of postzygotic epidermal migration; does not follow nerve, dermatome, or vascular pattern	Linear epidermal nevus, incontinentia pigmenti, hypomelanosis of Ito
Bulla	Clear, fluid-filled lesion >1 cm with intact roof	Immunobullous diseases, impetigo, lymphedema, drug
Carbuncle	Several coalescing furuncles	Staphylococcus aureus infection, hidradenitis suppurativa
Chancre	Well-circumscribed ulcer on genital skin	Syphilis, herpes, chancroid
Cicatrix	Scar	Hypertrophic or keloid scar
Comedone	Plugged pilosebaceous unit with keratinocytes, sebum, and bacteria. Closed comedone is white with intact epidermis over top. Open comedone is black (due to oxidized fats and dirt) with an open roof	Acne, Favre-Racouchot disease
Corymbiform	Grouped arrangement that consists of a central cluster of lesions, beyond which are scattered individual lesions (like an explosion)	Syphilis, sarcoidosis, tuberculosis, Hansen's disease
Crust	Dried serum, inflammatory cells, red cells, platelets, fibrin	"Scab"

Cyst	Fluid- or keratin-filled, solitary, encapsulated with epithelial lining	Follicular cyst, epidermal inclusion cyst, tricholemmal cyst, steatocystoma, eruptive vellus hair cyst, median raphe cyst
Darier's sign	Urticarial wheal reaction when lesion is stroked or rubbed	Urticaria pigmentosa, solitary mastocytoma
Dermatome	Limited to the area innervated by a specific level of the spinal cord	Herpes zoster, focal hyperhidrosis (from spiral cord lesion)
Dimple sign	Application of lateral pressure with the thumb and index finger results in the formation of a depression (dimple) characteristic of a dermatofibroma	Dermatofibroma
Eczema	"Boiling over." Characterized histopathologically by spongiosis of the epidermis (intercellular edema)	Atopic dermatitis, contact dermatitis, nummular dermatitis, id reaction
Erosion	Loss of epidermis with intact dermis	Trauma, superficial blistering disease (pemphigus, impetigo)
Eschar	Thick, adherent crust with early scarring, dermal fibrosis	Anthrax, ecthyma, ecthyma gangrenosum, recluse bite
Excoriation	Superficial excavation of epidermis and sometimes dermis caused by scratching or other means	Neurotic excoriation, delusions of parasitosis, pruritic skin condition, neuropathic pruritus
Fissure	Deep, linear cracks through epidermis to dermis	Chronic eczematous dermatitis, hand and foot contact dermatitis
Furuncle	Deep necrotizing form of folliculitis with pus accumulation	Furunculosis, hidradenitis suppurativa, Staphylococcus aureus infection
Hemangioma	Vascular proliferation of endothelial cells forming channels and spaces filled with blood	Infantile hemangioma, pyogenic granuloma, kaposiform hemangioendothelioma, tufted angioma

Continued

TABLE 10-6. DERMATOLOGY TERMS AND DEFINITIONS—*cont'd*

TERM	DEFINITION	EXAMPLES
Herpetiform	Grouped or clustered in pattern characteristic for Herpes	HSV, dermatitis herpetiformis, varicella zoster
Hirsutism	(Only in females) increased amount of hair in a male pattern	Gonadal tumors, familial, 21-hydroxylase deficiency 17-beta hydroxylase deficiency, medications
Hutchinson's sign	1. Pigment on nail fold secondary to melanoma of digit 2. Herpes zoster lesion on nasal tip indicating eye involvement	1. Melanoma 2. Varicella zoster
Hutchinson's triad	Hutchinson's teeth, keratitis, deafness	Congenital syphilis
Hypertrichosis	Increased amount of hair in normal distribution	Porphyrias, cyclosporin, familial, hypertrichosis lanuginosa
Ichthyosis	Fishlike pattern of scale on dry skin	Ichthyosis vulgaris, lamellar ichthyosis, x-linked ichthyosis, epidermolytic hyperkeratosis
Immunobullous disease	Immunoreactants targeting specific cutaneous antigens leading to erosions, blisters, bulla, and often scarring	Bullous pemphigoid, pemphigus vulgaris, epidermolysis bullosa acquisita, paraneoplastic pemphigus, mucous membrane pemphigoid, bullous SLE
Immunofluorescent studies	Direct immunofluorescence: Counterstaining tissue with known antibodies to IgG, IgA, IgM, complement components, or fibrin in pathologic tissue mounts to determine in vivo antibodies, which are present in the tissue. Indirect immunofluorescence uses patient's serum to stain known antigens.	Immunobullous diseases fluoresce in epidermis or at the dermoepidermal junction. SLE has IgG at the dermoepidermal junction. Early LCV (Henoch-Schönlein purpura has IgA in vessels). Vessels fluoresce with IgG in porphyria

Keratotic	Hard, rough-surfaced, keratin-derived debris	Actinic keratosis, seborrheic keratosis, warts
Koebner (isomorphic) phenomenon	Formation of new, similar lesions at areas of trauma	Psoriasis, lichen planus, lichen nitidus, warts
KOH (potassium hydroxide) test	Dissolves keratinocytes but not hyphal walls (diagnosis of tinea)	Tinea
Lichenification	Accentuated skin lines and dermatoglyphics with thickening of the epidermis and usually with slight elevation, usually caused by chronic rubbing or scratching	Lichen simplex chronicus, chronic contact dermatitis
Light	Near UV: 300-400 nm. Far UV: 200-300 nm. Visible light: 400-760 nm. Infrared: 760-100,000 nm	UVC: 200-290 nm (germicidal). UVB: 290-320 nm (erythemogenic). UVA: 320-400 nm (long wave UV, “black light” from Wood’s lamp)
Macule	<1 cm, flat, usually well-circumscribed, of different color or texture than surrounding skin	Solar lentigo, junctional nevus, vitiligo, pityriasis alba
Nikolsky’s sign	Sheetlike removal of epidermis by gentle lateral torsional pressure	Toxic epidermal necrolysis (TEN), staphylococcal scalded skin syndrome
Nodule	>1 cm, but less than 3 cm, palpable, solitary, well-circumscribed lesion (may be subcutaneous)	Furuncle, follicular cyst, other benign and malignant tumors of the skin
Nummular	Coin-shaped	Nummular eczema, mycosis fungoides
Palpable purpura	Nonblanching, red/purple, macule/papule with palpable/nodular quality indicating vasculitic process with extravasated red blood cells (RBCs)	Leukocytoclastic vasculitis
Papule	<1 cm, raised, palpable, solitary lesion	Benign and malignant skin tumors, inflammatory papules

Continued

TABLE 10-6. DERMATOLOGY TERMS AND DEFINITIONS—*cont'd*

Term	Definition	Examples
Patch	>1 cm, flat, of different color or texture than surrounding skin	Melasma, vitiligo, café-au-lait macules, nevus depigmentosus
Patch testing	Placement of chemically impregnated patches on skin to determine allergen	Allergic contact dermatitis
Petechiae	Nonblanching, flat, red/purple pinpoint macules caused by extravasated red blood cells in upper dermis	Thrombocytopenia, leukocytoclastic vasculitis, primary systemic amyloidosis, chronic pigmented purpura
Photodistribution	Dorsal hands/forearms, face, sparing submental, upper lip, eyes	Photocontact dermatitis, photodrug, connective tissue disease
Photopatch testing	As above but with irradiation after contactant applied to determine photocontact allergen	Photocontact dermatitis
Phototesting or minimal erythema dose (MED) testing	To determine lowest dose of UV light needed to produce erythema	Before UV light treatment of psoriasis and other disorders, diagnosis of photosensitivity
Plaque	>1 cm, raised, palpable, often formed from confluent papules	Psoriasis, mycosis fungoides, tinea corporis, pityriasis rosea
Poikiloderma	Combination of atrophy, hyperpigmentary and hypopigmentary changes, and telangiectases	Poikiloderma of Civatte, dermatomyositis, mycosis fungoides, radiation dermatitis, Rothmund-Thompson syndrome
Port-wine stain	Vascular/capillary malformation (no abnormal proliferation of vessels) with dilated vessels just beneath epidermis forming confluent purple/pink patch	Port wine stain, vascular birth marks, nevus flammeus, Sturge-Weber syndrome, nevus phakomatosis pigmentovascularis

Pseudocyst	Fluid-filled, solitary, without epithelial lining	Digital mucous cyst, pseudocyst of the auricle, mucocele
Purpura	Nonblanching, flat, red/purple macules or patches caused by extravasated RBCs in upper dermis	Solar purpura, thrombocytopenia, scurvy, leukocytoclastic vasculitis, trauma
Pustule	Pus (neutrophil/granulocyte)-filled lesion with intact roof	Staphylococcus aureus infection, acne, Behçet's disease, tinea, pustular psoriasis, acute generalized exanthematous pustulosis
Reticular	Lacelike or netlike	Cutis marmorata, livedo reticularis, antiphospholipid syndrome, medium to large vessel vasculitis, physiologic
Scar	Dermal fibrosis caused by injury and increased collagen deposition in layered pattern. Hypertrophic scar: Overabundant production of collagen at site of injury. Keloid scar: As above but with extension of scar beyond the borders of initial injury	Secondary to trauma or inflammation
Sclerosis	Hardening or induration of the skin	Lichen sclerosus, radiation dermatitis, morphea, scleroderma
Serpiginous	Snakelike	Subacute cutaneous lupus, tinea, urticaria, deep gyrate erythema, cutaneous larva migrans
Telangiectasia (telangiectases)	Abnormal permanent dilation of vessels (usually venules) with distinct visible vessels in the upper dermis	CREST, scleroderma, hereditary hemorrhagic telangiectasia, ataxia telangiectasia, rosacea, telangiectasia macularis eruptive perstans, generalized essential telangiectasia
Tumor	>3 cm, palpable, solitary, well-circumscribed	Benign and malignant skin tumors

Continued

TABLE 10-6. DERMATOLOGY TERMS AND DEFINITIONS—*cont'd*

Term	Definition	Examples
Tzanck smear	Shows keratinocytes with enlarged nuclei, molding, peripheral chromatin margination, and multinucleation	HSV, VZV
Ulcer	Loss of epidermis and part of dermis	Venous stasis ulcer, neuropathic ulcer, arteriopathic ulcer, malignant neoplasm
Verrucous	Wartlike, papillomatous	Wart, seborrheic keratosis, verruciform xanthoma, epidermal nevus, verrucous carcinoma
Vesicle	Clear, fluid-filled lesion <1 cm with intact roof	Miliaria crystallina, HSV, varicella, eczema, contact dermatitis, dermatitis herpetiformis, polymorphous light eruption, porphyria
Wheal	Urticarial reaction with an edematous, transient or moving, evanescent, pale pink to erythematous papule or plaque, often with halo of erythema and central pallor, and sometimes arranged in arcuate, gyrate, annular patterns or singly without pattern, usually without surface epidermal changes	Urticaria (acute and chronic), urticarial vasculitis physical urticarias, iodine reaction, anaphylaxis, urticarial bullous pemphigoid, drug eruption
Zosteriform	Dermatomal distribution	VZV, reflex sympathetic dystrophy, segmental neurofibromatosis

PMHx: Noncontributory.

PSHx: Noncontributory.

Childhood History: Normal childhood illnesses.

Occupational History: Noncontributory.

Travel History: Noncontributory.

Animal or Insect Exposures History: Noncontributory.

Medications, Allergies: Oral contraceptive pills, occasional ibuprofen, no known drug allergies (NKDA).

Family History: Noncontributory.

Health Maintenance: Patient wears sunscreen daily.

Psychosocial History: Nonsmoker, social drinker, homemaker, lives with husband.

Condition does not affect work.

Review of Systems: Noncontributory.

Physical Exam: Multiple purple, planar, polygonal papules distributed bilaterally and symmetric over the volar wrists and dorsal ankles, with scattered lesions slightly proximal in location. No oral mucosal lesions noted. No genital lesions noted.

11

EMERGENCY MEDICINE (TRAUMA ASSESSMENT FOCUS)

Eric H. Hanson, MD, MPH, Sam Galvagno, DO, and Roy DiLeo, MD

EMERGENCY MEDICINE (FOCUS ON TRAUMA) AREAS COVERED

I. Primary Survey: ABCDE
II. Resuscitation Phase
   ABCs Reassessment
      Shock Parameters
      Oxygen Delivery
      Guidelines
III. Secondary Survey
   AMPLE History
   Head-to-Toe Examination
IV. Acronyms and Abbreviations
V. Definitions
VI. Sample H&P Write-Up

I. PRIMARY SURVEY

The primary survey takes the place of the chief complaint and history of present illness in trauma patients and in all patients requiring resuscitation. ABCDEs of the primary survey.

ABCDEs OF PRIMARY SURVEY.	
Airway	Open the airway. Head tilt/chin lift or jaw thrust. Foreign object removal. Oral airway placement if indicated
Breathing	If not breathing, two slow breaths via face mask or bag-valve-mask (BVM) with 100% high-flow oxygen
Circulation	Is a carotid pulse present? No, call for defibrillator and start closed-chest compressions. Yes, assess hemodynamic status
Disability	Assess level of consciousness and Glasgow Coma (GCS)
Exposure/events	Cut off all clothing. Protect for hypothermia. Obtain brief history of events

A. Airway

1. Ensure cervical spine (C-spine) control, especially with blunt trauma above the clavicle.
2. Maintain airway patency.
   - a. Position the airway: When there is no threat of neck injury, perform jaw thrust by lifting the chin and tilting the head.
   - b. Position the airway: With suspected neck injury, lift the chin by placing the fingers behind the mandible and displace forward (i.e., chin lift). If there is no chest movement or there is a possible foreign body, reposition and apply suction (if patient is conscious) or sweep (if the patient is unconscious).
3. Intubate.
   - a. If the patient is unresponsive and you are unable to clear or maintain a patent airway.
   - b. If there is central nervous system depression.
   - c. If the patient's upper airway is obstructed, and the patient has cyanosis, gurgling, or stridorous breathing.
   - d. If patient's respiratory efforts are inadequate even with strong inspiratory efforts and use of accessory respiratory muscles.
4. Considerations for difficult airway maintenance:
   - a. Teeth, blood, or debris in the mouth.
   - b. Facial trauma or possible cribriform plate fracture. Avoid nasotracheal intubation.
   - c. Neck injury victim. Orotracheal intubation with inline cervical stabilization is considered safe and effective.
   - d. Cricothyrotomy. Recommended if unable to intubate or with severe maxillofacial injuries or laryngeal fractures.
   - e. Intubate at the site of open tracheal injuries.
5. Rapid-sequence intubation.
   - a. Used for definitive airway control.
   - b. Sequence of events.
     - (1) Preoxygenate with 100% oxygen.
     - (2) Establish cricoid pressure.
     - (3) Administer anesthetic and/or paralytic agent of choice.
     - (4) Intubate patient.
     - (5) Confirm breath sounds and end-tidal CO_2.
     - (6) Obtain post-intubation chest x-ray (CXR).

B. Breathing

1. CPR breathing rates (if victim has a pulse).
2. Intubated patient: Is Yankhauer or dental suction present? Follow-up endotracheal tube (ETT) placement with auscultation and CXR. Confirm adequacy of ventilation with serial arterial blood gases (ABGs).
3. Oxygen: All patients with altered level of consciousness receive 100% oxygen.

C. **Circulation**
   1. Pulse assessment: Carotid, femoral, radial, and brachial pulses. Quality, rate, and regularity. Carotid pulse represents approximately 60 mmHg systolic pressure, and radial represents approximately 80 mmHg systolic pressure.
   2. Perfusion: Level of consciousness and skin color.
   3. Shock indicators: Skin assessment (cool or warm, pale, diaphoretic), delayed capillary refill (>2 seconds), tachycardia, cerebral insufficiency, hypotension, and oliguria.
   4. Hemorrhage control: External, exsanguinating hemorrhage should be controlled during the primary survey (e.g., direct pressure, pressure points, tourniquets). Classes of hemorrhage are summarized in Table 11-1.

D. **Disability Evaluation**

RAPID MINI-NEURO EVALUATION SUMMARY	
1. State of consciousness	4. Respiratory pattern
2. Pupillary size and reactivity	5. Reflexes
3. Glasgow Coma Scale (GCS)	

   1. Determine state of consciousness.
      a. Assess patient for altered level of consciousness: Changes in patient's awareness or wakefulness that interfere with a normal response to external stimuli or internal need.
      b. Assess patient with coma for altered level of consciousness: Patient is neither awake nor aware and cannot be awakened, made aware, or aroused by verbal or physical stimulus.
      c. Assess patient without coma for altered level of consciousness: Patient may be awakened but is not fully aware.
         (1) Awake: Patient has awareness of self and environment. Patient is alert and oriented times four: oriented to person, place, time, and condition.
         (2) Lethargic: Patient is wakeful but has depressed awareness of self and environment globally.
         (3) Obtunded: Patient is aroused by verbal stimulus or shaking stimulus.
         (4) Stuporous: Patient is unresponsive and is aroused only with noxious stimuli and does not return to normal (baseline) awareness of self or environment.
         (5) Comatose: Patient is in a state of unresponsiveness that cannot be aroused by verbal or physical stimulus.

Table 11-1. CLASSES OF HEMORRHAGE.

Class of Hemorrhage	Blood Loss in mL (%)	Pulse/Heart Rate	Blood Pressure (Systolic/Diastolic)	Capillary Refill	Central Nervous System (CNS)	Urine Output	Respiratory Rate
Class I	750 (15%)	72-84 Normal	≥120/80 Normal	(<2 seconds) Normal	Anxious	Normal	Normal
Class II	1000-1250 (20-25%)	100 Normal	110/80 Normal	Poor	Anxious	Normal	High
Class III	1500-1800 (30-35%)	>120	70-90/50-60	Poor	Confused	Low	High
Class IV	over 2000	>140	>60 sys	Poor	Lethargic	Low	Higher

2. Assess pupillary size and reactivity.
   - **a.** Note pupil size, reactivity, and direct and consensual accommodation response. Rule out congenital anisocoria, false eye, and direct trauma.
   - **b.** Focality may suggest level of involvement.
   - **c.** Evaluate eye movement.
     - **(1)** Nystagmus: Assess further with oculovestibular response.
     - **(2)** Disconjugate or fixed gaze, roving eyes.
     - **(3)** Corneal reflex (afferent is cranial nerve [CN] V, efferent is CN VII).
     - **(4)** Fundi: Assess for hemorrhages, papilledema, and venous pulsations.
3. Glasgow Coma Scale (GCS) (Table 11-2). Useful in trauma patients only.
4. Assess respiratory patterns (Table 11-3).
5. Evaluate reflexes.
   - **a.** Physiologic deep tendon reflexes (DTRs): Evaluate for horizontal and vertical symmetry; spasticity, or flaccidity.
   - **b.** Pathologic reflex (Babinski): Upper motor neuron (brain and spinal cord) lesion assessment. Monitor for change or progression; evaluate for symmetry.

E. Exposure/Events

1. The patient must be completely undressed.
2. Hypothermia must be treated or prevented.
3. At this point, focused questions should be asked regarding mechanism of injury and events leading to injury.

F. Additional Areas to Consider in the Primary Survey: Has the patient ingested any illicit, poisonous, or toxic drugs?

1. When was the substance taken? How much? Was an antidote given?
2. Evaluate pharmacologic effects, side effects, and metabolism of drug.
3. Assess for immediate, potential, or no danger.
   - **a.** Decontaminate, block absorption, enhance elimination, specific antidotes, and supportive care.
   - **b.** Degree: Core temperature assessment with hypothermia and hyperthermia.
   - **c.** Database: Ensure that all vital information and procedures are documented.
   - **d.** Exposure: Remove and save all clothing (possible evidence and personal effects).
   - **e.** Family and friends: Keep the families up to date whenever possible, and also look for additional history.

Table 11-2. GLASGOW COMA SCALE.

Eye Opening Response (4 points)	Score	Verbal Response (5 points)	Score	Best Upper Limb Motor Response (Pain Applied to Nailbed: 6 points)	Score
Spontaneous	4	Oriented	5	Obeys commands	6
To voice	3	Confused	4	Localizes	5
To pain	2	Inappropriate	3	Withdraws	4
Unresponsive	1	Incomprehensible	2	Abnormal flexion (decorticate)	3
		None	1	Extensor response (decerebrate)	2
				No movement	1

Add the scores from each of the three sections

Table 11-3. RESPIRATORY PATTERNS AND POSSIBLE SITES OF NEUROLOGIC LESIONS.

Pattern Descriptor*	Pattern	Possible Site of Neurologic Lesion
Cheyne-Stokes	Alternating between hyperpnea and apnea	Deep bilateral hemisphere lesion with structural or metabolic etiology
Central neurogenic hyperventilation	Regular-depth to rapid, deep breathing	Midbrain structural lesions
Apneustic breathing	Two- to three-second pause on inspiration. Long, ineffective expiratory phase	Pontine structural lesions
Ataxic breathing	Totally disorganized pattern. Periods of apnea alternating with series of shallow breaths	Medullary respiratory center lesion, forerunner of agonal respirations

**General principle:* The less regular, less periodic, less predictable the respirations are, the lower down the brainstem the abnormality exists.

II. RESUSCITATION PHASE

A. ABCs Reassessment

1. Airway.
   a. C-spine and full-spine immobilization procedures in place.
   b. Tube placement: Reassess patent airway; oral airway ETT placement and position.
2. Breathing.
   a. Monitoring of respiratory rate, ABGs, pulse oximetry, end-tidal CO_2 detector.
   b. Ventilation/oxygenation guidelines.
      (1) Low-flow oxygen systems and delivery devices (do not meet total patient demand).
      (2) High-flow oxygen systems and delivery devices (high airflow with oxygen enrichment [HAFOE], which meets total oxygen demands of the patient).
3. Circulation.
   a. Frequent blood pressure (BP) and pulse assessments.
   b. Persistent shock despite intravenous (IV) fluids.
      (1) Persistent shock despite IV fluids indicates either continuing occult hemorrhage or another cause of shock.

(2) Consider additional studies, labs, procedures, and therapies. For example:
  - (a) Chest x-ray: Rule out hemothorax/pneumothorax.
  - (b) Peritoneal lavage, laparotomy: Rule out abdominal hemorrhage.
  - (c) Pericardiocentesis or thoracotomy: Rule out cardiac tamponade.
  - (d) Emergency urography: Rule out renal trauma.

III. SECONDARY SURVEY

A. History Mnemonic (AMPLE)

- **A** Allergies
- **M** Medications
- **P** Past Medical/Surgical History (PMHx/PSHx)
- **L** Last meal and dose of medication(s)
- **E** Events preceding

B. Sources of Information

1. At the scene of event, ask involved individuals, "What do you think is wrong?"
2. Request specific information about the accident from police and paramedics.
3. Search through patient's available personal belongings, such as wallet or address book, to obtain health and contact information. Look for a Medic Alert bracelet or card.
4. Contact patient's family physician.
5. Obtain hospital or clinic medical records.
6. Contact family members or friends.

C. Accident Information

1. Fall from 20 feet or more (special trauma care is probably indicated in these cases).
2. Motor vehicle accident (MVA).
   - a. Vehicle speed estimate and size of car. Ask if accident occurred at greater than 20 mph (special trauma care is probably indicated in these cases).
   - b. Position in car (e.g., bent steering wheel, windshield damage, dashboard intact).
   - c. Passenger compartment intrusion of 15 inches on victim's side of car (special trauma care is probably indicated in these cases).
   - d. Pedestrian struck by a moving vehicle/child younger than 12 years struck by a car (special trauma care is probably indicated in these cases).
   - e. Death of other passenger(s) (special trauma care is probably indicated in these cases).
   - f. Restraint mechanisms. Seat belts fastened, airbags, and neck rest present.
   - g. Ejected or thrown from vehicle (special trauma care is probably indicated in these cases).

h. Predisposing factors/environment.
3. Motorcycle accident (special trauma care is probably indicated in these cases).
4. Blunt trauma: Direction of impact determines patterns of injuries: front, rear, side, and ejection.
5. Penetrating trauma: Region of body is important.
   a. Chest (special trauma care is probably indicated in these cases): Rule out pneumothorax, myocardial contusion, aortic rupture, tracheobronchial tear, esophageal and diaphragm perforation, to guide subsequent interventions.
   b. Abdomen or groin (special trauma care is probably indicated in these cases): Use diagnostic peritoneal lavage (DPL) indications and results.
   c. Head (special trauma care is probably indicated in these cases): Evaluate for signs of increased intracranial pressure (ICP), altered mental status, emesis, and papilledema.
   d. Spinal injuries: Immobilize and determine spinal level.
   e. Extremities: Rule out commonly missed fractures, fractures of two or more long bones (special trauma care is probably indicated in these cases), major amputation (above the ankle or wrist: special trauma care is probably indicated in these cases), severe burns (>20% body surface area, >15% of face and/or airway burns: special trauma care is probably indicated in these cases).

D. Additional Diagnostic Imaging, Labs, and Studies to Consider

1. Diagnostic imaging: Use judiciously and should not delay resuscitation (which should be completed).
   a. C-spine: In addition to lateral C-spine, obtain open-mouth odontoid and swimmer's view (if required).
   b. Anteroposterior (AP) chest/abdomen/thoracolumbar/pelvis films.
   c. Extremity films as indicated.
   d. Computed tomography (CT) or magnetic resonance imaging (MRI).
2. Laboratory evaluations: Complete blood count (CBC), toxicology screen, alcohol levels, thyroid studies, cortisol, methemoglobin, creatine kinase (CK), pregnancy test, prothrombin time/partial thromboplastin time (PT/PTT), liver function tests (LFTs), metabolic panel, cholesterol panel, if not previously obtained.
3. Studies: For example, thoracentesis, pericardiocentesis, DPL, lumbar puncture.

E. Secondary Survey (Head-to-Toe Examination)

1. Vital signs and monitor readings.
   a. Level of consciousness (alert, lethargic, obtunded, stuporous, comatose).
   b. Respiratory rate (RR).
   c. Pulse oximetry (SAO_2).

d. Pulse (quality, rate, and regularity).
e. Blood pressure.
f. Cardiac rhythm monitor.
g. Temperature: Monitor to prevent hypothermia.
h. Urinary output (adults 50 mL/hr and children 1 mL/kg/hr are desirable).
i. Odors (e.g., alcohol, almond with cyanide poisoning).

2. Skin.
a. Temperature.
b. Color.
c. Turgor.

3. Neck and spine.
a. Inspect for blunt or penetrating injury, stoma, neck vein distention, and tracheal deviation.
b. Palpate entire length of spine for point tenderness, swelling, spasm, and deformity.
c. Auscultate for bruits, reassess C-spine and back board immobilization, traction (inline manual traction).

4. Head and skull (maxillofacial).
a. Inspect for scalp or facial lacerations, contusions, or ecchymoses (mastoid).
b. Palpate for skull deformities, tenderness, and swelling (facial bones stability: zygomas, nasal bridge, maxilla and mandible).
c. Reassess pupil size, equality, and reaction (direct and consensual); visual acuity (with Jaegher or Snellen chart or 4 × 4 package writing or IV bag writing); external eye hemorrhages (look for contact lenses and remove); fundoscopic evaluation—hemorrhage, retinal or lens detachment.
d. Ears (mastoid bruising, external auditory canal [EAC] bleeding).
e. Assess for cerebrospinal fluid (CSF) leakage and hemotympanum.
f. Nose (septal deviation, assess for CSF leakage or bleeding).
g. Mouth: Inspect for debris, swelling (obstruction), tongue lacerations, avulsed teeth, odors, and bleeding.

5. Lungs and chest wall.
a. Inspect chest wall and back for ecchymoses, penetrating injury, deformity, accessory muscle use, equal expansion.
b. Auscultate and percuss apices (rule out pneumothorax), lung fields, and bases (rule out hemothorax).
c. Assess air entry, breath sounds, and expiration.
d. Palpate for tenderness, deformity (flail segments), and crepitation.
e. Assess for sternal fracture, ecchymoses, and tenderness.

6. Cardiac examination.
   a. Heart sounds (distant?, rate, rhythm, murmurs, rubs, or gallops).
   b. Jugular venous distention (JVD).
   c. Peripheral pulses (quality, rate, regularity; carotid pulse represents at least 60 mmHg, radial pulse represents at least 80 mmHg).
7. Abdomen.
   a. Inspect for ecchymoses, lacerations, or penetrating injuries.
   b. Assess flanks bilaterally.
   c. Auscultate bowel sounds.
   d. Palpate for tenderness, guarding or rebound, distention, rigidity, masses, and hepatosplenomegaly (HSM).
8. Perineum, rectum, and vagina.
   a. Inspect perineum for urethral bleeding, lacerations, contusions, or scrotal/vulvar hematomas, rectum for laceration or bleeding.
   b. Assess anal sphincter tone, bowel wall integrity, pelvic fractures, and prostate position.
   c. Check stool for occult blood.
   d. Inspect vaginal mucosa and vaginal vault for lacerations or bleeding.
   e. Perform manual examination.
9. Musculoskeletal.
   a. Inspect extremities for ecchymoses, contusions, penetrating injury, lacerations, and deformity.
   b. Palpate extremities for tenderness, crepitation, and sensation.
   c. Palpate peripheral pulses and assess capillary refill.
   d. Evaluate for signs of compartment syndrome.
   e. Full assessment of the pelvis, including inspection and palpation of landmarks and stability by AP pressure to bilateral anterior-superior iliac spines (ASIS) and pubic symphysis.
   f. Neurologic assessment of extremities as indicated with motor, sensory, cerebellar, deep tendon reflexes (DTRs), and pathologic reflex assessment (Babinski).
   g. List of commonly missed fractures (basilar skull, zygoma/orbital, C6-T1 fractures, odontoid, posterior shoulder dislocation, scaphoid/lunate, radial head, seatbelt fracture, femoral neck, pelvic, posterior hip dislocation, tibial plateau, and talus).
10. Neurologic.
    a. Level of consciousness.
    b. Glasgow Coma Scale (GCS) score.
    c. Reevaluate pupils.

d. Reevaluate respiratory pattern.
e. Cranial nerve assessment, motor sensory, reflexes, cerebellar assessment as indicated.
f. Evaluate for evidence of paralysis or paresis.

IV. ACRONYMS AND ABBREVIATIONS (Table 11-4)

V. DEFINITIONS (Table 11-5)

VI. SAMPLE H&P WRITE-UP

CC: "My chest hurts."

HPI: H.S. is a 55-year-old white male who presents complaining of chest pain after sustaining a blunt impact to the steering wheel of his 4 × 4 late-model pick-up truck during a motor vehicle crash. He is a reliable source. He complains of chest pain and difficulty breathing. During the initial primary survey, his condition deteriorates and he becomes unresponsive.

Accident Information: His vehicle collided with a compact passenger car, both traveling approximately 60 miles per hour. He was wearing a seat belt but there was no air bag deployment. The passenger in the other vehicle was ejected and pronounced dead on the scene. EMS personnel reported extensive dashboard damage, a bent steering wheel, and intact windshield. Based on the position of the vehicles, a head-on collision was thought to be most likely.

MHx: The patient denies any medical problems.

SHx: No prior surgeries.

Medications: Denies use of medications, OTC products, or supplements.

Social History: Unable to illicit from the patient (unresponsive).

Family History: Unable to illicit from the patient (unresponsive).

FOCUSED HHYSICAL EXAMINATION

Vitals: T 98.8°F P 110 BP 90/66 RR 24 Weight 120 kg.

Primary Survey: The patient is received with the cervical spine in the neutral position and fully immobilized with a collar and long rigid board. The airway is patent. Respirations are shallow and rapid. No tracheal deviation is noted. No subcutaneous air is palpated. JVD is evident. There are no signs of obvious external injury. Accessory muscle use is not noted. Examination of the chest reveals equal lung sounds bilaterally without dullness or hyperresonance to percussion. No external bleeding is identified. The radial pulse is rapid and weak. The patient's skin color is pale and diaphoretic with delayed capillary refill (5 seconds). The patient moans to a deep sternal rub. Pupils are equal and briskly reactive bilaterally.

Secondary Survey

General: Unresponsive white male; appears in severe distress.

HEENT: No evidence of contusions, abrasions, deformity, or penetration to the cranium. Pupils equal and reactive to light. Conjunctiva and sclera intact. Facial bones intact.

Neck: JVD to 8 cm. The JVD increases when the patient inspires spontaneously. Trachea midline. No subcutaneous emphysema.

Table 11-4. TRAUMA ACRONYMS AND ABBREVIATIONS.

Acronym or Abbreviation	Definition	Acronym or Abbreviation	Definition
ABC	Airway, Breathing, Circulation	**GCS**	Glascow Coma Scale
ABCDE	Airway, Breathing, Circulation, Disability, Exposure/Events	**HSM**	Hepatosplenomegaly
ACLS	Advance Cardiac Life Support	**I-E ratio**	Inspiratory-expiratory ratio
AP	Anterior/Posterior	**IO**	Intraosseous (refers to intraosseous puncture or infusion)
ASIA	Anterior superior iliac spine	**JVD**	Jugular venous distention
ATLS	Advanced Trauma Life Support	**LPM or L/min**	Liters per minute
AVPU	Alert, verbal, pain, unresponsive	**MAST**	Military antishock trousers
BVM	Bag-valve-mask	**Mg**	Magnesium
C-spine	Cervical spine	**mg/kg**	Milligrams per kilogram
Ca	Calcium	**mmHg**	Millimeters of mercury
CBC	Complete blood count	**mL**	Milliliters
CC	Cubic centimeter	**mL/kg**	Milliliters per kilogram
CK	Creatine kinase	**MVA**	Motor vehicle accident
CM H_2O	Centimeters of water	**NGT**	Nasogastric tube
CN	Cranial nerve	**OR**	Operating room

COPD	Chronic obstructive pulmonary disease	**PALS**	Pediatric Advance Life Support
CO_2	Carbon dioxide	**PASG**	Pneumatic antishock garment
CSF	Cerebral spinal fluid	**PEEP**	Peak and expiratory pressure
CT	Computed tomography scan	**PMH**	Past medical history
CVP	Central venous pressure	**PO_4**	Phosphorous level
CXR	Chest x-ray	**PSH**	Past medical history
DONT	Dextrose, oxygen, naloxone, thiamine	**PT**	Prothrombin time
DPL	Diagnostic peritoneal lavage	**PTT**	Partial thromboplastin time
DTR	Deep tendon reflex	**RR**	Respiratory rate
EAC	External auditory canal	**RSI**	Rapid-sequence intubation
ECG	Electrocardiogram	**SCIWORA**	Spinal cord injury without radiographic abnormality
ED	Emergency Department	**SAO_2**	Oxygen saturation
ETOH	Ethanol level	**Sys**	Systolic blood pressure
ETT	Endotracheal tube	**T + C**	Type and cross
FAST	Focused abdominal sonography for trauma	**TBI**	Traumatic brain injury
FIO_2	Fraction of inspired oxygen	**TEE**	Transesophageal echocardiography
GCS	Glasgow Coma Scale		

EMERG

Table 11-5. DEFINITION OF TRAUMA TERMS.

Term	Definition
Axial unloading	Longitudinal compression of the spinal segments; common in falls
Battle's sign	Ecchymosis over the mastoid process; a sign of basilar skull fracture
Beck's triad	Muffled heart sounds, increased venous pressure (e.g., JVD), and decreased arterial pressure
Brown-Sequard syndrome	Hemisection of the spinal cord; manifests as ipsilateral motor loss, loss of position sense, and contralateral sensory loss one to two levels below the injury
Burst fracture	Fracture of the vertebral body following an axial load
Cauda equina syndrome	Injury to lumbar, sacral, and coccygeal peripheral nerve roots, producing "saddle anesthesia," bowel and bladder dysfunction, and variable motor and sensory loss in the lower extremities
Cervical cape	The area overlying the pectoralis muscle, innervated by the supraclavicular nerves (C-2 through C-4)
Contrecoup injury	Contusions occurring on the opposite side of the brain as the result of head trauma
Decompressive trephination	Also known as "burr holes"; involves drilling holes through the skull to decrease ICP
Flail chest	Free-floating segment of ribs no longer connected to the rest of the thorax; results from multiple rib fractures
Hamman sign	Crunching sound heard over the heart during systole in patients with pneumomediastinum
Hangman's fracture	Fracture of posterior elements of C-2 (e.g., pars articularis)
Kussmaul's sign	Associated with cardiac tamponade; a rise in venous pressure with inspiration, manifested by increased JVD with inspiration
LeFort fractures	Four categories used to describe maxillary fractures

Table 11-5—cont'd

Term	Definition
Marcus-Gunn pupil	Pupil dilates rather than constricting when exposed to light; may occur in periorbital or orbital trauma
Massive hemothorax	Defined as 1500 mL (or more) of blood in the pleural space
Monro-Kellie doctrine	Pertains to the ICP; states that the volume of intracranial contents remains constant
NEO complex	The naso-ethmoidal-orbital complex of bones in the medial orbital area
Postconcussive syndrome (PCS)	Vague complaints such as dizziness, memory changes, or headaches occurring as long as one year after a traumatic brain injury
Raccoon eyes	Periorbital ecchymosis; a sign of facial or skull fracture
Rapid-sequence intubation	Use of sedatives, paralytics, and other drugs to produce a temporary state of anesthetic induction to facilitate intubation
Rotary subluxation	More common in children; a rotation of C-1 resulting in persistent rotation of the head, usually secondary to trauma or other causes
Submental-vertex view	Also known as the "jug-handle" view; shows the base of the skull and zygomatic arches on a skull radiograph
Telecanthus	Widening of the intercanthal distance; normal distance is 35 to 40 mm in adults
Towne view	Radiographic view on a skull film that shows the mandibular ramus, condyles, and base of the skull
Tripod fracture	A serious zygoma fracture: involves the frontal, maxillary, and temporal bones

EMERG

Lungs: Clear to auscultation without adventitious sounds. Equal and bilateral chest rise noted.

Cardiovascular: Heart sounds are muffled and difficult to assess.

Abdomen: Soft, nontender with no palpable masses. No contusions, abrasions, penetrations, or deformities.

Genitourinary: Rectal examination is heme negative with normal sphincter tone.

Extremities: No edema. MILD contusions to both forearms. A contusion to the left shoulder is noted. No other contusions, abrasions, penetrations, or deformities.

Neurologic: The patient is responsive only to a deep sternal rub. Pupils as above. Glasgow Coma Score is 10.

Differential Diagnosis

Pericardial tamponade, hemothorax, traumatic disruption of the aorta, myocardial contusion, tension pneumothorax

Laboratory Studies and Diagnostic Evaluation

CBC, chemistries, cardiac enzymes, CXR, ECG, echocardiography.

12

ENDOCRINOLOGY

Tom J. Sauerwein, MD, Bryan Kahl, MD, Sharon Harris, MD, and Thomas S. Neuhauser, MD

I. HISTORY OF PRESENT ILLNESS

The three most common endocrine presentations are Type 2 diabetes mellitus, hyperthyroidism, and hypothyroidism.

A. Type 2 Diabetes Mellitus (DM)

1. Do you have any of these symptoms/signs? Character (qualitative and quantitative assessments).
   a. Polyuria.
   b. Polydipsia.
   c. Polyphagia.
   d. Weight loss.
   e. Fatigue.
   f. Blurry vision.
   g. Foot ulcers.
   h. Paresthesia.
   i. Frequent fungal or bacterial infections.
2. Short-term and long-term complications (either microvascular or macrovascular complications): Do you have any of the following symptoms/signs?
   a. Cardiac symptoms.
   b. Autonomic postural hypotension.
   c. Gastroparesis.
   d. Diarrhea.
   e. Constipation.
   f. Urinary retention.
   g. Impotence.
   h. Lower extremity pain.
   i. Numbness.
3. When did your symptoms begin? Have you been diagnosed previously? What treatments, if any, have you received? Have you had gestational diabetes?
4. What aggravates your symptoms (precipitators or exacerbators)? Infections may worsen or precipitate symptoms. Chronic poor control predisposes to complications.
5. What has relieved your symptoms? Relieving factors (relievers) may include the level of glycemic control and current tracking of glycemic control. Improved glycemic control decreases sign/symptoms.

6. Are symptoms associated with any related symptoms or conditions? Autoimmune diseases may predispose patient to Type 1 DM. Type 2 DM is associated with obesity, hypertension (HTN), hyperlipoproteinemia (HLP), coronary disease, and renal disease. Gestational diabetes is associated with pregnancy.
7. Have you received any treatments? Medications specifically for this condition (e.g., sulfonylureas, biguanides, thiazolidinediones, alpha-glucosidase inhibitors, and insulin therapy), health care received for complications (e.g., hospitalizations, surgical procedures, laser photocoagulation), DM education (e.g., dietary, exercise, general knowledge).
8. What clinical monitoring and preventive assessments do you receive? Hgb A1c levels quarterly or semiannually? Annual albumin/creatinine ratio (24-hour microalbumin)? Annual serum creatinine? Lipid profile annually, along with liver function testing? Retinal examinations annually? Diabetic foot evaluations with each clinic visit? Occasionally, a fructosamine may aid if the Hgb A1c is not valid).

B. Hyperthyroidism

1. Do you have any of these symptoms/signs? Character (quality and quantitative assessments).
   a. Fatigue.
   b. Restlessness or irritability.
   c. Weight loss.
   d. Heat intolerance.
   e. Tachycardia.
   f. Palpitations.
   g. Diarrhea.
   h. Tremor.
   i. Dry, irritable eyes.
   j. Menstrual irregularities.
   k. Hair loss.
   l. Exercise intolerance.
   m. Sleep disturbance.
   n. Decreased concentration.
2. Where are the symptoms located (distribution, radiation(s), local vs. systemic)? Specific organs that might be involved include eyes (exophthalmos), skin (pretibial myxedema), neck (pain, enlargement), and nails (onycholysis).
3. When did the symptoms begin? What, if any, previous diagnoses and treatments have you received?
4. Are there any aggravating factors (precipitators or exacerbators)? Heat intolerance, for example, is most often present in summer months, and associated with exercise, aspirin use, and recent iodine loads (kelp, contrasted radiologic studies).
5. Any factors that relieve symptoms? Pregnancy may induce temporary remission.

6. Any associated symptoms or conditions? Postpartum thyroiditis, other autoimmune diseases, thyroid nodules, and periodic paralysis?
7. What treatments have you received? Radioactive iodine, antithyroid drugs, or beta-blockers?

C. Hypothyroidism

1. Do you have any of these symptoms/signs? Character (quality and quantitative assessments).
   a. Fatigue.
   b. Slow thinking.
   c. Depression.
   d. Cold intolerance.
   e. Weight gain.
   f. Constipation.
   g. Dry skin.
   h. Menstrual irregularities.
   i. Weakness.
   j. Decreased libido.
   k. Infertility.
   l. Paresthesia.
   m. Bradycardia.
   n. Hypothermia.
   o. Myxedema.
   p. Decreased pulse pressure.
   q. Delayed deep tendon reflexes (DTRs).
   r. Loss of lateral third of eyebrows.
2. Where are the symptoms located (distributions, radiations, local vs. systemic)?
3. When did the symptoms begin? Have you been previously diagnosed with thyroid disease? What treatment did you receive? Did you undergo surgery?
4. Are there any aggravating factors (precipitators or exacerbators)? These may include infection, surgery, iodine deficiency, and medication noncompliance.
5. Any factors that relieve symptoms? Thyroid hormone replacement may relieve symptoms.
6. Any associated symptoms or conditions? Vitiligo? Other autoimmune diseases?
7. What treatments have you received? Thyroid hormone replacement?

II. PAST MEDICAL AND SURGICAL HISTORY

A. Past Medical History

1. With what other conditions have you been diagnosed? Evaluate unrelated diseases that comprise syndromes (e.g., polyglandular disease and autoimmune diseases).
2. Anticipate possible endocrine complications from other medical conditions (e.g., osteoporosis from hypogonadism in

male patient treated for prostate cancer or from steroid use in cases of chronic obstructive pulmonary disease), hypothyroidism from neck x-ray therapy (XRT) for cancer therapy.

B. Past Surgical History

1. Have you had a surgical procedure that involved removing an endocrine gland? Rule out hypofunction of an endocrine gland(s) secondary to accidental removal (e.g., hypoparathyroidism after thyroidectomy and accidental removal of parathyroids) or intentional removal (adrenal insufficiency after bilateral adrenalectomy for bilateral pheochromocytomas).
2. What surgical procedures have you undergone? Surgical history may identify possible endocrine diseases (e.g., hemigastrectomy with vagotomy for recurrent ulcers, gastrinoma of multiple endocrine neoplasia [MEN 1]).

C. Emergency and Trauma History

1. Have you had any head trauma? This can result in both diabetes insipidus and growth hormone deficiency.
2. Other trauma, infection, surgical procedures? Significant stress from infection, surgery, or trauma may produce abnormal thyroid function tests without thyroid disease; "euthyroid sick," or more appropriately called nonthyroidal illness (NTI).
3. Have you ever experienced paralysis? Hyperthyroidism can cause periodic paralysis.
4. Have you been treated for shock? Adrenal insufficiency can cause shock.

D. Childhood History

1. Were you exposed to radiation as a child? Childhood radiation exposure is an important risk factor for thyroid nodules and cancer.
2. Was your sexual development normal? Precocious puberty? Premature thelarche? What was your age at adrenarche and menarche?
3. Were you of normal height and weight? Growth charts showing height and weight are needed to evaluate short stature and possible childhood metabolic disease.

E. Occupational History

1. Have you been exposed to radiation in your work? Prior occupational exposure such as ionizing radiation increases thyroid cancer risk and the development of thyroid nodules.
2. Have you been exposed to heavy metals (e.g., cadmium, zinc, arsenic, lead)? Exposure is associated with male infertility.
3. Were you exposed to Agent Orange while serving in the military? Vietnam exposure to Agent Orange has been associated with increased risk of Type 2 DM.

F. Travel History

1. Have you traveled? In the United States? Foreign countries? Must rule out nonendocrine source of disease (e.g., fever and tachycardia from infection and not thyrotoxicosis).

2. Did you consume any unusual foods? Hypoglycemic poisoning is associated with eating unripe Jamaican aki aki fruit.

III. MEDICATIONS, ALLERGIES, AND ADVERSE REACTIONS

A. Medications

1. Are you taking any prescription medications? List all medications, doses, and indication for use. Many drugs may significantly alter laboratory studies (e.g., steroid use during a cortrosyn stimulation study or spironolactone use while undergoing a hyperaldosterone work-up).
2. Do you use any over-the-counter (OTC) medications (including those from other countries, Mexico in particular), herbal preparations, or supplements? Herbal preparations and supplements for weight loss may contain thyroid hormone extract or ephedra.

B. Allergies and Adverse Reactions

1. What medications have you stopped using? Why? List discontinued medications and reason for stoppage.
2. Was your reaction a true allergy or an adverse effect (e.g., gastrointestinal upset)? Consider use of another medication without the adverse effect (e.g., angiotensin-converting enzyme inhibitors [ACE-I] produce a cough, whereas angiotensin receptor blockers [ARBs], which provide blood pressure control and renal protection in DM patients, do not).

IV. HEALTH MAINTENANCE

A. Prevention

1. What, if any, immunizations have you had?
   a. Pneumococcal immunization? Diabetic patients should receive pneumococcal vaccination at initial diagnosis. Booster shot should be given at age 65 years if it has been at least 6 years since initial vaccination.
   b. Annual influenza shot? All diabetic patients should have these.
2. What precautions have you taken in your home to prevent falls? Fall risk precautions should be discussed with all osteoporosis patients.

B. Diet

1. What type of diet do you follow (e.g., diabetic, Mediterranean, low-fat, low-carbohydrate, Zone diet)?
2. How many calories do you consume each day? Ask patients complaining of weight gain.
3. Do you take any medications with food or with other medications? Concomitant use of Levothyroxine or bisphosphonate may significantly reduce absorption.
4. How much and what type of calcium is included in your usual diet (with or without food)? Ask of patients with osteoporosis.
5. Are you taking any homeopathic therapies? These may contain thyroid extract (produce thyrotoxicosis) or have hypoglycemic properties.

C. **Exercise/Recreation:** Do you exercise regularly? How much, how often, at what intensity, and at what time of day? (Purpose: weight and glycemic control.)

D. **Sleep Patterns**

1. Do you have difficulty falling asleep at night? Are you unable to? This may be caused by agitation from thyrotoxicosis (hyperthyroidism or taking levothyroxine at bedtime) or pheochromocytoma.
2. Are you unable to remain asleep? Frequent waking from night can result from thiazide diuretic use, back pain from osteoporotic compression fractures, or nocturnal hypoglycemia.
3. Do you snore? Snoring in hypogonadal men since reduction in testosterone is adaptive in sleep apnea. Treatment with testosterone worsens sleep apnea.

E. **Social Habits**

1. Do you drink alcohol? What type? How much and how often? Use in evaluation of hypoglycemia, hypertriglyceridemia, and osteoporosis.
2. Do you use tobacco? What form? How much? For how long? Tobacco use exacerbates Graves' eye disease, erectile dysfunction, and osteoporosis. Tobacco also increases coronary events in diabetic patients.

V. FAMILY HISTORY

A. **First-Degree Relatives' Medical History**

1. Have any of your first-degree relatives had an autoimmune disease? Thyroid disease? Premature ovarian failure? These are more common in first-degree relatives.
2. Have any first-degree relatives had medullary thyroid carcinoma or MEN syndromes? Medullary thyroid carcinoma can be, and MEN syndromes are familial.
3. Do any first-degree relatives have DM? Patients who have a first-degree relative with DM have a significant increased risk of developing DM themselves.
4. Do any first-degree relatives have hyperparathyroidism or hypocalciuric hypercalcemia? First-degree relatives' serum calcium and urine calcium can help make the diagnosis between confusing cases of primary hyperparathyroidism and familial hypocalciuric hypercalcemia.

B. **Three-Generation Genogram:** Useful with patients who have MEN and familial medullary carcinoma.

VI. PSYCHOSOCIAL HISTORY

A. **Personal and Social History**

1. Where were you born? Birth country may help identify iodine deficiency and related thyroid diseases.
2. What is your ethnic background (include race)? Race or ethnicity may identify increased risk of disease (e.g., diabetes in Hispanic patients, increased risk of end-stage renal disease and

need for dialysis in African-American patients, 21-OH deficiency in patients of Mediterranean descent).

3. Describe the physical layout of your residence. This is important for advising patients with osteoporosis about precautions to take against falling (e.g., night lights, throw rugs, slip guards in tub, stairs, extension cords).
4. Will you be able to afford medications or therapy (e.g., metformin, glyburide)?
5. What level of education have you attained? This is important when assessing the ability of a patient with DM to count carbohydrates for tight glucose control or to self-titrate insulin with a supplemental scale.

B. **Current Illness Effects on the Patient**

1. Are you aware of, and do you understand, possible complications of your illness? Discuss diabetic complications and their effect on the patient's autonomy (e.g., blindness, need for dialysis, heart attack, or lower extremity amputation).
2. Discuss death and dying issues in patients with endocrine manifestations of nonendocrine cancers: hypercalcemia from breast or squamous cell carcinoma (e.g., have you considered power of attorney? a living will? consulted a lawyer about a will?).

C. **Interpersonal and Sexual History:** Assess morning erections and libido in patients with hypogonadism and diabetes (e.g., Do you still have an interest in sex? Has your interest/frequency changed since the onset of symptoms? Has your partner noticed any change?).

D. **Family Support**

1. Are family members available to provide assistance? Assess familial support for patients with DM who are visually impaired, patients with amputations, and patients with frequent hypoglycemia.
2. Are any family members knowledgeable about your condition and treatment? Ensure that the family is educated on indications and procedures for glucagon injections with diabetic patients.
3. Follow-up for other family members to assess impact of illness on family and discuss possible inheritance of some disease processes (e.g., MEN syndrome, DM).

E. **Occupational Aspects of the Illness**

1. Does your job involve driving or operating machinery? Hypothyroid patients should avoid driving or operating heavy machinery if condition is not under control.
2. How flexible is your work schedule regarding break and lunch times? Diabetic patients should have flexible schedules to eat at specific times to avoid hypoglycemia.

VII. REVIEW OF SYSTEMS (Tables 12-1 to 12-3)

Many symptoms observed with endocrine disease are nonspecific (e.g., fatigue, weight gain, increased urination), which creates an enormous differential diagnostic list. The diagnosis becomes straightforward when a constellation of symptoms coalesce (e.g., polyuria, polydipsia, polyphagia in an obese, middle-aged male with a family history of diabetes mellitus is clearly diabetes mellitus).

Table 12-1. GENERAL ENDOCRINOLOGY SYMPTOMS BY SYSTEM.

SYSTEM	SYMPTOMS
General	Fatigue, change in weight, heat or cold intolerance, headache, hypoglycemic symptoms
HEENT	Red, dry, and/or scratchy eyes, change in vision (double/loss of vision), hearing loss, increased tongue size (macroglossia), change in voice: deepening (only in women)
Neck	Pain, tenderness, thyroid enlargement, difficulty swallowing or choking sensation when lying flat
Cardiovascular	Palpitations, tachycardia, chest pain, dyspnea on exertion (DOE), orthopnea, paroxysmal nocturnal dyspnea (PND)
Chest	Breast development, enlargement, pain or tenderness, nipple discharge
Gastrointestinal	Polyphagia, polydipsia, diarrhea, constipation, emesis, nausea
Genitourinary	Polyuria, blood in urine (kidney stones), loss of libido (hypogonadism), erectile dysfunction in men, morning erections, infertility, testicular pain
Obstetrics/ Gynecologic	Age of onset of menstruation; regularity, duration, and quantity of menstrual flow; prior pregnancy, change in libido, infertility, secondary sexual characteristics
Lymphatic	Neck lymphadenopathy
Musculoskeletal	Proximal muscle weakness (e.g., difficulty climbing stairs or getting out of a chair)
Skin	Striae, easy bruising, hirsutism (women): distribution of hair growth, rash, change in pigmentation (hyper/hypopigmentation), dry skin or hair
Extremities	Tremor; increase in ring, shoe, or hat size; paresthesia, ulcers, numbness

Table 12-2. NONSEPECIFIC SYMPTOMS AND ASSOCIATED ENDOCRINOLOGIC DISEASES.

Symptom	Diseases
Abdominal pain	Addisonian crisis, diabetic ketoacidosis, hyperparathyroidism
Amenorrhea or oligomenorrhea	Adrenal insufficiency, congenital adrenal hyperplasia, anorexia nervosa, Cushing's syndrome, hyperprolactinemic states, hypopituitarism, hypothyroidism, menopause, ovarian failure, polycystic ovaries, pseudohermaphroditic syndromes
Anemia	Adrenal insufficiency, gonadal insufficiency, hypothyroidism, hyperparathyroidism, panhypopituitarism, renal insufficiency
Anorexia	Addison's disease, diabetic ketoacidosis, hypercalcemia (e.g., hyperparathyroidism), hypothyroidism, malignancy
Constipation	Diabetic neuropathy, hypercalcemia, hypothyroidism, pheochromocytoma
Depression	Adrenal insufficiency, Cushing's syndrome, hypercalcemic states, hypoglycemia, hypothyroidism
Diarrhea	Hyperthyroidism, metastatic carcinoid tumors, metastatic medullary thyroid carcinoma, vasoactive intestinal peptide adenoma (VIPoma), Zollinger Ellison syndrome, diabetes mellitus
Fever	Adrenal insufficiency, hyperthyroidism (severe: thyroid storm), hypothalamic disease
Hair changes	Decreased body hair (e.g., hypothyroidism, hypopituitarism, Cushing's syndrome, thyrotoxicosis), hirsutism (e.g., androgen excess states, Cushing's syndrome, acromegaly)
Headache	Hypertensive episodes with pheochromocytoma, hypoglycemia, pituitary tumors, Paget's of the skull
Hypothermia	Hypoglycemia, hypothyroidism, hypothalamic dysfunction

Continued

Table 12-2. NONSEPECIFIC SYMPTOMS AND ASSOCIATED ENDOCRINOLOGIC DISEASES—*cont'd*

SYMPTOM	DISEASES
Libido changes	Adrenal insufficiency, Cushing's syndrome, hypercalcemia, hyperprolactinemia, hyperthyroidism, hypokalemia, hypopituitarism, hypothyroidism, poorly controlled diabetes mellitus
Nervousness	Cushing's syndrome, hyperthyroidism, pheochromocytoma
Polyuria	Diabetes insipidus, diabetes mellitus, hypercalcemia, hypokalemia
Skin changes	Acanthosis nigricans (obesity, polycystic ovaries, severe insulin resistance, Cushing's syndrome, acromegaly), acne (androgen excess), hyperpigmentation (adrenal insufficiency, Nelson's syndrome), dry (hypothyroidism), hypopigmentation (panhypopituitarism), striae, plethora, bruising, ecchymoses (Cushing's syndrome), vitiligo (autoimmune thyroid disease, Addison's disease)
Weakness and fatigue	Addison's disease, Cushing's syndrome, diabetes mellitus, hypokalemia (e.g., primary aldosteronism, Bartter's syndrome), hypothyroidism, hyperthyroidism, hypercalcemia (e.g., hyperparathyroidism, panhypopituitarism, pheochromocytoma)
Weight gain	Central nervous system disease, Cushing's syndrome, hypothyroidism, insulinoma, pituitary tumors, acromegaly, hypothalamic dysfunction
Weight loss	Adrenal insufficiency, anorexia nervosa, endocrine cancer, hyperthyroidism, insulin dependent diabetes mellitus, panhypopituitarism, pheochromocytoma

Modified and reprinted by permission of the publisher from Baxter JD. Introduction to endocrinology. In Basic and Clinical Endocrinology, ed 5. New York: Appleton & Lange, 1997;29.

Table 12-3. COMMON ENDOCRINOLOGIC DISEASES AND THEIR SYMPTOMS.

DISEASE	SYMPTOMS
Diabetes mellitus	Polyuria, polydipsia, polyphagia, weight loss, fatigue, blurry vision, foot ulcers, paresthesia
Hyperthyroidism	Fatigue, restlessness, irritability, weight loss, heat intolerance, tachycardia, palpitations, diarrhea, tremor, dry irritable eyes, hair loss, exercise intolerance, sleep disturbance
Hypothyroidism	Fatigue, slow thinking, depression, cold intolerance, weight gain, constipation, dry skin, menstrual irregularities, weakness, decreased libido, infertility, paresthesia

VIII. PHYSICAL EXAMINATION

Endeavor to be comprehensive. Many endocrine glands exist throughout and affect the entire body.

A. Endocrine Physical Examination by System (Table 12-4)

B. Thyroid Examination

1. The thyroid is butterfly-shaped with two laterally placed lobes connected medially by the isthmus, located just inferior to the cricoid cartilage. The thyroid is the only endocrine gland that can be reproducibly palpated in the physical examination.
2. Examination technique.
   a. While observing the patient's neck from front, have patient drink sips of water. The thyroid will move up along with the trachea because it is fixed to the pretracheal fascia.
   b. Patient's neck should be slightly extended to raise the thyroid from the supraclavicular region and press it against the subcutaneous structures.
   c. Observe for general enlargement (goiter) or nodules.
   d. Palpate the neck from behind or to the side of the patient. The neck should be slightly flexed forward to relieve tension on the sternocleidomastoid muscles.
   e. Locate the cricoid cartilage with your right index finger. The cricoid cartilage is a small protrusion just below the thyroid cartilage.
   f. Place your index finger just inferior to the cricoid cartilage, and have the patient take a sip of water. As the patient swallows, you should feel the isthmus pass beneath your finger. Note its consistency, size, and any tenderness.

Text continued on p. 195.

Table 12-4. FINDINGS OF PHYSICAL EXAMINATION AND POSSIBLE DIAGNOSES.

System	Physical Examination Finding	Diagnoses
Vital Signs		
Pulse	Tachycardia	Thyrotoxicosis, pheochromocytoma: volume contraction (any etiology)
Blood pressure (BP)	Orthostatic	Pheochromocytoma, adrenal insufficiency; autonomic neuropathy (diabetes mellitus), isolated aldosterone deficiency
	Hypertension	Pheochromocytoma, hyperaldosteronism, Cushing's; congenital adrenal hyperplasia (CAH)
	Widened pulse pressure (increased systolic BP, decreased diastolic BP)	Thyrotoxicosis
	Hypotension	Adrenal insufficiency, diabetic ketoacidosis (DKA)
Weight	Centripetal obesity	Cushing's syndrome
	Gradual weight gain	Hypothyroidism, acromegaly, insulinoma
	Rapid weight loss	Thyrotoxicosis, adrenal insufficiency, diabetes mellitus
Height	Short stature	Turner's syndrome, growth hormone deficiency, delayed puberty, familial short stature
HEENT		
Head	Frontal bossing (prominent supraorbital ridge)	Acromegaly
	Prognathism (enlarged chin)	Acromegaly

	Skull/facial deformities	Paget's disease
	Loss of outer half of eyebrow (Queen Anne's sign)	Hypothyroidism
Eyes	Conjunctival injections	Hyperthyroidism, Graves' disease
	Blue sclera	Osteogenesis imperfecta
	Exophthalmos (bulging eyes)	Graves' disease
	Lagophthalmos (inability to close eyes)	Graves' disease
	Periorbital edema (swelling around eyes)	Graves' disease
	Lid lag (from up to down gaze during EOM)	Thyrotoxicosis (any cause)
	Retraction of upper eyelid (chronic stare)	Thyrotoxicosis (any cause)
	Visual field defects (bitemporal hemionopsia)	Pituitary macroadenoma
	Dot and blot hemorrhages, hard exudates, microaneurysms, and cotton-wool spots on retinal examination (diabetic patients)	Diabetic retinopathy
	Lipemia retinalis	Hypertriglyceridemia
Ears	Decreased hearing (CN VIII entrapment)	Paget's disease
	Prominent low-set, deformed ears	Turner's syndrome
Nose	Broad nasal bridge	Acromegaly
Mouth	Macroglossia (enlarged tongue)	Acromegaly, hypothyroidism
	Interdental separation (space between teeth)	Acromegaly
	Tongue tremor	Thyrotoxicosis (any cause)
	Buccal hyperpigmentation	Addison's disease
	Gingival hyperpigmentation	Addison's disease
	Orange tonsils	Tangier's disease

Continued

Table 12-4. FINDINGS OF PHYSICAL EXAMINATION AND POSSIBLE DIAGNOSES—*cont'd*

System	Physical Examination Finding	Diagnoses
Face	Facial plethora (fullness)	Cushing's syndrome
	Plethoric suffusion of the face with raised hands (Pemberton's sign)	Substernal goiter
Neck		
Thyroid	Goiter (any enlargement of the thyroid)	Simple goiter, Graves' disease, multinodular goiter
	Nodule	95% benign, 5% malignant
	Multiple nodules	Multinodular goiter, Hashimoto's thyroiditis
	Thyroid bruit	Graves' disease
	Tender firm enlarged thyroid	Subacute thyroiditis
Posterior neck	Increased posterior fat pad (buffalo hump)	Cushing's syndrome
	Short neck, broad-based with web appearance	Turner's syndrome
Lungs		
	Assess for lung carcinoma (dullness to percussion, decreased breath sounds, wheezes)	Ectopic adrenocorticotropic hormone, ACTH (Cushing), carcinoid
Chest	Gynecomastia (male patients)	Hypogonadism
	Galactorrhea	Hyperprolactinemia
	Wide-spaced nipples	Turner's syndrome
	Shield like chest	Turner's syndrome

Cardiovascular	Tachycardia	Hyperthyroidism, diabetic autonomic neuropathy, pheochromocytoma
	Hyperdynamic precordium	Hyperthyroidism
Abdomen	Violaceous striae (purple stretch marks 1 cm wide)	Cushing's syndrome
Genitourinary		
Male	Small testis	Central hypogonadism; Klinefelter's syndrome
Female	Clitoromegaly	Virilization (adrenal or ovarian tumor), congenital adrenal hyperplasia
Skin		
	Eruptive xanthomas	Hypertriglyceridemia (any cause)
	Hyperpigmented velvety skin (has appearance of dirty skin)	Acanthosis nigricans (insulin resistance, diabetes mellitus; acromegaly, Cushing's syndrome)
	Tuberous xanthomas (cobblestone appearance, extensor surfaces)	Dysbetalipoproteinemia
	Thick/oily skin: doughy	Acromegaly
	Skin tags	Acromegaly
	Numerous ecchymoses (easy bruising)	Cushing's syndrome
	Dry skin	Hypothyroidism, diabetic neuropathy

Continued

Table 12-4. FINDINGS OF PHYSICAL EXAMINATION AND POSSIBLE DIAGNOSES—*cont'd*

System	Physical Examination Finding	Diagnoses
Extremities	Tendonous xanthomas (found on extensor surfaces, particularly the Achilles tendon)	Familial hypercholesterolemia
	Large spade like hands with sausage-shaped digits	Acromegaly
	Clubbing (nail enlargement, thyroid acropachy)	Graves' disease
	Onycholysis	Thyrotoxicosis
	Pigmentation of palmar creases	Addison's disease, carotenemia of hypothyroidism
	Short fourth metacarpal	Pseudohypoparathyroidism, Turner's syndrome
Neurologic	Trousseau's sign (carpal pedal spasm with insufflation of blood pressure cuff)	Hypocalcemia
	Chvostek's sign (percussion of facial nerve causing facial spasm)	Hypocalcemia
	Peripheral neuropathy	Hypothyroidism, hyperthyroidism, DM
Deep tendon reflexes (DTRs)	Hyperreflexia	Thyrotoxicosis
	Delayed relaxation phase	Hypothyroidism

g. Once the isthmus is palpated, slide your fingers laterally from it to palpate the left lobe of the thyroid.
h. Place the first two fingertips of your right hand on the lateral aspect of the trachea, and gently rub in a circular or up-and-down pattern to feel the left lobe. Have the patient take another sip of water and feel for any nodules. Again note the size, gland consistency, and location of any nodules.
i. Palpate for a thrill in thyrotoxic patients. Perform the same examination on the right side of the gland with your left hand. After both lobes have been evaluated separately, palpate them simultaneously to compare the size and constancy. Use your right hand to palpate the right lobe and your left hand to palpate the left lobe, again from behind the patient.
j. After palpation is complete, auscultate to assess for bruits or venous hums in any patient who presents with thyrotoxicosis.

C. Lid and Orbital Lag Examination and Technique

1. Place index finger approximately 2 feet from patient's eyes.
2. Initially move finger upward so patient is staring up, then move your finger downward (not too rapidly), concentrating on the upper eyelid.
3. Look for the appearance of any white sclera between the iris and the upper lid margin. Lid lag is present if the sclera becomes visible.
4. Orbital lag is done in the same fashion but in the opposite direction. With the patient looking downward, move your finger vertically, again observing for white sclera between the iris and the upper lid.
5. Orbital lag is present if the lid retracts quickly and the orbit is slow to follow. Both findings are seen in thyrotoxicosis of any etiology.

D. Diabetic Foot Examination

1. Assess feet for discoloration, cracks, and areas of erythema.
2. Note any signs of current or previous ulceration.
3. Examine the nail and interdigital spaces for macerated skin or pressure lesions predisposing to infections. Determine if foot is clean, dry, or moist (dry, cracked skin is suggestive of autonomic neuropathy).
4. Observe the shape of the foot. Look for claw toes (autonomic neuropathy) or Charcot arthropathy (collapsed arch of midfoot). Palpate pulses and note whether present, diminished, or absent.
5. Assess deep tendon reflexes, vibratory sense, and proprioception.
6. Perform the sensory examination with a 10-gram monofilament (see Figure 12-1). The monofilament should be placed perpendicularly to the plantar surface of the foot and enough

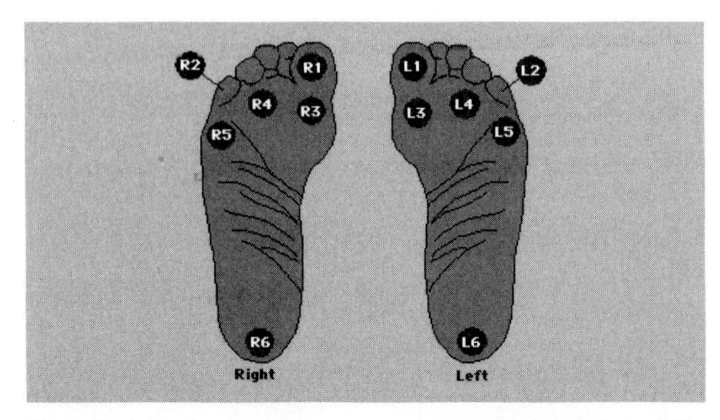

Figure 12-1 Testing sites for pressure sensation in evaluation of diabetic foot. The monofilament used to evaluate pressure sensation should be tested at each of the 12 sites shown, which represent the most common sites of ulcer formation. Failure to detect cutaneous pressure at any site indicates that the patient is at high risk for future ulceration.

Reprinted by permission of the publisher from David K McCulloch: Evaluation of the Diabetic Foot. Chevy Chase, MD: UpToDate Inc., Copyright 27 Jul 1999 by UpToDate Inc.

pressure applied to buckle the monofilament (a known amount of pressure). Repeat the test at all 12 sites. Any decrease in sensation markedly increases the patient's risk for future ulceration.

IX. DIFFERENTIAL DIAGNOSIS (Table 12-5)

Table 12-5. PATHOLOGIC DIAGNOSIS OF ENDOCRINE SYSTEM.

DISEASE/SYSTEM	PATHOLOGIC DIAGNOSES
Anterior pituitary disease	Hyperfunctioning adenomas: microadenoma [<1.0 cm] and macroadenoma [>1.0 cm] (prolactinoma, acromegaly, Cushing's syndrome, thyroid stimulation hormone/TSH secreting tumors, and gonadotrophic adenomas). Hypopituitarism (secondary to mass effect, radiation therapy or post surgical ablation)
Posterior pituitary disease	Diabetes insipidus. Suprasellar: Craniopharyngioma, Rathke's pouch cyst, sarcoid, Langerhan's cell histiocytosis (LCH), lymphocytic hypophysitis, glial neoplasm, hamartoma

Table 12-5—cont'd

DISEASE/SYSTEM	PATHOLOGIC DIAGNOSES
Thyroid disease	Hyperthyroidism (Graves' disease, toxic nodule, toxic multinodular goiter, thyroiditis), hypothyroidism (Hashimoto's thyroiditis, postablative and postsurgical removal), benign thyroid nodules, thyroid neoplasm (papillary, follicular, medullary, anaplastic carcinoma, and lymphoma) and goiter
Parathyroid	Hyperparathyroidism (parathyroid adenoma, hyperplasia, carcinoma, first-, second-, third-degree hyperparathyroidism). Hypoparathyroidism (postsurgical)
Adrenal	Hyperfunctioning adenoma (hyperaldosteronism, Cushing's syndrome, virilizing adrenal adenoma, pheochromocytoma, congenital adrenal hyperplasia).
Adrenal insufficiency	(Addison's disease, steroid-induced [actually third-degree not first-degree], bilateral hemorrhage [as in Waterhouse-Friderichsen syndrome], adrenal leukodystrophy)
Pancreas	Diabetes mellitus, insulinoma, VIPoma, gastrinoma, glucagonoma, and carcinoid
Lipids	Familial hypercholesterolemia (FH), dysbetalipoproteinemia, hypertriglyceridemia, familial combined hyperlipidemia and polygenic hypercholesterolemia
Genitourinary	Hyperfunctioning tumors (virilizing ovarian tumors, polycystic ovarian syndrome [PCOS]). Hypogonadism (first- and second-degree), Klinefelter syndrome, Turner's syndrome
Bone	Osteoporosis, Paget's disease, rickets, osteomalacia

ENDO

X. LABORATORY STUDIES AND DIAGNOSTIC EVALUATIONS

A. Laboratory Studies

1. Serum chemistries.
   - **a.** Insulin like growth factor (IGF-1), also called somatomedin C (acromegaly).
   - **b.** Pituitary hormones (overproduction and underproduction).
   - **c.** Measurement of specific hormone levels (e.g., 17 hydroxyprogeterone levels in congenital adrenal hyperplasia, insulin if suspect insulinoma, follicle stimulating hormone

[FSH] and luteinizing hormone [LH] for assessment of hypogonadism).

d. Electrolytes: Levels affected by multiple endocrine disease processes and their treatments.

e. Serum osmolarity: Useful in work-up for diabetes insipidus and syndrome of inappropriate antidiuretic hormone secretion (SIADH).

f. Aldosterone: Useful for assessment of hyperaldosteronism.

g. Parathyroid hormone and parathyroid-related protein: Useful for assessment of parathyroid disease.

h. Additional useful chemistries: Glucose (e.g., DM, acromegaly), hemoglobin A1c/glycohemoglobin (DM), lipid profile (e.g., acromegaly, DM), calcium (e.g., acromegaly, parathyroid disease, thyrotoxicosis, Addison's disease, and pheochromocytoma).

i. Thyroid function tests (e.g., T3, T4, TSH, T3RU): Useful for assessment of thyroid function.

2. Urine.

a. Urinary free cortisol: Useful for evaluation for Cushing's syndrome/disease.

b. Urine osmolarity: Useful in work-up for diabetes insipidus.

c. Urine vanillylmandelic acid (VMA): Assessment for pheochromocytoma.

3. Endocrine tests.

a. Dexamethasone suppression test: Useful for evaluation for Cushing's syndrome/disease.

b. Cortrosyn stimulation test: Assessment of hypothalamic-pituitary-adrenal axis (e.g., adrenal insufficiency).

c. Glucose tolerance test: Used for assessment of acromegaly and DM (including treatments/compliance).

4. Biopsy: Fine-needle aspiration (FNA) is useful for assessment of thyroid lesions.

B. Radiologic Studies

1. Magnetic resonance imaging (MRI) and computed tomography (CT): Useful for assessment of lesion(s) (e.g., pituitary, adrenal gland, but only after a biochemical diagnosis has been confirmed).

2. Bone-density scan: A noninvasive way to measure bone density and identify people at risk for osteoporosis and nontraumatic fractures. Many methods are available that measure either peripheral sites (heel ultrasound and distal forearm dual-energy x-ray absorptiometry [DEXA]) or central sites (quantitative CT of the spine and DEXA of hip and AP spine). DEXA scans of the hip and AP spine are most commonly used.

3. Radioactive iodine uptake: A radioisotope (I^{123}) is useful for determining the amount and pattern of iodine uptake in the thyroid. This study is essential for determining the cause of hyperthyroidism.

4. Whole-body scan: A radioisotope scan (I^{131}) that is useful for determining recurrence of differentiated thyroid cancers (follicular and papillary) and need for further surgery or radioactive iodine ablation. It can also be used after a radioactive iodine ablative dose to determine efficacy of treatment and exact location of recurrent carcinoma that was treated.

C. Additional Studies

1. Colonoscopy: Assess for polyps (acromegaly).
2. Sleep studies: Rule out sleep apnea (acromegaly and obese hypogonadal males).
3. Echocardiography: Assessment for ventricular mass and left ventricular hypertrophy in acromegaly.
4. Visual field testing: Useful for assessment of pituitary disease.

XI. ACRONYMS AND ABBREVIATIONS (Table 12-6)

XII. DEFINITIONS (Table 12-7)

XIII. SAMPLE H&P WRITE-UP

CC: "I feel like my heart is racing a mile a minute, and I have lost 15 pounds in the past month."

HPI: T.H. is a 30-year-old white female who presents as a new patient for evaluation of thyrotoxicosis. She presented to her primary care manager 4 days ago with complaints of an increased heart rate, nervousness, tremor, and a 15-pound weight loss. Her symptoms began approximately 4 weeks before evaluation and have progressed over that time period. She denies any recent illness, pregnancy, medication use, or history of thyroid problems.

In addition, she did not menstruate last month and has not started her cycle. She has noted some new hair growth over her chin and upper arms and now has at least three bowel movements per day (normal is one every other day). She denies fevers, diplopia, eye pain, muscle weakness, or periodic paralysis. Her neck is not tender and she has no dysphagia.

PMHx: She denies any chronic medical conditions. She has not had any contrasted imaging studies.

PSHx: She denies prior surgeries.

MEDICATIONS: She was recently started on Propranolol 10 mg po qid by her primary MD. Before that, she took a multivitamin (MVI) qd.

HEALTH MAINTENANCE

Prevention: Immunizations up to date.

Diet: Regular diet with no restrictions. She denies recent consumption of shellfish or kelp.

Exercise: She has not been able to exercise secondary to extreme fatigue, palpitations, and a very rapid pulse.

Sleep Patterns: She has had great difficulty getting to sleep and once asleep, usually wakes several times during the night.

Social Habits: She denies smoking or tobacco use. She does drink on occasion (socially). She denies illicit drug use.

Table 12-6. ENDOCRINE ACRONYMS AND ABBREVIATIONS.

Acronym or Abbreviation	Definition	Acronym or Abbreviation	Definition
ACE-I	Angiotensin-converting enzyme inhibitor	**IGF-1**	Insulin like growth factor-1
ACTH	Adrenocorticotropic hormone	**IHA**	Idiopathic hyperaldosteronism
ADH	Antidiuretic hormone	**IPSS**	Inferior petrosal sinus sampling
AGE	Advanced glycosylation end-product	**ITT**	Insulin tolerance test
AKA	Above-the-knee amputation	**IVF**	In vitro fertilization
APA	Aldosterone-producing adenoma	**LDL**	Low-density lipoprotein
ARB	Angiotensin receptor-blocker	**LH**	Luteinizing hormone
AVP	Arginine vasopressin	**LT4**	Levothyroxine
APUD	Amine precursor uptake and decarboxylation cell	**MEN**	Multiple endocrine neoplasia
BKA	Below-the-knee amputation	**MNG**	Multinodular goiter
BMI	Body mass index	**MTC**	Medullary thyroid carcinoma
BMD	Bone mineral density	**NTI**	Nonthyroidal illness
BMR	Basal metabolic rate	**OGTT**	Oral glucose tolerance test
CAH	Congenital adrenal hyperplasia	**OHSS**	Ovarian hyperstimulation syndrome
CRH	Corticotropin-releasing hormone	**OI**	Ovulation induction
DCCT	Diabetes care and complications trial (study of type 1 DM)	**PCOS**	Polycystic ovarian syndrome
DDAVP	Desmopressin	**PET**	Positron emission tomography
DEXA/DXA	Dual-energy x-ray absorptiometry	**PGE**	Polyglandular endocrinopathies
DHEA-S	Dehydroepiandrosterone sulfate		

DI	Diabetes insipidus	**POF**	Premature ovarian failure
DKA	Diabetic ketoacidosis	**PPAR**	Peroxisome proliferator-activated receptor
DM	Diabetes mellitus	**PTH**	Parathyroid hormone
ED	Erectile dysfunction	**PTHrP**	Parathyroid hormone-related protein
FBS	Fasting blood sugar	**PTU**	Propylthiouracil
FCH	Familial combined hyperlipidemia	**RIA**	Radioimmunoassay
FFA	Free fatty acid	**RAIU**	Radioactive iodine uptake
FH	Familial hypercholesterolemia	**SIADH**	Syndrome of inappropriate antidiuretic hormone secretion
FHH	Familial hypocalciuric hypercalcemia	**SERM**	Selective estrogen receptor modulator
FNA	Fine-needle aspiration	**SHBG**	Sex hormone–binding globulin
FSH	Follicle-stimulating hormone	T_3	Tri-iodothyronine
GDM	Gestational diabetes mellitus	T_4	Thyroxine
GH	Growth hormone	**T3RU**	T_3 resin uptake
GnRH	Gonadotropin-releasing hormone	**TBG**	Thyroxine-binding globulin
GRHA	Glucocorticoid-remediable hyperaldosteronism	**TMNG**	Toxic multinodular goiter
HDL	High-density lipoprotein	**TPO, anti-**	Thyroperoxidase antibody
HCTZ	Hydrochlorothiazide	**TRH**	Thyrotropin-releasing hormone
HPA	Hypothalamic-pituitary-adrenal	**TSH**	Thyroid-stimulating hormone
HRT	Hormone replacement therapy	**TSI**	Thyroid-stimulating immunoglobulin
HTN	Hypertension	**VDDR**	Vitamin D–dependent rickets
HLP	Hyperlipoproteinemia	**VIP**	Vasoactive intestinal polypeptide
HHS	Hyperglycemic hyperosmotic syndrome	**VLDL**	Very low-density lipoprotein
ICSI	Intracytoplasmic sperm injection	**VMA**	Vanillylmandelic acid
IDL	Intermediate-density lipoprotein	**WBS**	Whole-body scan

Table 12-7. COMMON ENDOCRINE TERMS.

TERMS	DEFINITIONS
Acanthosis nigricans	Papillomatous (wartlike) hyperplasia of the skin
Apoplexy, pituitary	Acute life-threatening intrapituitary hemorrhage, which may result in loss of anterior pituitary function
BIDS therapy	Bedtime insulin, daytime sulfonylurea therapy for Type 2 DM
Chvostek's sign	Percussion of facial nerve causing facial spasm
Cushing's disease	Cushing's syndrome resulting from a benign pituitary adenoma
Cushing's syndrome	A disease of excessive glucocorticoids from any source
Dawn phenomenon	Increased hepatic gluconeogenesis in early morning hours secondary to surge of counter-regulatory hormones
Diabetes insipidus	A disorder caused by deficiency of, or resistance to, vasopressin
Exophthalmos	Abnormal protrusion of the eyeball secondary to disease
Galactorrhea	Persistent flow of milk-like discharge from breast
Goiter	Any enlargement of the thyroid gland
Gynecomastia	Overdevelopment (hypertrophy) of the male breast
Hemoglobin A1c	A measure of glycosylated hemoglobin-A used to determine a 2- to 3-month average glycemic control for patients with diabetes
Hyperthyroidism	Excess thyroid hormone production from the thyroid gland
Hypothyroidism	A state of deficient thyroid hormone production (autoimmune disease, ablation, or surgical removal)
Intensive insulin regimen	Three to four shots per day insulin regimen with frequent monitoring
Jod-Basedow syndrome	Thyrotoxicosis resulting from excess iodine load
Lagophthalmos	Inability to completely close eyes, secondary to exophthalmos
Myxedema coma	A life-threatening condition characterized by exaggerated manifestations of severe hypothyroidism

Table 12-7—cont'd

TERMS	DEFINITIONS
Osteomalacia	Inadequate mineralization of newly formed mature bone
Osteopenia	Low bone mass defined by the World Health Organization (WHO) as a T-score between −1 and −2.5 standard deviations below the mean
Osteoporosis	A disease characterized by low bone mass and microarchitectural deterioration of bone tissue, leading to enhanced bone fragility
Osteopetrosis	A heterogeneous group of disorders characterized by an increase in bone density (marble bone disease)
Pemberton's sign	Plethoric suffusion of the face with raised hands
Plummer's nail	Distal separation of the nail plate from the underlying bed
Polydipsia	Abnormal thirst that leads to drinking large quantities of fluids
Polyuria	The production of large quantities of dilute urine
Pretibial myxedema	Edematous, indurated plaques over the pretibial area in patients with Graves' disease
Queen Anne's sign	Loss of outer half of eyebrow
Thyroiditis	Acute or chronic inflammation of the thyroid gland
Thyrotoxicosis	Excess thyroid hormone from any source
Trousseau's sign	Carpal pedal spasm with insufflation of blood pressure cuff
Wolff-Chaikoff effect	A transient inhibition of thyroid hormone production by iodine

ENDO

FAMILY HISTORY

First-Degree Relatives' Medical History: The patient's father has hypertension. Her mother has a thyroid problem and is currently on medication. She is unsure what her mother's diagnosis was. She has one younger sister who is healthy without any medical problems.

REVIEW OF SYSTEMS: As indicated by HPI.

PHYSICAL EXAMINATION

Vitals: T 98.6°F P 104 BP 140/84 RR 18 Weight 122 lbs.

HEENT: Mild conjunctival injections, stare and lid lag. No periorbital edema, lagophthalmos, or exophthalmos. Few terminal hairs on chin and cheek.

Neck: Twice normal size thyroid, symmetric, nontender with a soft bruit and palpable thrill. No nodules palpated.

Lungs: Clear to auscultation bilaterally.

Cardiovascular: Tachycardic rate with normal S1, S2, and rhythm. Occasional premature beats. Grade II/VI systolic ejection murmur at left upper sternal border (LUSB). Easily palpable point of maximum impulse (PMI).

Abdomen: Soft and nontender.

Skin: Moist with a fine rash over the abdomen.

Extremities: Positive for tremor. No clubbing of her digits, fingernail changes, or skin changes over the front of her shin.

Neurologic: 3+/4 DTR hyperreflexia throughout. No focal sensory or musculoskeletal deficits.

13

GASTROENTEROLOGY

Gregory R. Owens, MD, and Thomas S. Neuhauser, MD

I. CHIEF COMPLAINT

A. Chief Complaint: Why is patient here and seeking help/advice at this time? Try to use the patient's own words.

B. Identifying Data: Obtain age, sex, medical record number, and race/ethnicity of each patient you evaluate.

II. HISTORY OF PRESENT ILLNESS

A. HPI for Systemic Gastroenterology Complaints, Signs, and Symptoms

1. Swallowing.
   - **a.** Do you have difficulty swallowing with solids, liquids, or both (dysphagia)? Differentiate from globus.
   - **b.** Do you have pain with swallowing (odynophagia)? Association with medications such as nonsteroidal antiinflammatory drugs (NSAIDs), tetracycline, or alendronate?
   - **c.** Do you choke or cough with meals, recurrent aspiration?
   - **d.** Do you have heartburn or substernal chest pain?
   - **e.** Have you had any strictures, prior esophageal dilations, or prior radiation to chest?
2. Stool habits.
   - **a.** Are you experiencing diarrhea or constipation? For how long?
   - **b.** How often do you have bowel movements? Of what volume? What are the characteristics of the stool (color, consistency)?
   - **c.** Is there any blood, mucous, or pus?
   - **d.** Has there been a change in stool caliber? Intermittent or progressive?
   - **e.** Any associated pain, urgency, tenesmus, or sense of incomplete evacuation?
   - **f.** When do you have bowel movements? Timing in relationship to meals?
   - **g.** Do you experience nocturnal awakening related to bowel movements? Incontinence or soiling?
   - **h.** Do you use laxatives, cathartics, or herbals?
   - **i.** Have you had irritable bowel syndrome (IBS) or inflammatory bowel disease (IBD)?
   - **j.** When did you have your last bowel movement?
3. Vomiting.
   - **a.** Are you vomiting? How often? How much? Characteristics?

   b. Is vomiting associated with nausea? Is it spontaneous?
   c. Does it occur before, after, or during meals? Relationship/timing with meals.
   d. Regurgitation or rumination present? Undigested food present?
   e. Do you experience early satiety? Postprandial bloating or distension?
   f. Have you had bulimia or other eating disorder?

4. Gastrointestinal (GI) bleeding: Distinguish from epistaxis, hemoptysis.
   a. Have you had ulcers, esophageal varices/cirrhosis, hemorrhoids, diverticulosis?
   b. Do you use NSAIDs? Antiplatelet medications or "blood thinners"?
   c. Have you had anemia or iron deficiency?
   d. Recent endoscopic or invasive procedures (e.g., colonoscopy with polypectomy)?
   e. Upper GI (defined as proximal to the ligament of Trietz): Hematemesis? Coffee-ground emesis, melena (question regarding use of iron or bismuth-containing products, which can cause dark stool)? Orthostatic symptoms? Prior abdominal aortic aneurysm (AAA) repair?
   f. Lower GI: Hematochezia? Painless or with pain? Blood alone or blood with stool? Blood coating stool or mixed with stool? Blood present at beginning of bowel movement or only at end? Orthostatic symptoms?

5. Abdominal pain.
   a. Where is your pain located (by quadrants)? Upper, lower? Right- or left-sided?
   b. Well or poorly localized? Radiation?
   c. What is the character and intensity of your pain?
   d. Is it related to meals (e.g., during, immediately following, several hours after)?
   e. Any relationship to bowel movements (e.g., during, immediately following, several hours after)?
   f. What makes the pain worse or better (aggravating and alleviating factors)?
   g. What, if any, medications aggravate or alleviate the pain?
   h. Have you had any ulcers, gallstones, pancreatitis, neoplasms, or trauma?
   i. Are there any associated symptoms (e.g., nausea/vomiting, fever/chills, altered bowel habits, jaundice)?

6. Hepatobiliary.
   a. Have you had hepatitis, cirrhosis, blood transfusions (before 1990), jaundice, clay-colored stools, dark urine, pruritis, increased abdominal girth, fever, or chills?

b. Do you have right upper quadrant (RUQ) pain (especially postprandial or after fatty meals), or a history of gallstones?
c. Have you been exposed to any chemicals or toxins? Do you use acetominophen? Have symptoms occurred after an alcohol binge? Do you take estrogen or an oral contraceptive?
d. Have you recently traveled? Have you received vaccinations for hepatitis A or B?
e. Are symptoms associated with use of any prescribed or over the counter (OTC) medications, supplements, or herbs?

7. Pancreatic.
a. Personal or family history of pancreatitis?
b. Postprandial pain, history of gallstones, jaundice, nausea/vomiting?
c. Association with alcohol (ETOH) binge, prior ETOH abuse?
d. Floating/oily stools (i.e., steatorrhea), undigested meat in stools (i.e., azatorrhea), weight loss, history of diabetes mellitus?
e. Association with medications, abdominal trauma, or viral syndrome?
f. History of lipid disorders, parathyroid disease?

B. **Characteristics of GI Symptoms:** For each presenting symptom, obtain additional information by asking the following questions:

1. Area/location involved.
a. Where are your symptoms located? Where do you have pain (radiation or referred pain)?
b. Where are associated symptoms, if present, located?
c. Are the symptoms associated with any physiologic function (e.g., menses, bowel movements, stress, eating)?

2. Chronology.
a. How long have you had the symptoms and how often do you have them? Total duration and frequency of symptoms.
b. Is there a pattern to your symptoms? Are they constant or episodic, regular or sporadic, abrupt or gradual in onset; increasing, decreasing, or static in frequency; waxing or waning in intensity?
c. Do you have the symptoms now (at time of examination)?

3. Quality/character (descriptive terms useful).
a. What type of pain do you have? Sharp, dull, burning, stabbing, tearing, throbbing, squeezing?
b. What is the color of your (symptomatic) blood, urine, stool, or other fluid? Brown, maroon, bright red, black, clay-colored, coffee-grounds, yellow-green (bilious)?
c. What is the consistency of your (symptomatic) stool, blood, urine, or other fluid? Tarry, sticky, hard, watery, soft, formed, soupy, or gelatinous?

4. Quantity/intensity.
   a. Body fluid examples: Quantify with familiar measures (e.g., cupful, 2 teaspoons, 1 tablespoon, one-half liter is more useful than "large amount").
   b. Pain examples: Rate on scale (include when at worst, best, and present).
5. Aggravating factor(s).
   a. Are your symptoms made worse with activity (e.g., when jogging) or while resting?
   b. Do any positions or postures (e.g., supine) aggravate it?
   c. Are visceral functions (e.g., postprandial) aggravating factors?
   d. At what time (e.g., nocturnal) do your symptoms worsen?
   e. What is going on in your life? What psychologic stressors are present (e.g., check for anxiety, depression)?
6. Alleviating factors.
   a. Are your symptoms better with activity or with rest?
   b. Do symptoms improve with any positions or postures (e.g., when upright)?
   c. Visceral functions (e.g., after defecation) alleviate?
   d. Do your symptoms improve at a particular time (e.g., early morning)?

III. PAST MEDICAL AND SURGICAL HISTORY

A. Past Medical History

1. Have you been diagnosed with a chronic medical condition? When did the illness begin? How is the condition now? What responses to interventions did you have? Any complications or sequelae?
2. Were you ever hospitalized? For what reason? When?
3. Have you had any injuries, fractures? Have you been in any accidents? Dates and sequelae?

B. Past Surgical History

1. What, if any, surgical procedures have you had? When?
2. Did you have any operative or postoperative complications (e.g., infection, obstruction, dumping syndrome)?
3. What type of anesthesia was used, if known? Any complications?

C. Emergency and Trauma History

1. Have you ever been treated at an emergency room? What was the cause? When?
2. Injuries/accidents with dates, sequelae (e.g. esophageal or biliary atresia, cystic fibrosis, annular pancreas).

D. Childhood History

1. What childhood illnesses did you have?
2. Did you have any hereditary or congenital disorders (e.g., esophageal or biliary atresia, cystic fibrosis, annular pancreas)?

E. Occupational History

1. What occupations have you had (include military service)? When?
2. Were you ever exposed to hepatotoxins?
   a. Factory work (e.g., exposure to aniline dyes, hydrocarbons, yellow phosphorus, carbon tetrachloride)?
   b. Farm work (e.g., mycotoxins from aprophytic fungi: aflatoxin)?
   c. Mushrooms (e.g. *Amanita phalloides*)?
   d. Thorium thiazide was used until mid-1950s. Although no longer used, it has lifelong liver storage; some patients may still be affected and increases risk of cholangiocarcinoma.
3. Have you worked in the health care field? Exposure to infectious agents such as viral disease (e.g., hepatitis, human immunodeficiency virus [HIV]), bacteria (e.g., campylobacter, shigella, yersinia, cholera, salmonella, tuberculosis), and chemical agents (e.g., formalin, radiation, radioactive agents/reagents).
4. Have you been a day care worker? Exposure to young children and infectious agents?

F. Travel History

1. Where have you traveled? In the United States? In foreign countries? For how long? Were prophylaxes taken?
2. When did the travel occur (some disease processes such as parasites may not be recognized until decades following the trip)?
3. What was your diet while traveling?
   a. Did you drink the local water?
   b. Did any beverages consumed contain ice cubes made with local water?
   c. Did you consume any unwashed fruits or vegetables?
   d. Did you drink untreated water (e.g., from streams or rivers)?

IV. MEDICATIONS, ALLERGIES, AND ADVERSE REACTIONS

A. Medications

1. Are you taking any prescription medications? When did you begin taking them? What is the current dosage and schedule? Some drugs can be hepatoxic: Anabolic steroids, oral contraceptives, tranquilizers/anticonvulsants (phenytoin, valproic acid), diuretics (chlorothiazide), chemotherapeutics (tetracycline, isoniazid, erythromycin, methyldopa), anesthetics (halothane), arsenicals.
2. Are you taking any OTC medications (e.g., vitamins, NSAIDs, laxatives), herbal preparations, or supplements?

B. Allergies to Medications and Side Effects/Adverse Reactions

1. What, if any, allergic or adverse reactions have you had to medications? What treatments did you receive with what response?
2. Consider interactions if patient is taking multiple medications.

V. HEALTH MAINTENANCE

A. Prevention

1. Screening status: Have you had prior colorectal cancer screening? When? Results?
2. Surveillance programs: Surveillance for Barrett's esophagus? Colon dysplasia in IBD? Cancer screening?
3. Treatment programs: In-house program for alcohol dependence versus outpatient program (e.g. Alcoholics Anonymous [AA])?

B. Diet/Nutrition

1. Have you had any unintentional weight gain or loss?
2. Do your symptoms have any relationship to meals? Do they become better or worse with meals?
3. Are your symptoms provoked by specific foods (e.g., fatty, spicy, meats, citrus, dairy products)?
4. What is your usual diet? Having patients keep food journals may be beneficial.
5. Do you consume any unusual items (e.g., hair, clay, ice)?
6. Are you anorexic? Early satiety?
7. When was your last meal?

C. Exercise

1. Have you made any recent changes in your exercise routine?
2. Have you recently started exercising?

D. Sleep Patterns: Have your sleep patterns changed recently?

E. Social Habits

1. Do you use tobacco? What type? How much and for how long (in pack-years: packs per day times number of years).
2. Do you drink alcohol? How much and how often? Have you had any physical or legal problems related to drinking?
3. Do you use any illicit drugs? Which ones? How often? In what form?

VI. FAMILY HISTORY

A. First-Degree Relatives' Medical History

1. Are there any familial syndromes? Polyposis of the gastrointestinal tract may be part of a syndrome (e.g., Gardner's syndrome, hereditary polyposis syndrome) and predispose to adenocarcinoma.
2. Have any family members had cancer? Some cancers run in families (e.g., hereditary nonpolyposis colonic adenocarcinoma).
3. Any metabolic disorders? Hereditary hemochromatosis (iron overload)?

B. Three-Generation Genogram: Gastrointestinal disease processes can be traced back many generations (e.g., polyposis syndromes).

VII. PSYCHOSOCIAL HISTORY

A. Personal and Social History

1. Where were you born (city and country)? What is your race/ethnic background?
2. Are you married? Any children?

3. What level of education have you attained (e.g., years of schooling, college and advanced degrees)?
4. Are you involved in any social groups? What leisure activities (e.g., hobbies, sports) do you pursue? Assess social involvement.
5. Any financial difficulties or stressors? *Helicobacter pylori* is more prevalent in lower socioeconomic levels.

B. **Current Illness Effects on the Patient**
1. Have you missed work because of your condition? How many days?
2. Are you unable to perform desired activities?
3. Do you need to remain close to a restroom?

C. **Interpersonal and Sexual History**
1. Do you engage in anal intercourse?
2. Do you have multiple sexual partners?

D. **Family Support:** Are family members supportive and able to provide assistance?

E. **Occupational Aspects**
1. Are symptoms worse at work? During which specific job activities?
2. Will this illness prevent you from returning to your current job? Consider whether rehabilitation will be required.

VIII. **REVIEW OF SYSTEMS (Tables 13-1 to 13-3)**

Text continued on p. 216.

Table 13-1. GENERAL GASTROINTESTINAL SYMPTOMS BY SYSTEM.

SYSTEM	SYMPTOMS
General	Unintended weight gain or loss, fever/chills/sweats, fatigue
HEENT	Hoarseness, prior head/neck cancers, radiation, dental erosions or caries, globus
Respiratory	Wheezing, chronic cough, recurrent aspiration pneumonia, progressive dyspnea, pulmonary fibrosis
Cardiovascular	Chest pain, heart failure, orthopnea, dyspnea on exertion, palpitations, history of dysrhythmias, paroxysmal atrial fibrillation, venous thromboses, claudication, peripheral vascular disease, pedal edema
Genitourinary (GU)	Frequent urinary tract infections, pneumaturia, dark or golden urine kidney stones, renal failure, polycystic kidney disease, malignancies

Continued

GI

Table 13-1. GENERAL GASTROINTESTINAL SYMPTOMS BY SYSTEM—*cont'd*

System	Symptoms
Obstetrics/ gynecologic	Last menstrual period, pregnancy status, recent, endometriosis, chronic pelvic pain, menorrhagia, uterine, gynecologic malignancies, any radiation treatments
Hematologic	Easy bleeding/bruising, anemia, hereditary blood dyscrasias
Infectious disease/ immunologic	Tuberculosis or exposure, human immunodeficiency virus (HIV), recurrent parasitic infections
Endocrine	Polyuria, polydipsia, polyphagia, history of glucose intolerance, hypoglycemia, fasting diaphoresis/weakness, heat/cold intolerance, thyroid disease, weight gain/loss, hair, thyroid nodules or cancer, increasing ring/hat size, weight gain, coarsening of facial features, history of acromegaly, amenorrhea, impotence, loss of libido, galactorrhea, kidney stones, hypercalcemia, history of parathyroid disease, history of pituitary problems
Neuropsychiatric	Depression/anxiety disorders, psychoses, seizures, Parkinson's, Alzheimer's, other dementias, prior strokes, myasthenia gravis, difficulty concentrating, memory problems, somnolence, paresthesias, numbness/tingling in extremities, ataxia
Dermatologic	Rashes, nonhealing sores, painful nodules, urticaria or hives, cutaneous flushing, history of psoriasis
Musculoskeletal/ rheumatologic	Conditions requiring chronic NSAID use, acetaminophen use, back pain/stiffness, joint pain/swelling, sclerodactyly, Raynaud's, sicca syndrome, premature or severe osteoporosis, history of spine/hip fractures

Table 13-2. NONSPECIFIC SYMPTOMS AND THEIR GASTROENTEROLOGIC DISEASES.

Symptom	Diseases
Arthritis	Ankylosing spondylitis in inflammatory bowel disease (IBD), reactive arthritis associated with infectious colitis, amyloid liver in rheumatoid arthritis
Bruising/bleeding	Coagulopathy caused by chronic liver disease, NSAID use, Henoch-Schönlein purpura, vitamin K malabsorption in steatorrhea
Chest pain	Esophageal or upper abdominal sources may mimic angina but always exclude cardiac etiology
Cough (chronic)	Associated with reflux esophagitis
Cutaneous flushing	Carcinoid
Dark urine	Possible jaundice, acute intermittent porphyria (AIP)
Dental caries	Could indicate severe reflux or bulimia
Depression/anxiety	Increased prevalence in patients presenting with IBS or other functional GI disorders
Dyspnea on exertion	May occur in hereditary hemochromatosis, GI carcinoids, large hepatic hemangiomas, anemia from occult blood loss/iron or B_{12} malabsorption
Hematuria/ pneumaturia	Could indicate enterovesicular fistula caused by diverticulitis, Crohn's disease, colorectal cancer
Hoarseness (chronic)	May indicate chronic reflux or esophageal tumor
Libido loss	Hemochromatosis
Odynophagia	Pill esophagitis, infectious esophagitis (e.g., herpes, candida)
Painful skin lesions	Erythema nodosum or pyoderma gangrenosum with IBD, dermatitis herpetiformis in celiac disease
Paresthesias/ataxia	Consider B_{12} deficiency
Pedal edema	Could be caused by liver disease, GI malignancy with lymphatic obstruction
Psoriasis	Increased liver disease with methotrexate therapy
Psychosis	Wilson's disease, acute porphyria

Continued

GI

Table 13-2. NONSPECIFIC SYMPTOMS AND THEIR GASTROENTEROLOGIC DISEASES—*cont'd*

SYMPTOM	DISEASES
Raynaud's	Scleroderma associated with esophageal dysmotility, chronic intestinal pseudoobstruction, bacterial overgrowth
Recurrent aspiration	Gastroparesis or gastric outlet obstruction, achalasia, tracheoesophageal fistula from tumor
Seizures	Wilson's disease or acute intermittent porphyria (AIP)
Sicca syndrome	Sjögren's associated with primary biliary cirrhosis, pancreatitis
Somnolence	Encephalopathy in cirrhotics
Spine/hip fracture	Cholestatic liver disease (vitamin D malabsorption)
Urticaria/hives	Hepatitis B or C
Weight change (unexpected)	Gain may precipitate reflux, loss may suggest malignancy or malabsorption/ maldigestion

Table 13-3. COMMON GASTROENTEROLOGIC DISEASES AND SYMPTOMS.

DISEASE	SYMPTOMS
Bowel obstruction	Projectile vomiting, colicky abdominal pain, abdominal distension, obstipation
Cholelithiasis/ choledocholithiasis	Episodic noncolicky RUQ pain (postprandial), nausea/vomiting, jaundice
Cirrhosis	Increased abdominal girth, jaundice, difficulty concentrating or somnolence, easy bleeding
Colonic ischemia	Acute-onset crampy abdominal pain followed by passage of blood/clots
Esophagitis	Substernal chest pain, "heartburn," regurgitation, nocturnal wheezing, intermittent dysphagia
Hemochromatosis	Jaundice, RUQ fullness, polyuria/ polydipsia (diabetes), impotence, decreased libido, joint pain/swelling, bronze skin pigmentation, dyspnea, pedal edema

Table 13-3—cont'd

DISEASE	SYMPTOMS
Hepatic encephalopathy	Stage 1: irritability, personality changes, impaired concentration Stage 2: drowsiness, poor memory, behavioral changes Stage 3: somnolence, confusion, amnesia Stage 4: stupor, coma
Hepatocellular carcinoma	New ascites, increased encephalopathy, hypoglycemia, RUQ pain, anorexia
Hepatitis	Nausea and/or vomiting, RUQ pain or fullness, jaundice, "dark" urine, altered taste, fever, malaise
Infectious diarrhea	
Bacterial	Fever/chills, blood/pus in stool, abdominal pain, tenesmus
Viral	Fever/chills, myalgias, nausea/vomiting, watery stool, abdominal cramping
Parasitic	Nausea, bloating, abdominal cramping, watery stool, blood in stool (entamoeba)
Inflammatory bowel disease	Bloody mucoid diarrhea, fecal urgency, tenesmus, fever, fatigue, weight loss, crampy abdominal pain, joint pain, back pain, eye discomfort or blurred vision
Irritable bowel syndrome	Chronic/recurrent LLQ abdominal pain (relieved by defecation), altered stool frequency or consistency (constipation/ diarrhea/both), mucous in stool, bloating
Malignancies of hollow viscous	Weight loss, anorexia, early satiety, progressive dysphagia, colicky abdominal pain, vomiting, hematochezia, melena, change in stool caliber, fatigue (anemia)
Pancreatic adenocarcinoma	Painless jaundice, constant epigastric pain radiating to back, weight loss, anorexia, steatorrhea
Pancreatitis, acute	Acute abdominal pain radiating to back, nausea/vomiting, orthostasis, anorexia, obstipation, abdominal distension
Peptic ulcer disease	Dull epigastric pain/discomfort exacerbated or improved by meals, nausea, hematemesis, melena, fatigue (anemia)

IX. PHYSICAL EXAMINATION

A. Physical Examination by System (Table 13-4)

B. Physical Examination of the Abdomen

1. Inspect for visible peristalsis (e.g., bowel obstruction), obvious masses or abnormal contour (e.g., hernias, tumors, aortic aneurysm, organomegaly), distension (e.g., ascites), abnormal discolorations (e.g., flank ecchymosis in acute pancreatitis with retroperitoneal hemorrhage).
2. Auscultate each quadrant for bowel sounds (presence or absence; rushes, tinkles, gurgles) and bruits; check for succussion splash (if vomiting present).
3. Palpate each quadrant for masses (pulsatile masses need timely evaluation), tenderness (note area of maximal tenderness), splenomegaly, or hepatomegaly (note distance in cm below left or right costal margins, respectively); note presence or absence of Murphy's sign if RUQ is tender; check for presence or absence of peritoneal signs (rebound: pain on palpation worsens when released suddenly, slapping heel or shaking bed elicits tenderness) and guarding.
4. Percuss liver and spleen and note span of dullness in cm for each; assess for flank dullness, fluid wave, shifting dullness (if ascites suspected), and costovertebral angle (CVA) for tenderness.
5. Perform digital rectal examination (DRE): Inspect perianal area, assess sphincter tone, note hemorrhoids if present, palpate for masses, palpate prostate in men for nodules, note presence or absence of stool in rectum, color and consistency of stool, and presence or absence of blood with a hemoccult test.

X. DIFFERENTIAL DIAGNOSIS (Table 13-5)

XI. LABORATORY STUDIES AND DIAGNOSTIC EVALUATIONS

A. Serum Studies

1. Aspartate aminotransferase (AST)/alanine aminotransferase (ALT): Increased with hepatocellular damage.
2. HBsAg, anti-HBs, anti-HBc, anti-HBe, anti-HD, HAV, HCV: Assessment for possible current or past viral hepatitis.
3. Bilirubin (direct and indirect): Increased with hepatic disease, biliary disease, and hemolysis.
4. Vitamins B_{12} and folate: Assess for deficiencies (e.g., malabsorption, diet).
5. Albumin, calcium, cholesterol, magnesium, iron, chloride: Diet, malabsorption, protein-losing enteropathies.
6. Albumin: Liver disease.
7. Ferritin: Assessment for iron deficiency (multiple etiologies, including chronic blood loss or malabsorption).
8. Ammonia, alkaline phosphatase: Increased with liver disease.

Text continued on p. 223.

Table 13-4. FINDINGS OF PHYSICAL EXAMINATION AND POSSIBLE DIAGNOSES.

System	Physical Examination Finding	Diagnoses
General	Note general body habitus and position of comfort	Acute abdomen: supine, still
Vital Signs		
Pulse	Tachycardia	GI bleeding; volume depletion in pancreatitis, vomiting, diarrhea
Blood pressure	Orthostatic vital signs, if necessary Hypotension	GI bleeding; volume depletion in pancreatitis, vomiting, diarrhea
Respiratory rate	Hyperpnea	Liver failure
	Tachypnea	Intraabdominal sepsis, anion-gap metabolic acidosis (perforation, mesenteric ischemia, diarrhea)
Weight	Obesity Cachexia	GERD, nonalcoholic steatohepatitis (NASH) internal malignancy, malabsorption/ maldigestion
HEENT		
Eyes	Kayser-Fleischer rings	Liver disease (Wilson's disease)
	Scleral icterus, conjunctival pallor, uveitis	Liver disease, anemia, inflammatory bowel disease
Nose	Evidence of epistaxis	GI bleeding

Continued

Table 13-4. FINDINGS OF PHYSICAL EXAMINATION AND POSSIBLE DIAGNOSES—*cont'd*

System	Physical Examination Finding	Diagnoses
Mouth	Teeth erosions	Frequent emesis (bulimia, severe reflux)
	Oral lesions	Thrush, aphthous ulcers, macular spots, Peutz-Jegher's, Crohn's, Behcet's
	Cheilitis, glossitis, macroglossia	Vitamin deficiencies, malabsorption
Face	Sebaceous adenoma, keratoacanthoma	Colorectal cancer
Neck		
Thyroid	Goiter	Hyperdefecation (Grave's)
	Nodule	Multiple endocrine neoplasia (MEN-1)
Anterior neck	Adenopathy	Lymphoma, AIDS
Posterior neck	Adenopathy	Mononucleosis, lymphoma
Supra-clavicular	Adenopathy	Lymphoma, metastasis from GI malignancy (Virchow's node)
Lungs	Wheezes	Reflux-related asthma
	Inspiratory crackles	Scleroderma
	R-sided rales, rhonchi	Aspiration
	Percussion dullness	Left pleural effusions in acute pancreatitis
Chest	Gynecomastia	Alcoholic liver disease, spironolactone
Cardiovascular	Rate, rhythm, murmurs, any extra heart sounds, jugulovenous distension (JVD), peripheral pulses, note presence/absence of pedal edema	

Abdomen	Visible peristalsis	Bowel obstruction
	Obvious masses or abnormal contour	Hernias, tumors, abdominal aortic aneurysm (AAA), organomegaly
	Distension	Ascites
	Abnormal discolorations, flank ecchymosis	Acute pancreatitis with retroperitoneal hemorrhage
	Note tenderness (note maximal areas of tenderness), splenomegaly or hepatomegaly (note distance in cm below left or right costal margins, respectively); auscultate each quadrant for bowel sounds (presence or absence, rushes, tinkles, gurgles) and bruits; check for succussion splash (if vomiting present); (if ascites suspected) costovertebral angle (CVA) for tenderness; perform digital rectal examination (DRE: inspect perianal area, assess sphincter tone, note hemorrhoids if present, palpate for masses, palpate prostate in men for nodules, note presence/absence of stool in rectum and color/consistency)	
	Palpate each quadrant for masses. Pulsatile masses need timely evaluation.	Tumor(s) (benign and malignant), aneurysm
	Note presence or absence of Murphy's sign if RUQ is tender, check for presence/absence or peritoneal signs (rebound: pain on palpations worsens when released suddenly; slapping heel or shaking bed elicits tenderness) and guarding	Cholecystitis, peritonitis
	Percuss liver and spleen and note span of dullness in cm for each; assess for flank dullness, fluid wave, shifting dullness	Ascites, hepatomegaly

Continued

Table 13-4. FINDINGS OF PHYSICAL EXAMINATION AND POSSIBLE DIAGNOSES—*cont'd*

System	Physical Examination Finding	Diagnoses
GENITOURINARY		
Male	Testicular atrophy	Hereditary hemochromatosis
Female	Genital ulcers	Behcet's
SKIN	Pallor, jaundice, hyperpigmentation, petechiae, purpura, ecchymoses	Bleeding dyscrasias or use of NSAIDs, Henoch-Schönlein purpura
	Note presence of any rashes (characterize by color/location and distribution/shape/size)	Dermatitis herpetiformis (celiac disease), systemic vasculitis with bleeding or mesenteric ischemia, livedo reticularis with mesenteric ischemia from emboli
	Spider angiomas on chest/abdomen and palmar erythema	Liver disease
	Nevi or irregular moles	GI tract a frequent site for metastatic melanoma
	Telangiectasias	Blue rubber bleb nevus syndrome with GI bleeding, hereditary telangiectasias commonly associated with occult/overt GI bleeding
	Recent development of numerous seborrheic keratoses	Associated with GI malignancy
	Sebaceous adenomas or keratoacanthomas	Associated with colon cancer

Lymphatics	Mass(es) of neck, under arms, in groin	Lymphoma
Extremities and spine	Joint swelling, tenderness, warmth, and erythema	IBD suspected, Reiter's, shigellosis
	Spine for range of motion	Ankylosing spondylitis
	Sacroiliac joint tenderness, nail/fingertip color changes	Raynaud's may indicate scleroderma with accompanying esophageal disorders
	Tender nodules	Rheumatoid arthritis, erythema nodosum in IBD
Neurologic	General level of consciousness and orientation	Liver disease or dementia syndromes-hepatic encephalopathy
	Cranial nerve examination	Dysphagia/swallowing complaints
	Focal or generalized muscle weakness	Stroke, muscular dystrophies, myasthenia gravis, in patients younger than 40 years; assess for focal deficits that might suggest Wilson's disease
	Vibratory and position sense	Vitamin B_{12} deficiency
	Asterixis	Liver disease
	Romberg's test	B_{12} deficiency (e.g., pernicious anemia, Crohn's disease)
	Peripheral neuropathy with pinprick, touch sensation	Diabetics, if present, GI complications such as gastroparesis, intestinal, and colonic dysmotility, are more likely

Table 13-5. DIFFERENTIAL DIAGNOSES OF GASTROENTEROLOGIC CONDITIONS AND SYMPTOMS.

CONDITION/ SYMPTOM	DIAGNOSES
Abdominal pain, upper	Cholelithiasis/choledocholithiasis/cholecystitis, PUD, NUD, mesenteric ischemia, pancreatitis, MI, pneumonia, AAA, splenic infarct, acute intermittent porphyria (AIP), malignancy (distal esophagus, gastric, pancreatic), bowel obstruction
Abdominal pain, lower	Diverticulitis, appendicitis, mesenteric ischemia, ureterolithiasis, IBS, Crohn's disease, colon cancer, AIP, bowel obstruction, ovarian cyst, PID, ectopic pregnancy, GU malignancy, ischemic colitis
Dysphagia	Bulbar neuropathies, Parkinson's, myasthenia gravis, goiter, thyroglossal cyst, esophageal neoplasms, GERD, peptic stricture, Schiatzki's ring, esophageal web, esophageal achalasia, Chaga's disease
Vomiting	Achalasia, bulimia, pyloric stenosis (acquired versus congenital), gastroparesis, gastric outlet obstruction (PUD versus malignant obstruction), bowel obstruction, pancreatitis, infectious gastroenteritis, gastric bezoar, functional vomiting, cyclic vomiting syndrome, intestinal migraine, intracerebral hemorrhage, intracranial neoplasm
Hematemesis	Variceal hemorrhage, Mallory-Weiss tear, PUD, epistaxis, esophageal malignancy, portal gastropathy, Dieulafoy's lesion, aorto-esophageal fistula
Melena	Variceal hemorrhage, PUD, Mallory-Weiss tear, Dieulafoy's lesion, portal gastropathy, NSAID enteropathy/colopathy, small bowel leiomyoma, Meckel's diverticulum, aortoenteric fistula, hemosuccus pancreaticus, hemobilia
Hematochezia	Massive UGI Bleeding, hemorrhoids, rectal varices, anal fissure, diverticulosis, colon polyp, angiodysplasia/arteriovenous malformations, colon cancer, solitary rectal ulcer syndrome, ulcerative colitis, ischemic colitis, colonic leiomyoma

9. Glucose: Most notably increased with diabetes mellitus (pancreatic disease, insulin resistance). May be low with hepatic failure and hepatocellular carcinoma.
10. Coagulation factors, prothrombin time (PT), partial thromboplastin time (PTT): May be affected by liver disease.
11. Glutamyl transpeptidase (GGT): Increased with liver disease.
12. 5′-Nucleotidase: Associated with obstructive liver (biliary) disease.
13. Certain drug levels (e.g., FK503 and cyclosporine in transplant patients).
14. Amylase/lipase: Assessment for pancreatic disease.
15. Hormone levels (gastrin, insulin, glucagon, vasoactive intestinal peptide (VIP), somatostatin): Pancreatic disease and tumors.

B. **Culture:** Assessment for infectious disease processes.

C. **Stool**
1. Assess for inflammatory cells: Infection, enterocolitis.
2. Fat content: Assess for steatorrhea such as in pancreatic disease, malabsorption/maldigestion.
3. Assess for undigested meat fibers: Pancreatic disease.

D. **Liver Biopsy:** Assists in differential diagnosis and prognosis of liver disease; assesses liver damage (necrosis, fibrosis), stage fibrosis, and grade inflammatory component.

E. **Tumor Markers** (carcinoembryonic antigen [CEA], alpha fetoprotein [AFP], carbohydrate antigen [CA 19-9]): Assessment for some malignancies and recurrence.

F. **Endoscopy (Flexible Sigmoidoscopy, Colonoscopy, Esophagostomy):** Used for screening; assess etiology of bleeding; biopsy and confirm diagnosis; assist in treatment (control bleeding, dilate stricture in esophagus); screen for premalignancy (Barrett's esophagus); remove foreign bodies.

G. **Radiologic Studies**
1. Ultrasound: Assessment of gallbladder for stones, volume, contractility; assess liver for texture, lesions, ductal dilation, and portal/hepatic flows.
2. Radioisotope scans (HIDA): Identification of cystic duct obstruction, assessment of bile ducts.
3. Esophageal motility studies: Aid in assessment for achalasia, esophageal spasm, scleroderma, other motor disorders, preoperative before fundoplication.
4. Barium studies: Assessment of luminal GI tract for lesions, ulcers, deformities, or thickening.
5. Computed tomography (CT), magnetic resonance imaging (MRI): Assessment for intraabdominal lesions, deformities.
6. Angiography: Assessment of ischemia, hemorrhage, and vascular abnormalities.
7. Endoscopic retrograde cholangiopancreatography (ERCP): Visualization of pancreaticobiliary tract; allow for biopsy and cytology studies, stone removal, stenting strictures.

XII. EPONYMS, ACRONYMS, AND ABBREVIATIONS (Tables 13-6 and 13-7)

Table 13-6. SELECTED GASTROENTEROLOGY EPONYMS.

Eponym	Description
Aaron's sign	A sensation of pain in the epigastric or precordial area on pressure over McBurney's point in appendicitis
Auenbruger's sign	Bulging in epigastric area caused by extensive pericardial effusion
Chauffard's point	Point of tenderness situated under the right clavicle in gallbladder disease
Cole's sign	Deformation of the duodenal contour as seen in the x-ray, associated with duodenal ulcer
Duchene's sign	Sinking in of the epigastrium on inspiration in paralysis of the diaphragm or in certain cases of hydropericardium
Federici's sign	Cardiac sounds can be heard during auscultation of the abdomen in cases of intestinal perforation and with presence of gas in the peritoneum
Henning's sign	Angular deformity of the angulus of the stomach in which it forms a Gothic arch shape, a sign of gastric ulceration
Lennhoff's sign	Furrow appearing on deep inspiration below lowest rib and above echinococcal cyst in liver
McBurney's point	Situated about one third the distance between the anterior superior iliac spine and the umbilicus, corresponding to the normal position of the base of the appendix. Tender in appendicitis
Mackenzie's point	Tenderness in gallbladder disease in the upper segment of the rectus muscle
Munro's point	Midway between the umbilicus and the left anterior iliac spine; used for performing abdominal puncture
Murphy's sign	Sign of gallbladder disease consisting of interruption of deep inspiration when the examiners' fingers are pressed deeply beneath the right costal arch, below the hepatic margin

Table 13-6—cont'd

EPONYM	DESCRIPTION
Psoas sign	Flexion of or pain on hyperextension of the hip caused by contact between an inflammatory process and the psoas muscle; a sign often seen in appendicitis
Robson's point	Point of greatest tenderness in gallbladder inflammation, situated opposite the junction of the middle and lower third of a line drawn from the right nipple to the umbilicus
Rosenbach's sign	Absence of the abdominal skin reflex in inflammatory disease of the intestines

XIII. DEFINITIONS (Table 13-8)

XIV. SAMPLE H&P WRITE-UP

CC: "My belly is swollen."

HPI: M.D. is a single, 58-year-old African-American male with a long history of alcohol abuse and a history of hepatitis C. He initially was referred to the gastroenterology clinic 1 year ago with complaints of bright red blood per rectum and "a severe hemorrhoid problem." Work-up at that time showed elevated liver function tests with AST and ALT as high as 300 and 350, respectively, as well as positive titers for hepatitis C antibody. Liver biopsy at that time was significant for stage 3/4 fibrosis. although he enrolled in a voluntary in-house alcohol treatment program, he left after 1 week for job-related problems. Since then he admits to multiple attempts to cut back, and achieved sobriety for up to only 1 week. Over the last 4 months, he has admitted to a gradual increase in his abdominal girth, accompanied by a vague, diffuse, dull abdominal pain as well as overall fatigue. He continues to experience occasional bleeding per rectum that "turns the water in the toilet bright red," and admits to several days of "black, tarry, smelly" stools. This is different from his usual bowel movements of 1 to 2 movements per day. He also relates difficulty concentrating in last several months. He denies problems with swallowing, nocturnal awakening, incontinence, nausea/vomiting/hematemesis, early satiety, nose bleeds, fever/chills, history of ulcers, drug use, history of gallstones, floating/oily stools, weight loss, abdominal trauma. He does admit to daily aspirin as needed for abdominal pain and headache, and noticing "funny-colored eyes" when he looked in the mirror.

PMHx: Diagnosis of hepatitis C and alcohol dependence made approximately 1 year before this visit. He has no history of delirium

Table 13-7. GASTROENTEROLOGY ACRONYMS AND ABBREVIATIONS.

Acronym or Abbreviation	Term	Acronym or Abbreviation	Term
AAS	Acute abdominal series	**IEM**	Ineffective esophageal motility
AFP	Alpha fetoprotein	**LDH**	Lactate dehydrogenase
AIP	Acute intermittent porphyria	**LFTs**	Liver function tests
ALT	Alanine aminotranferase	**LGIB**	Lower gastrointestinal bleeding
AST	Aspartate aminotransferase	**NAFLD**	Nonalcoholic fatty liver disease
BE	Barium enema	**NASH**	Nonalcoholic steatohepatitis
CD	Crohn's disease	**NSAID**	Nonsteroidal antiinflammatory drug
DRE	Digital rectal examination	**NUD**	Nonulcer dyspepsia
GGT	Glutamyl transpeptidase	**PBC**	Primary biliary cirrhosis
GERD	Gastroesophageal reflux disease	**PPI**	Proton pump inhibitor
H_2RA	H_2 receptor antagonist	**PSC**	Primary sclerosing cholangitis
HBV	Hepatitis B virus	**PSE**	Portosystemic encephalopathy
HCV	Hepatitis C virus	**PUD**	Peptic ulcer disease
HH	Hiatal hernia	**SBP**	Spontaneous bacterial peritonitis
HP	Helicobacter pylori	**SBFT**	Small bowel follow-through
IBS	Irritable bowel syndrome	**UC**	Ulcerative colitis
IBD	Inflammatory bowel disease	**UGIB**	Upper gastrointestinal bleeding

Table 13-8. GASTROENTEROLOGY TERMS.

Term	Definition
Asterixis	Periodic dropping of hands when wrists dorsiflexed and arms fully extended in the "stop traffic" posture with prompt recovery of position; may be seen in hepatic encephalopathy
Azatorrhea	Loss of protein in stool (protein-losing enteropathies)
Dysphagia	Difficulty swallowing
Globus	Foreign-body sensation in throat noted on swallowing ("lump in throat")
Henoch-Schönlein purpura	Pediatric vasculitis that may cause abdominal pain as well as GI perforation, bleeding, or obstruction
Kayser-Fleischer rings	Copper deposits within Descemet's membrane of the eyes that may be found in Wilson's disease
Korsakoff's syndrome	Anterograde and retrograde amnesia with confabulation; associated with alcoholic and nonalcoholic polyneuritis
Ligament of Trietz	Approximate anatomic location of transition from duodenum to jejunum
Moulage sign	A waxy cast appearance of bowel segments, a radiographic (x-ray) sign of celiac disease
Murphy's sign	Sudden cessation of inspiration during palpation of the RUQ; shown to be highly specific for acute cholecystitis
Odynophagia	Pain on swallowing
Raynaud's phenomena	Reversible ischemia of the digits; may be part of CREST syndrome or scleroderma associated with esophageal disorders
Romberg's test	Assessment of ability of patient to maintain balance with feet together and eyes closed (may be positive in B_{12} deficiency)
Sclerodactyly	Long, thin digits; may be part of CREST syndrome or scleroderma associated with esophageal disorders
Serum-ascites Albumin gradient (SAAG)	Difference between the serum albumin and the ascitic albumin as measured on paracentesis; useful in determining the etiology of ascites

Continued

Table 13-8. GASTROENTEROLOGY TERMS—*cont'd*

TERM	DEFINITION
Steatorrhea	Excessive fat in stool; may be qualitative (>100 fat droplets/HPF on Sudan stain) or quantitative (72-hr stool collection with >7 grams fat/day)
Trousseau's syndrome	Paraneoplastic syndrome manifested by systemic hypercoagulability associated with internal malignancies, particularly gastric and pancreatic adenocarcinomas
Wernicke's syndrome	Characterized by confusion, apathy, drowsiness, ataxia or gait, nystagmus, most commonly resulting from alcohol abuse, and frequently associated with Korsakoff's syndrome
Zollinger-Ellison syndrome	Clinical triad of gastric acid hypersecretion, recurrent peptic ulcers, and non-beta islet cell tumors (gastrinomas)

tremens or withdrawal seizures. Otherwise, no medical problems the patient can recall.

PSHX: No prior surgeries, with the exception of the liver biopsy performed 1 year ago and an appendectomy as a child.

Emergency and Trauma History: The patient was seen in the Emergency Department approximately two years ago for a one-vehicle accident (car versus tree). He was released to the police after 24 hours of observation for driving under the influence (DUI). This culminated in suspension of his driver's license for 1 year.

Childhood History: Chicken pox at age 4. He denies any other childhood illnesses.

MEDICATIONS: Aspirin for the past 2 days for mild headaches and abdominal discomfort. He denies use of herbal supplements/vitamins and any allergies/adverse reactions to medications.

HEALTH MAINTENANCE

Prevention: The patient has never had a colonoscopy or any type of cancer screening. He failed to keep his scheduled appointment with a psychiatrist following discharge from the alcohol rehabilitation facility.

Diet: Patient admits to an irregular diet, comprised primarily of fast food and canned goods. He admits to a weight gain of up to 15 pounds over last 3 months. His last meal was approximately 3 hours before this interview.

Exercise: The patient does not exercise.

Sleep Patterns: The patient wakes up multiple times to void, especially after an evening of particularly heavy drinking. Sometimes he "cannot make it in time." He recently woke up early in morning because of an immediate urge to defecate, productive of a dark, tarry stool.

Social Habits: The patient denies smoking or tobacco use. He admits to drinking up to a 12-pack per night. He initially started drinking heavily in college. He did not drink at all a few years after graduating, but started drinking regularly sometime in his early 20s.

FAMILY HISTORY

First-Segree Relatives' Medical History: The patient's father was reported to be healthy "until he died of old age." The patient's mother is alive with adult-onset diabetes. He has no siblings.

PSYCHOSOCIAL HISTORY

Personal and Social History: The patient is African-American. He is single and lives in an apartment. He was divorced in his early 30s due to "irreconcilable differences" and admits it may be in part because of his heavy drinking. He has one son who is estranged. The patient admits to recently receiving reprimands from his boss for being late to work or failing to show up. He is not currently living with anybody and has had multiple sexual partners over the last few years.

REVIEW OF SYSTEMS

General: 15-pound weight gain in last 3 months and positive for fatigue. No fever, chills, or sweats.

HEENT/Neck: No hoarseness, history of radiation, cancers, or epistaxis. Positive for dental caries and scleral icterus.

Respiratory: No cough, dyspnea, shortness of breath, or wheezing.

Cardiovascular: No tachycardia, palpitations, orthopnea, paroxysmal nocturnal dyspnea, chest pain, claudication, pedal edema.

Gastrointestinal: As above.

Genitourinary: No dysuria, urinary urgency, urinary tract infections, or malignancies. Positive for occasional dark urine.

Hematologic/Lymphatic: No easy bruising or bleeding tendencies or anemia.

Endocrine: No polyuria, polydipsia, polyphagia, thyroid disease, or hair loss. Positive for recent problems with impotence.

Skin: No rash or pigmentary changes. Positive for intermittent diffuse itching.

Neuropsychiatric: Intermittent headaches and occasional bouts of depression. Also admits to forgetfulness, difficulty concentrating, and occasional blackouts. No history of seizures, somnolence, paresthesias, numbness/tingling in extremities, or ataxia.

Musculoskeletal: Occasional back discomfort. No weakness.

Extremities: Mild foot edema over the past week.

PHYSICAL EXAMINATION

Vitals: T 99.0°F P 92 BP 138/90 RR 18 Weight 179 lbs.

General: Slightly anxious black male with protuberant abdomen.

HEENT: Obvious scleral icterus and slightly injected conjunctivae. No nystagmus. Pupils equal and reactive to light. Teeth with multiple apparent erosions. No oral lesions, cheilitis, or glossitis.

Neck: No thyroid enlargement.

Lungs: Clear to auscultation bilaterally.

Chest: Apparent mild hypertrophy of bilateral breasts, otherwise unremarkable.

Cardiovascular: Normal S1 and S2. Regular rate and rhythm. No murmur, JVD. Positive 1+ bilateral pedal edema.

Abdomen: Marked abdominal distention with protruding umbilicus. No abnormal discolorations or palpable masses. Spleen and liver not palpable. No Murphy's sign/rebound. No bruits. Fluid wave and dullness to percussion bilateral flanks. No CVAT. DRE positive for marked hemorrhoids and obvious dry blood. No masses. Sphincter tone normal.

Skin: Mild jaundice noted of palms and soles. No petechiae, rashes, or telangiectasias. Spider angiomas noted of the face.

Extremities: 1+ pitting edema.

Neurologic: Oriented to person, place, and time. Cranial nerve examination normal to direct confrontation. No focal sensory deficits noted. Mild asterixis demonstrated.

14

GYNECOLOGY

Jamal Mourad, DO, Michael R. Foley, MD, and Ingrid Skop, MD

I. CHIEF COMPLAINT

A. **Chief Complaint:** Use the patient's own words for the major complaint or reason for admission, duration, and other relevant signs and symptoms.

B. **Identifying Data:** Name, age, race/ethnicity background, and gravity/parity/abortions (G/P/A).

II. HISTORY OF PRESENT ILLNESS

A. **Pain Description:** Obtain a detailed description of patient's complaint with special attention to chronology. For example, if the patient is complaining of pain, use questions referring to palliation, quality, radiation, severity, and timing (PQRST).

1. Palliation (P): What makes it better? What makes it worse? What were you doing when it happened?
2. Quality (Q): Does it feel like pressure? Is it sharp?
3. Radiation (R): Does it radiate anywhere? Is it localized or generalized?
4. Severity (S): On a scale of 1 to 10 (1 being mild and 10 being severe), how bad is it now?
5. Timing (T): How long have you had the pain? When did it start? How long does it last? Has it improved or worsened since the onset?

B. **Gynecologic History**

1. How old were you when you first had your period (menarche)?
2. How old were you when you first noticed breast development (thelarche)?
3. How old were you when you first noticed pubic hair growth (adrenarche)?
4. When was your last Papanicolaou (Pap) smear? What was the result?
5. Have you ever had an abnormal Pap smear? Did it require any treatment? If so, what type of treatment?
6. Did your mother take any medications (e.g., diethylstilbestrol [DES]) when she was pregnant with you?
7. Have you ever had or been exposed to any sexually transmitted diseases (STDs)? If so, what type of infection? Were you and/or your partner treated?
8. Have you had any gynecologic diagnostic procedures such as vulvar, vaginal, cervical, or endometrial biopsies; dilation and curettage; laparoscopy; or hysteroscopy?

C. **Menstrual History**

1. At what age did you start menstruating (menarche)?
2. When was the first day of your last menstrual period (LMP)?
3. When was the first day of your last normal menstrual period (LNMP)?
4. Are your menstrual periods regular?
5. How frequent are your menstrual periods?
6. How long do your periods last; does the flow quantity or quality change during your period? Do you have excessive clotting (i.e., use more than 8 pads or tampons in a 24-hour period)?
7. Do you have associated pelvic pain, breast tenderness, mood alterations, bloating, or other symptoms before or during your menstrual period?

D. **Sexual History**

1. Do you have any discomfort with intercourse? If so, describe.
2. Do you use any kind of lubrication during intercourse?
3. How many times per month do you have intercourse?
4. Have you noticed a change in your sexual drive?
5. Are you in a monogamous relationship?
6. Do you have sex with men, women, or both?
7. What method of contraception do you currently use? What have you used in the past?
8. At what age did you become sexually active?
9. How many sexual partners have you had?
10. Have you ever been sexually abused?
11. Have you experienced any sexual dysfunction or difficulty with orgasms?

E. **Obstetric History**

1. How many times have you been pregnant?
2. Have you had any spontaneous or elective abortions (<20 weeks' gestation)? At how many weeks' gestation did these occur? Did you have any complications or require surgical intervention (e.g., dilation and curettage [D&C]) with these abortions? If more than two miscarriages, have you had any evaluation for the cause? If elective abortions, how were these performed?
3. Have you had any ectopic (tubal) pregnancies? If so, how were you treated?
4. How many deliveries (>20 weeks' gestation) have you had? At how many weeks gestation did you deliver? How much did each infant weigh at delivery? What gender was each infant? What type of delivery did you have with each pregnancy? Were there any maternal or neonatal complications with each delivery?
5. How many living children do you currently have?

III. **PAST MEDICAL AND SURGICAL HISTORY**

A. **Past Medical History**

1. Have you received regular medical care and preventive screenings (e.g., Pap smears)?

2. What is the patient's past medical history (e.g., diagnoses, date of onset, progression, responses to interventions, complications or sequelae)?
3. Are any advanced and untreated diseases present (typically infectious disease, such as tuberculosis or hepatitis, or other chronic conditions like diabetes, asthma, hypertension or cardiac disease)?
4. Any hospitalizations for medical conditions?

B. Past Surgical History

1. Have you had any previous operations (diagnoses, procedures, responses to interventions)? Where (e.g., hospital or outpatient)? When (date of procedure[s])?
2. Any operative or postoperative complications?
3. Type of anesthesia and any complications or adverse effects with use? Is there a history of prolonged anesthesia?

C. Emergency and Trauma History

1. Have you ever had a blood transfusion? If yes, for what reason and how many units did you receive (if known)? Complications? What was done?
2. Have you been tested for HIV if the transfusion occurred between 1977 and 1991?

D. Childhood History

1. Have you had any childhood illnesses? If so, what were they?
2. Any childhood developmental abnormalities (e.g., testicular feminization syndrome, clitoromegaly, ambiguous genitalia)?

E. Occupational History

1. What is your occupation?
2. Are you exposed to any chemicals, radiation, or other toxins at your workplace?

F. Travel History

1. Have you traveled recently? If so, where have you traveled?
2. Have you been exposed to any individuals who may have been infected with a disease endemic to a particular area (e.g., tuberculosis)?

G. Animals and Insects Exposure History

1. Do you have any pets?
2. Have you had reactions in the past to bites or stings?

IV. MEDICATIONS, ALLERGIES, AND ADVERSE REACTIONS

A. Medications

1. Do you currently take any prescribed or over-the-counter (OTC) medications? If so, what are they?
2. What, if any, vitamins or supplements do you take?
3. Have you taken any medications since your last menstrual period?

B. Allergies and Adverse Reactions: Have you ever had an allergic or adverse reaction to a medication? If so, what type of reaction did you have?

V. HEALTH MAINTENANCE

A. Prevention

1. Did you receive immunizations during your childhood and adolescence? If so, for what types of diseases did you receive immunizations? Hepatitis B series is particularly important if has high-risk sexual partners or history of intravenous (IV) drug use. Measles/mumps/rubella (MMR) and documentation of rubella immunity are important if considering pregnancy.
2. Have you had yearly Pap smears since the age of 18 (or at the onset of sexual activity)?
3. Do you examine your breasts regularly/monthly?
4. Do you receive regular clinical breast examinations by a health care provider? All women older than 40 years should receive an annual clinical breast examination.
5. Mammograms? Women older than 40 years should have mammograms every 1 to 2 years.
6. If patient is 50 years or older, ask whether she has had a colonoscopy. A screening colonoscopy should occur every 5 years starting at the age of 50.
7. Have you had a bone-density testing? Women at increased risk for osteoporosis (i.e., family history, postmenopausal) or women at or approaching menopause should be clinically evaluated for bone densiometry testing.
8. Do you perform Kegel exercises? These exercises involve alternating contraction and relaxation of perineal muscles for prevention of urinary stress incontinence.

B. Diet: What is your regular diet (including caloric intake, fiber intake, hydration, use of multivitamins and calcium supplements)? Caffeine may worsen breast tenderness, Vitamin E and B supplementation may help. A diet high in soy phytoestrogens may improve estrogen deficiency symptoms after menopause.

C. Exercise: Do you exercise? If so, what type and how often? How long do you exercise and at what intensity? Recommend at least 20 minutes at 80% of maximum of heart rate 3 to 4 times per week. Exercise can improve premenstrual symptoms and dysmenorrhea.

D. Sleep Patterns

1. Do you have any difficulties falling asleep? Staying asleep?
2. Have you experienced any changes in your sleep pattern?
3. Do you think your sleep pattern abnormality is related to your occupation, stress, or medications?
4. Have you had chills or felt flushed? Insomnia is common in menopausal women experiencing estrogen deficiency symptoms.

E. Social Habits

1. Do you use tobacco products? If so, what type, how much, and for how long? Tobacco may worsen dysmenorrhea.

2. Do you use alcohol? If yes, how often and how much?
3. Do you use illicit drugs? If yes, what drugs, how much, and how often?

VI. FAMILY HISTORY

A. **First-Degree Relatives' Medical History**
1. Is there a history of breast, ovarian, colon, or endometrial cancer in any first-degree relatives?
2. Do any of your relatives have bleeding disorders (especially important for patients who have had menorrhagia since menarche)? Hypercoagulability?
3. Is there a family history of fibroids, endometriosis, osteoporosis, or premature menopause?

B. **Three-Generation Genogram:** Are there any inherited illnesses, recurrent miscarriages, adverse pregnancy outcomes, mental retardation, or congenital malformations in family members?

VII. PSYCHOSOCIAL HISTORY

A. **Personal and Social History**
1. What is your place of birth (country and city)? Religious and race/ethnicity background?
2. Are you married? Any children?
3. What level of education have you attained (e.g., years of schooling, college and advanced degrees)?
4. Where do you currently live?
   a. With whom do you live?
   b. What is the physical layout of your home and living conditions (e.g., 3 bedrooms, 1 bath, 8 occupants)?
5. Do you have any financial difficulties or stressors?

B. **Current Illness Effects on the Patient**
1. How is this problem affecting your daily activities?
2. Does it interfere with work?
3. Does it prevent you from interacting socially?
4. Is your illness affecting your relationships with family and friends?

C. **Interpersonal and Sexual History**
1. Are you now, or have you ever been, in a relationship that involves domestic violence?
2. Are you sexually active? If so, how many partners do you have? Of what gender?
3. Do you use any contraception? If so, what type and how often?
4. Do you practice safe sex?
5. Have you ever had, or been exposed to, an STD? If so, what type, when, and what treatment have you received?

D. **Family and Friends Support**
1. Do you have relatives or friends in town?
2. Are family members available to assist you, if necessary?

E. **Occupational Aspects of Current Illness**
1. Has your pain prevented you from performing your duties at work or school?

2. Have you had to miss work or school because of your pain? How often?

VIII. REVIEW OF SYSTEMS (Tables 14-1 to 14-3)

Table 14-1. GENERAL GYNECOLOGIC SYMPTOMS BY SYSTEM.

SYSTEM	SYMPTOMS
General and systemic	Fatigue, weight changes, hypertension, diabetes mellitus, collagen vascular disease (systemic lupus erythematosus [SLE])
HEENT/neck	Visual changes, epistaxis, teeth hygiene, neck swelling (thyroid), sore throat (gonococcal pharyngitis)
Respiratory	Cough, dyspnea, asthma
Cardiovascular	Palpitations, tachycardia, irregular rhythms, mitral valve prolapse (MVP), congenital heart disease with/without repair, Marfan's syndrome, rheumatic heart disease
Chest/Breasts	Tenderness, masses (mobile or fixed), retractions, nipple discharge (white, milky or clear vs. bloody, black, green or purulent, bilateral vs. unilateral), asymmetry, supernumerary nipples or accessory breast tissue, inverted nipples
Gastrointestinal	Nausea, vomiting, hyperemesis gravidarum, gastroesophageal reflux disease (GERD), peptic ulcer disease (PUD), cholelithiasis, constipation, appetite changes, bowel disease, hepatitis
Genitourinary	Dysuria, urinary frequency, urinary urgency, urine loss (accompanied by stress, a sense of urgency, or both), nocturia, retention, hematuria, history of urinary tract infections (UTIs), vaginal discharge, vaginal bleeding or spotting, vaginal or vulvar discoloration and/or itching, dyspareunia, pelvic cramping or pain. Also, see history section for obstetric/gynecologic review
Hematologic	Easy bruising/bleeding tendencies, tendency to form blood clots, thrombophlebitis, deep venous thrombosis (DVT), varicosities, sickle cell disease/trait, thalassemia
Lymphatic	Lymphadenopathy
Neurologic	Seizure disorder, migraines/headaches worsening with menses

Table 14-1—cont'd

System	Symptoms
Musculoskeletal and extremities	Arthritis, muscle weakness, back pain, peripheral edema, tremor, paresthesias, numbness
Skin	Rash, pigmentary changes, striae, spider angiomata, hirsutism, acne, jaundice
Psychiatric	Mood disorders, substance abuse, depression, anxiety, emotional lability (especially premenstrual and around menopause)

Table 14-2. NONSPECIFIC SYMPTOMS AND GYNECOLOGIC DISEASES.

Symptom	Diseases
Abdominal or pelvic pain	Physiologic dysmenorrhea, endometriosis, fibroids, ovarian cysts (rupture or torsion), ovarian torsion, uterine fibroids, adenomyosis, adhesive disease, infections (e.g., pelvic inflammatory disease [PID]), salpingitis, tuboovarian abscesses [TOAs], ectopic pregnancy or threatened abortion, pelvic congestion, ovarian hyperstimulation after fertility medications, and postoperative adhesions). Nongynecologic causes to consider are appendicitis, mesenteric adenitis, diverticulitis, irritable bowel syndrome (IBS), fibromyalgia, adhesive disease, appendicitis, cholelithiasis
Amenorrhea	Pregnancy, hypogonadotropic hypogonadism, exercise induced, ovarian failure, menopause, Asherman's syndrome (synechiae within the endometrial cavity, often causing amenorrhea and infertility), Sheehan's syndrome (postpartum pituitary necrosis syndrome)
Ascites	Ovarian cancer
Back pain	Referred from pelvic processes, hydronephrosis from ureteral obstruction secondary to large fibroids or invasion from malignancy or endometriosis, pyelonephritis, nephrolithiasis

Continued

Table 14-2. NONSPECIFIC SYMPTOMS AND GYNECOLOGIC DISEASES—*cont'd*	
SYMPTOM	DISEASES
Dyspareunia	Endometriosis, vaginismus, vaginal atrophy, vestibulitis, uterine fibroids
Dyspnea	Pulmonary embolus, compression from large abdominal tumor, metastases from gynecologic malignancies
Fever	Pelvic inflammatory disease (PID), tumor necrosis (fibroid or malignancy), tuboovarian abscess, endometritis, septic abortion, toxic shock syndrome, septic pelvic thrombophlebitis
Hirsutism	Polycystic ovarian syndrome, hyperandrogenism, congenital adrenal hyperplasia
Musculoskeletal	Joint pain may be secondary to gonorrhea
Nipple discharge	Galactorrhea, physiologic discharge, breast cancer
Pelvic pressure	Pelvic floor prolapse, rectocele, cystocele, uterine prolapse
Skin changes	Hyperpigmentation, melasma, spider angiomata, and varicosities may be secondary to hormones. Ulcers may be secondary to herpes, lymphogranuloma venereum, chancroid, chancre, granuloma inguinale, or syphilis. Rash may be candidiasis or syphilis. Raised lesions may be condylomas or molluscum contagiosum. Lymphedema may be caused by pelvic tumor, particularly gynecologic malignancies
Urinary leakage	Stress urinary incontinence, detrusor instability, neurogenic bladder
Vaginal bleeding	Menses, atypical menses, threatened abortion or ectopic pregnancy, uterine fibroids, endometritis, endometrial hyperplasias, uterine or other gynecologic malignancies, polyps (uterine or cervical), anovulation, lower genital tract lesion or laceration, foreign body, or oral contraceptive pills or hormone replacement therapy taken incorrectly
Vaginal discharge	PID, gonorrhea, chlamydia, herpes, bacterial vaginosis, candidiasis, trichomonas, atrophic vaginitis, contact or irritant dermatitis, fallopian tube malignancy, or physiologic discharge
Vaginal lesions	Herpes, syphilis, molluscum contagiosum, condyloma, Bartholin's gland cyst

Table 14-3. COMMON GYNECOLOGIC DISEASES AND SYMPTOMS.

DISEASE	SYMPTOMS
Anovulation	Rare or irregular menses, sometimes associated with hirsutism, obesity, and glucose intolerance (polycystic ovarian syndrome [PCOS])
Bacterial vaginosis	Vaginal discharge, odor after intercourse
Cervical cancer	Vaginal bleeding, pelvic pain, back pain
Cervical dysplasia	Irregular or postcoital bleeding, often asymptomatic
Cystocele	Vaginal pressure, urinary incontinence
Detrusor instability	Frequency, urgency and urge incontinence
Ectopic pregnancy	Pelvic/abdominal pain, vaginal bleeding
Endometrial cancer	Vaginal bleeding
Endometriosis	Cyclical pelvic pain, infertility, dyspareunia, dysmenorrhea, pelvic masses, low sacral backache, patients with urinary or gastrointestinal involvement may present with hematuria and hematochezia
Ovarian torsion	Severe intermittent pelvic pain
Pelvic inflammatory disease (PID)	Pelvic pain, vaginal discharge, irregular bleeding, odor, burning sensation, dyspareunia, sometimes fever and systemic symptoms
Pelvic prolapse	Types: Cystocele, rectocele, uterine prolapse, vaginal vault prolapse, enterocele. Pressure, pain, sensation of tissue protruding from the vagina, urinary retention or incontinence, constipation, splinting to achieve defecation
Polycystic ovarian syndrome (PCOS)	Weight gain, hirsutism, amenorrhea, and infertility
Rectocele	Vaginal pressure, rectal fullness, incomplete evacuation
Stress urinary incontinence	Urinary leakage on sneezing, laughing, or coughing. Frequency, urgency, urge incontinence, and a postvoid sensation of fullness are common
Trichomonas	Copious green, frothy discharge, vaginal pain, and dysuria
Urinary tract infection (UTI)	Frequency, urgency, and dysuria. Occasionally hematuria and fever

Continued

GYN

Table 14-3. COMMON GYNECOLOGIC DISEASES AND SYMPTOMS—*cont'd*

DISEASE	SYMPTOMS
Uterine fibroids	Pelvic pain, pelvic masses, infertility, pressure, dyspareunia, abnormal uterine bleeding, urinary incontinence, constipation
Yeast infection	Thick, white vaginal discharge, pruritus

IX. PHYSICAL EXAMINATION (Table 14-4)

This examination should always be conducted with a chaperone present.

Table 14-4. FINDINGS OF PHYSICAL EXAMINATION AND POSSIBLE DIAGNOSES.

SYSTEM	PHYSICAL EXAMINATION FINDING	POSSIBLE DIAGNOSES
Vitals		
Pulse	Tachycardia	PID, TOA, Ruptured ectopic pregnancy, thyroiditis
Blood pressure	Hypotension	Acute abdomen (ruptured ectopic, ruptured hemorrhagic ovarian cyst), sepsis (disseminated gonococcal infection, ruptured TOA)
Respiratory rate	Tachypnea	Postoperative complication (pulmonary embolus, pulmonary edema)
Weight	Rapid weight loss	Malignancy
Height	Decrease in height	Osteoporosis
Temperature	Fever	PID, TOA
HEENT		
Eyes	Exophthalmos	Graves' disease of the thyroid
	Argyll Robertson (pupils accommodate but they do not react)	Syphilis

Table 14-4—cont'd

System	Physical Examination Finding	Possible Diagnoses
Face	Hirsutism	Polycystic ovarian disease (PCOS), congenital adrenal hyperplasia (CAH)
Neck		
Thyroid	Thyroid enlargement, goiter, or nodule	Thyroiditis, thyroid cancer
Lungs	Inspiratory effort, rales, rhonchi, wheezes	Gynecologic metastases or pulmonary embolus
Chest	Nipple discharge	Galactorrhea (physiologic/pituitary adenoma)
	Peau d'orange changes from edema	Breast cancer or malignancy
	Lump/mass	Breast cancer
Cardiovascular	Murmur	Consider SBE prophylaxis if surgical procedure planned
Abdomen		
	Blue umbilicus (Cullen's sign)	Hemoperitoneum
	Fluid wave	Ascites or hemoperitoneum
	Generalized pain	Fibromyalgia, endometriosis
Genitourinary		
Female	Labial swelling	Bartholin's gland cyst
	Vulvar pigmentation	Vulvar dysplasia, cancer
	Urethral mass	Urethral diverticulum
	Vaginal mass	Cystocele, rectocele, uterine prolapse
	Fixed uterus	Endometriosis, uterine fibroids
	Pelvic mass	
Skin	Facial melasma	Oral contraceptive use
	Hyperpigmentation	Hormonally induced changes

Continued

GYN

Table 14-4. FINDINGS OF PHYSICAL EXAMINATION AND POSSIBLE DIAGNOSES—*cont'd*

System	Physical Examination Finding	Possible Diagnoses
	Upper lip or chin hair growth	(PCOS)
	Rash	Paget's disease (intraductal carcinoma) with scaly, eczematous lesion of the nipple signaling underlying malignancy; toxic shock syndrome if associated with fever and systemic symptoms
	Pubic hair: Typical female pattern is inverted triangle over mons pubis	Diamond pattern may indicate excessive androgen activity
Lymphatics	Lymphadenopathy	Sexually transmitted disease (e.g., lymphogranuloma venereum [LGV]), GU cancer
Extremities	Homan's sign: calf spasm with knee dorsiflexion	Deep venous thrombosis
Neurologic	Loss of position sense, wide-based gait, postural instability, ataxia, and pain	Tertiary syphilis (tabes dorsalis)

A. **External Genitalia:** Lesions, discoloration, atypical moles, ulcers, hyperplastic dystrophy (thickening), lichen sclerosis, clitoromegaly, excoriations, normal development.
B. **Vulva:** Skin discoloration, condyloma or molluscum contagiosum, lesions, clitoris, presence of hymen, atrophy.
C. **Vagina:** Color, presence of rugae, discharge with pH, saline mount, potassium hydroxide (KOH) evaluation, lesions, cystocele, rectocele, enterocele, lesions, mucosal integrity, inflammation or enlargement of Skene's or Bartholin's glands, fistulas.
D. **Cervix:** Nulliparous versus parous, lesions, inflammation, transformation zone, discharge, cervical motion tenderness (i.e., Chan-

delier sign), bluish discoloration (i.e., Chadwick's sign), white plaque, punctations, or abnormal vessels may signify human papilloma virus (HPV) or dysplasia, nabothian cysts.

E. **Uterus:** Size in weeks, uterine softening in early pregnancy (i.e., Hegar's sign), position (anteflexed, anteverted, mid, retroverted, retroflexed); version applies if uterus and cervix are on the same axis, flexion applies if the fundus is displaced but the cervix is on the usual axis), lateral displacement may occur if adhesions are present, contour (regular/irregular), mobility, prolapse (categorized as stage I if minimal descent, stage II if descends to introitus, and stage III if descends through introitus, procidentia if uterus completely extruded from vagina).

F. **Adnexa:** Fullness, masses, tenderness, mobility, position.

G. **Pelvic Adequacy:** Diagonal conjugate, ischial spines, sacral prominence, subpubic arch, pelvic type (gynecoid, android, anthropoid, platypelloid).

H. **Rectovaginal (RV) Examination:** Evaluate the integrity of the RV septum, uterosacral ligaments, and uterine position.

X. DIFFERENTIAL DIAGNOSIS (Table 14-5)

GYN

Table 14-5. GYNECOLOGIC DIFFERENTIAL DIAGNOSIS.

Symptom	Possible Diagnoses
Amenorrhea	Pregnancy, polycystic ovarian syndrome, hypogonadotropic hypogonadism, anorexia, prolactinemia
Dysuria	Acute cystitis, acute urethritis, or vulvovaginitis
Endometriosis	Physiologic dysmenorrhea, fibroids
Fibroids	Pregnancy, sarcoma, ovarian masses
Infections	Tumor necrosis, physiologic discharge, atrophic vaginitis, tuberculosis
Hirsutism and virilization	Exogenous or iatrogenic, pregnancy (luteoma), polycystic ovarian syndrome, stromal hyperthecosis, ovarian tumors, adrenal tumors, Cushing's syndrome, adult-onset congenital adrenal hyperplasia
Ovarian cyst	Benign neoplasm, malignancy, corpus luteum, ovulatory follicle, ectopic pregnancy
Ovarian mass (Benign)	Simple follicular cyst, corpus luteum cyst, theca lutein cysts, benign cystic teratoma (dermoid cyst), endometriomas, fibroma, Brenner tumors, cystadenofibromas
Malignancies	Ovarian cysts or benign neoplasms, fibroids, endometriosis, TOA

Continued

Table 14-5. GYNECOLOGIC DIFFERENTIAL DIAGNOSIS—*cont'd*

Symptom	Possible Diagnoses
Pelvic pain	Ovarian cyst, ovarian torsion, ectopic pregnancy, endometriosis, pelvic inflammatory disease
Pelvic pressure	Uterine fibroids, large ovarian mass, pelvic floor prolapse
Recurrent pregnancy loss	Chromosomal abnormality, antiphospholipid syndrome, lupus, hypothyroidism, uterine anomalies (myomas, uterine septum, bicornuate uterus)
Urinary incontinence	Detrusor instability, genuine stress incontinence, intrinsic sphincter dysfunction, overflow incontinence, reflex incontinence, urge incontinence, and extraurethral incontinence (fistulas)
Vaginal discharge	Physiologic discharge, bacterial vaginosis, yeast infection, trichomoniasis, gonorrhea, fallopian tube cancer

XI. LABORATORY TESTS AND STUDIES

A. Tests Performed in Clinic

1. Pap smear: Routine cytology.
2. Liquid-based cytology: More sensitive, able to perform HPV subtyping.
3. Cultures can be obtained for infectious organisms.
4. Wet mount.
   a. White blood cells indicate cervicitis and possible gonococcal disease (GC)/chlamydia.
   b. Clue cells indicate bacterial vaginosis, trichomonads indicate trichomonas, and lactobacilli are present in a normal environment.
   c. KOH: Lyses cells so hyphae or yeast spores can be identified.

B. Laboratories and Studies

1. BHCG: Human chorionic gonadotropin (pregnancy test).
2. CA 125 is elevated in most epithelial ovarian malignancies.
3. Alpha fetoprotein (AFP) is elevated (along with BHCG) in germ cell tumors.
4. Estradiol and progesterone have limited usefulness because of cyclic fluctuations (but progesterone can tell if ovulation has occurred).
5. Gonadotropins (follicle-stimulating hormone [FSH], luteinizing hormone [LH]).

6. Thyroid-stimulating hormone (TSH).
7. Prolactin.
8. Dehydroepiandosterone sulfate (DHEAS).
9. Testosterone (free and total).
10. Antiphospholipid antibodies, lupus anticoagulant, anticardiolipin antibodies.
11. Rapid Plasma Reagin (RPR), Venereal Disease Research Laboratory (VDRL), Micro-Hemagglutinin-Treponema Pallidum (MHATP): Tests for syphilis.
12. Gonorrhea and chlamydia DNA probes.
13. Endometrial, cervical, and vulvar biopsies.

C. **Radiology Studies**
1. Pelvic ultrasound.
2. Mammograms.

XII. ACRONYMS AND ABBREVIATIONS

Table 14-6. COMMON GYNECOLOGY TERMS.

Term	Definition
Adrenarche	Age at first notice of pubic hair growth
Amenorrhea	Absence of menses during the reproductive years
Dysfunctional uterine bleeding	Excessive uterine bleeding with no demonstrable organic cause
Dysmenorrhea	Painful menstruation
Dyspareunia	Painful intercourse
Hydrosalpinx	A collection of watery, sterile fluid in the fallopian tube
Induced abortion	Intentional medical or surgical termination of pregnancy before 20 weeks' gestation
Menarche	Age at first menstruation
Menometrorrhagia	Prolonged uterine bleeding occurring at irregular intervals
Menorrhagia (hypermenorrhea)	Prolonged (more than 7 days) or excessive (more than 80 mL) uterine bleeding occurring at regular intervals
Metrorrhagia	Uterine bleeding occurring at irregular but frequent intervals
Polymastia	More than two breasts
Polymenorrhea	Uterine bleeding occurring at regular intervals of less than 21 days
Polythelia	More than two nipples
Thelarche	Age at first notice of breast development
Vaginismus	Involuntary spasm of vaginal, introital, and levator ani muscles causing painful sexual intercourse or preventing penetration

XIII. DEFINITIONS

Table 14-7. GYNECOLOGY ACRONYMS AND ABBREVIATIONS.

Acronym or Abbreviation	Definition	Acronym or Abbreviation	Definition
AROM	Artificial rupture of membranes (amniotomy)	**LGV**	Lymphogranuloma venereum
AFP	Alpha-fetoprotein	**LMP**	Last menstrual period
ART	Artificial reproductive technologies	**LTCS**	Low transverse cesarean section
BTL	Bilateral tubal ligation	**MMK**	Marshall-Marchetti-Kranz retropubic urethropexy
BSO	Bilateral salpingoophorectomy	**OCP**	Oral contraceptive pill
BV	Bacterial vaginosis	**PCO**	Polycystic ovaries
CIN	Cervical intraepithelial neoplasia	**PCOS**	Polycystic ovarian syndrome
CIS	Carcinoma in situ	**PID**	Pelvic inflammatory disease
CVS	Chorionic villus sampling	**PMS**	Premenstrual syndrome
D&C	Dilation and curettage	**PROM**	Premature rupture of membranes
DES	Diethylstilbestrol	**PPROM**	Preterm premature rupture of membranes

DIC	Disseminated intravascular coagulopathy	**SAB**	Spontaneous abortion
DUB	Dysfunctional uterine bleeding	**STD**	Sexually transmitted disease
EBL	Estimated blood loss	**SROM**	Spontaneous rupture of membranes (at term, in labor)
EGBUS	External genitalia; Bartholin's, urethral, and Skene's glands	**TAB**	Therapeutic abortion
EMB	Endometrial biopsy	**TAH**	Transabdominal hysterectomy
HSG	Hysterosalpingogram	**TOA**	Tuboovarian abscess
HPV	Human papilloma virus	**TOP**	Termination of pregnancy
IUD	Intrauterine device	**TSS**	Toxic shock syndrome
IUP	Intrauterine pregnancy	**TVH**	Transvaginal hysterectomy
IVF	In vitro fertilization	**UPT**	Urine pregnancy test
HRT	Hormone replacement therapy	**UTI**	Urinary tract infection
HSV	Herpes simplex virus	**VDRL**	Venereal disease research laboratory
LAVH	Laparoscopically assisted vaginal hysterectomy	**VBAC**	Vaginal birth after cesarean
LEEP	Loop electrosurgical excision procedure		

XIV. SAMPLE H&P WRITE-UP

CC: Pelvic pain.

HPI: J.R. is a 22-year-old gravida 0 (G0), who presents to the emergency room complaining of progressively worse right-sided pelvic pain for the past 3 days. The pain is characterized as sharp, intense, and radiating to the back. She also reports right shoulder pain. The patient recalls two episodes of emesis, moderate vaginal bleeding, no fever or diarrhea. On further questioning, the patient admits to vaginal spotting one week ago, reports being sexually active, and uses contraception occasionally. Her menstrual cycles are very irregular, ranging from 32 to 60 days, and she does not recall when her last period was.

Past Obstetrical History: None.

Previous GYN History: Menarche at age 10, menses have been irregular since. Her last Pap smear was normal. She has taken oral contraceptives in the past. Currently she is sexually active, has 2 partners, and uses barrier contraception (condom) almost all the time. She has had chlamydia in the past, which was treated appropriately.

Past Medical History: The patient gives a history of childhood asthma (resolved). She denies any chronic medical problems.

Past Surgical History: Tonsillectomy and adenoidectomy at age 3.

Emergency and Trauma History: The patient reports being involved in a motor vehicle accident 2 years ago with blunt trauma to the abdomen that required hospitalization for observation and pain management.

Childhood History: Noncontributory.

Occupational History: The patient is a junior in college and works at a local bar as a waitress.

Medications and Allergies: The patient has been taking 800 mg of ibuprofen every 6 hours for the past 2 days due to intense abdominal/pelvic pain. Denies intake of any other medication. She is not allergic to any medication.

Social History: The patient is a college student, works as a waitress part-time. She reports occasional use of tobacco and alcohol and denies the use of any illicit drugs.

Review of Systems

General: Feeling weak for almost 1 week.

Respiratory: No cough or shortness of breath.

Cardiovascular: Palpitations and chest discomfort (heaviness).

Gastrointestinal: Generalized abdominal pain, and 2 episodes of vomiting. No diarrhea.

Genitourinary: Mild vaginal spotting for the past 1 week, progressing to heavier bleeding a few days ago. Severe pelvic pain for 2 to 3 days.

Physical Examination

Vital signs: T 37°C (98.6°F) HR 140 BP 82/38 RR 28 Weight 57 kg (125 lbs.) Height = 163 cm (5′4″).

HEENT: No abnormalities.

Lungs: Clear to auscultation and percussion.

Chest: No masses or tenderness. No nipple discharge.

Cardiovascular: Tachycardia, regular rhythm, no murmurs.

Abdomen: Soft, not distended, tender to palpation (R > L), +rebound, +guarding, distant bowel sounds.

Pelvic examination: EGBUS – Normal female genitalia, TANNER V, no lesions noted.

Speculum examination: Vaginal mucosa pink and ruggated, no lesions, cervical os nulliparous with bright red blood. Clots noted in vaginal vault.

Bimanual examination: Exquisite tenderness to palpation, uterus small, anteverted, and mobile, right adnexal fullness noted, otherwise difficult to assess secondary to discomfort.

Skin: Pale, no rashes.

15

HEMATOLOGY

Thomas S. Neuhauser, MD, and Michael Osswald, MD

I. CHIEF COMPLAINT

A. Chief Complaint: Use the patient's own words.

B. Identifying Data: Obtain the patient's age, sex, medical record number, and race/ethnicity.

II. HISTORY OF PRESENT ILLNESS

A. Most Common Hematologic Symptoms

1. Fatigue and decreased energy levels (e.g., anemias).
2. Bleeding or bruising disorders (congenital or acquired deficiencies or abnormal function of blood components; platelets and coagulation factors).
3. Excessive clotting disorders and sequelae (e.g., thromboembolic diseases).

B. Characteristics of Symptoms

1. How long have you had this symptom? A symptom that has been present for many years is more likely to be benign or congenital.
2. Have you received treatment for a hematologic disease?
3. What work-ups, if any, have already been done?
4. How do these symptoms affect your daily life? Assess the patient's current performance and activity levels.
5. What is your race/ethnicity? Some hemoglobinopathies (e.g., glucose-6-phosphate deficiency [G-6-PD]) are more common in certain ethnic groups, and some disease processes (e.g., sickle cell anemia) are related to race.

III. HEMATOLOGIC DISEASE PROCESSES

There are three general categories of hematologic disease processes: (1) diseases of blood components—red blood cells (RBCs), white blood cells (WBCs), platelets, and coagulation factors; (2) diseases of blood-forming tissues—congenital or acquired, transient or permanent; and (3) hematologic diseases secondary to other conditions.

A. Have You Been Diagnosed with a Disorder of RBCs?

1. Do you have anemia? Anemia is a manifestation of a disease, not a disease in itself. Symptoms include:
   - a. Weakness?
   - b. Fatigue?
   - c. Malaise?
   - d. Decreased energy level?
   - e. Pale skin?
   - f. Numbness/coldness in hands or feet?

2. Hemoglobinopathies.
   a. Joint pain?
   b. Fatigue?
   c. Yellow eyes?
   d. Itching/pruritus? Hemoglobinopathies may be associated with joint pain (e.g., sickling disorders), fatigue, yellow sclera (e.g., jaundice), and itching/pruritis (e.g., thalassemia major, hemoglobin H disease). They may be brought to attention in asymptomatic patients through screening (e.g., sickle dex positive) or unexplained complete blood count (CBC) abnormalities (e.g., thalassemia trait, hemoglobin variants such as C, D, E, and hereditary persistence of fetal hemoglobin [HPFH]).

B. **Have You Been Diagnosed with a Platelet Disorder?** Disorders of platelets may be associated with coagulopathies (hypercoagulability or hypocoagulability associated with many disease processes), congenital dysfunction (e.g., von Willebrand's disease, storage pool defects), or acquired decrease thrombocytopenia (e.g., idiopathic thrombocytopenic purpura [ITP], aplastic anemia).
   1. Blood clots?
   2. Limb pain or swelling?
   3. Shortness of breath?
   4. Ischemia? Thromboembolic diseases are associated with blood clots, limb swelling, shortness of breath (e.g., deep venous thrombosis [DVT], pulmonary emboli [PE]), and sometimes ischemia (e.g., heparin-induced thrombocytopenia [HIT]).
   5. Easy bruising?
   6. Bleeding problems? Congenital bleeding disorders (e.g., von Willebrand's) are associated with easy bruising, excessive bleeding (e.g., abnormal menstrual and rectal bleeding, excessive bleeding following trauma/surgery, bleeding from gums, history of bleeding from umbilical cord stump, frequent and long-lasting nose bleeds).
   7. Disseminated intravascular coagulation (DIC): A manifestation of many disease processes; depending on stage, associated with oozing from wounds/surgical sites, skin and mucus membrane bleeding, acrocyanosis, thrombosis (as above).

C. **Have You Been Diagnosed with a Disorder of Coagulation Factors?**
   1. Joint disease?
   2. Ecchymosis?
   3. Easy bruising?
   4. Vision loss?
   5. Anemia?
   6. Neurologic or psychiatric problems?
   7. Hematuria? Disorders of coagulation factors may be associated with scarring of the joints or joint disease, ecchymosis, easy

bruising, vision loss from bleeding into the eye, chronic anemia from blood loss, neurologic or psychiatric problems, and hematuria (e.g., hemophilias A and B).

8. Clotting or bleeding problems? May be associated with propensity to clot (e.g., factor V Leiden deficiency; decreased/dysfunctional proteins C, S, and antithrombin III). May be associated with propensity to bleed, but less severely than hemophiliacs (e.g., afibriniginemia, dysfibrogenemia).
9. Bleeding history questions.
   a. Duration of bleeding?
   b. Where and type (umbilical cord, mucous membranes, skin, joint, gastrointestinal (GI), and genitourinary (GU) tract)?
   c. How long (acute, lifelong)?
   d. Appearance of petechiae on body? Ecchymosis? New limb swelling?

D. Have You Been Diagnosed with Abnormal White Blood Count (WBC)?

1. Congenital or cell-mediated immune impairment?
   a. Frequent severe infections?
   b. Hematopoietic malignancy? Congenital humoral and/or cell-mediated immune impairment (e.g., severe combined immunodeficiency [SCID], DiGeorge's syndrome); lifelong propensity to develop severe infections and hematopoietic malignancy.
2. Acquired immune deficiency?
   a. Severe, life-threatening infections?
   b. Malignancy? Acquired immune deficiency (e.g., patient's infected by human 1 immunodeficiency virus [HIV], neutropenia caused by chemotherapy/drugs). Vulnerable to severe life-threatening infection(s). HIV patients have propensity to develop different types of malignancy with time (e.g., non-Hodgkin's lymphoma, Kaposi's sarcoma).
   c. Lack of immune globulin?
      (1) Recurrent infections? Some patients may have problems with recurrent infection.
      (2) Severe anaphylactic reaction?
      (3) Pulmonary edema?
      (4) Shortness of breath?
      (5) Fever? Lack of immune globulin (e.g., IgA deficiency). Patients may come to clinical attention because of severe anaphylactic reaction to blood transfusion: Pulmonary edema, shortness of breath, fever. This must be documented in chart, and patient must always receive blood products deficient in IgA.

E. Have You Been Found to Have Any Abnormalities of Cellular Function?

1. Have you been diagnosed with a recurrent infection with a catalase-positive organism? Neutrophils cannot mount a respiratory burst (e.g., chronic granulomatous disease [CGD]); patients have propensity to develop recurrent infections with catalase-positive organisms (e.g., pseudomonas, aspergillus, staphylococcus, and chromobacterium).
2. Do you frequently develop infections? Abnormalities of lysosome function (e.g., Chediak-Higashi syndrome): Propensity to develop infections.
3. Have you been diagnosed with an enzyme deficiency?
   - **a.** Any progressive neurologic dysfunction?
   - **b.** Visceromegaly?
   - **c.** Skeletal abnormalities?
   - **d.** Marked deformations?
   - **e.** If a child, any degeneration of acquired abilities? Accumulation of material in lysosomes caused by enzyme deficiency (e.g., Gaucher's disease, Nieman-Pick disease).
     - **(1)** Manifestation varies with type, but in general, patients may manifest progressive neurologic dysfunction, visceromegaly, skeletal abnormalities, marked deformations, and degeneration of acquired abilities (children).
     - **(2)** Spectrum of illness with some forms; some may present in adulthood with minimal symptoms.

F. Have You Been Diagnosed with a Disease of Blood-Forming Tissue?

1. Have you had bone marrow disease or bone marrow failure?
   - **a.** Fever?
   - **b.** Cachexia?
   - **c.** Malaise?
   - **d.** Weakness? Bone marrow disease/failure: Signs/symptoms may be general (e.g., fever, cachexia, malaise, weakness) or reflect underlying disease process (e.g., aplastic anemia: associated with myasthenia gravis; replacement: associated with high-stage breast and prostate cancer).
2. Bone marrow replacement or loss: Malignancy (metastatic disease, fibrosis, primary hematopoietic neoplasia), aplastic anemia (primary/idiopathic, secondary).
3. Transient arrest of bone marrow production (e.g., transient erythroblastopenia of childhood: associated with viral infection; erythropenia: associated with thymoma, vitamin deficiency, heavy metal toxicity; neutropenia: associated with infectious disease processes, idiopathic reaction to medications).

G. Have You Had Splenic Disease? Signs/symptoms may be referable to underlying disease process involving spleen and/or reflect splenomegaly itself.

1. Have you had an enlarged spleen? A splenectomy? Hypersplenism: Defined as cytopenias caused by an enlarged spleen, which recover following splenectomy. Bleeding disorders, resulting sequestration of platelets by the spleen.
2. Have you had a splenic rupture? Splenic rupture with subsequent hemoperitoneum (infection [e.g., infectious mononucleosis, malaria], extramedullary hematopoiesis [e.g., thalassemia major, bone marrow replacement], tumor(s) [e.g., metastasis, primary hematopoietic malignancy, benign and malignant neoplasm(s)]). This is a surgical emergency!
3. Portal hypertension? Signs/symptoms of portal hypertension caused by diversion of blood supply to enlarged spleen.
4. Have you had an autosplenectomy or traumatic splenectomy? Autosplenectomy (e.g., sickling disorders) or traumatic splenectomy (e.g., motor vehicle accident, splenectomy performed for hypersplenism/malignancy), predisposing to infections with encapsulated bacterial organisms.

H. Thymic Disease

1. Do you have a congenital development condition? Congenital maldevelopement/aplasia (e.g., DiGeorge's syndrome) may be associated with T-cell disorders, predisposing to infection.
2. Have you had a malignancy? Airway obstruction? Chest discomfort? Involved by malignancy (e.g., precursor T-cell acute lymphoblastic lymphoma [ALL], thymic carcinoma), associated with general signs/symptoms of hematopoietic disease as well as local disease (e.g., airway obstruction, chest discomfort).
3. Systemic disease? Hyperplasia (e.g., thymoma) may be associated with systemic disease (e.g., signs/symptoms of myasthenia gravis or erythroid maturational arrest).

I. Hematologic Diseases/Manifestations Secondary to Other Conditions (see Past Medical History)

1. Do you have anemia?
2. Are you experiencing any bleeding?
3. Have you been diagnosed with thromboembolic disease?
4. Do you have an infection?

IV. PAST MEDICAL AND SURGICAL HISTORY

A. Past Medical History

1. Have you had any major illnesses? Some illnesses can influence hematologic processes or be underlying causes of blood or blood-forming disorders.
2. Have you been hospitalized for similar problems (e.g., recurrent sickle cell crisis for sickling disorders, bleeding in hemophiliac patient caused by factor inhibitors)?
3. What infections have you had? How many? How treated? Sequelae?

B. Past Surgical History

1. What surgical procedures have you had? When? For what reason?

Table 15-1. DIFFERENTIAL DIAGNOSES OF ETIOLOGY FOR SELECTED HEMATOLOGIC CONDITIONS.	
CONDITION ASSOCIATIONS	POSSIBLE UNDERLYING CAUSES AND
Anemia	Trauma, element/vitamin deficiency (e.g., iron, B_{12}, folate) whatever the etiology (e.g., poor diet, bleeding, malabsorption), congenital (hemoglobinopathy, abnormal red cells [e.g., spherocytosis, elliptocytosis]), hemolysis (e.g., burn, DIC, transfusion reaction, enzyme deficiency (glucose-6-phosphate deficiency [G-6-PD]), chronic disease, aplastic anemia (thymoma with or without myasthenia gravis, transient erythropenia of childhood, drug effect, idiopathic), heavy metal poisoning (e.g., arsenic, lead)
Coagulation/ bleeding	DIC, congenital coagulation factor deficiency/ dysfunction, hemolytic uremic syndrome: thrombotic thrombocytopenic purpura (HUS-TTP) liver disease, idiopathic thrombocytopenic purpura (ITP), transfusion reaction, aplastic anemia
Thromboembolic disease	DIC, underlying malignancy, congenital coagulation disorder, Virchow's triad (trauma, stasis, propensity to clot), lupus anticoagulant (LA), anti-cardiolipin antibody (ACA), homocysteinemia, plasminogen deficiency, HUS-TTP, paroxysmal nocturnal hemoglobinuria (PNH)
Recurrent infections	Congenital immune deficiency (usually lifelong difficulties), acquired immune deficiency (infection, drug induced, bone marrow transplant/replacement), splenectomy (congenital [rare] and acquired: autosplenectomy as in sickle cell or following trauma/surgery)

2. Have you had a splenectomy? This can predispose to certain infections (e.g., encapsulated organisms such as pneumococcus) and may cause abnormalities in CBC and on the peripheral smear (thrombocytosis, red blood cell [RBC] inclusions).
3. Have you had any bleeding following surgery, treatment, or complications?

4. History of cardiac valve replacement? This may cause schistocytes to be present on a blood smear.

C. **Emergency and Trauma History**

1. Have you had blood transfusions? Any reactions to the transfusions? Known alloantibodies? An antibody specific for an alloantigen? Alloantigens are antigenic differences that will cause an immune response to allografts because of species differences in alleles (are allogeneic).
2. How many transfusions have you had? Multiple transfusions predispose to formation of alloantibodies. Important in oncology patients, who frequently utilize numerous blood products.

D. **Childhood History**

1. Do you have any congenital conditions?
   a. Down's syndrome.
   b. Fanconi's anemia: Autosomal-recessive disorder involving defection DNA repair.
   c. Li-Fraumeni syndrome: Rare autosomal-dominant syndrome in which patients are predisposed to cancer.
2. Hemoglobinopathies? Inherited disorders or traits (e.g., hemoglobin C, D, E traits; hereditary persistence of fetal hemoglobin [HPFH]) usually asymptomatic.
3. Did you ever have excessive bleeding?
   a. At birth from the umbilical stump.
   b. Following tooth extraction(s) or brushing teeth.
   c. Frequent epistaxis.
   d. Long-term abnormal pattern of menses.

E. **Occupational History**

1. Do you take necessary safety precautions at work?
2. Are you exposed to hazardous materials or chemicals at your workplace?
3. Are you exposed to infectious agents (e.g., health care workers) at your workplace?

F. **Travel History**

1. Have you recently traveled? In the United States? To foreign countries? Some geographic areas can predispose to stasis/thrombosis (Virchow's triad: stasis, hypercoagulability, trauma).
   a. Did you consume local water?
   b. Did you eat any unwashed fruits? Doing so may expose to infectious agents; some bacterial organisms produce hemolysins (e.g., staphylococcus, streptococcus).
2. Have you served in the military overseas? Older vets exposed to hookworms may still be infected, with chronic blood loss and eosinophilia.

G. **Animals and Insects Exposure History:** Have you been exposed to any animals or insects? Bites from certain venomous snakes and insects (e.g., spiders) may cause bleeding diathesis.

V. MEDICATIONS, ALLERGIES, AND ADVERSE REACTIONS

A. Medications

1. What prescription medications are you currently taking? Some medications are clearly linked to bleeding (e.g., nonsteroidal antiinflammatory drugs [NSAIDs], Coumadin, aspirin). The actions of some drugs may potentiate the actions of others. Others may lead to hemolysis (e.g., penicillin, alpha-methyldopa).
2. What over the counter (OTC) products are you currently taking?
3. Do you take any herbal preparations or supplements?

B. Allergies to Medications and the Side Effects

1. Have you had any allergic reactions to medications? Which ones? What treatment with what response? Some medications can result in bone marrow suppression/various cytopenias (e.g., aplastic anemia with chloramphenicol, neutropenia with OTC antacids).
2. Have you had an adverse side effect to medications?

HEME

VI. HEALTH MAINTENANCE

A. Prevention: Have you had regular immunizations? Immunizations are especially important if patient is immunocompromised/ post-splenectomy.

B. Diet

1. What is your typical diet? Some foods and chemicals may have anticoagulant activity.
2. Assess iron intake.
   a. Diets low in iron (e.g., strict vegetarianism) could lead to iron deficiency, and high in iron could lead to overload.
   b. Long-term poor eating habits (e.g., alcoholics) may lead to B_{12}/folate deficiency.
   c. Prolonged diet of milk without supplementation in infants may lead to iron deficiency.
3. Assess protein intake. Low protein leads to anemia.

C. Exercise/Recreation

1. Have you experienced any changes in exercise tolerance?
2. Have you had exposure to hazardous chemicals or agents (e.g., exposure to heavy metals in homemade moonshine) in your exercise or recreational activities?

D. Sleep Patterns: Any change in sleep pattern? Night sweats? Chills?

E. Social Habits

1. Does the patient use tobacco products? How many packs per day for how many years (pack-years)?
2. Does the patient consume alcohol? Clearly related to B_{12}/folate deficiencies as well as liver disease/factor deficiencies.
3. Illicit drug use: How long? How often?

VII. FAMILY HISTORY

A. First-Degree Relatives' Medical History

1. Family history of bleeding in males or females.

2. History of blood clots: Deep vein thromboses (DVTs), pulmonary emboli (PE), or spontaneous abortions.
3. History of congenital disease (e.g., Down syndrome, G-6-PD deficiency).
4. History of hematopoietic disease (e.g., sickle cell disease, hemoglobinopathy(ies), cancer-associated syndromes).
5. History of iron overload, refractory anemias, diabetes mellitus, arthritis, heart/liver disease.
6. History of malignancy (e.g., lymphoma or leukemia, colon cancer).

B. **Three-Generation Genogram:** Help distinguish autosomal-dominant from autosomal-recessive pattern, linkage to sex chromosomes.

VIII. PSYCHOSOCIAL HISTORY

A. Personal and Social History

1. What social support/resources does the patient have? Cancer, hemochromatosis, some hemoglobinopathies (e.g., sickle cell anemia), coagulopathies (e.g., hemophilia), and their treatments can place an incredible social, financial, and time burden on patients and their families.
2. Referral(s) may be necessary for home health care/assistance and transportation.

B. Current Illness Effects on the Patient

1. Does the patient understand why he or she is here?
2. Assess patient's understanding of possible disease(s) complications and long-term prognosis.
3. Will the patient be able to maintain daily routine? What changes will have to be made, if any?

C. Interpersonal and Sexual History

1. Is the patient married? Single? In a relationship?
2. Is the patient sexually active? Monogamous or multiple partners? Take appropriate precautions?

D. Family Support

1. Be mindful of hopes and fears of the patient and of his or her family. Give the family understanding of the patient's illness(es).
2. Genetic counseling may be necessary for family as well as patient.

E. **Occupational Aspects of the Illness:** How will the illness/treatment affect employment?

IX. REVIEW OF SYSTEMS (Tables 15-2, 15-3, and 15-4)

Table 15-2. GENERAL HEMATOLOGY SYMPTOMS BY SYSTEM.

SYSTEM	SYMPTOMS
General/systemic	Performance status, weakness, fevers, malaise
HEENT	Headache, pallor, epistaxis, mouth ulcers, icterus, loss of taste, neck masses/enlarged lymph nodes, bleeding from gums
Respiratory	Shortness of breath
Cardiovascular	Palpitations, tachycardia
Gastrointestinal	Nausea, vomiting, abdominal distention, dyspepsia, diarrhea, rectal bleeding
Genitourinary	Hematuria
obstetric/ Gynecologic	Menstruation or cessation thereof, pregnancy
Hematopoietic	Fatigue, infections, easy bruising
Lymphatic	Lymphadenopathy
Musculoskeletal	Contractures, arthritis (MCP joint affected in hemochromatosis)
Dermatologic	Rashes, bruising, ecchymosis, petechiae
Central nervous system (CNS)	Headache, photophobia, nausea, weakness, mental status changes
Psychiatric	Depression, insomnia, mania, restlessness, mood changes

Table 15-3. NONSPECIFIC SYMPTOMS AND ASSOCIATED DISEASE PROCESSES.

SYMPTOMS	DISEASES
Bruising (easy)	Trauma, coagulopathy, inherited bleeding disorder
Rectal bleeding	Trauma, hemorrhoids, mass lesions, abnormal vessels, coagulopathy, diverticulae, infarction, bleeding "upstream" (esophagus, stomach), swallowed blood
Abnormal/heavy menstruation	Stress, menopause, hormone/drug effect, coagulopathy, hereditary bleeding disorder, malignancy
Petechiae	Thrombocytopenia of any etiology (e.g., idiopathic thrombocytopenic purpura [ITP], bone marrow pathology, disseminated intravascular coagulation [DIC])
Lymphadenopathy	Infection, hematopoietic malignancy, metastasis

Table 15-4. COMMON HEMATOLOGIC DISEASES AND THEIR SIGNS/SYMPTOMS.

DISEASE	SYMPTOMS
Anemia	Fatigue, weakness, dyspnea, decreased exercise tolerance, chest pain (if underlying cardiovascular disease), pallor, orthostatic hypotension, tachycardia, glossitis (iron, folate, B_{12} deficiency), koilonychias (iron deficiency), jaundice (hemolytic anemia), splenomegaly (thalassemia, chronic hemolytic anemia), neurologic abnormalities (B_{12} deficiency), low back/abdominal pain, cheilosis (iron deficiency)
Hemochromatosis	Symptoms of end-organ damage: Hepatic/renal/cardiac failure, diabetes, hypogonadism, arthropathy, bronze/slate gray skin
Hemophilia	Bleeding into joints, contractures, ecchymosis
Leukemia/ lymphoma, myelodysplastic syndrome, myeloproliferative disorders	Fever, night sweats, lymphadenopathy, bone pain, recurrent infections, lymphadenopathy, painful/bleeding gums (hyperplasia), headache (CNS involvement), symptoms associated with anemia
Plasma cell malignancies	Fever, night sweats, chills, dyspnea, bone pain, weight loss, recurrent infections
von Willebrand's disorder	Bleeding from gums/following tooth extraction, easy bruising

X. PHYSICAL EXAMINATION (Table 15-5)

Table 15-5. HEMATOLOGY-FOCUSED PHYSICAL EXAMINATION.

SYSTEM	PHYSICAL EXAMINATION FINDING	POSSIBLE DIAGNOSES
General or systemic	Delay of growth/ failure to thrive	Sickling disorders, thalassemia major
	Performance status	Decrease with advancing stages of malignancy

Table 15-5—cont'd

System	Physical Examination Finding	Possible Diagnoses
Vital Signs		
Temperature	Fever	Infection, malignancy
Pulse	Increased, hyperdynamic state	Severe anemia
Respiratory rate	Increased	Thromboembolus, fever, infection
Weight	Unexpected weight loss	Malignancy
HEENT		
Eyes	Scleral icterus	Chronic hemolysis
	Retinal infarct, arteriovenous abnormalities, vitreous hemorrhage	Sickling disorders
Nose	Bleeding	Coagulation/platelet abnormalities (many) etiologies), mass
Mouth	Bleeding gums/ extraction sites	Platelet disorder (e.g., von Willebrand's, ITP)
	Gum swelling	Scurvy
	Angular stomatitis	Iron-deficiency anemia
	Glossitis	Iron-deficiency anemia, folate deficiency
	Smooth, beefy red tongue	B_{12} deficiency
	Cheilosis	Folate deficiency
Face	Deformity	Thalassemia major
Neck	Lymphadenopathy	Malignancy, infection
Lungs	Pleuritic pain	Sickle crisis, thromboembolic disease
Chest	Pain on palpation	Sickle crisis
Cardiovascular	Hyperdynamic state, murmur	Severe anemia
Abdomen	Cholelithiasis	Chronic hemolytic disease processes

Continued

Table 15-5. HEMATOLOGY-FOCUSED PHYSICAL EXAMINATION—*cont'd*

SYSTEM	PHYSICAL EXAMINATION FINDING	POSSIBLE DIAGNOSES
	Splenomegaly	Malignancy, storage disease, hemophilia, hemoglobinopathy (e.g., severe thalassemias), liver disease, chronic hemolysis
	Jaundice	Chronic hemolysis (many etiologies)
	Pain	Bleeding, thrombosis, malignancy, sickle crisis
Genitourinary		
Male	Scrotal gangrenous changes	Thrombosis (many etiologies)
	Engorgement of penis	Sickle crisis
Female		
Skin	Pallor	Anemia
	Bruising, ecchymosis	Coagulation disorder (factor deficiency), vascular disorder (e.g., Ehlers-Danlos syndrome)
	Rashes/discoloration (Henoch-Schönlein purpura)	Certain food/drug allergies, some upper respiratory infectons
	Hyperkeratosis	Scurvy
	Petechiae	Coagulation disorder (platelet disorder, whatever etiology)
	Bleeding at catheter sites	DIC, platelet disorder, anticoagulants
	Jaundice	Chronic hemolysis
	Cyanosis	Vitamin K deficiency, methemoglobinemias (e.g., carbon monoxide poisoning, high oxygen affinity hemoglobins), severe anemia/acute blood loss, heavy metal poisoning

Table 15-5—cont'd

System	Physical Examination Finding	Possible Diagnoses
	Ulceration	Patients started on coumadin without preceding heparin with protein C/S deficiency, sickling diseases
Lymphatics	Lymphadenopathy	Infection, malignancy (all types)
Musculoskeletal or extremities	Sternal tenderness or bony tenderness elsewhere	Malignancy involving bone, markedly increased hematopoiesis
	Koilonychia (spoon nails)	Iron deficiency
	Arthritis	History of bleeding (e.g., hemophilia), infarction (sickling disorder), sickle crisis
	Swelling weight-bearing joint (hemarthrosis)	Hemophilia, thrombosis (many etiologies)
	Gangrenous changes	Thrombosis (many etiologies)
	Contracture	Hemophilia
Neurologic	Lower extremity weakness, decreased sensation, abnormal reflexes	Retroperitoneal hematoma
	CNS/mentation changes	Malignancy, bleeding (many etiologies), thrombosis (many etiologies)
	Peripheral neuropathy, ataxia, gait abnormalities	B_{12} deficiency
	Abnormal (pathologic) reflexes	B_{12} deficiency
Rectum	Bright red blood per rectum (BRBPR)	GI malignancy, Vitamin K deficiency (many etiologies, e.g., liver disease, biliary disease), transfusion reaction

XI. DIFFERENTIAL DIAGNOSIS (Table 15-6)

Table 15-6. FINDINGS OF PHYSICAL EXAMINATION AND LABORATORY STUDIES AND POSSIBLE DIAGNOSES.

Finding	Possible Diagnoses
Anemia, microcytic	Iron deficiency, anemia of chronic disease, thalassemia, hemoglobinopathy
Anemia, macrocytic	B_{12}/folate deficiency (all etiologies), myelodysplastic syndrome (MDS), recovering marrow (associated with reticulocytosis), hypothyroidism, autoimmune hemolytic anemia, cold agglutinin disease
Anemia, normocytic	Chronic disease, blood loss, DIC, burn, spherocytic anemia
Bone pain	Trauma, tumor, metastasis
Lymphadenopathy	Infection, malignancy (metastatic versus primary/lymphoma)
Splenomegaly	Infection (e.g., infections mononucleosis), extramedullary hematopoiesis (bone marrow pathology), mass (primary, secondary/metastatic), ITP, lymphoma/leukemia, congestion, storage disease

XII. LABORATORY STUDIES AND DIAGNOSTIC EVALUATIONS

Laboratory analysis plays an important role in evaluation of hematologic disease processes.

A. Complete Blood Count (CBC)

1. Enumerates WBCs, performs differential count (most automated machines).
   a. Details increase or decrease in WBCs and subsets.
   b. May prompt examination of a peripheral smear.
2. Performs RBC count and expresses overall measurement of size (mean corpuscular volume [MCV]) and degree of variation in size (red cell distribution width [RDW]) and hemoglobin content (mean corpuscular hemoglobin [MCH]).
   a. Allows for determination of type of anemia, thereby narrowing differential.
   b. Newer machines can give reticulocyte count, and even degree of maturity: Useful for measurement of bone marrow recovery, response to anemia.
3. Performs platelet count: Newer machines detail variation in size (platelet distribution width [PDW]).

4. Many new machines may analyze presence or absence of nucleated red blood cells (NRBCs).
   a. Depending on the age of patient, this may prompt examination of peripheral smear.
   b. NRBCs never normal in adult patients.
   c. In older automated machines, likely counted as WBCs.

B. **Peripheral Blood Smear**
1. Verify findings of CBC.
2. Assess WBC morphology.
3. Assessment/assistance in classification of hematopoietic neoplasia (e.g., count blasts).
4. Examine blood for organisms (e.g., filaria, spirochetes).
5. Examine RBCs for inclusions (e.g., Howell-Jolly bodies, Heinz bodies), parasites (e.g., malaria), and abnormal forms (e.g., target cells, schistocytes, ovalocytes).

C. **Coagulation**
1. Coagulation factors.
   a. Assess amount (expressed as percent activity) and function.
   b. Assess for inhibitors (common in hemophiliacs, sometimes acquired in association with chronic disease processes, sometimes no associated underlying disease process).
   c. Mixing study: Initial assessment for inhibitor versus factor deficiency.
2. Prothrombin time (PT), partial thromboplastin time (PTT).
   a. Measurement of intrinsic PTT and extrinsic PT coagulation pathways.
   b. Assessment of function of anticoagulants: Coumadin PT and heparin PTT.
3. Lupus anticoagulant (LA) and factor V Leiden, proteins C and S, anti-thrombin III levels/activity: Assessment of patients with thrombus formation (DVT, PE).
4. D-Dimers/fibrinogen degradation products: Useful for assessment of disseminated intravascular coagulation (DIC).

D. **Serum Studies**
1. Lactate dehydrogenase (LDH), haptoglobin, Coombs, bilirubin, reticulocytes: Useful for assessment of hemolysis.
2. B_{12}, folate, thyroid function tests (TFTs), liver function tests (LFTs), and renal studies: Useful for assessment of macrocytosis.
3. Ferritin, iron, total iron binding capacity (TIBC): Assessment of iron.
4. Serum protein electrophoresis/urine protein electrophoresis (SPEP/UPEP): Assessment for monoclonal spike and subclassification of plasma cell malignancies.
5. Blood urea nitrogen (BUN)/Creatinine (Cr): Assessment for uremia.
6. Cold agglutinins: Used for assessment of cold agglutinin disease/syndrome, which may cause severe hemolysis.

E. **Hemoglobin Electrophoresis:** Useful for assessment of hemoglobinopathies.

F. **Bone Marrow Biopsy**

1. Assessment of bone marrow elements (e.g., cellularity, increases/decreases in normal elements, assessment of cellular morphology).
2. Subclassification of hematopoietic malignancies.
3. Assessment for space-occupying lesions (e.g., malignancy, granulomas, fibrosis).
4. Assessment of iron stores.
5. Assessment for infection.

G. **Sickle Dex**

1. Screen for sickling disorders.
2. May be false negative if severely anemic (hematocrit <20%) or falsely positive for some hemoglobin variants (G-Coushatta).

H. **Flow Cytometry**

1. Useful for assessment of hematopoietic neoplasia of bone marrow, blood, body fluids, some solid tissues.
2. Assessment for ploidy (abnormal DNA content, associated with some tumors).
3. Assessment of abnormal RBCs (e.g., paroxysmal nocturnal hemoglobinuria).
4. Hemoglobin F levels.

I. **Cytochemical Studies** (bone marrow): Useful in classification of acute hematopoietic malignancies.

J. **Molecular Studies/Gene Testing**

1. Certain chromosomal translocations associated with various malignancies.
2. Some translocations/abnormalities associated with specific disease processes (e.g., hemochromatosis).

K. **Tissue Examination**

1. Diagnosis of pathologic conditions (e.g., malignancy, hemochromatosis).
2. Iron: Measure dry weight, increased in hemochromatosis.

L. **Radiologic Studies**

1. Skeletal assessment for infarction, indirect evidence of increased hematopoiesis, lesions.
2. Computed tomography (CT)/magnetic resonance imaging (MRI): Assessment for lesions, organomegaly.
3. May be used for assessment of tissues of patients with known disease, to assess for relapse/recurrence.

M. **Thromboelastograph (TEG):** Determination of possible procoagulant deficiencies/hypercoagulable states as well as suggest treatments (e.g., blood products, coagulation); most useful for operating room and critical care patients.

XIII. ACRONYMS AND ABBREVIATIONS

Table 15-7. HEMATOLOGY ABBREVIATIONS AND ACRONYMS.

Acronym or Abbreviation	Term	Acronym or Abbreviation	Term
ACA	Anti-cardiolipin antibody	**MCH**	Mean corpuscular hemoglobin
ALL	Acute lymphocytic leukemia	**MCHC**	Mean corpuscular hemoglobin concentration
AML	Acute myelogenous leukemia	**MCV**	Mean corpuscular volume
CBC	Complete blood count	**MDS**	Myelodysplastic syndrome
CD	Cluster of differentiation	**NRBC**	Nucleated red blood cell
CGD	Chronic granulomatous disease	**OB**	Occult blood
CGL	Chronic granulocytic leukemia	**PDW**	Platelet distribution width
CML	Chronic myelogenous leukemia	**PNH**	Paroxysmal nocturnal hemoglobinuria
DIC	Disseminated intravascular coagulation	**PRBC**	Packed red blood cells
dRVVT	Dilute Russell viper venom time	**PT**	Prothrombin time, physical therapy
DVT	Deep venous thrombosis	**PTT**	Partial thromboplastin time
EBL	Estimated blood loss	**RBC**	Red blood cell
FFP	Fresh frozen plasma	**RDW**	Red (cell) distribution width
HCT	Hematocrit	**T&C**	Type and cross
HCL	Hairy cell leukemia	**T&H**	Type and hold
Hgb	Hemoglobin	**T&S**	Type and screen
HUS	Hemolytic uremic syndrome	**TRAP**	Tartrate resistant alkaline phosphatase
Ig	Immunoglobulin	**TT**	Thrombin time
ITP	Idiopathic thrombocytopenic purpura	**TTP**	Thrombotic thrombocytopenic purpura
LA	Lupus anticoagulant	**WBC**	White blood cells

XIV. DEFINITIONS

Table 15-8. DEFINITIONS OF HEMATOLOGY TERMS AND EPONYMS.

Term	Definition
Ataxia-telangiectasia	Autosomal-recessive genetic disorder characterized by cerebellar ataxia, oculocutaneous telangiectasia, and immunodeficiency
Cheilosis	Noninflammatory condition of lips, characterized by chapping and fissuring
Chronic granulomatous disease	Neutrophils and monocytes cannot mount respiratory oxidative burst following phagocytosis with catalase-positive organisms; X-linked recessive pattern of inheritance
Coagulopathy	Abnormal bleeding/clotting
Corrigan's sign	Purple line at the junction of the teeth and gum in chronic copper poisoning
D'Espine's sign	Normally, pectoriloquy ceases at the bifurcation of the trachea (adults) and 7th cervical vertebra (infants). Heard lower than this, indicative of enlargement of the bronchial lymph nodes.
DiGeorge's syndrome	Isolated T-cell deficiency associated with maldevelopment of 3rd and 4th pharyngeal pouches; may have severe impairment of humoral immunity
Ecchymosis	Bruising
Ehlers-Danlos syndrome	Associated with fragile blood vessels, resulting in bleeding, aneurysm formation, hemorrhage
Fanconi's anemia	Rare autosomal-recessive disorder characterized by defects in DNA repair; multiple congenital abnormalities, anemia, increased risk of hematopoietic malignancies.
Glucose-6-phosphate deficiency	Deficiency of enzyme with role in hexose monophosphate shunt, rendering RBC susceptible to lysis during oxidative stress; X-linked trait
Kehr's sign	Severe pain in left shoulder in some cases of rupture of the spleen

Table 15-8—cont'd

TERM	DEFINITION
Lupus anticoagulant	Antiphospholipid antibody, associated with propensity to clot/form thrombi and associated with recurrent (habitual) spontaneous abortions
Li-Fraumeni syndrome	Rare autosomal-dominant syndrome resulting from germline mutations in the p53 gene. Characterized by high risk of developing many hematopoietic and nonhematopoietic malignancies at an early age. Up to 50% of affected patients will experience the onset of invasive malignancy before the age of 30
Hemoglobinopathies	Hemoglobin variants or decreased production of constituents of normal hemoglobins; frequently result in CBC abnormalities and changes in electrophoretic mobility
Hemarthrosis	Bleeding into joint, common in hemophilia
Henoch-Schönlein purpura	Anaphylactoid purpura associated with vasculitis, seen in some food/drug allergies and upper respiratory infections (e.g., streptococcal)
HUS-TTP syndrome	Syndrome comprising renal failure, neurologic abnormalities, microangiopathic hemolytic anemia, thrombocytopenia, and fever
Koilonychia	Brittle, spoon-shaped, coarsely ridged fingernails; seen with chronic iron deficiency
Mosler's sign	Sternal tenderness associated with acute myeloblastic leukemia
Petechiae	Skin rash characterized by confluent purple punctuations; form on extremities of individuals with thrombocytopenia
Plummer-Vinson syndrome	Hypochromic anemia, with cracks/fissures at corners of mouth, atrophy of tongue mucosa, and dysphagia caused by esophageal webs/stenosis

Continued

Table 15-8. DEFINITIONS OF HEMATOLOGY TERMS AND EPONYMS—*cont'd*

Term	Definition
Thalassemia	Decreased production of globin chains, leading to anemia and abnormalities of CBC
Virchow's triad	Trauma, stasis, propensity to clot/hypercoagulability
X-linked agammaglobulinemia	Variable loss of immunoglobulins in males resulting from maldevelopment of mature B-cells, predisposing to severe infection(s)

XV. SAMPLE H&P WRITE-UP

CC: "My dentist told me I had to see you because of a bleeding problem."

HPI: A.N. is a 25-year-old white male who recently had 4 impacted wisdom teeth extracted. His dentist told him he had more bleeding than expected but did not require a blood transfusion. He was subsequently referred to hematology. A.N. admits to excessive bleeding as a child upon loosing his baby teeth and frequent nosebleeds. He also recalls his mother telling him he had a lot of bleeding from his umbilical cord stump soon after he was born. He denies a history of unexplained skin rashes, and otherwise states he is in perfect health.

MHx: Patient denies any chronic medical problems. The patient denies any known exposure to infectious disease processes.

SHx: History of appendectomy at 20 for appendicitis, to which the patient recalls the surgeon complaining of "excessive oozing" the next day.

Emergency and Trauma History: Patient has never been hospitalized, had a blood transfusion, or any trauma-related injuries.

Childhood History: Chicken pox at age 4 and numerous ear infections until age 7. He denies any other childhood illnesses. He had all the childhood immunizations given at the time (influenza, diphtheria, pertussis, tetanus, polio, measles, mumps, rubella). He cannot remember the time of his last tetanus diphtheria toxoid.

Occupational History: Computer software programmer since graduating college 4 years previously. No chemical or hazardous material exposure.

Travel History: Frequent travel across the continental United States to assist customers. No history of travel overseas.

Pets: One cat, that lives at home with the patient.

MEDICATIONS: Variable/irregular use of acetominophen for a "sore back," but none in the past week. Patient denies use of any other medications or any kind of supplements. No known allergies to foods or medications.

HEALTH MAINTENANCE

Prevention: Patient received all of the usual childhood immunizations, including MMR.

Diet: Regular diet. Eats approximately 3 times each day. Drinks one cup of coffee per day, and denies consumption of tea or sodas.

Exercise: Patent bikes in the gym 3 times per week for about an hour, and jogs 4 to 5 miles each weekend.

Sleep Patterns: Rarely wakes up to void at night. No recent changes.

Interpersonal and Sexual History: Patient has been married approximately 1 year. There have been no other sexual contacts other than his wife over that time.

Social Habits: Patient denies smoking or tobacco use. The patient drinks approximately 2 beers per night and denies illicit drug use.

FAMILY HISTORY

First-Degree Relatives' Medical History: Patient's father has a history of myocardial infarction and had problems with "oozing" following a quadruple bypass surgery 6 years ago. The patient does not recall if his father had any other surgeries or problems as a child. The patient's mother and 4 siblings are healthy, although one had problems with frequent nosebleeds as a child. All grandparents are alive and well.

Three-Generation Genogram: No known history of genetic traits or diseases within the patient's family.

PSYCHOSOCIAL HISTORY

Personal and Social History: Patient is white (non-Hispanic); family emigrated from Iceland two generations ago. He lives with his wife of one year. He completed four years of college and graduated with a BS in computer science. The couple does not have children.

Interpersonal History and Sexual History: Patient is in a monogamous relationship. As far as he can recall, his wife is healthy.

Understanding of Potential Illness: Patient understands he is being evaluated for a possible inherited bleeding disorder, which will likely entail laboratory testing. He is also aware his wife may additionally need to be tested pending the outcome of the evaluation.

REVIEW OF SYSTEMS

HEENT/Neck: No visual changes or scotomata. Frequent episodes of epistaxis as a child, but now on average once every other month. No history of head trauma. Hearing normal without tinnitus. No nasal obstruction or discharge. Denies sinus/head pain. Gums normal with the exception of occasional bleeding following brushing. Denies neck lesions/masses. Last dental examination 1 week before this evaluation.

Respiratory: No cough, dyspnea, or shortness of breath. Sputum clear.

Cardiovascular: No tachycardia, palpitations, orthopnea, or paroxysmal nocturnal dyspnea. Denies leg swelling.

Gastrointestinal: Denies nausea, vomiting, diarrhea, bright red blood per rectum, or hematemesis. No history of abdominal pain.

Genitourinary: No dysuria, urinary urgency, discharge, or hematuria.

Hematologic/Lymphatic: No easy bruising or masses in neck, axilla, or groin.

Skin: No rashes, pigmentary changes, or lesions.

Neurologic: No history of seizures or weakness.

Musculoskeletal: Occasional back discomfort. No arthritis or muscle weakness.

Extremities: No joint pain or loss of range of motion, swelling, muscle weakness, or deformities.

Psychiatric: No history of mental status changes.

PHYSICAL EXAMINATION

Vitals: T 98.7°F P 82 BP 123/77 RR 12 Weight 205 lbs.

General: Well-nourished, relaxed Caucasian male, approximately 6′1″ and proportionate weight.

HEENT: No sinus tenderness. Neck with normal range of motion and supple. No lymph nodes detected. Sclerae normal, pupils equally round and reactive to light. Normal fundoscopic examination without retinal lesions. Nose patent without discharge or blood. Gums with obvious tooth extraction sites and bloody oozing and moderately inflamed.

Lungs: Clear to auscultation bilaterally.

Cardiovascular: Regular rate and rhythm and without extra heart sounds.

Abdomen: Soft, nontender, without organomegaly.

Genitourinary: No CVA tenderness. Normal circumcised male.

Skin: No rash, petechiae, or jaundice. Nevi noted on chest and back.

Extremities: Normal strength and range of motion without joint swelling or tenderness. All pulses 2 to 3+.

Neurologic: Normal reflexes, gait, and station.

16

INFECTIOUS DISEASE

Patricia A. Meier, MD, and Thomas S. Neuhauser, MD

I. CHIEF COMPLAINT

A. **Chief Complaint:** Use the patient's own words when possible. Chronology is often included: Onset (acute, subacute or chronic), duration (minutes, hours, days, weeks, months or years), and frequency of symptom(s).

B. **Identifying Data:** Obtain patient's name, age, race/ethnic background.

C. **Fever:** Fever is the most common symptom that leads patients and physicians to consider a diagnosis of infection. For this reason, the focus of this section is the work-up of the febrile patient.

1. Fever refers to a pyrogen-mediated elevation of body temperature above the expected normal daily variation. In contrast, hyperthermia is an abnormality of thermoregulation that is not driven by pyrogenic cytokines, and therefore, unlike fever, is not ameliorated by antipyretic medications. For most patients, the temperature at which clinical evaluation of fever is indicated is 38.0°C (100.4°F).
2. Fever as a clinical symptom/sign of infection is neither sensitive nor specific. The absence of fever does not exclude infection, particularly in an immunocompromised, debilitated, or elderly patient.
3. Conversely, the presence of fever does not equate to infection because fever can be the initial manifestation of noninfectious maladies, including collagen vascular disease and malignancy.
4. A variety of terms are used to describe fever in terms of its pattern (e.g., intermittent versus remittent), duration (fever of unknown origin), and unique host characteristics (neutropenic fever). The more commonly used terms are summarized in Table 16-1.
5. Although specific fever patterns are not pathognomonic, a review of the patient's fever curve may provide diagnostic clues about the etiologic agent. Selected fever patterns and putative etiologic agents are summarized in Table 16-2.

D. **Appropriate Febrile Patient Triage:** The goals of triage are to expedite patient care while minimizing the unnecessary exposure of susceptible staff, patients, and family members.

1. Decide if the patient requires an immediate intervention, such as fluid resuscitation or empiric antibiotic therapy. For example,

Table 16-1. DEFINITION OF TERMS REGARDING FEVER.

TERM	DEFINITION
Fever	Fever is an elevation of temperature above the peak normal daily variation. The normal oral temperature range is 36.0-37.8°C (96.8-100.0°F)
Continuous fever	Persistent elevation of temperature with minimal fluctuations
Intermittent fever	Daily fever spikes with return to normal body temperature
Remittent fever	Fever spikes without return to normal body temperature between spikes
Relapsing fever	Cyclical pattern of alternating fever and normal temperature
Factitious fever	Fever produced artificially by the patient
Fever of unknown origin (FUO), classic definition	Illness of more than three weeks' duration. Documented fevers above 101°F (38.3°C) on several occasions. Lack of specific diagnosis after 1 week of inpatient investigation
Classic FUO, revised definition	As above, but investigation now revised to three hospital days or three outpatient visits
Neutropenic fever	A single oral temperature of $>38.3°C$ (101.0°F) or $>38.0°C$ (100.4°F) over at least 1 hour, in patient with a neutrophil count $<500\,mm^3$ or $<1000\,mm^3$ with predicted decline to less than $500\,mm^3$

a patient with acute bacterial meningitis should have antibiotics started before further diagnostic testing is completed.

2. Determine if empiric isolation precautions are warranted. The clinical syndromes for which empiric isolation precautions are advised by the Centers for Disease Control and Prevention (CDC) are summarized in Table 16-3.

II. HISTORY OF PRESENT ILLNESS

A. Infectious Diseases

1. The study of the relationship between a patient, an infectious agent(s), and the environment.
2. Once you have completed your initial triage, you are ready to proceed with an orderly, systematic review of the patient's unique susceptibilities and exposures.

Table 16-2. DIAGNOSTIC SIGNIFICANCE OF FEVER PATTERNS.

FEVER	CAUSES
Single fever spike	Manipulation of a colonized or infected mucosal surface, transfusion of blood/ blood products, infusion-related sepsis (contaminated infusate), temperature error, not a systemic infectious disease
Double quotidian fevers (twice daily)	Adult Still's disease, visceral leishmaniasis, miliary tuberculosis, mixed malarial infections, right-sided gonococcal endocarditis
Tertian fevers (every third day)	Malaria (*Plasmodium vivax*)
Quartan fevers (every fourth day)	Malaria (*Plasmodium malariae*)
Intermittent fevers	Gram-negative or gram-positive sepsis, abscess (renal, abdominal, pelvic), acute bacterial endocarditis, Kawasaki disease, malaria, miliary tuberculosis, antipyretics, peritonitis, toxic shock syndrome
Remittent fevers	Viral upper respiratory infections, *Plasmodium falciparum* malaria, acute rheumatic fever, Legionella/Mycoplasma infection, tuberculosis, subacute bacterial endocarditis (SBE)
Continuous or sustained fevers	Central fevers, roseola infantum (HHV6), brucellosis, Kawasaki disease, psittacosis, rocky mountain spotted fever, scarlet fever, subacute bacterial endocarditis, typhoid fever, drug fever
Biphasic (camelback) fever	Colorado tick fever, dengue fever, leptospirosis, brucellosis, lymphocytic choriomeningitis, yellow fever, polio, smallpox, rat-bite-fever (*Spirillum minus*), Chikungunya fever, African hemorrhagic fevers (Marburg, Ebola, Lassa), Echovirus infection
Relapsing fever	Relapsing fever (*Borrelia recurrentis*), yellow fever, smallpox, ascending cholangitis, brucellosis, dengue, chronic meningococcemia, malaria, rat-bite-fever

Table reproduced with permission from Cunha BA. Clinical approach to fever. In SL Gorbach, JG Bartlett, NR Blacklow (eds), Infectious Diseases, ed 2. Philadelphia: WB Saunders, 1998;86.

ID

Table 16-3. EMPIRIC ISOLATION PRECAUTIONS*.

Nonspecific Symptoms		Potential Pathogens[†]	Empiric Precautions
Diarrhea			
Acute diarrhea with a likely infectious cause in an incontinent or diapered patient		Enteric pathogens[‡] *Clostridium difficile*	Contact Contact
Diarrhea in an adult with a history of recent antibiotic use		*Neisseria meningitidis*	Droplet
Meningitis	Petechial/ecchymotic with fever	*Neisseria meningitidis*	Droplet
Rash or exanthems generalized, etiology unknown	Vesicular	Varicella	Airborne and contact
	Maculopapular with coryza and fever	Rubeola (measles)	Airborne
	Upper lobe pulmonary infiltrate in an HIV-negative patient or a patient at low risk for HIV infection	*Mycobacterium tuberculosis*	Airborne
Cough/Fever	Pulmonary infiltrate in any lung location in a HIV-infected patient or a patient at high risk for HIV infection	*Mycobacterium tuberculosis*	Airborne
	Paroxysmal or severe persistent cough during periods of pertussis activity	*Bordetella pertussis*	Droplet
	Respiratory infections, particularly bronchiolitis and croup, in infants and young children	Respiratory syncytial or parainfluenza virus	Contact

	History of infection or colonization with multidrug-resistant organisms[§]	Resistant bacteria[§]	Contact
Risk of multidrug-resistant microorganisms	Skin, wound, or urinary tract infection in a patient with a recent hospital or nursing home stay in a facility where multidrug-resistant organisms are prevalent	Resistant bacteria[§]	Contact
	Abscess or draining wound that cannot be covered	*Staphylococcus aureus,* group A streptococcus	Contact
Skin or Wound Infection			

Infection control professionals are encouraged to modify or adapt this table according to local conditions. To ensure that appropriate empiric precautions are implemented always, hospitals must have systems in place to evaluate patients routinely according to these criteria as part of their preadmission and admission care.

*Patients with the syndromes or conditions listed below may present with atypical signs or symptoms (e.g., pertussis in neonates and adults may not have paroxysmal or severe cough). The clinician's index of suspicion should be guided by the prevalence of specific conditions in the community, as well as clinical judgment.

†The organisms listed under the column "Potential Pathogens" are not intended to represent the complete, or even most likely, diagnoses, but rather possible etiologic agents that require additional precautions beyond Standard Precautions until they can be ruled out.

‡These pathogens include enterohemorrhagic *Escherichia coli* O157 : H7, *Shigella,* hepatitis A, and rotavirus.

§Resistant bacteria judged by the infection control program, based on current state, regional, or national recommendations, to be of special clinical or epidemiologic significance.

Reproduced from Garner JS. Hospital Infection Control Practices Advisory Committee. Guideline for isolation precautions in hospitals. Infect Control Hosp Epidemiol 1996;17:53-80, and Am J Infect Control 1996;24:24-52.

B. **Symptoms**
1. May be localized or systemic.
2. It is critical to be thorough in performing the entire history and physical (H&P).

C. **Historical Clues That May "Break the Case":** These clues generally fall into two categories: (1) those that delineate potential exposures to infectious agents, and (2) those that describe the patient's susceptibility to infection (Table 16-4).

D. **Important Questions for a Febrile Patient**
1. What is the duration and magnitude of fever? This will allow you to answer the important question, "Is this disease process acute or chronic?"
2. When did the fever begin? Quickly ascertain the onset of the fever because some disease processes dictate immediate treatment (e.g., acute bacterial meningitis).
3. Is there a pattern to the fever? (See Tables 16-1 and 16-2.) For some diseases (e.g., malaria), the periodicity of the fever can be a helpful clue. (Fever patterns also provide interesting material for questions during clinical rounds.)
4. Is there a specific part of your body that is bothering you/painful (e.g., determine localized vs. systemic infection)? When examining the febrile patient, evaluate all localizing symptoms so as not to overlook a potential infectious disease emergency, such as an invasive soft tissue infection.
5. Determine whether the patient is immunocompromised (Table 16-5). What is the specific immune defect? Certain host defects are associated with susceptibility to specific organisms or groups of organisms, some of which require immediate therapy. When caring for immunocompromised patients, it is important to remember that infection with more than one agent may occur simultaneously.
6. Has the patient traveled outside the United States recently? The febrile returning traveler should be evaluated expediently for life-threatening infections, such as malaria. A careful travel history is critical in establishing a differential diagnosis that takes into consideration details of travel itinerary, conditions of travel, prior immunizations, antibiotic prophylaxis, and exposure history.
7. Has the patient been hospitalized recently?
8. Has the patient taken any medications that may alter the fever?
9. Does the patient have occupational exposures or hobbies that make him or her susceptible to infection?
10. Has the patient been exposed to animals, raising the possibility of a zoonotic infection (Table 16-6)?

Text continued on p. 283.

Table 16-4. HOST FACTORS THAT INFLUENCE EXPOSURE, INFECTION, AND DISEASE.

Factors that Influence Exposure to Infectious Agents	Factors That Influence Infection and the Occurrence and Severity of Disease for the Patient
Animal exposure, including pets Behavioral factors related to age, drug usage, and alcohol consumption Blood or blood product recipient Child day care attendance Closed living quarters: military barracks, dormitories, homeless shelters, facilities for the elderly and mentally handicapped, prisons Food and water consumption Familial exposures Gender Hospitalization or outpatient medical care Hygienic practices Occupation Recreational activities, including sports and recreational injecting drug use Sexual activity: heterosexual and homosexual, type and number of persons School attendance Socioeconomic status Travel, especially to developing countries Vector exposure	Age at the time of infection Alcoholism Anatomic defect Antibiotic resistance (agent) Antibiotic use (host) Coexisting noninfectious diseases, especially chronic Coexisting infections Dosage: amount and virulence of the organism to which the host is exposed Duration of exposure to the organism Entry portal of organisms and presence of trauma at the site of implantation Gender Genetic makeup Immune state at the time of infection, including immunization status Immunodeficiency (specific or nonspecific): natural, drug induced, or viral (HIV) Mechanism of disease production: inflammatory, immunopathologic, or toxic Nutritional status Receptors for organism on cells needed for attachment or entry of the organism

Table reproduced with permission from Osterholm MT, Hedberg, CW, Moore KA. In Mandell GL, Bennett JE, Dolin R (eds), Principles and Practice of Infectious Diseases, ed 5. Philadelphia: Churchill Livingstone, 2000;163.

Table 16-5. CONDITIONS RESULTING FROM IMMUNE DEFECTS AND ASSOCIATED INFECTING ORGANISMS.

Defects	Conditions	Associated Infecting Organisms
Neutropenia	Leukemia, cytotoxic chemotherapy, AIDS, systemic lupus erythematosis (SLE), Felty syndrome, drugs	*Escherichia coli* *Klebsiella pneumoniae* *Pseudomonas aeruginosa* *Staphylococcus aureus* *Staphylococcus epidermidis* Streptococci species Yeasts Aspergillus and other fungi
Defective chemotaxis	Diabetes, alcoholism, renal failure, SLE, Hodgkin's disease, trauma, lazy leukocyte syndrome	Staphylococci, streptococci, and yeasts
Defective neutrophil killing	Chronic granulomatous disease, Down syndrome myeloperoxidase deficiency	Catalase-positive bacteria (e.g., *S. aureus, E. coli,* Candida spp.).
B-lymphocyte defects	Congenital and acquired agammaglobulinemia, burns, enteropathies, myeloma, lymphocytic leukemia	Encapsulated organisms (e.g., *Streptococcus pneumoniae, Haemophilus influenzae,* Neisseria spp.; also Salmonella and Campylobacter spp.)
T-lymphocyte defects	Congenital immunodeficiencies, AIDS, lymphoma, sarcoidosis, Epstein-Barr virus (EBV) infection, SLE, cytomegalovirus infection (CMV)	Intracellular infections with bacteria, mycobacteria, viruses, parasites, fungi
Complement components	Congenital absence	Miscellaneous bacterial infections

Reproduced with permission from Zinner SH. Treatment and prevention of infections in immunocompromised hosts. In Gorbach SL, Bartlett JG, Blacklow NR (eds), Infectious Diseases, ed 2. Philadelphia: WB Saunders, 1998;1252.

Table 16-6. ANIMAL ASSOCIATIONS AND ZOONOTIC DISEASE RISK.

Disease/ Animal	Aquatic Mammal	Bird	Cat	Cattle	Dog	Fish	Goats Sheep	Horse	Nonhuman Primate	Rabbit Hare	Rodent	Snakes Lizard	Swine	Wildlife
Anthrax			X	X	X		X	X					X	X
Bartonellosis			X											
Brucellosis			X	X	X		X	X		X			X	
Campylobacteriosis		X	X	X	X		X		X				X	
Capnocytophaga canimorsus					X									
Cryptosporidiosis			X	X	X	X	X	X					X	
Erysipiloid	X	X				X							X	
Giardiasis	X								X					
Hanta virus											X			
Hepatitis A									X					
Herpes B									X					X
Histoplasmosis		X												X
Lymphocytic choriomeningitis											X			
Leptospirosis			X	X	X		X	X			X		X	X
Listeriosis		X		X	X		X		X	X	X		X	
Mycobacterium spp.				X					X				X	X

Continued

Table 16-6. ANIMAL ASSOCIATIONS AND ZOONOTIC DISEASE RISK—*cont'd*

Disease/ Animal	Aquatic Mammal	Bird	Cat	Cattle	Dog	Fish	Goats Sheep	Horse	Nonhuman Primate	Rabbit Hare	Rodent	Snakes Lizard	Swine	Wildlife
ORF							X							
Ornithosis		X												
Pasteurellosis		X	X		X								X	
Rat-bite-fever											X			
Plague			X		X					X	X			X
Q fever			X	X			X			X				
Rabies			X	X	X		X	X		X	X		X	X
Salmonellosis		X	X	X	X		X	X	X	X	X	X	X	X
Streptococcus iniae					X									
Shigellosis									X					
Toxoplasmosis			X								X			X
Tularemia		X	X		X					X	X		X	
Vibriosis					X	X								
Viral hemorrhagic fever											X			X
Yersiniosis				X	X		X	X	X				X	

Table reproduced with permission from Weinberg AN. Zoonoses. In Mandell GL, Bennett JE, Dolin R (eds), Principles and Practice of Infectious Diseases, ed 5. Philadelphia: Churchill Livingstone, 2000;3242.

III. PAST MEDICAL AND SURGICAL HISTORY

A. Past Medical History

1. What diseases have you had? How were they treated? Certain disease processes and treatments may alter immune function.
2. Do you have any deficiencies? Determine whether they are natural, induced (chemotherapy), or viral (human immunodeficiency virus [HIV]).
3. Have you had a chronic disease process or paralysis?
4. Have you recently been hospitalized or received inpatient medical care? Consider recent outbreaks of hospital-acquired (nosocomial) infections.
   a. Have you had an infection? Involving the urinary tract, lungs, surgical wound, blood? The most common sites of nosocomial infections are the urinary tract, lung (pneumonia), surgical wound, and bloodstream (sepsis).
   b. Eliciting a history of recent hospitalization is helpful for both planning the diagnostic evaluation and for selecting empiric therapy.
   c. Hospital-acquired pathogens are often more drug resistant than community-acquired pathogens (e.g., vancomycin-resistant enterococcus, methicillin-resistant Staphylococcus species), and may require a modification of the usual empiric therapy for a given infection.

B. Past Surgical History

1. Have you had any surgical procedures that involved implanting foreign bodies (e.g., mesh, joints, screws/hardware, tooth implants, heart valves, pacemaker, breast implants)?
2. Did you undergo surgery to repair an anatomic defect (natural or acquired)?
3. Have you had a splenectomy?

C. Emergency and Trauma History

1. Have you ever been treated for trauma? Any damage to skin or mucous membranes?
2. Have you had a blood transfusion? The risk of a transfusion-transmitted infection has decreased considerably but has not been eliminated.

D. Childhood History

1. Development.
2. Illnesses (e.g., otitis media, respiratory infections, urinary tract infections [UTIs], seizures, and hospitalizations).
3. Child day care attendance.

E. Occupational History

1. What, if any, organisms or toxins are you exposed to at work?
2. Do you work in close proximity to co-workers (e.g., assess risk of exposure to co-workers)?

F. Travel History

1. Have you traveled within the United States? To foreign countries? Include geographic locations and dates.

2. Did you have a fever during or after your trip? Fever in the returning traveler requires an expedient evaluation to promptly recognize and treat potentially fatal diseases, such as malaria.
3. When taking a travel history, it is important to ask:
   a. Where did you go? For what duration? When did you return?
   b. What were the travel conditions (e.g., city versus remote)?
   c. Did you drink the local water?
   d. What exposures did you have to insects and animals?
   e. What types of food and drink did you consume?
   f. Did you have any sexual contacts? Was protection used?
   g. Obtain immunization and medication history, including those taken as prophylaxis.
4. Identify diseases that are capable of being transmitted to others, and for which isolation precautions are advised.

G. **Animal and Insects Exposure History** (See Table 16-6 for detailed list.)

1. What animals and insects have you recently been exposed to (including pets)? Have you been exposed to cats (toxoplasmosis, cat scratch disease) or pigeons (*Chlamydia psittacosis*)?
2. Have you had any reactions to bites or stings (envenomations)?

IV. MEDICATIONS

1. Are you taking any medications? Which ones? Note medications that may alter fever (e.g., nonsteroidal anti-inflammatory drugs [NSAIDs], medications containing NSAIDS, acetominophen).
2. Have you recently used antibiotics? For what reason? Antibiotics may alter disease manifestation and ability to culture etiologic agent.
3. Have you had any allergic or adverse reactions? Some patients may experience anaphylactic reactions to certain medications (penicillin and derivatives). Note specific agent and type of reaction. For some infections, desensitization may be required.

V. HEALTH MAINTENANCE

A. Prevention

1. What immunizations have you had?
   a. Childhood immunizations by type and/or age: Diphtheria, pertussis, tetanus, polio, measles, mumps, rubella, varicella, influenza, Hemophilus influenza type b, hepatitis B, meningococcus.
   b. Adult immunizations by type and/or age: Varicella, influenza, pneumococcus, tetanus-diphtheria toxoid, hepatitis A, hepatitis B, rabies, meningococcus, anthrax, yellow fever, cholera.
2. Hygiene practice: How often do you bathe? Do you brush your teeth daily? How often? How often and when do you wash your hands? How do you control menses (e.g., pads vs. tampons)? If you use tampons, how often do you change them? If a child, inquire about toilet training.

3. Prophylaxis: Do you take antibiotics on a daily basis or for specific procedures (e.g., before dental care in patients)? Ask about prophylactic antibiotic use if patient is immunocompromised (e.g., asplenic patients, HIV-infected patients) or has had surgery involving foreign body placement (e.g., cardiac valve replacement, hip replacement).
4. Do you use an insect repellent or take other precautions (e.g., covering head/face, tent)?

B. Diet: What food and water have you been exposed to recently? What is your usual diet? Evaluate nutritional status.

C. Exercise/Recreational Activities: In particular, note environmental exposures and zoonotic risks.

D. Sleep Patterns

1. Have there been any changes in your sleep pattern?
2. Have changes been caused by night sweats?

E. Social Habits

1. Do you use alcohol? How much and how often?
2. Do you use tobacco? What type? How much and for how long?
3. Do you use illicit or recreational drugs?

VI. FAMILY HISTORY

A. First-Degree Relatives' Medical History and Three-Generation Genogram: Look for a history of disease process(es) altering immune function (e.g., severe combined immune deficiency syndrome [SCIDS]).

B. Familial Exposure: Inquire about recent, potentially communicable, illnesses in family members.

VII. PSYCHOSOCIAL HISTORY

A. Personal and Social History

1. Where were you born (country and city)?
2. What is your religious affiliation?
3. What is your ethnic background?
4. Socioeconomic status: Describe your current residence. Whom do you live with? What is the physical layout? Note especially close-quarters facilities, such as military barracks, dormitories, homeless shelters, facilities for the elderly and mentally handicapped, and prisons.
5. Are you currently attending school?
6. Are you involved in a social club?

B. Current Illness Effects on Patient

1. Does the patient understand the illness?
2. Is counseling necessary (e.g., risk of transmission to others, any special precautions)?
3. Will the patient be able to continue current occupation?

C. Interpersonal and Sexual History

1. Are you sexually active? More than one partner? Do you use protection? Possible exposure to sexually transmitted disease (STD).

2. Do you now have, or have you had, an STD? Consider the need to report to appropriate authority(ies). Contact partners.

D. **Family Support**
1. Are family members available to provide any necessary assistance?
2. Consider whether it is necessary to counsel family members.
3. Does the patient require any special needs or arrangements (e.g., wheelchair, supplies for wound care, home health care)?

E. **Occupation Aspects of the Illness**
1. How will the rehabilitation requirements affect your employment (i.e., tertiary prevention)?
2. Will you be able to take necessary precautions (to protect self and co-workers)?

VIII. **REVIEW OF SYSTEMS (Tables 16-7, 16-8, and 16-9)**

Table 16-7. GENERAL INFECTIOUS DISEASE SYMPTOMS BY SYSTEM.

SYSTEM	SYMPTOMS
General	Weight loss, fatigue/weakness, chills (frequency, how long do they last?), night sweats, fever, and anorexia/loss of appetite
HEENT	Sinus pain, headache, conjunctivitis, icterus, eyes/ears/nose pain, bleeding or discharge, photophobia, sore throat, difficulty swallowing, drainage in back of throat, dentition
Neck	Any masses, pain on movement, stiffness
Cardiac	Angina, dyspnea, murmur
Respiratory	Cough (productive or nonproductive), hemoptysis, pleurisy, chest pain with or without radiation, shortness of breath
Gastrointestinal	Abdominal pain (location, quality, radiation), change in bowel habits/diarrhea, jaundice
Genitourinary	Flank pain, pain or burning on urination, discharge, hematuria
Obstetrics / gynecologic	Pelvic pain, dyspareunia vaginal discharge, last menstrual period (LMP), contraceptives
Hematopoietic	Anemia, easy bruising, bleeding
Skin	Color change (jaundice), easy bruising, rash
Neurologic	Loss of consciousness, change in mentation
Lymphatic	Neck, axillary, groin masses, drainage
Musculoskeletal	Trauma, pain, stiffness, swelling, backache, tumors/lesions

Table 16-8. NONSPECIFIC SYMPTOMS AND THEIR INFECTIOUS DISEASE CORRELATES.

Symptom	Disease
Abdominal pain (localized)	Appendicitis, abscess (peritoneal, subphrenic, of solid organs)
Abdominal pain (diffuse)	Peritonitis, gastroenteritis
Change in mentation	Meningitis (bacterial, fungal, viral, parasitic), anoxia (many etiologies)
Cough	Sinusitis, pharyngitis, bronchitis, pneumonia
Icterus	Many etiologies including hemolysis, liver/ biliary disease, malaria
Joint pain	Septic arthritis
Neck stiffness	Meningitis, osteomyelitis, soft tissue abscess
Pelvic pain	STD, PID
Photophobia	Meningitis
Pleurisy	Pleural effusion, irritation of diaphragm (abscess), pneumonia

Table 16-9. COMMON INFECTIOUS DISEASE SYNDROMES AND THEIR SYMPTOMS.

Syndrome	Symptoms
Sinusitis	Nasal discharge, cough, sinus pain, fever
Meningitis	Headache, photophobia, neck pain/stiffness, lethargy, fever, nausea, vomiting
Pneumonia	Fever, chills, rigors, headache, malaise, cough (may or may not be productive), hemoptysis, pleuritic chest pain, possible diarrhea, chest/back pain
Gastroenteritis	Fever, nausea, vomiting, variable abdominal pain (localized, diffuse, intermittent, colicky)

IX. PHYSICAL EXAMINATION (Table 16-10)

The physical examination of a patient with a febrile illness is no different from that of any other patient, with one exception: the need for empiric isolation precautions (Table 16-9). Because some infections are contagious, precautions may be needed to protect those who must interact with the patient.

A question that needs to be answered early in the triage of the febrile or infected patient is: "Does this patient have a disease that is

Text continued on p. 294.

Table 16-10. FINDINGS OF EXAMINATION AND POSSIBLE DIAGNOSES.

System	Physical Examination Finding	Possible Diagnoses
General	Chills	Septic shock (Gram-negative bacteria), localized infection, parasitemia
	Weight loss/emaciation	Undiagnosed abscess (e.g., subphrenic, perirenal, other deep seated), chronic infection (HIV, parasite)
Vital signs		
Pulse	Tachycardia	May be early sign of impending sepsis
Blood pressure	Hypotension	Septic shock
Respiratory rate	Tachypnea	Pneumonia
HEENT		
Eyes	Photophobia	Meningitis (e.g., viral, bacterial, fungal), syphilis
	Icterus	Many etiologies, including liver/biliary disease, hemolysis (malaria)
	Periorbital edema/redness	Periorbital cellulitis
	Injected conjunctivae	Conjunctivitis
	Failure to accommodate/react to light, weak extraocular muscles, ptosis	Botulism
	Corneal ulceration/lesions	Bacterial, viral, parasite (e.g., acanthamoeba)
	Subretinal hemorrhage	Trichinosis

Ears	Injected, immobile tympanic membranes	Otitis media
	Inflamed canal	Otitis externa
	Discharge	Bacterial, fungal, viral infection
Nose	Peripharyngeal/peritonsillar mass	Retropharyngeal/peritonsillar abscess
Mouth	Tonsillar exudate	Pharyngitis (e.g., strep throat)
	Whitish coloration	Thrush
	Induration/edema floor of mouth	Infection of sublingual/submandibular space
	Petechiae, erythema soft palate	Scarlet fever
	Koplik's spots	Measles
	Beefy red tongue	Scarlet fever
	Membrane	Diphtheria
	Gingival edema/bleeding	Gingivitis (e.g., bacterial)
	Sit forward with protrusion of mandible	Epiglottitis
	Fluid in sinus (transillumination)	Sinusitis
Face	Unilateral pain/swelling with overlying redness	Suppurative parotitis
	Bilateral swelling/pain	Viral (e.g., mumps)
	Pain/stiffness in jaw (risus sardonicus)	Tetanus
	Disfigurement	Hansen's disease, Leishmaniasis
Neck	Stiffness (e.g., Kernig's sign, Brudzinski's sign)	Meningitis, submastoid (Bezold's) abscess
General	Point tenderness/mass	Deep infection, osteomyelitis
	Thrombophlebitis jugular vein	Associated with Bezold's abscess
Lungs	Rales/rhonchi	Pulmonary edema (septic shock), bronchitis, pneumonia
	Dullness to percussion	Effusion, consolidation (e.g., pneumonia)
	Respiratory obstruction	Mediastinal abscess

Continued

Table 16-10. FINDINGS OF EXAMINATION AND POSSIBLE DIAGNOSES—*cont'd*

System	Physical Examination Finding	Possible Diagnoses
	Bronchophony, pectoriloquy, tracheal deviation	Pneumonia
	Left pleural effusion	Splenic/pancreatic/subphrenic abscess, pneumonia, empyema
	Right pleural effusion	Liver/subphrenic abscess, pneumonia, empyema, amebiasis
	Pain	Pneumonia, empyema, bronchitis
Chest	Friction rub	Pericarditis
Cardiovascular	New onset murmur	Endocarditis
	Decreased heart sounds	Tamponade (pericarditis)
Abdomen	Fluid wave	Peritonitis (e.g., spontaneous bacterial peritonitis [SBP])
	Pain, right lower quadrant (McBurney's point)	Appendicitis, abscess, PID
	Dullness to percussion	Ascites/peritonitis
	Mass, right upper quadrant	Liver abscess (e.g., amoebic, bacterial), echinococcal cyst, PID
	Rigidity	Peritonitis
	Hepatomegaly	Abscess
	Vague, variable, nonlocalized discomfort	Bacterial infection, "food poisoning" (e.g., enterotoxin), protozoal (e.g., Giardia)
	Splenomegaly	Abscess, parasitemia (e.g., malaria, schistosomiasis)
	Lower abdominal pain	Appendicitis, PID

	Distension	Organomegaly (e.g., abscess) some pneumonias, peritoneal effusion
	Rebound	Peritonitis, appendicitis, gastroenteritis
Flank	Pain	Retroperitoneal abscess, pyelonephritis, gastroenteritis
Genitourinary	Perineal pain, tender prostate	Prostatitis
Male	Urethral pain, meatal erythema	STD
	Testicular pain	Epididymitis, STD
	Ulceration(s)	STD
	Scrotal edema	Parasitemia (e.g., filariasis)
Female	Vaginal "fullness"/tenderness	Retrofascial abscess
	Pelvic pain during examination/cervical movement	PID
	Adnexal mass/fullness	Tuboovarian abscess (TOA)
	Vulvar/vaginal/introitus erythema with or without white discoloration	Fungal (e.g., Candida)
	Vaginal discharge	Bacterial/fungal disease, STD, PID
	Ulceration(s)	STD, fungal, viral
	Cyanosis	Septic shock, pneumonia
Skin	Jaundice	Hemolysis (e.g., septic shock), biliary disease (cholangitis), liver disease (e.g., abscess, cyst: amoebic, echinococcal, viral)
	Redness, tenderness, swelling, heat	Dermal/subcutaneous infection
	Reddish streaks with lymphadenopathy	Lymphangitis
	Warts, papules	Viral (e.g., HPV)

Continued

Table 16-10. FINDINGS OF EXAMINATION AND POSSIBLE DIAGNOSES—*cont'd*

System	Physical Examination Finding	Possible Diagnoses
	Erythematous lesions	Impetigo, pyoderma, cellulitis
	Ulceration	Viral (e.g., HSV), bacterial (e.g., septic thrombi)
	Petechiae	Endocarditis
	Red rash	Scarlet fever
	Red rash, exfoliative dermatitis	Scalded skin syndrome, toxic shock syndrome
	Erythematous papule—eschar	Anthrax
	Marbling/bronzing of skin	Clostridium
	Petechiae, hemorrhages	Waterhouse-Friderichsen syndrome, DIC associated with sepsis
	Annular lesions	Lyme disease
	Targetoid rash on palms/soles	Syphilis (secondary)
	Maculopapular rash	Viral exanthems, trichinosis
	Vesicles (diffuse, dermatome distribution)	HSV, VZV
	Large skin folds	Onchocerciasis
	Lymphadenopathy	Infection of draining area, lymphangitis, parasitemia
Lymphatics	Suppurative lymphadenitis in groin	Lymphogranuloma venereum (LGV)
	Mass	Abscess
Extremities	Joint pain, swelling, redness	Septic arthritis
	Crepitus	Infection with gas-producing organism (emergency)

	Paronychia	Infection around nail
	Bone pain	Osteomyelitis
	Exquisite tenderness in distribution of tendon sheath/compartment with flexion	Suppurative tenosynovitis
	Hip/thigh pain, paresthesias	Retropsoas abscess
	Inguinal/iliac crest pain, pain with movement of hip	Retrofascial abscess
	Hyperreflexia	Tetanus
	Progressive weakness—paralysis	Botulism, viral (e.g., polio)
	Reduced reflexes	Botulism
	Massive edema	Parasitemia (e.g., filariasis)
	Severe pain, edema (compartment syndrome)	Gas gangrene (e.g., Clostridia)
	Splinter hemorrhages (nail)	Endocarditis, trichinosis
	Mental status changes	Meningitis, septic shock, parasitemia (e.g., Chagas' disease, trypanosomiasis), ruptured abscess
Neurologic	Radiculopathy, cranial neuritis	Lyme disease
	Chorea	Lyme disease
	Perirectal mass/pain, fistula(s)	Perirectal abscess
Rectum	Fullness/tenderness	Retrofascial abscess
	Vague to severe pelvic pain, relieved with defecation, anal/coccygeal pain	Supralevator (ischiorectal) abscess
	Erythema, exudates, ulceration, mucosal bleeding	Proctitis (e.g., STD: bacterial, viral)

potentially transmissible, and thus should isolation precautions be initiated?"

X. LABORATORY STUDIES AND DIAGNOSTIC EVALUATIONS

A. **Diagnostic Studies:** Microbiologic cultures, in particular, are an integral part of the work-up of a patient with a suspected infection.
   1. It is important to be familiar with the unique capabilities of your hospital laboratory and to communicate directly with laboratory personnel about your differential diagnosis.
      a. Some infections require unique methods of detection, and you must convey your suspicions to the laboratory personnel. For example, if you suspect a skin infection is caused by *Mycobacterium marinum*, the specimen should be cultured at 30°C to optimize growth.
      b. You should also alert lab personnel if you suspect the patient's infection is caused by an etiologic agent that may pose a danger to lab personnel if cultured (e.g., coccidioidomycosis).
   2. The diagnosis of an infection is typically made by the following method:
      a. Direct examination of a clinical specimen.
      b. Isolation of the microorganism(s).
      c. Measurement of the host's immune response to the organism.
   3. The proper collection, transport, and handling of specimens are critical to obtaining useful information (Table 16-11). The goal of proper specimen collection and handling is to minimize extrinsic contamination while facilitating growth of the pathogen.

B. **Radiologic Studies:** These may be critical for arriving at a correct diagnosis (chest x-ray for pneumonia, abdominal CT for abscess).

C. **Routine Tests:** In hospitalized patients with community-acquired pneumonia.
   1. Chest radiograph.
   2. Arterial blood gas (ABG) analysis.
   3. Complete blood count (CBC).
   4. Chemistry profile, including kidney and liver function tests (LFTs) and electrolyte levels.
   5. HIV serology (age 15 to 54 years).
   6. Blood culture.
   7. Sputum Gram stain and culture +/– acid-fast stain and culture, Legionella test (culture, direct fluorescent antibody stain, or urinary antigen assay), Mycoplasma immunoglobulin M.
   8. Pleural fluid analysis (if present): White blood cell (WBC) count and differential, lactate dehydrogenase (LDH), pH, protein, glucose, Gram stain, acid-fast stain; and culture for bacteria (aerobes and anaerobes), fungi, and mycobacteria.

Text continued on p. 299.

Table 16-11. SPECIMEN COLLECTION AND TRANSPORT FOR BACTERIOLOGY.

SPECIMEN	COLLECTION AND TRANSPORT	COMMENT
	BLOOD	
	Adults 1. 10 mL into each of two 100-mL vacuum bottles *or* 2. 5 mL into each of two 50-mL vacuum bottles and 10 mL into isolator, *or* 3. 10 mL into one 100-mL vacuum bottle and 10 mL into isolator 4. 10 mL into each of two BACTEC high-volume resin resin bottles	
	Infants 1. 1-3 mL into each of two 50- or 100-mL vacuum bottles, *or* 2. 0.5-1.0 mL into pediatric isolator and any remaining blood into 50- or 100-mL vacuum bottle	A minimum of two and a maximum of four cultures per septic episode are recommended
Intravascular catheter	Remove catheter aseptically, clip one (from 2- to 3-inch catheter) or two (from 8- to 24-inch catheter) 2-inch segments, and transfer into swab transport device (Culturette)	Catheter segments should be cultured semi-quantitatively
Exudate (transudate, drainage, ulcer)	Swab or sterile, screw-capped tube	Such specimens are rarely suitable for anaerobic culture
Feces	Freshly passed specimen in sealed container or rectal swab	Transport medium is recommended if delay is anticipated

Continued

Table 16-11. SPECIMEN COLLECTION AND TRANSPORT FOR BACTERIOLOGY—*cont'd*

Specimen	Collection and Transport	Comment
	Fluids	
Cerebrospinal fluid (CSF)	Sterile, screw-capped tube to be delivered to the laboratory immediately	Refrigeration may be harmful to *Neisseria or Haemophilus*
Peritoneal (including dialysate)	Inoculate 10 mL into blood culture bottles	Direct inoculation of blood culture systems has increased yield of bacteria from patients with spontaneous peritonitis and continuous ambulatory peritoneal dialysis-associated peritonitis
Pleural	Inoculate a portion of the specimen into an anaerobic transport system	Pleural or empyema fluid is a major source of anaerobic bacteria causing pleuropulmonary infection
	Genitourinary System	
For *Neisseria gonorrhoeae*	Send swab moistened with Stuart or Amies transport medium directly to laboratory (4-hour maximum transport time) or directly inoculate modified Thayer Martin medium into Transgrow or JEMBEC device	**Women** **Cervix:** Moisten speculum with water before inserting into vagina; insert swab into cervical canal **Anal swab:** Insert swab approximately 2 cm and move from side to side to sample crypts **Men** **Urethra:** Swab may be used when a discharge is present; otherwise, a sterile bacteriologic loop is inserted to obtain scrapings for smear and culture **Anal swab:** Same procedure as for women

Cervix, vagina, for other bacteria	Swab	Specimens from these sites are not suitable for anaerobic culture
	Urine	
Midstream catheter	Collect in sterile, screw-capped container, which must be transported to the laboratory within 2 hours unless refrigerated	
Suprapubic aspirate	Inject portion of aspirate into an anaerobic transport tube or vial	This is the only type of urine specimen that is acceptable for anaerobic culture
Abscess, traumatic or postoperative wound	Aspirate pus with syringe and needle and transport to laboratory by injecting aspirate into an anaerobic transport vial or taking syringe directly to the laboratory	A swab provides too little material for Gram-stained smear or aerobic and anaerobic cultures. If the amount of pus is limited, one may inject the area with 0.5 to 1.0 mL bacteriostat-free lactated Ringer's, and aspirate material
	Respiratory Tract	
For *Bordetella pertussis*	Use flexible-wire, calcium-tipped swab or soft rubber catheter to obtain nasopharyngeal specimen	Cough plate is not recommended
Throat	Swab posterior pharynx, tonsils, any areas of purulence or ulceration; dry swab acceptable if cultured within 2 hours; otherwise, moisten swab with Stuart or Amies transport medium	Avoid contamination with oral secretions. Ordinarily, testing for group A streptococci is sufficient. The laboratory must be notified in case of suspected diphtheria, pertussis, or gonococcal infection

Continued

Table 16-11. SPECIMEN COLLECTION AND TRANSPORT FOR BACTERIOLOGY—*cont'd*

Specimen	Collection and Transport	Comment
	Respiratory Tract	
Sputum	Obtain specimen by expectorating a deep cough into a sterile, screw-capped jar	Specimens should be screened cytologically and another specimen requested when >25 squamous epithelial cells are observed per low-power field
Transtracheal aspirate	Collect aspirate in a Lukens trap or inject into an anaerobic transport vial	Such specimens are suitable for anaerobic culture
Protected brush	The brush is severed from the inner cannula and transported to the laboratory in 1 mL of bacteriostat-free lactated Ringer's solution	Quantitative culture of the vortexed lactated Ringer's solution helps differentiate upper from lower respiratory tract bacterial origin
Bronchoalveolar lavage (BAL)	Obtain at least 40 mL for complete microbiologic examination	Cytocentrifuge smears should be made for Gram and other appropriate stains. Quantitative culture will help differentiate upper from lower respiratory tract bacterial origin
Tissue	Sterile, screw-capped container	A sufficient amount of tissue must be obtained for both histopathologic and microbiologic examinations

*Reproduced with permission from Isenberg HD. Clinical microbiology. In Gorbach SL, Bartlett JG, Blacklow NR (eds), Infectious Diseases, ed 2. Philadelphia: WB Saunders, 1998;125.

XI. EPONYMS, ACRONYMS, AND ABBREVIATIONS (Tables 16-12 and 16-13)

Table 16-12. SELECTED INFECTIOUS DISEASE–FOCUSED EPONYMS.

EPONYM	DESCRIPTION	ASSOCIATION(S)
Bezold's abscess	Abscess associated with mastoid disease	Mastoiditis
Biederman's sign	Dark red coloration of the anterior pillars of the throat	Seen in some patients with syphilis
Borsieri's sign (line)	When fingernail drawn along skin, a white line is left, which quickly turns red.	Associated with early stages of Scarlet fever
Brudzinski's sign	Flexion of the neck results in flexion of the hip and knee	Associated with meningitis
Brunati's sign	Opacities in the cornea	Appearance in the course of pneumonia or typhoid fever
Clavicular sign	Tumefaction of the inner third of the right clavicle	Associated with congenital syphilis
Filopovitch's (palmoplantar) sign	Yellow discoloration of the prominent parts of the palms/soles	Seen with typhoid fever
Guilland's sign	Brisk flexion of the hip when contralateral quadriceps are pinched	Associated with meningeal irritation
Hatchcock's sign	Tenderness on running finger toward angle of the jaw	Associated with mumps
Jackson's sign	Prolongation of expiratory sound over affected area	Pulmonary tuberculosis
Horn's sign	Pain produced on traction of right spermatic cord	Associated with appendicitis
Kernig's sign	When lying with knee on abdomen or when sitting, the leg cannot be completely extended	Associated with meningitis
Koplik's spots	Bright red spots on buccal/lingual mucosa	Measles
Lenhoff's sign	Furrow appearing on deep inspiration below the lowest rib and above cyst in liver	Echinococcal cyst of liver

Continued

Table 16-12. SELECTED INFECTIOUS DISEASE–FOCUSED EPONYMS—*cont'd*

Eponym	Description	Association(s)
McBurney's sign	Tenderness at a point two thirds of the distance from the umbilicus to the anterior superior spine of the ilium	Associated with appendicitis
Murat's sign	Vibration of the affected side of the chest with a feeling of discomfort when speaking	Associated with tuberculosis
Obturator sign	Hypogastric/adductor pain by passive internal rotation of the flexed thigh	Associated with appendicitis
Osler's sign	Painful, small erythematous swellings in the skin of the hands and feet	Associated with endocarditis
Parrot's sign	Dilation of the pupils when skin on the back of the neck is pinched	Seen with meningitis
Romberg's sign	Swaying of the body or falling when standing with feet close together and eyes closed	Seen with tabes dorsalis
Skoda's sign	Tympanic sound heard on percussing chest above large pleural effusion or lung consolidation	Pneumonia
Squire's sign	Alternate dilation and contraction of the pupil	Basilar meningitis
Waterhouse-Friderichsen	Meningitis with sudden onset, short course of fever, coma, collapse, cyanosis, petechial hemorrhages of skin and mucous membranes	Meningitis associated with bilateral adrenal hemorrhage (e.g., meningococcal disease)
Weill's sign	Absence of expansion in the subclavicular region of the affected side	Infantile pneumonia

Table 16-13. SELECTED INFECTIOUS DISEASE–FOCUSED ACRONYMS AND ABBREVIATIONS.

Acronym or Abbreviation	Term	Acronym or Abbreviation	Term
AIDS	Acquired immunodeficiency syndrome	**HIV**	Human immunodeficiency virus
ARDS	Adult respiratory distress syndrome	**HSV**	Herpes simplex virus
BAL	Bronchoalveolar lavage	**MAC**	Mycobacterium avium intracellulare complex
BCG	Bacilli Calmette-Guerin vaccine	**MRSA**	Methicillin-resistant *Staphylococcus aureus*
CGD	Chronic granulomatous disease	**PCP**	*Pneumocystis carinii*
CMV	Cytomegalovirus	**PID**	Pelvic inflammatory disease
CJD	Creutzfeldt-Jakob disease	**PML**	Progressive multifocal leukoencephalopathy
CVAT	Costovertebral angle tenderness	**RPR**	Rapid plasma reagin (serologic test for syphilis)
EBV	Epstein-Barr virus	**RSV**	Respiratory syncytial virus
EHEC	Enterohemorrhagic *E. coli*	**SBP**	Spontaneous bacterial peritonitis
EIA	Enzyme immunoassay	**SCIDS**	Severe combined immune deficiency syndrome
ELISA	Enzyme-linked immunosorbent assay	**SIRS**	Systemic inflammatory response syndrome
FUO	Fever of unknown origin	**STD**	Sexually transmitted disease
GVHD	Graft versus host disease	**TMP-SMX**	Trimethoprim sulfamethoxazole
HUS	Hemolytic uremic syndrome	**UTI**	Urinary tract infection
HAV, HBV, HCV	Hepatitis A, B, and C virus	**VRE**	Vancomycin-resistant enterococcus
		VZV	Varicella Zoster virus

XII. DEFINITIONS (Table 16-14)

Table 16-14. INFECTIOUS DISEASE–FOCUSED DEFINITIONS.

Term	Definition
Bacteremia	Bacteria present in blood, as confirmed by culture; may be transient
Hypotension	A systolic blood pressure of <90 mmHg or a reduction of >40 mmHg from baseline in the absence of another known cause for hypotension
Infection	Presence of an organism in a normally sterile site that is usually, but not necessarily, accompanied by an inflammatory host response
Refractory septic shock	Septic shock that lasts for more than 1 hour and does not respond to fluid administration or pharmacologic intervention
Sepsis	Describes the inflammatory response to infection. See clinical evidence of infection and evidence of systemic response, manifested by two or more of the following conditions: Temperature >38°C (100.4°F) or <36°C (96.8°F) Heart rate >90 beats per minute Respiratory rate >20 breaths/minute or arterial carbon dioxide tension of <32 mm White blood cell (WBC) count: >12,000 cells/mm^3, <4000 cells/mm^3, or >10% immature band forms These changes should represent an acute alteration from baseline in the absence of another known cause for the abnormalities
Sepsis syndrome	Sepsis plus evidence of altered organ perfusion, with at least one of the following: Hypoxemia, elevated lactate, oliguria, altered mentation
Septicemia	Same as bacteremia, but implies greater severity
Septic shock	Sepsis with hypotension despite adequate fluid resuscitation, with the presence of perfusion abnormalities that may include, but are not limited to, lactic acidosis, oliguria, or an acute alteration in mental status. Patients who are receiving inotropic or vasopressor agents may not be hypotensive at the time that perfusion abnormalities are measured

Table 16-14—cont'd

TERM	DEFINITION
Severe sepsis	Sepsis associated with organ dysfunction, hypoperfusion, or hypotension. Hypoperfusion and perfusion abnormalities may include, but are not limited to, lactic acidosis, oliguria, or altered mental status
Systemic inflammatory response syndrome	Response to a wide variety of clinical insults, which can be infectious, as in sepsis, but can be noninfectious in etiology (e.g., burns, pancreatitis)

Table adapted with permission from Young LS. Sepsis syndrome. In Mandell GL, Bennett JE, Dolin R (eds), Principles and Practice of Infectious Diseases, ed 5. Philadelphia: Churchill Livingstone, 2000; 690.

XIII. SAMPLE H&P WRITE-UP

CC: "I've got the worst headache of my life."

HPI: J.R. is an 18-year-old white male college student who presents with an acute onset of the worst headache of his life. He was in his usual state of excellent health until 12 hours before admission, when he developed fever, headache, and stiff neck.

PMHx: The patient denies any chronic medical problems. He states that two other students in his dormitory have similar symptoms and are being evaluated in the emergency room.

PSHx: History of an automobile accident at age 16, during which he suffered a ruptured spleen and required a splenectomy. No other hospitalizations or surgeries.

Emergency and Trauma History: No history of head trauma. No prior transfusions.

Childhood History: Varicella at age 7. He denies any other childhood illnesses.

Occupational History: Freshman in college; works at a local fast-food restaurant as a cook.

Travel History: No recent or remote history of travel.

Sexual History: Reports monogamous relationship with healthy female student.

MEDICATIONS: Ibuprofen during the past day for headache and fever. He has not taken any other medications. The patient denies any known allergies.

HEALTH MAINTENANCE

Prevention: The patient received all of the usual childhood immunizations. He does not recall receiving any additional immunizations following his splenectomy.

Diet: Regular diet with no restrictions. Eats meals in college cafeteria and at fast-food restaurant where employed. No ingestion of raw meats.

Exercise: The patient is on the college track team.

Sleep Patterns: Wakes at most once each night to void. Denies recent changes.

Social Habits: The patient denies tobacco use or illicit drug use. Drinks approximately one six-pack of beer per weekend.

FAMILY HISTORY

First-Degree Relatives' Medical History: The patient's father has hypertension and adult-onset diabetes mellitus. The patient's mother has a history of intermittent migraine headaches that respond well to medication. The patient's two siblings have no medical problems.

PSYCHOSOCIAL HISTORY

Personal and Social History: The patient is a white college student who lives in the freshman dormitory.

REVIEW OF SYSTEMS

General: Fever, chills, rigors, and severe headache over past 12 hours.

HEENT/Neck: Positive for headache, photophobia. No discharge, difficulty swallowing, or drainage in back of throat.

Respiratory: Denies cough or dyspnea.

Cardiovascular: No chest pain, dyspnea, or history of murmur.

Gastrointestinal: Mild abdominal pain "all over" without radiation. Reports several episodes of emesis after headache began. No diarrhea.

Genitourinary: No dysuria, urinary urgency, hematuria, or discharge.

Hematopoietic/Lymphatic: No bleeding or adenopathy.

Neurologic: No loss of consciousness (LOC) or change in mentation.

Skin: New onset of rash on legs and lower abdomen.

Musculoskeletal: Recent neck stiffness.

PHYSICAL EXAMINATION

Vitals: T (oral) 102°F P 99 BP 90/60 RR 22 Weight 170 lbs.

General: Agitated, well-developed, well-nourished Caucasian male who appears his stated age. Patient is oriented to person, place, time, and circumstances, but appears in moderate distress secondary to headache.

HEENT: Head is normocephalic without palpable defects. Mild sinus tenderness on percussion. Lids/sclera normal. Conjunctivae slightly injected. Pupils measure 3 mm bilaterally and react symmetrically to light. Photophobia present. Tympanic membranes are clear and mobile. Nares are patent with slight mucosal erythema and clear nasal discharge. Neck stiff with limited range of motion. Positive Kernig's and Brudzinski's signs. Trachea normal position. No JVD.

Tonsils slightly injected but otherwise within normal limits. No adenopathy appreciated.

Lungs: Clear to auscultation bilaterally.

Cardiovascular: Normal S1 and S2. Regular rate and rhythm. No JVD, murmur.

Abdomen: Well-healed surgical scar in the left upper quadrant. Soft with diffuse mild tenderness and no localizing signs. No organomegaly, flank pain (CVAT), or suprapubic tenderness.

Genitalia: Normal circumcised male. No penile lesions/discharge, testicular pain, or masses.

Rectum/Prostate: Normal external appearance. Guaiac negative. Prostate normal size with no tenderness on palpation.

Extremities: Normal range of motion. No weakness or muscle tenderness.

Skin: Multiple purpuric lesions noted on both lower extremities and lower abdomen.

Lymphadenopathy: "Fullness" noted bilateral neck (anterior cervical), but otherwise no adenopathy.

Neurologic: Normal mental status examination and gait.

17

INTENSIVE CARE UNIT AND ADULT CRITICAL CARE MEDICINE

Alan P. Marco, MD, MMM, and Thomas Papadimos, MD, MPH

Intensive Care Unit (ICU) and Critical Care medicine covers a broad range of topics in acute care. ICU patients may present with medical, surgical, or combined illnesses. Single systems, such as the cardiovascular system in the setting of an acute myocardial infarction, or multiple organs may be involved. Depending on the hospital, the ICU may treat mixed medical and surgical patients, or it may be a specialty unit for cardiac, pulmonary, surgical, neurologic, or burn care.

A system-focused assessment of critically ill patients is preferred over the traditional approach to the patient (history, physical examination, laboratory study sequence). In Critical Care, the focus should

ICU AND ADULT CRITICAL CARE MEDICINE OUTLINE

I. Chief Complaint
II. History of Present Illness
  A. Neurologic Assessment
  B. Cardiac Assessment
  C. Pulmonary Assessment
  D. Gastrointestinal Assessment
  E. Renal Assessment
  F. Infectious Disease and Wound Assessment
  G. Hematologic Assessment
  H. Endocrinologic Assessment
  I. Miscellaneous ICU Assessment Considerations
III. Past Medical and Surgical History
IV. Medications, Allergies, and Adverse Reactions
V. Health Maintenance
VI. Family History
VII. Psychosocial History
VIII. Review of Systems
IX. Differential Diagnosis
X. Eponyms, Acronyms, and Abbreviations
XI. Definitions
XII. Sample H&P Write-Up and Progress Note

be on organ systems followed by a final synthesis of the care plan. The history often cannot be obtained from the patient; therefore, the clinician must rely on the patient's medical record, chart, and family.

I. CHIEF COMPLAINT

A. Admitting Diagnosis: Review the previous 24 hours of physician and nursing notes and laboratory findings. The patient admitted yesterday, for example, with chronic obstructive pulmonary disease (COPD) exacerbation might now be having myocardial ischemia.

B. Identifying Data

1. Obtain patient's name, age, gender, race, and ethnicity.
2. Admitted to, or transferred from (e.g., emergency department, post-op, ward)? How (e.g., ambulance)?
3. Contact person or representative (especially if patient is not able to make medical decisions).

II. HISTORY OF PRESENT ILLNESS

In the ICU setting, this portion of the H&P is intensive and relies heavily on accurate history collection from available sources and thorough physical examination of numerous organ systems to compile an accurate record of the patient's current overall status and needs.

A. Neurologic Assessment (Tables 17-1, 17-2, and 17-3)

Table 17-1. NEUROLOGIC HISTORY AND PHYSICAL EXAMINATION.

Neurologic History	
Assessment	Symptoms, Signs, or Findings
Level of consciousness (LOC)	Sedation (know drugs used), changes in LOC
Central nervous system (CNS)	History of stroke: What kind, any residual deficits? Transient ischemic attacks: Frequency, pattern, causative agents, therapy Dizziness: Precipitating factors, frequency, "lightheadedness" versus vertigo (room spinning) History of seizures
Peripheral nervous system (PNS)	Numbness, weakness, paresthesias, known neuromuscular diseases: Myasthenia, multiple sclerosis, muscular dystrophy

Continued

Table 17-1. NEUROLOGIC HISTORY AND PHYSICAL EXAMINATION—*cont'd*

Neurologic Physical Examination (at the Bedside)	
Assessment or Disorder	Symptoms, Signs, or Findings
CNS	
Gross function	Alert, oriented, following commands to respond and open eyes, responds to name, oriented to place and time, follows commands (moves extremities/digits when asked), if intubated, ask to write answers/questions on paper, Glasgow Coma Scale (GCS) <8 is comatose Must distinguish from vegetative state and locked-in syndrome
Cranial nerve examination	Ptosis (III) Corneal reflex (V) Facial droop or asymmetry (VII) Hoarse voice (X) Articulation of words (V, VII, X, XII) Abnormal eye position (III, IV, VI) Abnormal or asymmetrical pupils (II, III)
Facial nerve	Look for asymmetry, ptosis
Pupils	Consider drug effects (such as atropine)
PNS	Check reflexes, motor strength, and sensation of extremities. If using epidural analgesia, check motor and sensory level

Intracranial monitoring	Intracranial pressure (ICP) in mmHg
	If cerebrospinal fluid (CSF) drainage system present, know the system in use
	  Intracranial injury and PEEP >15–20 cm H_2O may require ICP monitoring
	Cerebral perfusion pressure should be ≥60 mmHg
	Cerebral blood flow (CBF)
	  Transcranial Doppler measures velocity of flow in the circle of Willis
	Jugular venous saturation monitoring ($SvJO_2$): Surrogate marker for O_2 extraction
	$CMRO_2 = CBF \times [C(a-v)\ O_2/100]$
	(<50% equals increasingly poor outcomes)

Electrophysiologic monitoring	Visual evoked responses (VER) Auditory: Brainstem auditory evoked responses (BAER) Somatosensory evoked potentials (SSEP) Motor evoked responses electromyograph (EMG)

Table 17-1—cont'd

NEUROLOGIC PHYSICAL EXAMINATION (AT THE BEDSIDE)	
ASSESSMENT OR DISORDER	SYMPTOMS, SIGNS, OR FINDINGS
Respiratory pattern	Cheyne-Stokes respirations Hyperventilation Ataxic breathing indicates caudal brainstem site injury
Pupils	Normal = 3-4 mm in diameter, bilaterally equal in size, constrict briskly and symmetrically to light Slightly smaller reactive pupils present in the early stages of early herniation (i.e., thalamic compression) Midposition, dilated (5–7 mm), fixed and unreactive to light signifies damage at the midbrain or lower Pinpoint pupils (1–1.5 mm) indicate focal damage of pons
Extraocular movements	Full reflex eye movements mean brainstem integrity is intact from the pontomedullary to midbrain levels. Tested by: 1. Oculovestibular reflex ("doll's eyes" maneuver) or 2. Unilateral ice water irrigation against the tympanic membrane ("calorics"). A comatose patient with an intact brainstem will demonstrate full conjugate movement of both eyes to the side of ice water stimulation. Complete absence of response to "calorics" implies a diffuse lesion of the brainstem: metabolic or structural
Motor response to pain	Localizing: Patient reaches toward stimulus Decorticate: Flexion of arm at elbow, adduction at shoulder, and extension of trunk and legs, compression of thalamus, (i.e., increasing intracranial mass) Decerebrate: Extension at elbows with internal rotation at shoulders and forearm, together with lower extremity extension (lesions compromising brainstem)

Continued

Table 17-1. NEUROLOGIC HISTORY AND PHYSICAL EXAMINATION—cont'd

NEUROLOGIC PHYSICAL EXAMINATION (AT THE BEDSIDE)	
ASSESSMENT OR DISORDER	**SYMPTOMS, SIGNS, OR FINDINGS**
	No response to pain (occasionally some knee flexion) indicates pontine and medullary lesions)
Brain death	Cessation of: 1. Hemispheric function: Findings of coma with unreceptivity and unresponsivity 2. Brainstem function: Absence of pupillary light, corneal, occulocephalic, occulovestibular, oropharyngeal and respiratory reflexes 3. Irreversibility: Cause of coma must be known and must be adequate to account for the loss of brain function

Table 17-2. CAUSES OF COMA.

ETIOLOGY OR DISORDER	DESCRIPTION
Supratentorial lesions	Produce asymmetric signs and symptoms that precede the onset of coma. Brain is compromised in a rostral-caudal manner (hemispheres, then thalamus, then midbrain, pons, and medulla)
Subtentorial lesions (brainstem)	Alters consciousness early and suddenly
Metabolic insult	Progressive rostral-caudal, level-by-level dysfunction does not occur. Insult travels through bloodstream and affects the brain diffusely. The examination will be symmetric (with the occasional exceptions of hepatic encephalopathy and hypoglycemia)
Seizure disorders	Coma by epileptic discharge to contralateral hemisphere. Obvious motor signs and recovery of consciousness is rapid

Table 17-3. MOTOR STRENGTH ASSESSMENT.

GRADE	DESCRIPTION
0/5	No muscle movement
1/5	Visible muscle movement, but no movement at the joint
2/5	Movement at the joint, but not against gravity
3/5	Movement against gravity, but not against added resistance
4/5	Movement against resistance, but less than normal
5/5	Normal strength

B. **Cardiac Assessment:** Review the vital signs (respiratory rate, pulse, blood pressure, hemoglobin saturation with oxygen [SpO_2]), as well as temperature, cardiac rhythm, arterial blood gas, and chest radiography (Tables 17-4 and 17-5).

Table 17-4. CARDIAC HISTORY AND PHYSICAL EXAMINATION.

CARDIAC HISTORY	
ASSESSMENT OR DISORDER	SYMPTOMS, SIGNS, OR FINDINGS
Blood pressure disorders	Determine usual range and previous/current therapy for hypotension and hypertension (e.g., beta-blockers, calcium channel blockers, angiotensin-converting enzyme (ACE) inhibitors, diuretics, vasodilators)
Cardiac rhythm	Arrhythmias, palpitations, atrial fibrillation Pacemaker/internal defibrillator Medical therapy (digoxin, antiarrhythmics)
Ischemia	Angina: Frequency, intensity, duration, precipitating/relieving factors
	Myocardial infarction: When, residual deficits/limitations on activity, exercise tolerance, activity level
	Congestive heart failure: Compensated or not, dyspnea on exertion, orthopnea
	Therapy: Surgical (e.g., CABG, PTCA) or medical
Valvular disease	Murmurs, known valvular disease, such as mitral valve prolapse (MVP), valve replacement

Continued

ICU

Table 17-4. CARDIAC HISTORY AND PHYSICAL EXAMINATION—cont'd

CARDIAC PHYSICAL EXAMINATION (AT THE BEDSIDE)	
ASSESSMENT OR DISORDER	**SYMPTOMS, SIGNS, OR FINDINGS**
Electrocardiograph (ECG)	Rate, rhythm, axis, left ventricle (LV) hypertrophy (LVH) Lead II: Useful for rate assessment Lead V: Useful for ischemia assessment Check electrolytes
Monitors	Arterial line (location) Pulmonary artery catheter (PAC, Swan-Ganz) +/– continuous cardiac output (CCO) Consider influence of ventilatory settings on these readings (see Table 17-7) Mixed venous O_2 (SvO_2)
Fluid status	Urinary bladder catheter (Foley) as indicator of organ perfusion IV access (type, gauge, location) and type and volume of fluid used (e.g., crystalloid, colloid, blood products)
Medications	Know the medications in use, especially vasopressors, ionotropes, and antibiotics
Cardiac examination	Neck assessment for abnormal pulsations and/or carotid bruits Palpate point of maximal apical cardiac impulse, thrills, pulses: Document and assess quality Auscultate for systolic, diastolic and holosystolic murmurs, S_1, S_2, S_3, S_4, and pericardial friction rubs, bruits: Carotid, subclavian, abdominal, femoral

Table 17-5. PULMONARY ARTERY CATHETER MEASUREMENTS AND EQUATIONS.

MEASUREMENT	EQUATIONS
Pulmonary artery occlusion pressure (PAOP, "wedge" pressure)	Read at end expiration Ventilated patient: at the tracing trough Spontaneously breathing patient: at the tracing peak

Table 17-5—cont'd

MEASUREMENT	EQUATIONS
Peak end-expiratory pressure (PEEP)	Artificially increases PAOP (PCWP) Increasing PEEP may increase SpO_2 and functional reserve capacity (FRC), but will decrease cardiac output (CO)
O_2 delivery (DO_2)	$DO_2 = Q \times CaCO_2$ (Q = C.O.) $Q \times (1.34 \times Hb \times SAO_2) \times 10$ in mL/min/m^2 Normal = 520-570 mL/min/m^2
O_2 uptake	$VO_2 = Q \times 13.4 \times Hb \times (SAO_2 - SVO_2)$ Normal = 110-160 ml/min/m^2
O_2 extraction ratio (O_2ER)	O_2 ER = $VO_2/DO_2 \times 100\%$ (normal = 20-30%)
Cardiac index (CI)	CI = CO/BSA, target is 3 2.2 L/min/m^2
Mixed venous oxygen (SVO_2)	$SVO_2 = DO_2/VO_2 = (CO/VO_2) \times Hb \times SAO_2$ Normal @ 65-75% 5% change lasting more than 10 minutes is significant

C. **Pulmonary Assessment:** Determine level of respiratory support (ventilator, oxygen mask/nasal cannula, room air). Know the settings and FIO_2, vital signs (especially SAO_2), and recent arterial blood gas (ABG) findings (Tables 17-6 and 17-7).

Table 17-6. PULMONARY HISTORY AND PHYSICAL EXAMINATION.

PULMONARY HISTORY	
ASSESSMENT OR DISORDER	SYMPTOMS, SIGNS, DISORDERS, OR FINDINGS
Smoking history	Number of pack-years, acute/chronic bronchitis
Reactive airway disease (RAD)	COPD versus asthma Current and at-home therapy (e.g., O_2, beta-agonists, inhaled or systemic steroids, anticholenergics, aminophylline)
Infection	Pneumonia: Bacterial, viral, fungal indicators
Parenchymal lung disease	Interstitial fibrosis, occupational diseases (e.g., asbestosis, black lung, silicosis)
Previous respiratory failure	Prior intubation for respiratory failure (know when, why, and how long) Previous tracheostomy: Patent or closed

Continued

Table 17-6. PULMONARY HISTORY AND PHYSICAL EXAMINATION—cont'd

PULMONARY PHYSICAL EXAMINATION (AT THE BEDSIDE)	
ASSESSMENT OR DISORDER	**SYMPTOMS, SIGNS, DISORDERS, OR FINDINGS**
Chest examination	Palpate neck and chest for crepitus (air), hematomas, or defects (especially if fresh tracheostomy) Auscultate neck for air leaks Lung fields: Wheezes, crackles, evidence of infiltrates, pleural fluid, pneumothorax Note productive cough and character of expectorant
Respiratory pattern	Note tachypnea, tracheal "tugs," sternal retractions, or a "rocking boat" appearance to the patient's breathing pattern
Tubes	Endotracheal, chest, feeding: Know size, depth (especially endotracheal tube) Check for function, leaks, input/output

Table 17-7. VENTILATOR DATA.

ASSESSMENT	SETTINGS OR FINDINGS
Ventilator settings	FIO_2, tidal volume (TV), rate (mechanical and native), mode of ventilation (e.g., SIMV, AC, PC, PEEP, CPAP, APRV)
Peak end-expiratory pressure (PEEP)	PEEP >10 cm H_2O impairs CO, raises ICP, affects PAC readings
Peak inspiratory pressure (PIP)	Should be <40-45 cm H_2O
Plateau pressure	<30-35 cm H_2O
Static compliance	Plateau pressure-PEEP Normal is 100 mL/cm H_2O If <30-35 100 mL/cm H_2O, weaning difficult
PAO_2/FIO_2 ratio	If <238, extubation is difficult
Frequency-volume ratio (RR/V_T)	Normal <50 breaths/min/L If >100 breaths/min/L, will not wean
Ventilator trigger	Flow-by or negative pressure affects work of breathing
Arterial blood gases	Written as: pH/$PaCO_2$/PAO_2/HCO_3^- Normal range of values at sea level: PAO_2: 75-100 mmHg $PaCO_2$: 35-45 mmHg pH: 7.35-7.45 SAO_2: 94-100% HCO_3^-: 22-26 mEq/L

D. **Gastrointestinal Assessment:** In the ICU, hepatic and bowel function, infection, and metabolic issues are the most relevant aspects (Tables 17-8 and 17-9).

Table 17-8. GASTROINTESTINAL HISTORY AND PHYSICAL EXAMINATION.

Assessment	Symptoms, Signs, or Findings
	Gastrointestinal History
Bowel function	Note if patient is being fed and rationale if not (see Table 17-9). Note signs of obstruction or diarrhea
Hepatic function	Hepatitis (A, B, C, or drug/toxin exposure), residual function, presence of jaundice (suggests bilirubin >2 mg/dL), cirrhosis and/or ascites, hepatic encephalopathy
	Gastrointestinal Physical Examination (at the Bedside)
Assessment	**Symptoms, Signs, or Findings**
Function	Note flatus or stool (diarrhea: increased osmolality of nutritional feedings, rate of feedings, and *C. difficile* and elixir that contains sorbitol)
Abdomen	Size, bowel sounds, pain, tympani, organ size, masses
Tubes	Drains, ostomies, feeding tubes (nasogastric, gastrostomy, jejunostomy), rectal tubes

Table 17-9. NUTRITIONAL STATUS/FEEDING.

Assessment or Disorder	Symptoms, Signs, or Findings
Nutritional requirements	Basal energy expenditure (BEE) (Kcal/day) = 25 × wt (kg) Resting energy expenditure (REE) = 1.2 BEE (resting, but not fasting)
Total parenteral nutrition (TPN)	Peripheral (short term) Central (long term)
Enteral nutrition routes	Nasogastric/orogastric tube (14-16 French) Duodenal (8-10 French) Jejunostomy Confirm position of tubes by radiograph post-placement as needed

Continued

Table 17-9. NUTRITIONAL STATUS/FEEDING—*cont'd*

Assessment or Disorder	Symptoms, Signs, or Findings
Feeding	Infusions should be for 12–16 hrs/day (continuous infusions stress bowel) Determine gastric retention before starting. (Give water at the selected rate for 1 hour, clamp the tube, and measure the residual after 30 minutes. If <50%, proceed with feedings, if >50%, consider duodenal or jejunal route.)
Feeding tube occlusion	Warm, agitated water injected through tube with syringe or use of pancreatic enzyme
Pulmonary aspiration of feedings	Glucose concentration greater than 20 mg/dL in tracheal aspirate

E. **Renal Assessment:** In the ICU, renal function, its effects on electrolyte and fluid balance, and drug metabolism/excretion are most important (Tables 17-10 and 17-11).

Table 17-10. RENAL HISTORY AND PHYSICAL EXAMINATION.

Renal History	
Assessment or Disorder	**Symptoms, Signs, or Findings**
Renal function	Acute failure Chronic failure Note any intervention(s)
Concurrent medical conditions affecting renal function	Hypertension, diabetes, toxin (NSAIDS, aminoglycosides), polycystic disease, nephritis, UTIs, recent surgery on or near the kidney
Treatment	Hemodialysis, peritoneal dialysis, transplantation
Related issues	Electrolyte problems (Na^+ and K^+ balance), water restrictions, acid-base changes, coagulation status, infections, anemia, heart failure, hypertension, hyperglycemia, hyperparathyroidism

Table 17-10—cont'd

RENAL PHYSICAL EXAMINATION (AT THE BEDSIDE)	
ASSESSMENT	**SYMPTOMS, SIGNS, OR FINDINGS**
Fluid balance	All fluids, drains, Foley and nutrition, NG, rectal, skin turgor (sign of dehydration), peripheral edema, rales, S_3 gallop
Electrolytes	K^+, Na^+, Mg^{++}, Ca^{++}
Urine output	30 mL/hr or 0.25-0.5 mL/kg/hr minimum
Plasma osmolality (mosm/kg H_2O)	= 2 × (serum sodium mEq/L) + glucose (mg/dL)/18 + BUN(mg/dL)/2.8
Creatinine clearance (ml/min)	(140-age) × weight (kg)/(72 × serum creatinine) (mg/dL) For women, divide this number by 0.85 to account for less muscle mass
Fractional excretion of sodium	$\{U_{[Na^+]}/Plasma_{[Na^+]}\}/\{U_{[Cr]}/Plasma_{[Cr]}\} \times 100$ Diuretics alter FENa
Glomerular filtration	Tested by BUN (10-20 mg/dL), creatinine (0.7-1.5 mg/dL), and creatinine clearance (110-150 mL/min)
Tubular function	Tested by specific gravity (1.003-1.030), osmolality (40-1400 mosm/L) Urine sodium 1. >10 mmol/L may indicate diuretics, emesis, intrinsic renal diseases, Addison disease, hypothyroidism, or SIADH 2. >40 mmol/L of Na^+ and Cl^- suggests hypothyroidism, SIADH, or high intake 3. >40 mmol/L in oliguria suggests acute tubular necrosis 4. Low Na^+ excretion may be found with early obstructive uropathy, with oliguria of acute glomerulonephritis, and in some patients with x-ray contrast acute renal failure

Table 17-11. COMMON CAUSES AND DIAGNOSES OF RENAL FAILURE.

CLASSIFICATION	COMMON CAUSES	DIAGNOSIS
Prerenal	Congestive heart failure, hypovolemia	Urine specific gravity > 1.016 UNa < 20 mEq/L FENa < 1 % Urinary urea > 250 mmol/L Osmolality > 500 mosm/kg
Renal	Interstitial nephritis, vasculitis, acute tubular necrosis, acute glomerulonephritis	Urine specific gravity > 1.010 UNa > 40 meq/L FENa > 2 % Urinary urea < 185 mmol/L Isotonic urine 300-350 mosm/kg
Post-renal	Stones, Foley catheter obstruction, obstruction by tumor	Acute: prerenal values, chronic: renal values

F. **Infectious Disease and Wound Assessment:** Patients in both medical and surgical ICUs are at risk for infection from either their underlying diseases or iatrogenic sources such as invasive procedures (Tables 17-12 and 17-13).

Table 17-12. HISTORY AND PHYSICAL EXAMINATION FOR INFECTIOUS DISEASE AND WOUND ASSESSMENT.

INFECTIOUS DISEASE AND WOUND ASSESSMENT HISTORY	
ASSESSMENT	**SYMPTOMS, SIGNS, OR FINDINGS**
Underlying reason/conditions regarding ICU admission	Gives clues as to sources and risks of infection
Degree of infection	Localized or sepsis
Recent documented infections	Sites, organisms, treatments
Immune function	Immunocompromised from HIV, cancer, chemotherapy, steroids, transplant recipient
INFECTIOUS DISEASE AND WOUND ASSESSMENT PHYSICAL EXAMINATION (AT THE BEDSIDE)	
ASSESSMENT	**SYMPTOMS, SIGNS, OR FINDINGS**
Vital signs	Fever, tachycardia, tachypnea
Cultures	Know what was sent, results, organisms, antimicrobial sensitivities

Table 17-13. SOURCES OF INFECTIONS IN ICU PATIENTS.

Source	Symptoms, Signs, Findings or Disorders
Vector-borne	Pertinent to geographic location or recent travel (e.g., West Nile virus, Lyme disease, equine encephalopathy, Hanta virus)
Pulmonary	CXR for pneumonia, radiographs of sinuses (especially with nasotracheal intubation), dye/glucose testing of pulmonary secretions for aspiration, evidence of consolidation on auscultation
Vascular cannulation sites	Peripheral IVs, central lines, arterial lines Note presence or absence of induration, skin necrosis, pus, movement of catheter from original position (in or out), need for more frequent dressing changes
Wounds	Induration, pus, skin necrosis, fluctuance
Other invasive sites	Chest tubes, drains, stents: Investigate as mentioned previously
Urinary	Urine microscopic examination Consider presence of Foley catheter or urinary stents
Other causes	Pseudomembranous colitis, acalculous cholecystitis

G. **Hematologic Assessment:** The hematologic history and examination in the ICU setting focuses on coagulation ability and oxygen-carrying capacity (Tables 17-14 and 17-15).

H. **Endocrinologic Assessment:** In the ICU, diabetes, thyroid, neuroendocrine function, and steroid use are the most relevant (Table 17-16).

I. **Miscellaneous ICU Assessment Considerations**

1. Obstetrics.
   a. Consider possibility of pregnancy in patients at risk; determine first day of last menstrual period (LMP).
   b. Consider preeclampsia or eclampsia.
2. Cervical spine.
   a. A stable C-spine is likely in patients who are alert, aware, without mental status changes and neck pain, and who have no distracting injuries or neurologic defects.

ICU

Table 17-14. HEMATOLOGIC HISTORY AND PHYSICAL EXAMINATION.

Hematologic History	
Assessment or Disorder	**Symptoms, Signs, or Findings**
Bleeding/bruising in past	Congenital coagulopathy (hemophilia, von Willebrand's disease)
	Acquired coagulopathy (anticoagulant therapy: warfarin/heparin, antiplatelet drugs, disseminated intravascular coagulation)
Anemia	Sickle cell disease (SCD) or trait, thalassemia, hemorrhage, nutritional status
Recent transfusion	Amount/type of components, current type and screen or crossmatch available
Hematologic Physical Examination (at the Bedside)	
Assessment or Disorder	**Symptoms, Signs, or Findings**
Cardiac	Tachycardia, hypotension, murmurs, orthostasis
Urologic	Hematuria from Foley irritation
Skin	Color, ecchymoses, petechiae, bleeding from surgical or catheter sites

Table 17-15. TRANSFUSIONS ASSESSMENT.

Assessment or Disorder	Symptoms, Signs, or Findings
Transfusion trigger	Hemoglobin less than 7 g/dL in those with heart disease/dysfunction and/or cerebrovascular insufficiency Ongoing cardiac and/or cerebrovascular ischemia in patients with adequate blood volume, increased lactate levels, or VO_2 less than 100 mL/min/m^2 O_2 ER greater than 0.5 in those with adequate cardiac index/output
Red blood cells (RBCs)	Available as whole blood, packed RBCs, leukocyte-reduced RBCs (for those with antibodies to leukocytes or to minimize cytokine-related reactions), and washed RBCs (for hypersensitivity transfusion reactions)

Table 17-15—cont'd

ASSESSMENT OR DISORDER	SYMPTOMS, SIGNS, OR FINDINGS
Adverse reactions	Acute hemolytic reactions, febrile nonhemolytic reactions, allergic reactions, acute lung injury, transmission of infectious agents (viral and bacterial)
Blood products are available as:	Typed and crossed (preferred) Type specific, partially crossmatched Type specific, non-crossmatched "O" negative, universal donor

Table 17-16. ENDOCRINOLOGIC HISTORY AND PHYSICAL EXAMINATION.

ENDOCRINOLOGIC HISTORY	
ASSESSMENT OR DISORDER	SYMPTOMS, SIGNS, OR FINDINGS
Diabetes	Type 1 or 2 diabetes, normal treatment regimen and current treatment
Thyroid	Hyper/hypothyroid, replacement, symptoms (heat/cold intolerance, lethargy, weight gain, cardiac arrhythmias, dry skin)
Steroids	Indications, dose, timing of last dose
Neuroendocrine	Intracranial tumor, head trauma
ENDOCRINOLOGIC PHYSICAL EXAMINATION (AT THE BEDSIDE)	
ASSESSMENT OR DISORDER	SYMPTOMS, SIGNS, OR FINDINGS
Vital signs	Especially with thyroid disease: temperature
Blood glucose	Current levels and treatment, polyuria
Urine output	Osmotic diuresis from excessive glucose, SIADH

ICU

b. All other patients should have the following:
   (1) Lateral view of C-spine (include base of occiput to upper border of T_1).
   (2) Open-mouth odontoid view with lateral masses of C_1 vertebra and entire odontoid process.
   (3) Flexion/extension views of C-spine in those with neck pain and normal radiographs.

III. PAST MEDICAL AND SURGICAL HISTORY

A. Past Medical History

1. Neurologic: Stroke, transient ischemic attack (TIA), seizures, spinal cord injury.
2. Cardiac: Hypertension (HTN), myocardial infarction (MI), angina, valvular disease, congestive heart failure (CHF), paroxysmal nocturnal dyspnea (PND), dyspnea on exertion (DOE).
3. Pulmonary: COPD/asthma, prior intubation for respiratory failure, current pneumonia/bronchitis, other lung diseases.
4. Renal: Renal failure and end-stage renal disease (ESRD).
5. Endocrine: Diabetes (Type I or Type II), thyroid disease, syndrome of inappropriate antidiuretic hormone secretion (SIADH).

B. Past Surgical History: Prior surgical procedures and dates.

C. Emergency and Trauma History: Hospitalizations, transfusions, and injuries.

D. Childhood History: Congenital defects (cardiac), cerebral palsy, genetic diseases, or inborn errors of metabolism (cystic fibrosis, phenylketonuria [PKU]).

E. Occupational History: Type of work, occupational exposure to toxins (black lung, solvents, insecticides).

F. Travel History: Exposure to tropical diseases, parasites, insect and animal vectors.

IV. MEDICATIONS, ALLERGIES, AND ADVERSE REACTIONS

A. Medications

1. Prescription medications: Indications, last dose, duration of use, and possible drug interactions. Annotate date started and regimen changes. A medication list at the bottom of the HPI or within the past medical history section is helpful. Indicate on admission note all routine medications taken at home as well as current therapy.
2. Over-the-counter (OTC) medications: Analgesics, laxatives, sleeping medications, vitamins or supplements, herbal preparations, and diet pills.
3. Alternative medicine therapies.

B. Allergies and Adverse Reactions

1. What was the allergic reaction (e.g., respiratory or dermatologic manifestations)?
2. How was the allergic reaction treated?
3. What was the route of medication administration when the allergy occurred (e.g., po, IV, SQ)?

MEDICATION LIST EXAMPLE.

Medication	Dose and Route	Frequency	Indication
HOME MEDICATIONS			
Aspirin	(325 mg) two tabs po	prn (qd, bid, tid, qhs)	Headache
Cimetidine (Tagamet)	400 mg po	bid (qac and qhs)	Dyspepsia
CURRENT MEDICATIONS			
Dopamine	3 mg/kg/min	IV drip	Renal support

4. Differentiate between allergic manifestations and adverse reactions. Often an adverse effect does not represent a true IgE-mediated allergy, but rather intolerance to the medication (e.g., gastrointestinal upset with codeine).
5. Environmental allergies: Assess for history of reactive airway disease (RAD), hay fevers/allergic rhinitis, food allergies, and dermatologic reactions (e.g., nickel in earrings).

V. **HEALTH MAINTENANCE**

A. **Prevention:** Primary and secondary prevention are not typically a concern in ICU patients and are deferred to the primary care provider. Tertiary prevention (e.g., rehabilitation) needs to be addressed after patient is released from the ICU.

B. **Diet:** Preadmission diet not typically a concern in ICU patients.

C. **Exercise/Recreation:** Relevant only to determine exercise tolerance (cardiac function) and toxin/infectious disease exposure (e.g., *Chlamydia psittacosis* in pigeon fanciers and arboviruses in travelers).

D. **Sleep Patterns:** Assess for any awakening from sleep at night in pain or short of breath.

E. **Social Habit:** Alcohol, tobacco, and illicit drug use should be queried when possible.

VI. **FAMILY HISTORY:** Focus on cardiac risk factors.

VII. **PSYCHOSOCIAL HISTORY**

A. **Availability of Caregivers After Discharge:** Consider social worker involvement and early discharge planning.

B. **Living Will, Power of Attorney, and Do Not Resuscitate (DNR) Code Status:** These issues must be addressed.

C. **Restrictions on Care:** Patient's personal and religious preferences must be considered (e.g., no blood for Jehovah's Witnesses).

VIII. REVIEW OF SYSTEMS (Table 17-17)

Table 17-17. NONSPECIFIC SYMPTOMS AND DISEASE CONSIDERATIONS.

Symptom	Disease/Condition
Abdominal pain	Obstruction, ischemia, infarction, peritonitis, perforated viscus, gastric distension, ulcer disease/GI bleed, drugs, cholecystitis, metabolic disorders, tumors
Altered mental status	Drug effect (sedation/anesthesia) CVA, TIA, hypotension, CNS infection, CNS trauma, intracranial space-occupying lesion, postictal, ICU psychosis
Back pain	Trauma, bone fracture, aortic aneurysm, renal trauma/stone/infection, ruptured disc, metabolic (Paget's disease), tumors, systemic inflammatory disease, referred pain
Chest pain	MI, angina, esophagitis, rib/sternal fractures (blunt trauma or after CPR), pleuritic pain, pericarditis, pulmonary embolus, pneumonia
Dizziness	Hyperventilation, cardiac arrhythmia, stress, position change, head movement, drugs
Dyspnea	Anemia, asthma, COPD, restrictive lung disease, angina/CAD, CHF, bronchitis, pulmonary embolus, aspiration, anaphylaxis, pneumothorax, pain, airway obstruction, hypoxia, ventilator settings
Fever	Infections, collagen vascular disease, tissue injury (pulmonary embolus, sickle cell crisis, hemolysis), drugs, lymphoma, leukemia, familial Mediterranean fever, Fabry's disease, cyclic neutropenia
Headache	Vascular headache: Migraine, cluster, hypertension, alcohol, toxins, drugs, occlusive vascular disease Tension headache Traction-inflammation headache: Cranial arteritis, increased/decreased ICP, extracranial structural lesions, pituitary tumors Cranial neuralgias Extracranial structural lesions: Ocular lesions, sinusitis, tumor

Table 17-17—cont'd

SYMPTOM	DISEASE/CONDITION
Hypercarbia	Inadequate ventilator settings, bronchospasm, patient fatigue in setting of pulmonary compromise, metabolic alkalosis (e.g., induced by aggressive diuresis)
Hypertension	Pain, preexisting HTN, disruption of regulatory mechanisms (baroreceptors), withdrawal of routine medications, aggressive antihypotensive therapy (iatrogenic: too much vasopressor)
Hypotension	Volume depletion (inadequate input/excessive output, bleeding, GI losses), cardiogenic shock, spinal shock, sepsis
Hypoxia	CHF, pneumonia, interstitial lung disease, ARDS, atelectasis, sepsis, hepatic failure
Jaundice	Hepatic failure, acute cholecystitis/cholestasis, mobilization of hematoma (especially in trauma patients), transfusion reaction
Joint pain	Injury, arthritis (rheumatoid, osteoarthritis, infectious), infection, connective tissue disease, gout, pseudogout, hyperparathyroidism, hemochromatosis, hypophosphatemia, hypomagnesemia, myxedematous hypothyroidism, ochronosis
Malaise/fatigue	MI, anemia, drugs, viral/bacterial infection, Addison's disease, joint/muscle injury or inflammation, neuromuscular junction disease (myasthenia gravis, Lambert-Eaton), primary muscle disease
Myalgias	Viral or bacterial illness, drugs (succinylcholine, statins), inflammatory myopathies (dermatomyocytis, eosinophilia-myalgia syndrome), polymyalgia rheumatica, myxedema, myotonic disorders, necrotizing vasculitis, myoglobinemia, Vitamin B_{12} deficiency associated neuropathies, arsenic intoxication, alcoholism
Nausea	Toxins/drugs, MI, bradycardia, hypotension, pain, gastric retention, visceral perforation/inflammation/ischemia, high small bowel obstruction, peritonitis, metabolic disorders, intracranial disease or injury
Thirst	Diabetes mellitus, nonketotic hyperglycemia, hypovolemia/dehydration, hypernatremia, hypothalamic injury

Continued

Table 17-17. NONSPECIFIC SYMPTOMS AND DISEASE CONSIDERATIONS—*cont'd*

SYMPTOM	DISEASE/CONDITION
Tinnitus	Drugs, vascular tumors, aneurysm, vascular malformation, vascular compression, tumor (acoustic neuroma, cerebello-pontine angle tumor), brainstem ischemia/infarction, multiple sclerosis
Vertigo	Multiple sclerosis, labyrinthine concussion, ototoxicity, drugs, trauma, tumor (e.g., acoustic neuroma, cerebello-pontine angle tumor)
Weakness	Consider neuromuscular blockade, CVA, spinal cord injury, peripheral nerve injury, Guillain-Barré, autoimmune diseases (e.g., polymyalgia rheumatica)

IX. DIFFERENTIAL DIAGNOSIS (Table 17-18)

Table 17-18. ICU-FOCUSED DIFFERENTIAL DIAGNOSIS.

CONDITION/DISORDER	POSSIBLE DIAGNOSES
Bradycardia	Drugs, increased ICP, cardiac disease, acidosis, allergic reaction
Dyspnea	Chest wall disease (polio), COPD, granulomatous disease, asthma, aspiration, atelectasis, pneumonia, pneumothorax, pulmonary edema, pulmonary embolism, systemic illness (sepsis, shock, fever, acidosis, hypoxia)
Dysrhythmia	Hypovolemia, hypotension, anemia, hypoxia, hypercarbia, drugs, pain, myocardial disease, electrolyte abnormalities, endocrine disease, hypothermia, hyperthermia
Fever	Thrombophlebitis, infection, drugs, UTI, aspiration, atelectasis
Hypotension	Hypovolemia, acute blood loss, anaphylaxis, adrenal disease, arrhythmia, decreased ionotropy, hypoxia, sepsis, hypothermia, transfusion reaction, tension pneumothorax, pulmonary emboli (air, fat, clot), drugs, hypoglycemia

Table 17-18—cont'd

CONDITION/DISORDER	POSSIBLE DIAGNOSES
Hypoxia	Low FIO_2, hypoventilation, right-to-left cardiac shunts, V/Q mismatch, atelectasis, diffusion impairment, pulmonary edema, pulmonary embolus, pneumothorax, bronchospasm, low cardiac output, mechanical obstruction of endotracheal tube
Hypertension	Pain, hypoxia, hypercarbia, essential hypertension, hypothermia, drugs, bladder distension, autonomic hyperreflexia, fluid overload
Mental status changes	Hypoxia, pain, drugs, infection, hypoglycemia, hyponatremia, uremia, malignant hyperthermia, hypercalcemia, TIA, aneurysm, stroke
Tachycardia	Sepsis, cardiac disease, endocrine disease, hypovolemia, hypoxia, hypercarbia, fever, pulmonary embolus, pneumothorax, anemia, anxiety

X. EPONYMS, ACRONYMS, AND ABBREVIATIONS (Table 17-19)

XI. DEFINITIONS (Table 17-20)

XII. SAMPLE H&P WRITE-UP AND PROGRESS NOTE

A. ICU H&P

CC: Blunt trauma to the chest and abdomen, exploratory laparotomy with splenectomy, post-op day 1.

HPI: 63-year-old white male unrestrained passenger in motor vehicle accident with blunt trauma to the chest and abdomen. Awake and moving all extremities but hypotensive in the ED and ultrasound showed intraperitoneal blood. Exploratory laparotomy and splenectomy was performed. Blood loss was 3 liters, and the patient received 4 units PRBCs and 4 liters of crystalloid. Cefazolin was also administered intraoperatively. He was transferred to the ICU intubated and mechanically ventilated.

MHx: COPD, HTN, DM (type 2), renal insufficiency.

SHx: Right hip arthroplasty 3 years ago, right inguinal hernia repair 7 years ago, left ankle ORIF 3 years ago.

Medications: *Home medications:* ipratropium MDI, albuterol MDI, lisinopril, insulin (unknown doses). *Current medications:* cefazolin 1 g q6h, insulin drip 1-2 units/hour, albuterol and ipratropium MDI q4h, propofol 50 μg/kg/hr.

Allergies: None known.

Table 17-19. ICU EPONYMS, ACRONYMS, AND ABBREVIATIONS.

ACRONYM OR ABBREVIATION	DEFINITION	ACRONYM OR ABBREVIATION	DEFINITION
ABG	Arterial blood gas	F_{IO_2}	Fraction of inspired oxygen
AC	Assist control	**HTN**	Hypertension
APRV	Airway pressure release ventilation	**I/O**	Intake/output
ARDS	Adult respiratory distress syndrome	**IDU**	Intravenous drug use
BEE	Basal energy expenditure	**IJ**	Internal jugular (vein)
CABG	Coronary artery bypass graft	**MAP**	Mean arterial pressure
CAD	Coronary artery disease	**MDI**	Metered-dose inhaler (for administration of bronchodilators or inhaled steroids)
CBF	Cerebral blood flow (or coronary blood flow)	**MI**	Myocardial infarction
CHF	Congestive heart failure	**MV**	Minute ventilation
$CMRO_2$	Cerebral metabolic rate of oxygen consumption	**PAOP, PAWP, "wedge"**	Pulmonary artery occlusion pressure, pulmonary artery wedge pressure. The balloon-tipped PAC occludes the distal PA and the pressure recorded from the distal orifice is felt to reflect the left atrial and (by extension) the left ventricular filling pressures

CO	Cardiac output	**PAP**	Peak airway pressure
COPD	Chronic obstructive pulmonary disease	**PEEP**	Peak end-expiratory pressure
CPAP	Continuous positive airway pressure	**PIP**	Peak inspiratory pressure
CPP	Cerebral perfusion pressure, CPP = MAP – RAP or ICP, whichever is higher	**PRBCs**	Packed red blood cells
CVP	Central venous pressure	**PVR**	Pulmonary vascular resistance
CXR	Chest x-ray	**SIADH**	Syndrome of inappropriate antidiuretic hormone release
DIC	Disseminated intravascular coagulation	**SIMV**	Synchronized intermittent mandatory ventilation
EF	Ejection fraction	**SpO_2**	Oxygen saturation
ESRD	End stage renal disease	**SSEP**	Somatosensory evoked potential(s)
ETT	Endotracheal tube	**SvO_2**	Mixed venous O_2
FFP	Fresh frozen plasma	**TPN**	Total parenteral nutrition

Table 17-20. COMMON ICU TERMS.

TERM	DEFINITION
Advance directive	Varies by state, but includes Living Will, Do-not-Resuscitate (DNR) order, etc.
Cerebral blood flow (CBF)	Usually expressed as mL/100 g tissue
Cheyne-Stokes respiration	A pattern of breathing with gradually increasing depth followed by a decrease in depth to apnea. Seen with metabolic encephalopathy and coma or injury that affects respiratory centers
Crystalloid	Isotonic salt solutions for volume repletion such as normal saline (NS) or lactated Ringer's (LR)
Dead space	Areas of the lung that receive ventilation but no perfusion
ICU psychosis	Delirium seen in ICU patients. Diagnosis of exclusion, but may be related to multidrug therapy and sleep deprivation
Ionotropy	Vigorousness of cardiac contractility
Neuromuscular blockade	Chemical paralysis induced by drugs that block neuromuscular transmission (e.g., pancuronium, rocuronium, vecuronium, atracurium, cisatracurium)
Pulmonary artery catheter (PAC, Swan-Ganz)	Percutaneous, intravenous catheter used to measure cardiac output (thermodilution or continuous)
Shunt	Areas of lung that are perfused but not ventilated
V/Q mismatch	Imbalance between ventilation and perfusion, either a shunt or dead space

Social History: 2 pack per day × 40 years smoker, 1-2 drinks/day, no IDU or illicit drugs. Lives alone, office clerk, no advance directives,

Physical Examination: *General:* Weight today 70.6 kg, Right IJ 9 Fr sheath, 16 g IV both antecubital fossae, left radial arterial catheter, Foley catheter, hard cervical collar, intubated. *Neuro:* Sedated, moves all extremities to noxious stimulus, PERRL, no palpable step-off of cervical spine. *Pulmonary:* Breath sounds bilaterally coarse and with inspiratory rhonchi in all fields. Expiratory wheezes at bases. No spontaneous respiration ecchymoses right side.

ABG 7.25/48/65/25 on SIMV 10, V_T 700, FIO_2 0.8, PEEP 10, PS 5.

SAO_2 92 %, PAP 39, Plateau pressure 33, Static compliance 700/33 = 21.2 mL/cm H_2O, PAO_2/FIO_2 = 65/0.8 = 81.

No chest tubes.

CXR: Early bilateral pulmonary contusion, fracture right 5th and 6th ribs.

Cardiovascular: P 110, BP 95/60, supine CVP 5.

ECG: Tachycardia, LAD, nonspecific ST-T wave changes.

Regular rhythm, no murmurs, rubs, or gallops.

GI/nutrition: Abdomen with dressing, wound clean, no erythema or induration. No bowel sounds. NPO, no tube feeds/TPN/PPN.

Bilirubin, alkaline phosphatase, albumen, SGOT, SGPT, amylase, lipase pending.

Renal: I/O: 1250 LR in/ 350 urine out.

The common lab values are entered on a miniature chart. We have inserted the chart with labels and the values as they would be entered in real life:

Na^+	Cl^-	BUN	Glu
K^+	$HCO3^-$	Cr	

140	95	30	350
3.6	28	1.6	

Ca^{+2} 1.01, Mg^+ 1.9

Heme/ID: T_{IT} Hgb mission, $T_{current}$ 35.6°C

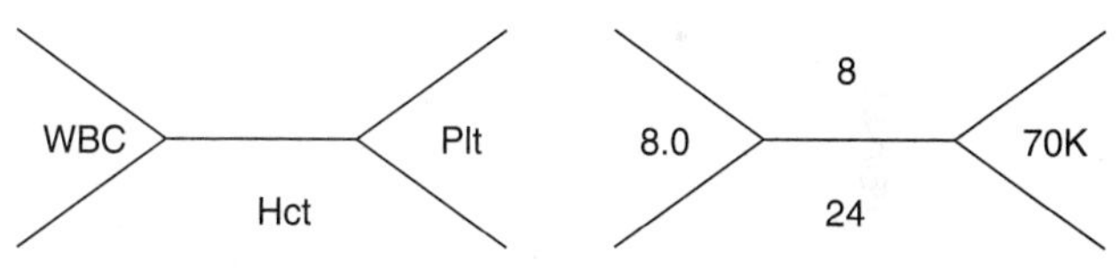

Cultures: none.

Lines: Right IJ day 1, arterial day 1.

Extremities: 4 limbs cool, delayed capillary refill, radial and femoral pulses palpable, pedal and posterior tibial pulses by Doppler, not palpated.

B. ICU Progress Note Format

1. Date:
2. Hospital/ICU day:
3. Physical examination numbers: T, BP, HR, RR, SpO_2; preop weight, yesterday, today
4. 24-hour events:
5. Neuro: Mental status/Glasgow Coma Scale (MS/GCS), deep tendon reflexes (DTRs), focal deficits.
6. Respiratory (Resp): Lung exam, tracheostomy, ventilator mode, fraction of inspired oxygen (FiO_2), rate (R), tidal

volume (TV), peak end-expiratory pressure (PEEP), minute volume (MV), peak inspiratory pressure (PIP), hydrogen ion concentration (pH), partial pressure (tension) of carbon dioxide (P_{CO_2}), partial pressure (tension) of oxygen (P_{O_2}), oxygen saturation (SAT), bicarbonate dissolved in blood (HCO_3^-). CXR: Weaning parameters (from the ventilator).

7. Cardiovascular (CV): Exam, HR, mean arterial pressure (MAP), central venous pressure (CVP), PAP, pulmonary capillary wedge pressure (PCWP), cardiac output (CO), systemic vascular resistance (SVR), peripheral vascular resistance (PVR), alveolar-arterial oxygen gradient (A-a D_{O_2}), oxygen delivery (D_{O_2}), oxygen consumption or uptake (V_{O_2}), electrocardiograph (ECG), cardiovascular medications (CV meds).
8. Nutrition/Metabolic: Electrolytes, calcium (Ca), magnesium (Mg), phosphorus (Phos), albumin (Alb), cholesterol (Chol), triglycerides (TG), glucose range, 24-hour insulin, nitrogen balance, diet, basal energy expenditure (BEE), calories (Kcal), protein, dextrose/fat ratio (Dex/fat).
9. Fluids/Lines: Arterial, nasogastric tube (NG), Foley, exam, edema.

   Inputs (Is): Total parenteral nutrition (TPN), intravenous (IV), per os or by mouth (PO) = total.

   Outputs (Os): Urine, nasogastric tube (NG), drains- = total.

   Net fluid balance=
10. Renal: Blood urea nitrogen (BUN), creatinine (Cr), hourly urine output (UOP), urine electrolytes: sodium (Na), potassium (K), chloride (Cl), serum/urine osmolarity (S/U Osm), creatinine clearance (Cr clearance).

    Urinalysis (UA): Specific gravity (Sp gr), protein (Pr), and list other parameters.
11. GI/Hepatic: Examination: Serum aspartate aminotransferase (ALT), serum alanine aminotransferase (AST) (ALT:AST ratio or SGPT/SGOT ratio), alkaline phosphatase (Alk phos), total/direct bilirubin (T/D Bili), albumin (Alb), total protein (TP).
12. Heme: White blood cells (WBC), hemoglobin and hematocrit (H/H), platelets (PLT), prothrombin time/partial prothrombin time (PT/PTT), thrombin time (TT), reticulocytes (Retic), fibrin (Fib), fibrin split products (FSP), blood products.
13. Skin: Examination, decubiti, dressings.
14. I.D.: Temperature (Temp), WBC, cultures/Gram stains, antibiotics (dose and day).
15. Radiology:
16. Other studies:
17. Medications:

18

INTERNAL MEDICINE AND FAMILY PRACTICE

Eric H. Hanson MD, MPH, and J. Eric Bermudez, MD

This chapter is an expanded version of the history and physical examination essentials presented in Chapter 1. This section focuses only on the H&P because of the breadth of topics covered by Internal Medicine and Family Practice, which are covered throughout the other specialty-focused H&P chapters.

INTERNAL MEDICINE AND FAMILY PRACTICE OUTLINE

I. Chief Complaint
II. Past History of Present Illness
III. Past Medical and Surgical History
   A. Past Medical History
   B. Past Surgical History
   C. Emergency and Trauma History
   D. Childhood History
   E. Occupational History
   F. Travel History
   G. Animals and Insects Exposure History
IV. Medications, Allergies, and Adverse Reactions
V. Health Maintenance
   A. Prevention
   B. Diet
   C. Exercise
   D. Sleep Patterns
   E. Social Habits
VI. Family History
   A. First-Degree Relatives' Medical History
   B. Three-Generation Genogram
VII. Psychosocial History
   A. Personal and Social History
   B. Current Illness Effects on the Patient
   C. Interpersonal and Sexual History
   D. Family Support
   E. Occupational Aspects of the Illness
VIII. Review of Systems
IX. Physical Examination
X. Eponyms, Acronyms, and Abbreviations
XI. Sample H&P Write-Up

I. CHIEF COMPLAINT

A. Chief Complaint

1. Chief complaint: Use the patient's own words. Ask open-ended questions and record the signs and symptoms that are most important to the patient.
2. Chronology is often included in the chief complaint: Onset (acute, subacute or chronic); duration (minutes, hours, days, weeks, months, or years); and frequency of symptom(s).
3. Example: J.L. is a 32-year-old married white female (MWF) with a complaint of (c/o) episodic "bandlike pain under my ribs" over a 12-hour period.

B. Identifying Data

1. Name.
2. Age and date of birth (DOB).
3. Sex.
4. Race/Ethnicity: Racial categories used in U.S. population estimates are Hispanic origin (of any race), White (not Hispanic), Black (not Hispanic), American Indian/Eskimo/Aleut, and Asian/Pacific Islander (not Hispanic). Ethnicity categories are Hispanic origin or not of Hispanic origin.
5. Place of birth (country and city).
6. Marital status: Married (M), divorced (D), widowed (W), or separated.
7. Occupation.
8. Religious preferences.
9. Source of history and reliability of the source (e.g., D.L., patient's son, who appears reliable).
10. Admission date, time, and site (emergency department, direct admit, or transfer [e.g., elective, urgent, or emergent]).
11. Patient's home address, phone number, and contact information of family or friends.
12. Name and phone number of patient's primary doctor.
13. Clarify patient's and/or families wishes for code and resuscitation status.

II. HISTORY OF PRESENT ILLNESS (HPI)

A. Characteristics of Symptoms, Conditions, or Disorders

1. Anatomic location.
2. Chronology (temporality).
   a. Onset: Acute, subacute, or chronic.
   b. Duration: Minutes, hours, days, weeks, months, or years.
   c. Frequency.
   d. Progression.
   e. Variations over time.
3. Quality of symptoms (e.g., sharp or dull).
4. Quantity of symptoms: Severity of pain can be assessed on a 1-10 scale. Provide the patient with a scale for comparison

(i.e., pain equal to 10 is the pain of having an extremity traumatically amputated).

5. Aggravating factors, including setting and context of symptom onset or precipitating factors.
6. Alleviating factors.
7. Associated or related symptoms and signs.
8. Past history of similar symptoms or disorders.
9. Current medications, treatments, or therapies.
   a. Responses to interventions.
   b. Recent regimen changes.
10. Allergic reactions and adverse reactions to medications or treatments.
11. Pertinent positives and negatives on conditions or disorders of interest picked up from the review of systems should be included in the HPI write-up.
12. Identify psychologic effects of the illness (e.g., significance, adaptation, family support).

III. PAST MEDICAL AND SURGICAL HISTORY

A. Past Medical History (PMHx)

1. Characterize patient's perception of general health status (excellent, good, fair, or poor).
2. Active and inactive medical problems: Differentiate between acute, subacute, and chronic problems. Acute diagnoses are usually included in the HPI (i.e., "see HPI").
3. Serious adult medical illnesses: Dates, diagnosis, degree, duration, doctor, hospital, treatment(s), medications, complications and sequelae, and response to interventions.
4. Psychiatric illnesses: Addictions, hospitalizations, recent treatments, or therapeutic regimens.

B. Past Surgical History (PSHx)

1. Surgical history: Diagnosis, procedure(s), responses to interventions, operative and postoperative complications or sequelae, month/year, hospital, anesthesia type (local, spinal, general), and anesthetic complications.
2. Obstetric surgical history: Method of delivery (vaginal or Caesarean), complications of labor and/delivery, anesthesia type (local, spinal, general), and anesthetic complications.

C. Emergency and Trauma History

1. Hospitalizations: Dates, diagnoses, degree or severity, duration, doctor, hospital, treatment, medications, complications and sequelae, and outcome.
2. Transfusions: Dates, total number, and known complications (e.g., HIV, hepatitis).
3. Trauma or injuries, including serious sprains or fractures. Document limitations of range of motion, deformities, disability, or weakness. Motor vehicle accidents (MVAs): Type of

vehicle, position in vehicle, speed of vehicle, deceleration force, use of restraints or other protective measures (e.g., air bags).

D. Childhood History

1. Childhood illnesses and injuries.
   a. Infectious diseases: Otitis media, respiratory infections, urinary tract infections (UTIs), meningitis, and febrile seizures. Patient is usually aware of most unusual childhood diseases, but may not remember the specific name (e.g., rheumatic fever, rubella).
   b. Congenital conditions: Respiratory or cardiac abnormalities.
   c. Emergency and trauma in childhood: Dates, conditions, and outcomes of hospitalizations and injuries.
2. Childhood development (see also the Pediatrics Specialty H&P section).
   a. Antenatal: Mother's history: gravida/para/abortions (G/P/A), prenatal care received, tobacco or alcohol complications. Intrauterine growth retardation (IUGR) indicators.
   b. Delivery: APGARs, birth weight, and complications.
   c. Postnatal/Newborn: Returned home with mom? Feeding problems. Illnesses: Respiratory problems, jaundice, or convulsions.
   d. Growth and development: Height and weight within 5% to 95% range (compare with family stature as well) and degree of consistency over time on growth charts.
   e. Social history: Behavioral problems or learning/school problems.
   f. Health maintenance: Immunizations, regular medical checkups.

E. Occupational History

1. Present occupation.
2. Prior occupations and jobs.
3. Chemical, hazardous materials, or noise exposures.
4. Occupational injuries or illnesses.

F. Travel History: Inquire about travel inside and outside country of residence (including geographic locations and dates).

G. Animals and Insects Exposure History

1. Cats (e.g., toxoplasmosis), pigeons (e.g., *Chlamydia psittacosis*), and other animal exposures.
2. Reactions in past to bites or stings (i.e., envenomations).

IV. MEDICATIONS, ALLERGIES, AND ADVERSE REACTIONS

A. Medications

1. Prescription medications, with dose, route, and frequency. Indications, last dose, duration of use, and consider possible drug interactions. Annotate date started and regimen changes. A medications list at the bottom of the HPI or within the past medical history section is helpful.

MEDICATION	DOSE AND ROUTE	FREQUENCY	INDICATION
Aspirin	(325 mg) two tabs po	prn (qd, bid, tid, qhs)	Headache
Cimetidine (Tagamet)	400 mg po	bid (qac and qhs)	Dyspepsia

2. Over-the-counter (OTC) medications: Analgesics, laxatives, sleeping medications, vitamins and supplements, herbal preparations, and diet pills.
3. Alternative medicine therapies.

B. Allergies and Adverse Reactions

1. Medication allergy information.
   a. What was the allergic reaction (e.g., respiratory or neurologic manifestations)?
   b. How was the allergic reaction treated?
   c. What was the route of medication administration when the allergy occurred (po, IV, SQ)?
2. Differentiate between allergic manifestations and adverse reactions. Often an adverse effect does not represent a true IgE-mediated allergy, but rather intolerance to the medication (e.g., gastrointestinal upset with codeine).
3. Environmental allergies: Assess for history of reactive airways disease (RAD), hay fever/allergic rhinitis, food allergies, and dermatologic reactions (e.g., reaction to nickel in earrings).

V. HEALTH MAINTENANCE

A. Prevention

1. Periodic health assessments and examinations: Frequency, evaluations, and screenings completed.
2. Preventive screenings.
   a. Females: Papanicolaou (Pap) smear, frequency and results; breast self-examination (BSE) and clinic examination frequency, mammogram frequency, and skin examinations.
   b. Males: Testicular examination frequency and skin examinations.
3. Safety counseling and injury prevention: Car seats, smoke detectors in home and workplace, poisonings, falls, drowning, choking, hot water safety, traffic safety, helmets, and seatbelts.
4. Prevention of unwanted pregnancies: Method(s) of birth control, appropriate use, and contraceptive options.
5. Immunizations.
   a. Childhood immunizations vary by type (Table 18-1) and age (Table 18-2). Common immunizations are diphtheria,

pertussis, tetanus; usually given as diphtheria and tetanus toxoids and acellular pertussis (DTaP); inactivated polio vaccine (IPV); measles, mumps, and rubella vaccine (MMR); varicella vaccine; Hemophilus influenza type b (Hib) conjugate vaccine; hepatitis B (Hep B); and heptavalent pneumococcal conjugate (PCV) vaccine. Hepatitis A vaccine (Hep A) is recommended for use in selected states and regions and for certain high-risk populations. Influenza vaccine is recommended for children 6 months of age or older with certain risk factors. Pneumococcal polysaccharide vaccine (PPV) is recommended in addition to PCV for certain high-risk groups.

Table 18-1. CHILDHOOD IMMUNIZATIONS BY TYPE.*

Immunization	Age
Hep B	#1 at birth (before hospital discharge) or up to 2 months if mother is HBsAg-negative, #2 at 1-4 months, #3 at 6-18 months
DTaP	#1 at 2 months, #2 at 4 months, #3 at 6 months, #4 at 15-18 months, #5 at 4-6 years
Td	Give Td if at least 5 years since last dose of tetanus and diphtheria toxoid-containing vaccine; subsequent Td boosters recommended every 10 years
Hib	#1 at 2 months, #2 at 4 months, #3 at 6 months, #4 at 12-15 months
IPV	#1 at 2 months, #2 at 4 months, # 3 at 6-18 months, #4 at 4-6 years
MMR	#1 at 12-15 months, #2 at 4-6 years
Varicella	Give at 12-15 months
PCV	#1 at 2 months, #2 at 4 months, #3 at 6 months, #4 at 12-15 months
Hep A	Recommended for use in selected states and regions and for certain high-risk populations
Influenza	Recommended for children 6 months of age or older with certain risk factors
PPV	Recommended in addition to PCV for certain high-risk groups

*Table does not include catch-up vaccination schedule or vaccines indicated for certain risk groups; additional detailed information available at www.aap.org/family/parents/immunize.htm.

Table 18-2. CHILDHOOD IMMUNIZATIONS BY AGE.*

AGE	IMMUNIZATIONS
Birth	Only monovalent Hep B vaccine can be used for the birth dose #1 (may be given by 2 months if mother is HBsAg-negative)
1-4 months	Hep B #2 (1-4 months); DTaP #1, Hib #1, IPV #1 and PCV #1 (2 months); DTaP #2, Hib #2, IPV #2 and PCV #2 (4 months)
6-18 months	Hep B #3, IPV #3 (6-18 months); DTaP #3, Hib #3 (6 months); Hib #4, MMR #4, PCV #4 (12-15 months); Varicella (12-15 months); DTaP #4 (15-18 months)
4-6 years	DTaP #5, IPV #4, MMR #2
11-12 years	Td (if at least 5 years since last dose of tetanus and diphtheria toxoid-containing vaccine; subsequent Td boosters recommended every 10 years)

*Table does not include catch-up vaccination schedule or vaccines indicated for certain risk groups; additional detailed information available at www.aap.org/family/parents/immunize.htm.

IM/FP

b. Adult immunizations vary by type and age (Table 18-3). Common immunizations include tetanus-diphtheria toxoid vaccine; influenza vaccine (age 50 years and older and certain high-risk groups); pneumococcal vaccine (age 65 years and older and certain high-risk groups); hepatitis B (adults at risk); measles, mumps, rubella vaccine; and varicella vaccine.

B. Diet

1. Typical food consumption patterns.
2. Food intake of last 24 hours.
3. Dietary restrictions.
4. Caffeine-containing beverages and foods.

C. Exercise

1. Types of exercise (aerobic).
2. Frequency.
3. Duration.
4. Intensity (how measured?).

D. Sleep Patterns

1. Time of awakening and going to sleep at night (usual pattern).
2. Average number of hours of sleep.
3. Napping patterns.
4. Products used to help fall asleep.
5. Difficulty in falling asleep or insomnia.
6. Awakening during the night (e.g., pain, micturition)?

Table 18-3. ADULT IMMUNIZATIONS.

Tetanus-diphtheria toxoid (Td)	Recommended for routine use in adults. Three intramuscular doses complete a primary series. Second dose is 4-8 weeks after first dose. Third dose is 6-12 months after the second dose. Boosters are recommended every 10 years, unless the patient suffers a tetanus-prone wound
Influenza vaccine	Inactivated (noninfectious) virus administered as a single intramuscular shot during the fall each year. November is the optimal time for organized vaccination campaigns, but patients seen routinely in October and December should be offered vaccines at that time. Protective antibody titers are achieved about two weeks after immunization and begin to decline after 4-6 months
Pneumococcal ploysaccharide vaccine (PPV)	A 23-valent polysaccharide vaccine. The 23 capsular types cause 88% of bacteremic pneumococcal disease. Administered as an intramuscular dose. Protective antibodies develop in 2-3 weeks. Immunization should be given at least two weeks before elective splenectomy or initiating immunosuppressive therapy. Patients at high risk for fatal pneumococcal infection (asplenia; groups with declining antibody levels—nephortic syndrome, renal failure and transplant patients; and HIV patients) should be revaccinated every 6 years. There is no evidence that routine revaccination is of benefit in other groups, and the CDC does not recommend it
Hepatitis B vaccine	Two types of HBV vaccines are available in the U.S.: recombinant HBV vaccine (Recombivax HBreg.) and plasme-derived HBV vaccine (Heptavax-B), which is a suspension of inactivated HBsAg protein. Heptavax-B is no longer produced in the U.S. and use is limited to hemodialysis patients, immunocompromised hosts, and persons with yeast allergy (used to produce Recombivax). Protective antibodies result in over 90% completing the series

E. Social Habits

1. Alcohol.
   a. Beer, wine, or hard alcohol.
   b. Drinks per day or week.
   c. Size of glass used.
   d. How many years?
2. Tobacco.
   a. Tobacco type (chew, snuff, cigarettes, cigars).
   b. Quantitative assessment of packs/day and numbers of years (pack-years).
3. Caffeine, tea, sodas, and diet pills.
4. Illicit or recreational drug use.
   a. Type (e.g., cocaine, crack, heroin, marijuana, mushrooms).
   b. Route (e.g., intravenous, snorting, smoking, ingestion).
   c. Frequency (per day or week) and duration of use (years).

VI. FAMILY HISTORY

A. First-Degree Relatives' Medical History

1. Record age, physical condition, state of health or cause of death, illnesses for parents, siblings, and children.
2. Illnesses that run in the family? Allergies, anemias, arthritis, asthma/reactive airways disease, autoimmune disorders, cancer (any kind), cataracts, cerebrovascular accidents (CVAs) or stroke, coronary artery disease (CAD) or peripheral vascular disease (PVD), diabetes mellitus, emphysema, epilepsy, hemochromatosis, hemophilias, hepatitis (or other liver disorders), hypertension (HTN), and neuropsychologic disorders (e.g., alcoholism or drug abuse, eating disorders, depression or other mental illnesses, multiple sclerosis, muscular dystrophy, sickle cell, Tay-Sachs).

B. Three-Generation Genogram: A simplified set of rules and guidelines for creating basic genogram structures.

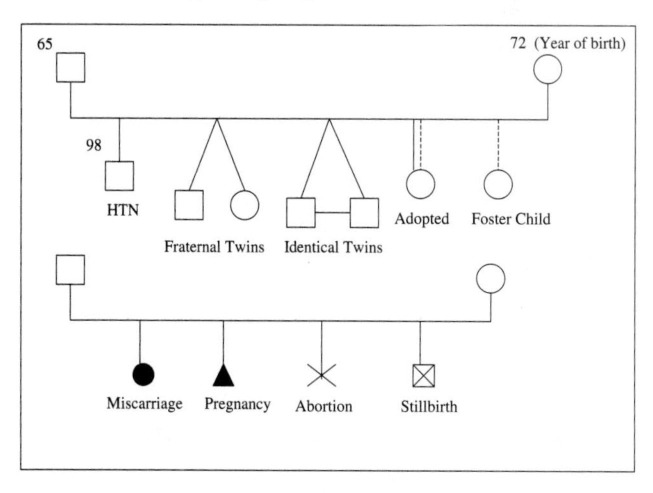

IM/FP

1. Males are depicted as square figures and circles note females. Males are placed to the left of the female in the father/mother dyad.
2. Record ages of living relatives inside the figures with specific disorders and the last two digits of the birth year to the upper left of the square or circle.
3. Marriage dates (last two digits of the year) are recorded above the line connecting the husband and wife. A separation is marked with one slashed line, and the date is recorded above the line connecting them (e.g., s. 97). A divorce is marked with two slashed lines (e.g., m. 97), and the date is recorded above the line connecting them. Liaisons or a couple living together are connected by a dashed line.
4. Deceased relatives are marked with an X or colored in with cause of death listed under or next to their square or circle.
5. Identify the patient (index person of the genogram) with a large arrow or with double lines around his or her circle.

VII. PSYCHOSOCIAL HISTORY

A. Personal and Social History

1. Place of birth (country and city), religious and race/ethnicity background.
2. Marital status and children.
3. Education level attained (e.g., years of schooling, college and advanced degrees).
4. Social involvement.
   - **a.** Leisure activities (e.g., hobbies, sports).
   - **b.** Religious involvement and activities.
   - **c.** Description of a typical day.
5. Current residence, including physical layout of the home and living conditions (e.g., 3 bedrooms, 1 bath, 8 occupants).
6. Socioeconomic status. Any financial difficulties or stressors?

B. Current Illness Effects on the Patient

1. Address the patient's perception of the severity of the illness.
2. Address death and dying issues as applicable.
3. Advanced directives in place (e.g., Living Will, durable power of attorney for health care [DPAHC])?

C. Interpersonal and Sexual History:

Ask only when applicable to the evaluation and use discreet questioning methods.

1. Does this disorder interfere with any part of your personal or sexual life?
2. Evaluate adverse medication effects as a source of sexual dysfunction.
3. Sexual orientation: Heterosexual, homosexual, or bisexual.
4. Abstinence, monogamous relationship, or promiscuous; history of sexually transmitted diseases (STDs) or concerns about STDs.
5. Birth control methods, type, and frequency of use.

D. **Family Support**
1. Significant others, sources of support, and emotions expressed at home.
2. Is the family informed about this illness?
3. Proximity of family and important phone numbers (helpful when information is needed or if information must be relayed to family).

E. **Occupational Aspects of the Illness**
1. How does this disorder affect your job (past, now, and in the future)? Stressors or problems with the job or other workers.
2. Does this patient need occupational therapy or physical therapy?
3. Past and present work, toxic exposures to occupational hazards (e.g., ocular, dermatologic, respiratory).

VIII. **REVIEW OF SYSTEMS**

1. General	11. Gastrointestinal
2. Head	12. Genitourinary
3. Eye	13. Gynecologic
4. Ear	14. Hematopoietic
5. Nose	15. Endocrine
6. Throat	16. Lymphatic
7. Neck	17. Musculoskeletal
8. Respiratory	18. Skin
9. Chest wall/breasts	19. Neurologic
10. Cardiovascular	20. Psychiatric

A. **General:** Most recent checkup, height, recent weight changes, normal weight, appetite, fatigue, weakness, insomnia/irritability, night sweats/chills.

B. **Head:** Headaches, tenderness, head trauma.

C. **Eyes:** Glasses, vision changes, diplopia, redness/inflammation, discharge, tearing, dryness, blind spots or blurring, photophobia, scotomata, glaucoma, last examination, and intraocular pressure (IOP).

D. **Ears:** Hearing changes, ringing in the ears (tinnitus), vertigo, earaches, discharge, otitis media or externa.

E. **Nose:** Diminished smell (olfaction), congestion, obstruction, runny nose (rhinorrhea), discharge, nosebleeds (epistaxis).

F. **Mouth:** Problems with teeth and/or gums, dentures, sore throats, hoarseness, difficulty swallowing, last dental examination.

G. **Neck:** Pains, decreased range of motion (ROM), masses, swollen glands, goiter.

H. **Respiratory:** Cough, sputum (color, quantity), hoarseness, hemoptysis, shortness of breath (SOB), pneumonia, reactive airway disease (RAD) or asthma, wheezing, bronchitis or emphysema, pulmonary embolus (PE), pain with breathing (pleurisy), tuberculosis (TB), positive PPD, last chest x-ray and result.

I. **Chest Wall/Breasts:** Clinical and breast self examinations (BSEs), breast masses or lumps, discharge from the nipples (galactorrhea), nipple inversion, pain, masses, fibrocystic disease (FCD), breast cancer, frequency of mammograms.

J. **Cardiovascular:** Chest pain, palpitations, murmurs, hypertension (HTN), stroke or transient ischemic attacks (TIAs), orthopnea, paroxysmal nocturnal dyspnea (PND), dyspnea on exertion (DOE), edema, leg pain or cramps, claudication, varicose veins, Raynaud's phenomenon (intermittent attacks of ischemia of fingers, toes, ears or nose), previous blood pressures (BP), previous electrocardiograph (ECG).

K. **Gastrointestinal (GI):** Nausea, vomiting, hematemesis, diarrhea, change in stools/pattern, dysphagia, heartburn, abdominal pain, hernias, constipation, hemorrhoids, melena, hematochezia or bright red blood per rectum (BRBPR), cholecystitis, stools that float (steatorrhea: frothy, foul-smelling stools that float because of high fat content/malabsorption), appendicitis.

L. **Genitourinary (GU):** Dysuria, unusual urine smell or color, sexually transmitted disease (STD), hematuria, frequency of urination, nocturia, reduced caliber or force of stream, flank pain, kidney stones, benign prostatic hyperplasia (BPH).

M. **OB/GYN:** Gravida/para/abortions/twins (number full term, premature, abortions, living), last menstrual period (LMP) or last normal menstrual period (LNMP), last Pap smear, menstruation characteristics (frequency/regularity, amount of flow, dysmenorrhea), age at menarche, age at menopause, miscarriages, spontaneous abortions (less than 20 weeks' gestation), postmenopausal bleeding, hot flashes, vaginal dryness, contraception, vulvar, cervical, endometrial disorder.

N. **Hematology:** Bleeding or bruising, coagulopathy, anemia, thalassemia, operations, transfusions, transfusion reaction.

O. **Endocrine:** Polyphagia, polydipsia, polyuria, enlarged thyroid, heat/cold intolerance, sweating, hyperlipidemia, dyslipidemia (e.g., low high-density lipoproteins [HDL]), changes in hair or skin texture or growth, change in hat/glove/shoe size.

P. **Lymphatics:** Enlarged lymph nodes, tenderness.

Q. **Musculoskeletal:** Joint pain, stiffness, swelling, soreness/inflammation, bone diseases, bony deformity, muscle tenderness, muscle weakness.

R. **Skin:** Rashes, dryness, pallor, itching (pruritis), pigmentation changes, jaundice, moles, bruises, or other lesions.

S. **Neurologic:** Numbness, tingling, burning, prickling, or hyperesthesia (paresthesias), unpleasant abnormal sensations (dysesthesias), involuntary movements, ataxia, tremors, vertigo (external world revolving around patient [objective vertigo] or patient revolving in space [subjective vertigo]), dizziness, loss of consciousness (syncope), seizures, epilepsy, memory loss, strokes.

T. **Psychiatric:** Use of medications, tension, anxiety, bizarre thoughts, paranoias, phobias, violent tendencies, insomnia, sexual dysfunction, reaction to illness, psychotherapy, depression screening tool mnemonic (SIG E CAPS).

U. **Symptoms of Depression ("SIG E CAPS"):** **S** = sleep, **I** = interests, **G** = guilt, **E** = energy, **C** = concentration, **A** = appetite (food and sex), **P** = psychomotor, **S** = suicide screen.

IX. PHYSICAL EXAMINATION

1. Vital Signs
2. General Appearance and Mental Status
3. Head and Neck (General)
4. Eyes
5. Ears
6. Nose
7. Mouth
8. Throat
9. Teeth
10. Chest
11. Lungs
12. Cardiovascular
13. Abdomen
14. Genitalia
15. Rectum and Prostate
16. Back and Spine
17. Extremities
18. Skin (Integument)
19. Lymphatics
20. Neurologic

A. Vital Signs

1. Temperature: Tympanic membrane (TM), rectal, or oral; <100.4°F = low-grade fever; >100.4°F = fever.
2. Respiratory rate (RR): Age dependent. RR range by age in the following table.

Newborns/ Neonates	1-6 Months Old	6 Months to One Year	1-2 Years Old	3 Years Old	5 Years Old	5 Years and Older and Adult
35-45	25-35	25-35	20-30	16-24	14-24	14-20

3. Pulse rate: Regular or irregular (if irregular note the apical impulse). Note the number of abnormal beats in 60 seconds.
4. Blood pressure: Extremity tested, time intervals used with orthostatics, supine, sitting, or standing.
5. Height and weight.

B. General Appearance and Mental Status

1. Age, gender, and race/ethnicity.
2. Mental status: Alert and oriented to person, place, and time (A&O ×3).
3. Body habitus and hygiene, nutrition, and state of health.
4. General description of comfort level (e.g., ill-appearing, mild discomfort, despondent, cooperative).

C. Head and Neck (General)

1. Head.
   a. Scalp, distribution and texture of hair, alopecia.
   b. Skull, facies.
   c. Sinus tenderness.
2. Neck.
   a. Range of motion (ROM), suppleness.
   b. Lymph nodes.
   c. Thyroid size, texture, and consistency. Presence of thyroid bruits, masses, or nodules.
   d. Carotid pulse or bruits.
   e. Jugular venous distention (JVD) or hepatojugular reflex (HJR).

D. Eyes

1. Inspect lids, conjunctivae, and sclerae.
2. Pupils equally round and reactive to light (PERRL), and accommodation (PERRLA), direct and consensual (PERRLADC).
3. Extraocular muscles intact (EOMI).
4. Visual fields normal to direct confrontation.
5. Visual acuity (Jaegher chart standard-size letters at 12 inches; Snellen chart has standard letters, normally viewed at a distance of 20 feet).
6. Ophthalmoscopic examination: Lenses, media, discs (cup-to-disc ratio <0.5), vessels, macula. Note presence of abnormalities (e.g., hemorrhages, exudates, microaneurysms, arteriovenous [A-V] nicking of retinal vessels, copper wiring, arteriolar narrowing).

E. Ears

1. Appearance of auricles and canals.
2. Tenderness to tragus traction.
3. Tympanic membranes (TMs): Color, landmarks, light reflex, and mobility with insufflation.
4. Hearing by rustling fingers or whispered voice.
5. Differentiation of conductive versus sensorineural hearing loss.

a. Weber tests lateralization of sound: Sound is louder on the side with a conductive disorder. Softer sound on one side indicates a sensorineural hearing disorder.

b. Rinne test: Bone conduction greater than air conduction (BC > AC) indicates conductive hearing loss. Air conduction greater than bone conduction (AC < BC) indicates sensorineural hearing loss.

F. **Nose**

1. Patency, appearance of mucosa (boggy or congested, normal, dry).
2. Septum midline: Specify absence of polyps, exudate, or discharge.
3. Sinus tenderness of maxillary and frontal sinuses to palpation.

G. **Mouth**

1. Lips and buccal mucosa appearance: Specify absence of ulcers, abnormal pigmentation, or leukoplakia. Salivary ducts and glands.
2. Tongue: Symmetry, size, texture, side-to-side motion (cranial nerve XII).

H. **Throat**: Tonsils, pharynx, uvula, and palate appearance. Specify absence of erythema or exudate.

I. **Teeth and Gums**

1. Dentition status, missing or carious teeth, bleeding or inflamed gums.
2. Ask patient to remove dentures and bridges. Examine under dental plates.

J. **Chest**

1. Thorax.
   a. Symmetry, anterior-posterior (AP) diameter, movement with respiratory excursion.
   b. Abnormal veins or pulsations.
   c. Gynecomastia (males).
2. Breasts (examine male and female).
   a. Contour, symmetry, retractions.
   b. Masses or tenderness.
   c. Nipple inversion or discharge.
   d. Lymph nodes.

K. **Lungs**

1. Clear to auscultation and percussion (CTAP), breath sounds equal bilaterally.
2. Equal diaphragmatic excursion posterior midscapular line.
3. Voice transmission tests.
   a. Tactile fremitus: Ask the patient to say "99" in a normal voice and palpate an area of the lung. Increased transmission in one area can be indicative of an area of consolidation or increased fluid in the lung. Decreased fremitus

indicates air or fluid outside the lung obstructing the transmission.

b. Whispered pectoriloquy: Ask the patient to whisper "99" and listen with the stethoscope. Faint sounds are normal, while increased transmission in one area can be indicative of an area of consolidation.

c. Egophony: Ask the patient to say "ee" several times. Listen with the stethoscope and you should hear a muffled "ee" sound. If you hear an "ay" sound, this is referred to as "E to A" or egophony.

4. Note adventitious (extra) lung sounds and diagram their locations.
   - a. Rales or crackles: Fine/coarse crackling sounds.
   - b. Rhonchi: "Snoring" or "gurgling" quality.
   - c. Rubs.
   - d. Stridor: Inspiratory wheeze usually associated with upper airway obstruction.
   - e. Wheezes: High-pitched and "musical" in quality.

L. Cardiovascular

1. Neck.
   - a. Jugular venous distension (JVD).
   - b. Hepatojugular reflex (HJR).
   - c. Carotid pulses and bruits.
2. Heart.
   - a. Intercostal space (ICS) of point of maximal impulse (PMI) at apex.
   - b. Location and character of lifts, heaves, thrills, or rubs.
   - c. Quality and splitting of first (S1) and/or second (S2) heart sounds.
   - d. S3 gallop: Third heart sound or ventricular gallop. Low volume and frequency (pitch). Best heard with the bell at the apex in the early diastolic period and is normal in children.
   - e. S4 gallop: Fourth heart sound or atrial gallop. Low volume and frequency. Best heard with the bell at the apex in the end-diastolic period.
   - f. Murmurs: Loudness (I-VI/VI), location and transmission, timing and duration (i.e., systolic or diastolic), components (e.g., opening snap, knocks), character and pitch (e.g., best heard with bell or diaphragm), position of patient for eliciting or accentuating murmurs.

M. Abdomen

1. Inspection: Distended, scars or striae, or dilated veins.
2. Auscultation: Bowel sounds and bruits.
3. Palpation.
   - a. Tenderness or masses. Rebound tenderness, rigidity, or guarding.
   - b. Fluid wave (positive or negative).

GRADING OF CARDIAC MURMURS.	
I/VI	Lowest intensity, often not heard by inexperienced listeners
II/VI	Low intensity, usually audible by inexperienced listeners
III/VI	Medium intensity without a thrill
IV/VI	Medium intensity with a thrill
V/VI	Loudest intensity that is audible when the stethoscope is placed on the chest and is associated with a thrill
VI/VI	Loudest intensity that is audible when the stethoscope is removed from the chest and is associated with a thrill

c. Aorta: Tenderness, size, bruits.
d. Liver: Size and position (centimeters below the right costal margin [RCM] at the midclavicular line [MCL]), texture, hepatojugular reflux (HJR).
e. Gallbladder: Tenderness to palpation (TTP), pain while palpating over the gallbladder with inspiration (i.e., Murphy's sign).
f. Spleen: Palpable or percussable, size, and position.
g. Kidneys: Size, bruits.
h. Bladder: Suprapubic tenderness.

N. Hernia (Male and Female)

1. Palpation with Valsalva or cough.
2. Bulge in abdominal wall versus palpable bowel in inguinal, femoral, or umbilical areas. Complete or incomplete.

O. Genitalia

1. Male.
   a. External appearance, penile lesions, discharge, or circumcised?
   b. Testicles: Descended bilaterally, tenderness, masses, consistency, varicocele, or hydrocele.
2. Female.
   a. Bartholin's glands, Skeen's glands, urethral meatus, vulva (BSUV).
   b. Vaginal mucosa, masses, discharge; cul-de-sac visualization.
   c. Rectocele, cystocele.
   d. Cervix: Parity, position, cervical motion tenderness, discharge, and Pap smear.
   e. Uterus: Size, position (anteverted or retroverted), and masses.
   f. Adnexa: Ovarian sizes if palpable, position, masses, tenderness.

P. Rectum and Prostate

1. External appearance, specify absence of fissures, fistulas, hemorrhoids. Diagram abnormalities using a clock designation.
2. Sphincter tone (normal or lax).
3. Guaiac test for blood in the stool: Positive or negative.
4. Prostate: Size, shape, texture, and consistency. Specify absence of masses, nodules, and enlargement (i.e., 1.5, 2, 2.5 times normal size). Also note symmetry.

Q. Back and Spine

1. Symmetry, kyphotic, and lordotic curvatures.
2. Range of motion (ROM).
3. Sacral edema, scars, or birthmarks/nevi.
4. Sacroiliac (SI) joint tenderness.
5. Costovertebral angle tenderness (CVAT).
6. Muscle atrophy or tenderness, and straight leg raise (SLR) result.

R. Extremities

1. Inspection: Bilateral symmetry, deformity, or weakness.
2. Range of motion (ROM): Active, passive, and specific joints.
3. Bone, joint, or muscle tenderness; swelling or inflammation; varicosities.
4. Vascular assessment.
   a. Pulses 0 to 4+ (0 absent; 1+ difficult to palpate, weak; 2+ normal; 3+ easily palpable, increased; 4+ bounding).
   b. Capillary refill (<2 seconds is considered normal).
   c. Clubbing, cyanosis, or edema (C/C/E), pitting edema: Bilateral measurement in millimeters documenting location.
   d. Lymphatics.

S. Skin (Integument)

1. Texture, temperature, and turgor (e.g., cool/warm, moist/dry).
2. Pigmentation, nevi, or nail abnormalities.
3. Location of petechiae, rashes, nevi, birthmarks, jaundice, telangiectasiae; clubbing, cyanosis, edema (C/C/E).

T. Lymphadenopathy

1. Occipital, auricular, submental, tonsillar, cervical (anterior and posterior), supraclavicular, axillary, epitrochlear, or inguinal lymph nodes.
2. Abnormal: >1 cm diameter. Specify location, number, size, fixed or mobile, and tenderness.

U. Neurologic (see neurologic examination outline)

1. Mental status examination: Attitude, reliability, general appearance, emotion (mood and affect), speech/language, thought processes, thought content, cognition, intelligence, insight, and judgment.
2. Cranial nerves (Table 18-4).

Table 18-4. FUNCTIONS OF CRANIAL NERVES.

Cranial Nerves		Function
I	Olfactory	Smell
II	Optic	Vision
III	Oculomotor	Levator palpebrae, superioris, superior, medial, and inferior recti muscles; parasympathetic to ciliary and pupillary constrictor muscles
IV	Trochlear	Superior oblique muscle
V	Trigeminal	Muscles of mastication; sensory for head and neck, sinuses, meninges, and external surface of tympanic membrane
VI	Abducens	Lateral rectus muscle
VII	Facial	Muscles of facial expression; parasympathetic to all glands of head except the parotid; sensory for ear and tympanic membrane, taste for the anterior two thirds of tongue
VIII	Vestibulocochlear	Hearing and balance
IX	Glossopharyngeal	Stylopharyngeus muscle; parotid gland; carotid body; sensation for the posterior one third tongue and internal surface of tympanic membrane; taste for the posterior one third tongue
X	Vagus	Muscles of the pharynx and larynx; parasympathetic to neck, thorax, and abdomen; sensory from pharynx, larynx and viscera, sensory from external ear
XI	Spinal Accessory	Trapezius and sternocleidomastoid muscles
XII	Hypoglossal	All tongue muscles except the palatoglossal

3. Motor: Strength, range of motion (ROM), and pronator drift (Table 18-5). Arms extended forward with palms up, eyes closed, and patient holds position while examiner taps arms briskly downward. Normal is arms returning to starting position. Abnormals, including pronation of one forearm or other changes, can indicate central nervous system (CNS) abnormality.

Table 18-5. GRADING OF MOTOR/MUSCLE STRENGTH.

Score	Reflex Response	Movement
0/5	Absent	No contraction detected
1/5	Trace	Slight contraction detected
2/5	Weak	Movement with gravity eliminated
3/5	Fair	Movement against gravity
4/5	Good	Movement against gravity and some resistance
5/5	Normal	Normal movement against gravity with full resistance

4. Sensory: Light touch, pin prick, proprioception, and vibratory.
5. Deep tendon reflexes (biceps C5-6, triceps C6-7, knee L2-4, ankle S-1): Grade 0 to 4+ (Table 18-6).

Table 18-6. GRADING OF DEEP TENDON REFLEXES.

Score	Reflex Response
0	No response
1+	Diminished
2+	Normal
3+	Increased
4+	Hyperactive

6. Babinski's sign: Extension of the great toe and abduction of the other toes instead of the normal flexion reflex to plantar stimulation, considered indicative of pyramidal tract involvement (positive Babinski). Down-going great toes bilaterally is a normal or negative Babinski test.
7. Cerebellar functions.
   a. Gait: Walking, tandem walking, walk on toes and heels.
   b. Station: Romberg test by having patient stand with feet together and eyes open.
   c. Coordination.
      (1) Rapid alternating movements (RAM): Hand pronation to supination on the thigh.
      (2) Heel to shin (H to S) testing: Tap heel three times on contralateral patella and move from knee to ankle (slowly) along the shin.
      (3) Finger to nose testing: Move fingertip between tip of nose and examiner's outstretched fingertip.

X. ACRONYMS, AND ABBREVIATIONS (Table 18-7)

XI. SAMPLE H&P WRITE-UP

Chief Complaint: "Shortness of breath and wheezing for the past 12 hours."

HPI: 23-year-old white female with past medical history significant for asthma presents to the Acute Care clinic with a 12-hour history of wheezing, refractory to home-administered metered-dose inhaler (MDI). Patient notes onset of rhinorrhea, mild cough, and malaise approximately 2 days ago. Symptoms were stable until late last evening, when she noticed onset of gradually worsening wheezing. She used her MDI every 2 hours throughout the evening but had an inadequate response, with persistent coughing, chest tightness, and wheezing.

PMHx: Significant for asthma starting at the age of 12, with rare, intermittent episodes after age 12. Patient had one admission approximately 1 year ago that lasted 3 days. She was treated with nebulizers and oral prednisone. Her usual peak flow meter reading is 350.

PSHx: None.

Occupational History: Homemaker. No toxic exposures.

Medications: Albuterol MDI with spacer up to every 2 hours as needed. Salmeterol MDI twice per day.

Allergies: NKDA.

Health Maintenance: Nonsmoker, nondrinker. Walks 2 miles around track by house every other day. No sleep disturbances.

Family History: No stroke, diabetes, heart disease, cancer, or asthma in any first-degree relative.

Three-Generation Genogram:

Mother: Alive, age 63, no medical problems.

Father: Alive, age 65, severe hypertension and peripheral vascular disease.

Maternal grandmother (MGM): Alive, age 82, rheumatoid arthritis.

Maternal grandfather (MGF): Deceased at age 90, brain tumor.

Paternal grandmother (PGM): Deceased at age 51, motor vehicle accident (MVA).

Paternal grandfather (PGF): Deceased at age 59, stroke.

Psychosocial History: Patient reports very good relations with her husband and one child (age 8). No domestic or marital discord or problems. She reports a satisfying sexual relationship with her husband. No financial difficulties. She appears to have an excellent social support network, as she is very active within her church and bowls on a ladies bowling league weekly. The patient reports that her asthma condition has had no limitations on her family or social life. Her asthma flare-ups are very infrequent, and she reports good relief with the medications that she has been prescribed previously.

Review of Systems: Patient denies fevers, chills, chest pain, palpitations, nausea, vomiting, rashes, or other significant symptoms.

Table 18-7. ACRONYMS, AND ABBREVIATIONS.

Acronym or Abbreviation	Definition	Acronym or Abbreviation	Definition
A&O × 3	Alert and oriented to person, place, and time	**MVA**	Motor vehicle accident
A&O × 4	Alert and oriented to person, place, time, and condition	**MWF**	Married white female
AC	Air conduction	**NABS**	Normal abdominal bowel sounds
AD	Right ear	**NAD**	No acute distress
AP	Anterior-posterior	**NCAT**	Normocephalic, atraumatic
AS	Left ear	**ND**	Nondistended
AU	Both ears	**NT**	Nontender
A-V	Arteriovenous	**O/P**	Oropharynx
BC	Bone conduction	**OD**	Right eye
BP	Blood pressure	**OS**	Left eye
BRBPR	Bright red blood per rectum	**OTC**	Over-the-counter medication
BSUV	Bartholin's gland, Skeen's gland, urethra, vagina	**OU**	Both eyes
C/C/E	Clubbing, cyanosis, edema	**PERRL (ADC)**	Pupils equal, round, reactive to light (accommodation: direct and consensual)
CMT	Cervical motion tenderness	**PMI**	Point of maximal impulse
CTAP	Clear to auscultation and percussion	**PND**	Paroxysmal nocturnal dyspnea

CTAB	Clear to auscultation bilaterally	**RAD**	Reactive airway disease
CVAT	Costovertebral angle tenderness	**RAM**	Random alternating movements
D	Divorced	**RCM**	Right costal margin
DOB	Date of birth	**ROM**	Range-of-motion
DOE	Dyspnea on exertion	**RR**	Respiratory rate
ECG	Electrocardiogram	**S**	Soft
EOMI	Extraocular muscles intact	**S1**	First heart sound
FROM	Full range-of-motion	**S2**	Second heart sound
G/R/R	Guarding, rebound, rigidity	**S3**	Third heart sound
HIV	Human immunodeficiency virus	**S4**	Fourth heart sound
HPI	History of present illness	**SLR**	Straight leg raise
HSM	Hepatosplenomegaly	**SQ**	Subcutaneous
HTN	Hypertension	**SSC**	Size, shape, and consistency
ICS	Intercostal space	**STD**	Sexually transmitted disease
IUGR	Intrauterine growth retention	**TB**	Tuberculosis
IV	Intravenous	**TIA**	Transient ischemic attack
JVD	Jugular venous distension	**TMs**	Tympanic membranes
LE	Lower extremity	**TTP**	Tenderness to palpation
LMP	Last menstrual period	**UE**	Upper extremity
M	Married	**VA**	Visual acuity
MCL	Midclavicular line	**W**	Widowed

PHYSICAL EXAMINATION

Vital Signs: T: 98.6°F, P 99, R 20, BP 125/70, Weight 150 lbs., Height 5′6″.

General: Well-nourished, well-developed white female in mild respiratory distress. Speaking in 5-word sentences. Moist mucous membranes.

HEENT: NCAT. PERRLA, EOMI, fundi benign bilaterally. Bilateral TMs: pearly, mobile. No sinus tenderness. Nares with clear nasal discharge. Normal pharynx without erythema, exudates, or enlarged tonsils. No carotid bruits. No JVD.

Lungs: Mild, diffuse, scattered wheezes bilaterally. Moderate excursion, with poor air movement. Some accessory muscle use. No crackles or rhonchi.

Heart: Regular rate and rhythm, with normal S1 and S2. No S3 or S4. No murmurs, rubs, or gallops.

Vascular: 2+ distal pulses in upper and lower extremities, bilaterally.

Abdomen: Normal abdominal bowel sounds, nontender, nondistended. No guarding, rebound, or rigidity. No masses or hepatosplenomegaly.

Genitourinary and Rectal: Deferred.

Extremities: No clubbing, cyanosis, or edema.

Skin: No rashes.

Neurologic: Cranial Nerves II-XII intact grossly; 5/5 strength in both upper and lower extremities; normal tone; patellar reflexes 2+ bilaterally; sensation intact grossly; no ataxia on finger-to-nose. Babinski: negative.

Peak Flow Meter Reading: 250.

19

NEONATOLOGY

Jorge L. Romeu Vélez, MD, MS, and Anne L. Naclerio, MD, MPH

I. CHIEF COMPLAINT

A. Source of History: Obtain the history from either the mother or the father if possible, the mother's obstetrics medical record, or the mother's next of kin. Areas of importance are relevant family medical genetic history, mother's history of prior pregnancies, and history of current pregnancy, including pertinent antenatal, natal, and perinatal events.

B. Identifying Data: Obtain the age, gender, medical record number, and race of all patients you evaluate.

II. HISTORY OF PRESENT ILLNESS

A. Mother's Past Medical History

1. Do you have any acute or chronic medical conditions?
2. Did you have any infections during pregnancy? TORCH is a useful acronym: **T**oxoplasmosis, **O**thers (syphilis, hepatitis B, coxsackie virus, Epstein-Barr virus [EBV], varicella-zoster virus [VZV], and human parvovirus), **R**ubella, **C**ytomegalovirus [CMV], and **H**erpes simplex virus [HSV]).
3. What is your typical diet? Did you take prenatal vitamins? Note any unusual dietary habits and/or use of prenatal vitamins.
4. Do you now, or have you used in the past, tobacco, alcohol, or illicit drugs?
5. Are there any illnesses or syndromes with genetic implications in your or your spouse's families?
6. Have you been exposed to any chemicals at your work?

B. History of Prior Pregnancies

1. At what age did you have your children? Women in their teens or older than age 35 have an increased risk of complications.
2. Gravidity: Is this your first pregnancy? If not, how many prior pregnancies?
3. Parity: If more than one pregnancy, how many were vaginal deliveries? How many were cesarean sections (C-sections)?
4. What is your blood type? ABO/Rh incompatibility, Rh_o (D) immune globulin?
5. What were previous pregnancy outcomes? Full term, premature, abortions, or living?

C. History of Current Pregnancy

1. When was the estimated date of conception (EDC)? Have you had an ultrasound during pregnancy? Estimated gestational age

by dates and by ultrasound if available; premature <37 weeks, term 37-42 weeks, post-term (a.k.a. post-dates) >42 weeks.

2. Did you have amniocentesis performed? For what reason? Results?
3. Have you had any screening tests before or during your pregnancy? Hepatitis B surface antigen (HBsAg), Rubella immune, antibody screen, maternal serum alpha-fetoprotein (MSAFP), human immunodeficiency virus (HIV), and group B streptococcus (GBS)?
4. Were any prior tests of fetal well-being (biophysical profiles or nonstress tests) done?
5. Did you have any pregnancy-related illnesses (e.g., urinary tract infections [UTIs], pregnancy-induced hypertension, gestational diabetes, preeclampsia-eclampsia, vaginal bleeding, or preterm labor)?

D. Labor and Delivery: This information is usually obtained from obstetrician or medical record.

1. Rupture of membranes (ROM): Spontaneous versus artificial rupture, duration, meconium staining, bloody, or foul odor.
2. Maternal fever, use of antibiotics, time of antibiotics before delivery.
3. Fetal distress: Talk to the delivering obstetrician.
4. Analgesia or anesthesia used (e.g., narcotics, epidural, spinal, general).
5. Other medications (e.g., magnesium sulfate, insulin, intravenous [IV] glucose).
6. Type of delivery: Normal spontaneous vaginal delivery (NSVD), C-section (first time or repeat), forceps assist, or vacuum extraction.
7. Condition of the baby at birth, resuscitation needed, and APGAR scores (see following section).

III. MOTHER'S PAST MEDICAL AND SURGICAL HISTORY

A. Past Medical History: Inquire about maternal disorders (Table 19-1).

Table 19-1. MATERNAL PAST MEDICAL HISTORY.

Disorder	Implications for Pregnancy
Infectious disease	Significant morbidity and mortality associated with syphilis, gonorrhea, chlamydia, bacterial vaginosis, genital herpes, cytomegalovirus, rubella, toxoplasmosis, AIDS, and tuberculosis
Cancer	The most common malignancies include cervical cancer, breast cancer, melanoma, ovarian cancer, leukemia/lymphoma, and colorectal cancer. Malignant metastasis to the fetus is extremely uncommon in all cancers. Teratogenesis from chemotherapy is the most important concern

Table 19-1—cont'd

DISORDER	IMPLICATIONS FOR PREGNANCY
Respiratory disease	Dyspnea of pregnancy is common in the third trimester
Cardiac disease	Mothers with functionally significant cardiac disease are at increased risk of having low-birth-weight and/or premature babies
Gastrointestinal and hepatobiliary diseases	Although uncommon, cholelithiasis may pose a surgical risk for the mother. Acute fatty liver of pregnancy is rare, but it may be severe and carries a high maternal mortality risk. Occurs late in pregnancy in primigravidas
Renal disease or hypertension	Renal disease is associated with an increased risk of first trimester spontaneous abortions and intrauterine growth restriction. Hypertension before pregnancy or development of hypertension may be an indicator of worsening renal disease
Urinary tract infections (UTIs)	UTIs increase the risk of preterm labor. *Escherichia coli* is the most common organism
Thromboembolic disorders	Phlebitis and pulmonary embolism. Morbidity in the fetus or neonate mostly due to medications used to treat the mother
Anemia	Iron-deficiency anemia (IDA) is the most common, but monitor for sickle cell anemia and thalassemia
Endocrine disease	Hyperthyroidism is frequently associated with Graves' disease. Hypothyroidism is rare during pregnancy, but you may encounter a mother who is on medication for this condition, which when untreated is associated with infertility. Hyperparathyroidism is extremely rare but associated with significant perinatal morbidity and mortality (low birth weight and neonatal tetany). Hypoparathyroidism is even more rare

Continued

Table 19-1. MATERNAL PAST MEDICAL HISTORY—*cont'd*

Disorder	Implications for Pregnancy
Glucose intolerance and diabetes mellitus	Infants of diabetic mothers are at increased risk of congenital anomalies, macrosomia (excessive fetal growth), neonatal hypoglycemia, hyperbilirubinemia, hypocalcemia and polycythemia, and respiratory distress syndrome. Poorly controlled mothers are at increased risk of spontaneous abortions, intrauterine fetal demise, and stillbirth
Neurologic disease	Fetal or neonatal morbidity are mostly associated with medications used to treat the mother. Use of Phenytoin during pregnancy is associated with fetal hydantoin syndrome (microcephaly, facial clefts and dysmorphism, limb malformations, and distal phalangeal and nail hypoplasia). Phenobarbital is associated with cleft lip and palate. Carbamazepine appears to be relatively safe. Most anticonvulsants are also associated with bone marrow suppression and depression of Vitamin K—dependent clotting factors
Dental disease	Emergency and routine dental care can be provided as usual. Local anesthetics without epinephrine offer little risk

B. **Past Surgical History:** What surgical procedures have you undergone? Risk of uterine rupture and associated fetal risk increases with a vaginal birth after C-section (VBAC).

C. **Emergency and Trauma History:** The fetus should be monitored as thoroughly as possible whenever a mother presents with a surgical condition. Abdominal trauma increases the risk of abruptio placenta. Talk to the obstetrician and prepare accordingly.

D. **Childhood History:** Is there a family history of childhood illnesses (e.g., asthma/reactive airway disease/atopy, Type I diabetes mellitus)? Important to ask when conditions have known genetic implications.

E. **Occupational History:** Were you exposed to any teratogens at work? Were there any occupational exposures to chemicals? What does your job entail (e.g., heavy lifting)?

F. **Travel History:** Although travel is not contraindicated, it is strongly discouraged in the late third trimester. This is not for medical reasons, but because the labor may occur away from health care providers who are knowledgeable about potential complications or high-risk pregnancies.

IV. MEDICATIONS

What medications, if any, did you take during pregnancy?

V. MOTHER'S HEALTH MAINTENANCE

A. **Prevention:** When did you begin receiving medical care for your pregnancy? How many prenatal visits have you had?

B. **Diet:** What is your typical diet? Look for any unusual dietary habits. Did you take prenatal vitamins?

C. **Exercise:** What type of exercise and how often do you exercise? Moderate exercise programs can be continued during pregnancy. Overly strenuous exercise, especially for prolonged periods, is discouraged. Discourage starting vigorous new exercise programs to mothers who are not used to exercising regularly.

D. **Sleep Patterns:** How much are you sleeping at night? During the day? Resting? It is beneficial to moderate physical activity and to allow for additional periods of rest.

E. **Social Habits:** Do you now use, or have you used in the past, tobacco, alcohol, or illicit drugs?

VI. FAMILY HISTORY

A. **First-Degree Relatives' Family History:** Any conditions with inheritable pattern?

B. **Three-Generation Genogram:** Useful to create if there are any suspected family illnesses/syndromes with genetic implications.

VII. PSYCHOSOCIAL HISTORY

A. Personal and Social History

1. What is your country of birth? Do you have access to a medical care facility and necessary equipment? What neonatal intensive care facility is nearest to your home?
2. What is your race/ethnicity? Ascertain parental beliefs, expectations, and desires.
3. Is the infant returning to a safe environment? Assess residential layout.
4. Will the parents be able to afford hospitalization of the potentially ill neonate?
5. What are the parents' levels of education? Are these teen parents? Will they understand what you are telling them? Avoid medical terminology as much as possible.

B. **Current Illness Effects on the Family:** Important to assess with extremely premature infants, severely ill neonates, or children with congenital anomalies. These conditions may impose tremendous emotional stressors on the family. Involve social workers, chaplains, and family members as necessary.

C. **Interpersonal and Sexual History:** Are you married to the infant's father? Are you sexually active at this time? Sexual activity is restricted or prohibited under certain circumstances, when it is known to have special risks (e.g., placenta previa, premature rupture of membranes [PROM], and preterm labor).

D. **Family Support**

1. Is there any significant social history such as domestic violence, spouse abuse, or child abuse?
2. Is there adequate support for the child at home? Is parent a single mom?
3. Do family members have adequate knowledge of the newborn's basic needs?

VIII. REVIEW OF SYSTEMS (Tables 19-2, 19-3, and 19-4)

Table 19-2. GENERAL NEWBORN SIGNS AND SYMPTOMS BY SYSTEM.

System	Signs and Symptoms
General	Appearance, weight, length, occipitofrontal circumference (OFC), dysmorphisms, syndromic features
CNS	Hypertonia, hypotonia, irritability, high-pitched cry, jitteriness, lethargy, hyper/hyporeflexic, seizure activity, posturing
Head	Macrocephaly, microcephaly, wide-opened fontanelles, craniosynostosis, cephalohematomas, caput succedaneum
Eyes	Placement, inflammation, discharge, subconjunctival hemorrhage, aniridia, leukochoria, gaze, light reflex
Ears	Placement, shape, hypoplastic ear(s), asymmetry, tags, pits
Nose	Unilateral or bilateral obstruction, discharge, septal deviation, nose irregularity, flaring
Oropharynx	Cleft lip, hard palate and/or soft palate, drooling, tongue thrusting
Neck	Torticollis, webbing, masses, tracheal deviation
Cardiovascular	Murmurs, decreased pulses, prolonged capillary refill
Chest and respiratory	Grunting, retracting, widened nipple space, pectus excavatum, decreased breath sounds (unilateral versus bilateral)
Gastrointestinal	Feeding intolerance, delayed meconium, meconium plug

Table 19-2—cont'd

SYSTEM	SIGNS AND SYMPTOMS
Genitourinary	Ambiguous genitalia, clitoromegaly, micropenis, cryptorchidism, hernias
Lymphatic	Enlarged lymph nodes (*extremely* rare in the newborn)
Musculoskeletal	Anatomical deformities, contractures, hypertrophy, atrophy
Skin	Jaundice, cyanosis, plethora, rash, petechiae, ecchymosis, calcifications, nevi (hyperpigmented or hypopigmented) café-au-lait spots
Extremities	Acrocyanosis, polydactyly, syndactyly
Hematologic	Anemia, bleeding, bruising, polycythemia

Table 19-3. NONSPECIFIC SIGNS/SYMPTOMS AND THEIR ASSOCIATED DISEASE PROCESSES.

SIGN OR SYMPTOM	DISEASE
Abdominal distention	Renal mass, small bowel obstruction, malrotation, posterior urethral valves with distended bladder
Anemia in the newborn	Decreased production (congenital [e.g., Diamond-Blackfan], nutritional [e.g., folate, iron]), sepsis, increased destruction (e.g., isoimmune [Rh, ABO, minor groups]), infection (viral versus bacterial), membrane disorders (e.g., hereditary spherocytosis, elliptocytosis, pyropoikilocytosis), enzyme disorders (e.g., glucose-6-phosphate defiency [G-6PD], hemoglobinopathy, disseminated intravascular coagulation (DIC), hemorrhage, prematurity (most common cause in this group is iatrogenic)
Feeding intolerance	Sepsis, hypoglycemia, duodenal atresia or stenosis, esophageal atresia, inborn errors of metabolism, congenital heart disease, prematurity, central nervous system (CNS) disorders
Hypothermia	Sepsis, prematurity, CNS disorders

Continued

Table 19-3. NONSPECIFIC SIGNS/SYMPTOMS AND THEIR ASSOCIATED DISEASE PROCESSES—*cont'd*

Sign or Symptom	Disease
Respiratory distress	Sepsis, congenital pneumonia, pneumothorax, acidosis, congenital heart disease
Skin findings	Vesicular rash (e.g., HSV, staphylococcus/ scalded skin syndrome [SSS], port-wine stain, Sturge-Weber, single large or multiple hemangiomas, blueberry muffin rash: cytomegalovirus [CMV])
Weight	Small for gestational age (e.g., symmetric versus asymmetric), large for gestational age: infant of diabetic mother, other syndromes

Table 19-4. COMMON NEWBORN CONDITIONS AND THEIR SYMPTOMS.

Condition	Symptom
Sepsis	Poor feeding, lethargy, hypo- or hyperthermia, abdominal distension, apnea, asphyxia (due to pneumonia)
Hypoglycemia	Lethargy, poor feeding, seizures, apnea, coma, pallor, tachycardia, sweating
Polycythemia	Hematocrit >65%, infant of diabetic mother, chronic fetal hypoxia, high altitude, post-mature, small for gestational age (SGA) > large for gestational age (LGA) > appropriate for gestational age (AGA), delayed cord clamping, twin-to-twin transfusion, trisomies (21, 18, 13), hyperthyroidism, hypothyroidism, Beckwith-Wiedemann syndrome
Transient tachypnea of the neonate (TTN)	Also known as respiratory distress syndrome (RDS) Type II; caused by slow absorption of fetal lung fluid, tachypnea, expiratory grunting, rarely retractions and cyanosis (resolved by oxygen), usually resolves within 72 hours
Meconium aspiration syndrome	Usually in post-term newborns and caused by distress in utero or more commonly after first breath. At birth newborn has respiratory distress, tachypnea, cyanosis, retractions, overdistended chest

Table 19-4—cont'd

CONDITION	SYMPTOM
GENETIC SYNDROMES	
Beckwith-Weideman	Hypoglycemia, macroglossia, large-size baby, visceromegaly (but mild microcephaly), omphalocele, characteristic ear lobe crease, increased incidence of tumors, increased insulin secretion, chromosome 11
Fragile X	X chromosome with a fragile site associated with a frequent form of mental retardation. After puberty these patients often exhibit large prominent ears, long narrow face, coarse facial features, and macroorchidism. Mental retardation in males is characteristic, although the manifestations of the syndrome are highly variable
Trisomy 21	Hypotonia, increased flexibility of joints, endocardial cushion defect, VSD, PDA, ASD, flat face and occiput, upslanting palpebral fissures, epicanthal folds, small ears, protruding tongue, single palmar crease (40%), extranuchal skin, clinodactyly, wide space between first and second toes
Trisomy 18	Prominent occiput, short sternum, congenital heart disease, clenched fists with the ndex finger overlapping the third and the fifth finger overlapping the fourth, rocker-bottom feet. High perinatal mortality. Majority die within first year of life. Survivors have severe mental retardation
Trisomy 13	Ophthalmologic abnormalities (e.g., microphthalmia, colobomas, retinal dysplasia), forebrain abnormalities, cleft lip and palate, posterior scalp defects, congenital heart disease, polydactyly, rocker-bottom feet. Most die in the first month. Survivors have severe mental retardation

IX. PHYSICAL EXAMINATION OF THE NEWBORN

A. General Principles

1. The newborn physical examination should be as extensive as the infant's condition and the environment in which the examination is performed will allow.

2. Resuscitate the sick newborn in accordance with the Neonatal Resuscitation Program protocol and before performing a complete and thorough physical examination.
3. Examine the infant under a radiant warmer to prevent hypothermia. The newborn's head accounts for a large proportion of the total body surface area and is a major source of heat loss.
4. Examine the infant immediately after birth (focus on ABCs: **A**irway, **B**reathing, **C**irculation).

B. APGAR Score (Table 19-5)

1. Used to determine integrity of cardiopulmonary systems.
2. Performed at 1 and 5 minutes of age (record every 5 minutes in severely depressed infants).
3. No predictive values for long-term outcomes. Serial scores help in describing severity of depression and quality of resuscitative efforts.
4. Evaluates five signs:
   a. Color: **A**ppearance
   b. Heart rate: **P**ulse
   c. Reflex irritability: **G**rimace
   d. Muscle tone: **A**ctivity
   e. Respiratory effort: **R**espiratory

C. Gestational Age: Use the new Ballard score to make an objective assessment of fetal maturation of the newborn.

D. Classification of Newborns by Weight, Length, Head Circumference, and Gestational Age

1. Appropriate for gestational age (AGA).
2. Small for gestational age (SGA, symmetric versus asymmetric).
3. Large for gestational age (LGA).

E. General Examination: Usually done in the nursery in a warm environment within the first 24 hours of life.

1. Observe the infant: While at rest in a quiet environment, then auscultate the chest, and lastly palpate the abdomen.
2. Heart rate: Normal newborn rate is 120 to 160 beats per minute. Evaluate rate and quality.
3. Respirations: Normal rate is 30 to 60 breaths per minute. Observe quality and effort.
4. Skin.
   a. Bruising, petechiae (common over infant's presenting part), ecchymosis, lacerations.
   b. Color: Cyanosis (central versus acrocyanosis), meconium staining, jaundice, and pallor.
   c. Plethora usually indicates polycythemia.
   d. Vernix (decreases as term approaches).
   e. Lanugo (fine hair covering the preterm infant's skin).
   f. Cracking and peeling (common in postterm infants).
   g. Edema.

Table 19-5. APGAR SCORES.

Score	Heart Rate	Respiratory Effort	Muscle Tone	Reflex Irritability	Color
0	Absent	Absent, irregular	Limp	No response	Blue, pale
1	<100 bpm	Slow, crying	Some flexion of extremities	Grimace	Acrocyanosis
2	>100 bpm	Good	Active motion	Cough or sneeze	Completely pink

NEO

NEWBORN MATURITY RATING & CLASSIFICATION

ESTIMATION OF GESTATIONAL AGE BY MATURITY RATING
Symbols: X—1st Exam O—2nd Exam

Side 1

Gestation by Dates__________wks

Birth Date ______Hour ______ am pm

APGAR________1 min______5 min

NEUROMUSCULAR MATURITY

	–1	0	1	2	3	4	5
Posture							
Square Window (wrist)	>90°	90°	60°	45°	30°	0°	
Arm Recoil		180°	140°–180°	110°–140°	90°–110°	<90°	
Popliteal Angle	180°	160°	140°	120°	100°	90°	<90°
Scarf Sign							
Heel to Ear							

MATURITY RATING

score	weeks
–10	20
–5	22
0	24
5	26
10	28
15	30
20	32
25	34
30	36
35	38
40	40
45	42
50	44

PHYSICAL MATURITY

Skin	Sticky; friable; transparent	gelatinous; red; translucent	smooth; pink; visible veins	superficial peeling &/or rash; few veins	cracking; pale areas; rare veins	parchment; deep cracking; no vessels	leathery; cracked; wrinkled
Lanugo	none	sparse	abundant	thinning	bald areas	mostly bald	
Plantar Surface	heel-toe 40–50 mm: –1 <40 mm: –2	>50 mm; no crease	faint red marks	anterior transverse crease only	creases ant. 2/3	creases over entire sole	
Breast	imperceptible	barely perceptible	flat areola; no bud	stippled areola; 1–2 mm bud	raised areola; 3–4 mm bud	full areola; 5–10 mm bud	
Eye/Ear	lids fused loosely: –1 tightly: –2	lids open; pinna flat; stays folded	sl. curved pinna; soft; slow recoil	well-curved pinna; soft but ready recoil	formed & firm; instant recoil	thick cartilage; ear stiff	
Genitals male	scrotum flat; smooth	scrotum empty; faint rugae	testes in upper canal; rare rugae	testes descending; few rugae	testes down; good rugae	testes pendulous; deep rugae	
Genitals female	clitoris prominent; labia flat	prominent clitoris; small labia minora	prominent clitoris; enlarging minora	majora & minora equally prominent	majora large; minora small	majora cover clitoris & minora	

SCORING SECTION

	1st Exam = X	2nd Exam = 0
Estimating Gest Age by Maturity Rating	____Weeks	____Weeks
Time of Exam	Date_____ Hour ___am pm	Date _____ Hour____am pm
Age at Exam	____ Hours	____ Hours
Signature of Examiner	________ M.D./R.N.	________ M.D./R.N.

Scoring system Ballare JL, Khoruy JC, Wedig K, Wang L, Eilers-Walsman BL, Lipp R, New Ballard Score, expanded to include extremely premature infants. *J Pediatr.* 1991; 119:417–423.

h. Birthmarks: Hemangiomas, Mongolian spots, café-au-lait spots, nevi (e.g., stork bites, angel kiss, salmon patches).
i. Milia (i.e., small subepidermal keratin cysts) versus miliaria (fever accompanied by an eruption of small, isolated, red pimples).
j. Erythema toxicum: Benign rash consisting of many small areas of red skin, with a yellow-white papule in the center.
k. Other pustules, papules, macules, or vesicles.

5. Head.
   a. Size (occipito-frontal circumference), shape, symmetry, fontanelles.
   b. Caput succedaneum versus cephalohematoma.

   c. Craniosynostosis.
   d. Facies.
6. Eyes.
   a. Size, symmetry, or evidence of trauma.
   b. Epicanthal folds.
   c. Widely spaced eyes.
   d. Clear versus cloudy cornea.
   e. Iris (coloboma, Brushfield's spots).
   f. Subconjunctival hemorrhages.
   g. Pupils: Red reflex, anisocoria, leukocoria, or congenital cataracts.
7. Ears.
   a. Size, shape, symmetry.
   b. Position: Low-set, posteriorly rotated.
   c. Tags or pits.
8. Nose.
   a. Size, shape.
   b. Air passage (pass a small suction or feeding tube to rule out choanal atresia; unilateral versus bilateral).
   c. Flaring (a sign of respiratory distress).
9. Mouth.
   a. Natal teeth (may be risk for aspiration).
   b. Epstein's pearls (multiple small, white epithelial inclusion cysts found in the midline of the palate in newborn infants).
   c. Cleft lip or palate.
   d. Tongue size.
   e. Syndromic features.
      (1) Pierre-Robin (small mandible and tongue with cleft soft palate).
      (2) Trisomy 21 and Beckwith-Wiedemann (prominent tongue).
      (3) Excessive drooling (think esophageal atresia).
10. Neck.
   a. Redundant skin or webbing (e.g., Turner's syndrome or Noonan's syndrome).
   b. Masses.
      (1) Midline (thyroid).
      (2) Anterior to sternocleidomastoid muscles (branchial cleft cysts).
      (3) Within the sternocleidomastoid (hematoma, torticollis).
      (4) Posterior to the sternocleidomastoid (cystic hygroma).
11. Chest and lungs.
   a. Look for any signs of respiratory distress (retractions, grunting).
   b. Look for any anatomic abnormalities (pectus, barrel chest).
   c. Listen for air entry bilaterally.

(1) Diminished breath sounds with respiratory distress: Pneumothorax, space-occupying lesion.

(2) Congenital diaphragmatic hernia (diminished breath sounds, bowel sounds on chest auscultation with respiratory distress, scaphoid abdomen: If suspected it needs immediate attention).

(3) Rales are commonly heard in the transitional period because of retained fetal lung fluid and are not of clinical significance at this age, unless persisting and associated with respiratory distress and oxygen requirement.

d. Feel for fractured clavicles (crepitus, bruising, tenderness).

12. Heart.

a. Heart murmurs are common in the transitional period (most often benign).

b. Severe congenital heart disease (CHD) may present with no murmur at all.

c. Cyanosis and abnormal pulses are most suggestive of CHD.

d. Diminished pulses at all sites suggest critical aortic stenosis or hypoplastic left heart.

e. Diminished lower extremity pulses suggest aortic coarctation or interrupted aortic arch.

f. Pulse oxymetry is not routinely done in the transitional period. When in doubt, do it.

13. Abdomen.

a. Newborn abdomens are prominent but soft (nondistended).

b. Observe for any obvious abnormalities.

(1) Prune belly syndrome (Eagle-Barret syndrome): Absent abdominal musculature with renal abnormalities.

(2) Gastroschisis (abdominal wall defect, intestines extruding).

(3) Omphalocele (membrane-covered herniation of abdominal contents into the base of the umbilical cord). Look for other associated anomalies (e.g., cardiac, gastrointestinal, chromosomal).

(4) Umbilical hernia (more common in African-American and Latino newborns).

c. Esophageal atresia may be ruled out by passing a soft catheter into the stomach and obtaining an x-ray to verify placement. ***Do not*** force the catheter if resistance is noted.

d. Most abdominal masses in newborns are associated with kidney disorders (e.g., multicystic, dysplastic, hydronephrosis).

e. Liver edge may be palpable 1-2 cm below the right costal margin.

f. Spleen: Check the size.

g. No urine in the first 24 hours of life suggests obstruction; a distended bladder suggests posterior urethral valves.

The most common cause of no urine in the first 24 hours of life is failure to record urine output from parents or nurses.

14. Genitals and anus.

a. Evaluate anatomy and maturity (using New Ballard maturity scores).

b. Ambiguous genitalia (do not assign sex to newborn until genetic studies reveal genotype).

c. In the male, examine the testis to rule out cryptorchidism. Evaluate for hydrocele versus scrotal hernia and examine the penis to rule out micro-penis, hypospadias, and epispadias.

d. In the female, a whitish vaginal discharge with or without blood during the first few days is normal.

15. Musculoskeletal.

a. Examine for obvious abnormalities (newborn position, movements, five fingers on each hand, five toes on each foot, club foot, webbing or fusion of fingers or toes, extra fingers or toes).

b. Assess for symmetry and range of motion. Rule out congenital hip dysplasia using the Ortolani-Barlow maneuver.

c. Rule out palsies or extremities fractures.

d. Examine the back and spine to rule out scoliosis, myelomeningocele, spina bifida. Investigate any pits, hair tufts, or other defects.

e. Multiple joint contractures (i.e., arthrogryposis) may be caused by limited motion in utero because of oligohydramnios or congenital neuromuscular disease.

16. Neurologic examination.

a. Evaluate newborn posture, symmetry of extremities, spontaneous movement (activity), facial expressions and symmetry, and eye movements and symmetry.

b. Primitive reflexes are present at birth depending on gestational age, but disappear in the first weeks to months of life. The most common reflexes are as follows:

(1) Rooting reflex: Newborn's head turns to side of facial stimulus.

(2) Palmar and plantar grasp, with placement of examiner's finger in the palm or plantar foot.

(3) Sucking reflex: Response to nipple or examiner's finger inside newborn's mouth.

(4) Moro (startle) reflex: Document presence and most important symmetry.

(5) Deep tendon reflexes: Several beats of ankle clonus and upgoing Babinski reflex may be normal.

(6) Other less commonly performed: Fencing, placing response; traction response; stepping response; Galant's reflex; and Perez's reflex.

X. DIFFERENTIAL DIAGNOSIS (Table 19-6)

Table 19-6. DIFFERENTIAL DIAGNOSIS OF CONGENITAL ANOMALIES.

Congenital Anomaly	Findings
Tracheoesophageal fistula	Excessive salivation, polyhydramnios, aspiration pneumonia. Unable to pass nasogastric tube into stomach
Choanal atresia	Respiratory distress while at rest in the delivery room. Unable to pass nasogastric tube through nares
Ductal dependent lesions	5T = tetralogy of Fallot (tricuspid atresia, truncus, transposition of great vessels, total anomalous pulmonary venous return); cyanosis, hypotension, metabolic acidosis, murmur
Diaphragmatic hernia	Respiratory distress, scaphoid abdomen, decreased breath sounds on the affected side, bowel sounds in the thoracic cavity
Intestinal obstruction	Bile-stained vomitus, polyhydramnios, cystic fibrosis
Potter syndrome (renal agenesis)	Oligohydramnios, pulmonary hypoplasia
Neural tube defects	Increased alpha fetoprotein, polyhydramnios
Gastroschisis, omphalocele	Polyhydramnios, intestinal obstruction
Pierre Robin	Micrognathia, cleft palate
Erb-Duchene paralysis	Injury at C5, C6. Adduction, internal rotation of arm with pronation of forearm, absent Moro ipsilaterally with normal hand grasp
Klumpke paralysis	Injury at C7, C8, and T1. Paralyzed hand, absent hand grasp. Ipsilateral ptosis and miosis if sympathetic fibers of T1 are involved
Large anterior fontanel	Hypothyroidism, prematurity, Vitamin D deficiency (rickets), hypophosphatasia, trisomies (21, 18, 13), rubella, hydrocephalus, osteogenesis imperfecta, achondroplasia, syndromes

XI. LABORATORY STUDIES AND DIAGNOSTIC EVALUATIONS (Table 19-7)

Table 19-7. SELECTED LABORATORY STUDIES AND DIAGNOSTIC EVALUATIONS.

TEST	USES
Cord blood arterial and venous gases	Provides additional information of the infant's conditions before delivery
Initial dextrose stix	Of paramount importance in infants that are large or small for gestational age, infants of diabetic mothers, and premature infants
Hematocrit	Used to rule out anemia or polycythemia
Complete blood count	Extremely important in sick infants. Useful to rule out neutropenia, leukocytosis, anemia, polycythemia, thrombocytopenia, or thrombocytosis
Newborn bilirubin screen	Useful to assess degree of hyperbilirubinemia and to determine when to start and stop phototherapy
Blood culture	Gold standard used to rule in or out bacteremia
Cerebrospinal fluid analysis	Useful to rule out meningitis in the critically ill neonate
Urine analysis	Useful to rule out urinary tract infection in the critically ill neonate
Newborn screen	Varies from state to state. Useful to rule out treatable conditions that are relatively common (examples include phenylketonuria, galactosemia, congenital adrenal hyperplasia)
Arterial blood gas	Useful to assess degree of acidosis, alkalosis, hypoxemia, and hyper- or hypocarbia
Pulse oxymetry	Useful to assess degree of hypoxia

XII. ACRONYMS AND ABBREVIATIONS (Table 19-8)

Table 19-8. NEONATOLOGY ACRONYMS AND ABBREVIATIONS.

Acronym or Abbreviation	Definition	Acronym or Abbreviation	Definition
AFOSF	Anterior fontanelle open, soft, and flat	**NR**	Nonreactive
AGA	Appropriate for gestational age	**NSVD**	Normal spontaneous vaginal delivery
AROM	Artificial rupture of membranes (Usually done by the friendly obstetrician)	**OFC**	Occipitofrontal circumference
ASD	Atrial septal defect	**PDA**	Patent ductus arteriosus
BF	Breast-feeding	**PNV**	Prenatal vitamins
BW	Body weight	**PPROM**	Prolonged premature rupture of membranes. ROM to delivery >18 hours Hypothermia is a core temperature <37.0°C (controversial)
CTA	Clear to auscultation	**PPV**	Positive pressure ventilation
FGR	Fetal growth restriction	**PROM**	Premature rupture of membranes
FROM	Full range of motion	**PTA**	Prior to admission
FTT	Failure to thrive	**PTD**	Prior to delivery

GC	Gonococcal	**ROM**	Rupture of membranes (amniotic sac)
HSM	Hepatosplenomegaly	**RW**	Radiant warmer
Is/Os	Fluid inputs (e.g., per oral, IV fluids) and outputs (e.g., stool, urine)	**SGA**	Small for gestational age. Birth weight is below the 10th percentile for gestational age or >2 standard deviations below the mean
IUGR	Intrauterine growth retardation (this was the old term). FGR for fetal growth restriction is now the proper term. It is defined as failure of normal fetal growth caused by multiple adverse effects	**SROM**	Spontaneous rupture of membranes (Nature's course)
LGA	Large for gestational age. Birth weight is 2 standard deviations above the mean weight for gestational age or above the 90th percentile	**SVD**	Spontaneous vaginal delivery
NABS	Normal active bowel sounds	**VLBW**	Very low birth weight
NAD	No acute/apparent distress	**VSD**	Ventricular septal defect
NICU	Neonatal intensive care unit	**WT**	Weight

XIII. DEFINITIONS (Table 19-9)

Table 19-9. NEONATOLOGY TERMS AND DEFINITIONS.

Term	Definition
Acrocyanosis	Bluish hands and feet only
Anisocoria	Asymmetry of the pupil size
Arthrogryposis	Persistent flexure or contracture of joint
Brushfield's spots	Small, white spots on the periphery of the iris, usually crescentic with concavity outward, frequently seen in children with Down syndrome
Café-au-lait spots	Pigmented light-brown macules, seen in neurofibromatoisis and Albright's syndrome
Caput succedaneum	Diffused edematous swelling occurring in and under fetal scalp during labor that extends across the suture line
Cephalohematoma	Subperiosteal hemorrhage that never extends across the suture line
Cherry red spot	Red circular area surrounded by gray-white retina, seen through the fovea centralis of the eye in the infantile form of Tay Sach's disease
Coloboma	Lack of appropriate development of choroids and retina; may occur in association with retinal detachment, trisomy 13, CHARGE syndrome, and de novo
Craniosynostosis	Premature closure of one or more sutures of the skull
Cryptorchidism	Undescended testis
Cyanosis	Bluish skin and/or tongue and lips
Dysmorphism	In neonatal medicine, refers to visually abnormal bodily development
Epispadias	Abnormal location (dorsally) of the meatus
Epstein's pearls	Keratin-containing cysts usually located on the hard and soft palate
Erythema toxicum	Benign rash consisting of many small areas of red skin, with a yellow-white papule in the center (they look like ant bites)
Flaring	Exaggerated opening of the nares during inspiration

Table 19-9—cont'd

TERM	DEFINITION
Fontanelles	Membrane-covered space in incompletely ossified skull of fetus or infant
Gravidity	Number of times the mother has been pregnant. Include miscarriages, spontaneous abortions, elective termination of pregnancy, and stillbirths
Hypospadias	Abnormal location (ventrally) of the meatus
Jaundice	Yellowish color caused by accumulation of bile
Leukocoria	Whitish reflex or mass in the pupillary area behind the lens (cat's eye reflex)
Macroglossia	Enlarged tongue
Meconium	First intestinal discharge of the newborn infant. It is composed of epithelial cells, fetal hair, mucus, and bile
Micrognathia	Smallness of jaws
Microphthalmia	Developmental defect characterized by small eyes; opacities of cornea and lens, scarring of the retina and choroid, and other abnormalities may also be present
Milia	Whitish, pinhead-sized, tiny, sebaceous retention cysts that are usually on the chin, nose, forehead, and cheeks
Miliaria	Syndrome of skin changes associated with sweat retention and extravasation of sweat occurring at different levels in the skin
Mongolian spots	Congenital melanocytic nevus characterized by a flat, smooth, bluish gray to gray-brown macular patch, most often located on the central lumbosacral area in Asian and dark-skinned races; usually disappears by 5 years of age
Mottling	Lacy red pattern
Oligohydramnios	Presence of less than 300 mL of amniotic fluid at term
Pallor	Washed out, whitish appearance
Parity	Number of times the mother actually delivered. Include stillbirths
Plethora	Deep, rosy red color
Polycythemia	Hematocrit >65% on two consecutive samples

Continued

Table 19-9. NEONATOLOGY TERMS AND DEFINITIONS—*cont'd*

Term	Definition
Polydactyly	Developmental anomaly characterized by extra digits on hands and feet
Polyhydramnios	Excess of amniotic fluid
Salmon patch	Salmon-colored nevus, flameus which is usually found over the eyelids, between the eyes, and on the mid-forehead, and commonly fades completely
Stork bite	Red mark on posterior aspect of neck
Syndactyly	Persistence of webbing between adjacent digits so more or less completely attached; most common (autosomal dominant) congenital abnormality
Torticollis	Contacted state of cervical muscles, producing twisting of the neck and an unnatural position of the head
Vernix	Whitish, cheesy, fatty substance covering the skin of the fetus. It is made of desquamated epithelial cells, lanugo hair, and sebaceous matter

XIV. SAMPLE H&P WRITE-UP AND CONSULTATION NOTE

A. Sample H&P

CC and HPI: The patient is an 1810 gram infant female product of a 34 0/7 wk gestation born via precipitous spontaneous vaginal delivery (SVD). The patient was born to a 29 yo G1P0 now P1, A pos/Abs neg, RI, RPR NR, HBsAg neg, HIV neg, GC/Chlamydia neg, PPD NR, GBS unknown. Pregnancy was unremarkable until one day PTD when mother complained of abdominal pain but denied having contractions. Mother presented to the hospital approximately 30 min after having PROM and an infant's foot was seen on vaginal exam. No history of maternal fever. Infant delivered, handed to Pediatrics limp, bruised, cyanotic, and with no spontaneous respirations. Infant placed under RW, dried, stimulated, suctioned, and positioned. PPV given briefly with rapid improvement of color, HR, and activity as well as spontaneous respirations (per resident's note). APGAR scores 5 at 1 minute (−2 color, −1 HR, −1 resp, −1 tone) and 9 at 5 minutes (−1 color). Infant was transferred to NICU for further evaluation and monitoring without problems.

Maternal History: Remarkable for mother with sickle cell trait.

PHYSICAL EXAMINATION

Vital Signs: T 35.9°C, HR 138, RR 40, BP RA 48/36 M 38; LA 48/28 M 35; RL 53/47 M 49; LL 70/35 M 49 O_2 sat >95% on room air.

BW 1810 g (40%), Length cm (>10%) OFC (45%).

Gen: Immature infant female under RW in NAD.

HEENT: NC. AFOSF. No cephalohematoma. Eyes normally placed. Ears, normal set/pos without tags or pits. Nares patent bilateral. Oropharynx moist, no cleft. Neck supple without mass.

COR: RR without murmurs, hemodynamically stable with +2 pulses (fem/brachial) bilateral. Cap refill <3 sec.

Chest/Lungs: Symmetric and CTA bilateral (CTAB).

Abdomen: Soft and ND without masses or HSM. NABS. 3-vessel cord.

Extremities: No anomalies, FROM × 4. No clavicular crepitus and no hip clicks/clunks.

Skin: Pink with marked bruising of entire left lower extremity and right below the knee. Normal turgor and perfusion.

Genitalia: Normal external female genitalia. No masses. Anus appears patent.

Neuro: Normal tone and activity. Normal grasp. Strong suck with gag present. Moro symmetric.

LABS: Initial D-stix 28.

CBC on admission: WBC 10.1 (31S, 5B, 47L, 13M, 4E), Hgb/Hct 15.7/45.6, Plt 121K.

B. Neonatology Consultation Note

CC: Patient is a 25-day-old Caucasian female with FTT and temperature instability.

HPI: Infant was born via cesarean section at 40 4/7 wk gestation to a 33 yo G2P2, A neg/Abs neg, RI, RPR NR, HBsAg neg, HIV neg, GC/Chlamydia neg, GBS negative. Cesarean section was performed secondary to history of HSV with many outbreaks during pregnancy (per report), although no outbreak at the time of delivery. Infant only required free-flow oxygen at delivery. APGAR scores 8/9 (−2 color and −1 color). Infant was stable and was discharged after 48 hours. Mother states infant was breast-feeding well (this is also on medical record) at the time of discharge.

Mother states infant was breast-feeding well approximately every hour for approximately 20 minutes. After the first week, infant appeared sleepier and mother reportedly started supplementing with formula (2 oz every 4 hours). Infant would sometimes sleep for 5 hours without waking to feed. Mother denies giving water, juice, or any other fluids to the baby. Mother reports that infant only had one stool from discharge to this admission (dark brown, "looked like peanut butter"). Infant was voiding >7x/day, although mother stated that diapers were not as wet as they are now in the hospital. Mother reports history of dribbling milk, but no history of emesis.

Infant seen at 2 weeks in Well Baby clinic and was noted to have ~20% weight loss from birth. Infant admitted for FTT and ROS work-up for temperature instability.

BW 3215 g (35%), LT 47.5 (28%), OFC 34 cm (32%).

MATERNAL PREGNANCY: Only remarkable for multiple HSV outbreaks during pregnancy, but no active lesions at delivery. Medications include PNV (occasionally) and Paxil. She denied use of tobacco, alcohol, illicit drugs, herbal, or other homeopathic products.

FAMILY HISTORY: Maternal history of anxiety/depression. There is a 5-year-old sister with chronic constipation but otherwise healthy. Father was reportedly a thin infant with problems with weight gain. There is a maternal uncle who died at 1-2 days (unknown cause). Negative family history of cystic fibrosis, galactosemia, sudden death, or other inheritable diseases.

PSYCHOSOCIAL HISTORY: Lives with both parents and an older sister. Unplanned pregnancy but parents happy about baby. No pets.

HOSPITAL COURSE: Has had temperature instability, but CBC is unremarkable and has had one negative urine culture (no blood culture done). Currently −6.7% from BW. On 120-130 kcal/kg/day (BF + 24 kcal/oz Enfamil every 3 hr). Voiding and stooling normally.

LABS: Most recent chemistry: Na 137, K 4.0, Cl 107, HCO_3 19, BUN/Cr 6/0.5, Glc 73, Ca 9.5, Mg 1.6, Phos 5.7.

Most recent CBC (19 June): WBC 8.2 (33S, 2B, 48L, 12M, 2E, 2Baso, 1ATL), Hgb/Hct 16.5/48.1, PLT 204K.

Most recent UA (19 June) specific gravity 1.015, pH 5.0, trace LE, rest negative (reducing substances not done.) UA culture no growth (June 18).

Initial Newborn Screen (2 June) was normal.

Extended newborn screen is pending.

PHYSICAL EXAMINATION

Vital Signs: Stable temperature now, and stable vital signs with no evidence of respiratory distress.

Admission: WT 2.84 Kg (<1% on 19 June 02) WT today 3.0 kg (7%)

Gen: Thin appearing, pale infant female in NAD.

HEENT: AFOSF. Sutures apposed. Eyes normally placed. Ears, normal set/pos with two preauricular tags on the left tragus. Nares patent bilateral. Mild micrognathia. Oropharynx moist, no cleft. Neck supple without mass.

COR: RR w/o murmurs, hemodynamically stable with +2 pulses (fem/brachial) bilateral. Cap refill <3 seconds.

Chest/Lungs: Symmetric and CTA bilateral.

Abdomen: Soft and ND without masses or HSM. NABS. 3-vessel cord at birth.

Extremities: No anomalies, FROM × 4. No clavicular crepitus and no hip clicks/clunks.

Skin: Pale without rash/petichiae. Normal turgor and perfusion.

Genitalia: Normal female external genitalia. No masses and no discharge. Anus patent.

Neuro: Normal activity when supine. Marked truncal hypotonia. Normal grasp/suck. Moro symmetric.

20

NEPHROLOGY

Irel Scott Eppich, MD, and Thomas S. Neuhauser, MD

I. CHIEF COMPLAINT

A. **Chief Complaint:** Use the patient's own words. Ask open-ended questions and record the signs and symptoms that are most important to the patient. Chronology is often included: Onset (acute, subacute, or chronic), duration (minutes, hours, days, weeks, months, or years), and frequency of symptom(s).

B. **Identifying Data:** Obtain patient's name, age, gender, race/ethnicity, and location of admission/evaluation.

II. HISTORY OF PRESENT ILLNESS

Persons with renal disease generally come to medical attention with one of the following presentations: Acute renal failure (ARF), chronic renal failure (CRF), and hematuria or proteinuria with normal renal function. It is incumbent upon the clinician to glean from the history the nature of the renal problem, its effects, and the potential for reversibility.

A. **Acute Renal Failure:** Approach the patient in a systematic way to determine if the insult is caused by prerenal, intrinsic renal, or postrenal factors (see Table 20-7).

B. **Chronic Renal Failure**

1. Patients with chronic renal failure who have not yet started renal replacement therapy are more likely to give a history of slowly progressive symptoms relating to progressive uremia.
2. Some patients may be totally asymptomatic.
3. Be aware that patients with chronic renal failure often present with acute worsening of their chronic renal failure.

C. **Hematuria and Proteinuria with Normal Renal Function**

1. Most patients with hematuria or proteinuria are asymptomatic.
2. It is vital to take a thorough history and review of systems in an effort to identify the source and severity of these findings.
3. The goals of the history (and subsequent physical examination and laboratory and radiologic data) are to:
   a. Identify the disorder as either primary to the kidney or secondary from a multisystem process with renal involvement.
   b. Identify the problem as being primarily nephritic or nephrotic.
4. Hematuria can result from bleeding anywhere along the urinary tract, from the glomerulus to the tip of the urethra.
5. It is necessary to determine where the hematuria is originating and if it is glomerular or nonglomerular.

6. Initially approach the patient with hematuria with the following questions:
   a. Has the hematuria ever been visible to you (e.g., gross hematuria)?
   b. Have you ever seen stones or blood clots in your urine?
   c. How long has the hematuria been present, or when was it first documented?
   d. Are there any accompanying symptoms (or historical clues)?
7. Protein in the urine may be caused by one of four different conditions. These should be kept in mind while taking the history to identify the pathophysiologic mechanism taking place.
   a. Altered glomerular permeability.
   b. Failure of the tubules to reabsorb filtered protein.
   c. Glomerular filtration of high quantities of low-molecular-weight protein.
   d. Increased secretion of uroepithelial mucoproteins in response to inflammation.
8. Initially approach the patient with proteinuria with the following questions:
   a. How long has the proteinuria been present, or when was it first documented?
   b. Is the proteinuria intermittent or persistent?
   c. What is the quantity of protein loss in a 24-hour period?
   d. Was the protein detected during physiologic stress (e.g., fever, exercise, acute Illness)?
   e. Do you have any accompanying symptoms (or historical clues)? (See Table 20-1.)

Table 20-1. GENERAL HISTORY QUESTIONS AND RATIONALE FOR ASKING.

GENERAL HISTORY	RATIONALE
Obtain objective evidence of previous renal function	Acute versus chronic renal failure
Recent urine output and urine characteristics, to include color, clarity, gross blood, odor	Etiology of oliguric versus nonoliguric renal failure
History of renal replacement therapy (dialysis)	Acute versus chronic renal failure

III. PAST MEDICAL AND SURGICAL HISTORY

A. Past Medical History

1. What other diseases or syndromes do you have? Autoimmune disease process such as systemic lupus erythematosus (SLE)? Genetic disease process such as von Hipple-Lindau, sickle cell disease, and polycystic kidney disease? Evaluate unrelated diseases that comprise syndromes.
2. Have you been diagnosed with a kidney disease? Evaluate acute and/or concomitant chronic disease processes that can involve kidneys (e.g., diabetes mellitus, vascular disease processes, hypertension, infection, scleroderma).
3. Have you had renal stones (i.e., nephrolithiasis)?
4. Have you been pregnant? Any complications (e.g., assess for preeclampsia)?
5. What, if any, infections have you had (e.g., glomerulonephritis [GN] following streptococcal pharyngitis)?
6. Have you had any malignancies? Some treatments may be nephrotoxic (e.g., radiation to kidneys, chemotherapeutic agents). Some neoplastic disease processes characteristically involve kidneys (e.g., amyloidosis).

B. Past Surgical History

1. Have you had cardiovascular surgery?
2. Genitourinary system surgery?
3. Other surgery? Note any surgery associated with excessive blood loss or hypotension because this may predispose patient to renal ischemia.

C. Emergency and Trauma History

1. Have you ever had acute blood loss (e.g., shock, ischemia)?
2. Abdominal/flank injury (e.g., concern for traumatic injury to viscera, bladder rupture)?
3. Assess hydration status: What happened before emergency visit? What fluids and how much infused in ambulance/emergency department/following admission?
4. Have you had blood transfusions (could be significant if considering kidney transplant down the road)?

D. Childhood History

1. Did you have any congenital anomalies (e.g., prune-belly syndrome, dysplastic kidneys)?
2. History of vesicoureteral reflux (VUR), frequent urinary tract infections (UTIs), and any sequelae?

E. Occupational History

1. What, if any, industrial chemicals have you been exposed to? Exposure to certain industrial chemicals (e.g., hydrocarbons) can predispose to genitourinary malignancies and be nephrotoxic.
2. Have you been exposed to heavy metals? Exposure to some heavy metals can be associated with chronic interstitial nephritis.

F. Travel History

1. Have you traveled to tropical regions? Certain tropical diseases can cause GN (e.g., leprosy, leptospirosis).
2. Certain organisms characteristically infect the urinary system (e.g., schistosomiasis can infect bladder and has been associated with GN and nephrotic syndrome).
3. Renal disease may be associated with systemic parasitemia (e.g., GN associated with malaria, nephrotic syndrome associated with malaria, filariasis, leprosy).
4. Some geographic regions are associated with kidney disease (e.g., Balkan nephropathy).

G. Animals and Insects Exposure History

1. What exposure to insects have you had? Some insects carry infectious agents that may affect the renal system as part of systemic disease (e.g., malaria).
2. Have you been bitten or stung? Bites or stings from certain insects/animals are associated with systemic collapse (e.g., some venom-producing snakes, scorpions, spiders, jellyfish). Some insects/animals are directly nephrotoxic (e.g., bee stings, fire ant bites).

IV. MEDICATIONS, ALLERGIES, AND ADVERSE REACTIONS

A. Medications

1. What prescription medications are you currently taking? Many medications may be nephrotoxic (e.g., aminoglycosides, amphotericin B, certain antineoplastic agents).
2. Are you taking any over-the-counter (OTC) medications (e.g., nonsteroidal antiinflammatory drugs [NSAIDs] may cause hemodynamically induced ARF, long-term use of analgesics can cause analgesic nephropathy).
3. Any herbal preparations?

B. Allergies to Medications and the Side Effects: Have you had allergic reactions to, or side effects from, medications? Acute interstitial nephritis is mostly associated with antibiotics, NSAIDs, and diuretics.

C. Adverse Reactions

1. Have you had any adverse reactions to medications? Some drugs, including OTC medications, can be associated with adverse kidney effects (e.g., papillary necrosis with some NSAIDs, nephrotic syndrome associated with organic gold).
2. Have you had any adverse reactions to radiologic contrast or anesthetic agent? These may be nephrotoxic.

V. HEALTH MAINTENANCE

A. Prevention: What cancer screenings have you had?

B. Diet: What is your usual diet? High-protein diets can potentially predispose to nephrolithiasis.

C. **Exercise/Recreation**

1. Do you exercise? What type? Vigorous exercise can be associated with hematuria, fluid loss predisposing to prerenal failure, and rhabdomyolysis-associated ARF.
2. At what level of intensity do you exercise? What specific activities?

D. **Sleep Patterns:** What is your usual sleep pattern? Has it changed in any way? Patient may experience nocturia if fluid overloaded (e.g., renal failure).

E. **Social Habits**

1. Do you use tobacco? This can predispose to genitourinary malignancies (e.g., bladder cancer) and is associated with cardiovascular disease.
2. Do you drink alcohol? This may predispose to liver disease and secondary renal dysfunction.
3. Do you use/abuse any IV drugs? Kidneys may be affected as part of systemic disease (e.g., hypertension associated with cocaine use, GN associated with infections) or directly affected (e.g., glomerular lesions and nephrotic syndrome associated with heroin use, HIV nephropathy).
4. Glue sniffing (toluene exposure)? This is associated with nephron injury.

VI. **FAMILY HISTORY**

A. **First-Degree Relatives' Medical History:** Have any first-degree relatives had renal disease, renal replacement/dialysis and transplantation, history of "passing" stones, or cardiovascular disease/hypertension?

B. **Three-Generation Genogram:** Look for conditions with familial inheritance (e.g., hematuria and/or deafness with Alport's syndrome).

VII. **PSYCHOSOCIAL HISTORY**

A. **Personal and Social History**

1. What is your country of birth? Birth country may indicate infectious exposure (e.g., tuberculosis [TB], schistosomiasis).
2. What is your ethnic background? Ethnicity may identify increased risk for certain disease processes (e.g., hypertension in African-Americans, diabetes in Hispanics).
3. Socioeconomic status affecting access to health care.
   a. Will you be able to afford medications or treatments (e.g., dialysis)?
   b. Describe your living situation and residence (e.g., exposure to lead).

B. **Current Illness Effects on the Patient:** Assess ability to conform to treatment regimens and to cope with stress associated with life changes caused by illness.

C. **Interpersonal and Sexual History:** Assess change in family dynamics associated with illness and treatments or potential treatments.

D. **Family Support:** Assess for future long-term treatments (e.g., dialysis or transplant).

E. **Occupational Aspects of the Illness:** Assess ability to perform professional duties with illness or exposure to potential nephrotoxins.

VIII. **REVIEW OF SYSTEMS (Tables 20-2 to 20-4)**

Table 20-2. GENERAL NEPHROLOGY SYMPTOMS BY SYSTEM.

System	Symptoms
General	Fatigue, weakness, thirst, nausea, fever, weight loss, anorexia
ENT	Nose bleeds (epistaxis)
Cardiovascular, pulmonary	Shortness of breath, orthopnea, paroxysmal nocturnal dyspnea (PND), hemoptysis, cough
Gastrointestinal (GI)	Anorexia, weight loss, nausea, vomiting, hiccups, bad taste, diarrhea, bleeding, abdominal pain
Genitourinary	Frequency, urgency, pain on urination (dysuria), hematuria, dribbling, anuria, malodorous urine, flank pain
Skeletal	Bone pain, fractures, swollen/painful joints, edema
Reproductive	Amenorrhea, menorrhagia/abnormal menstruation, pelvic pain, decreased libido
Neurologic	Apathy, confusion, impaired memory, narrowed span of attention, disorientation, irritability, depression, decreased sensation in extremities, burning feet, restless leg syndrome
Skin	Pruritis, pallor, rash, itching, photosensitivity, dry eyes
Immunologic	Fever, specific symptoms of infection

Table 20-3. COMMON NEPHROLOGY DISEASE PROCESSES AND ASSOCIATED SYMPTOMS.	
DISEASE PROCESS	SYMPTOMS
Acute interstitial nephritis	Skin rash, urticaria, fever, arthralgias, exposure to new medications
Acute renal failure	Thirst, nausea, orthostatic lightheadedness, vomiting, diarrhea, hemorrhage, abdominal pain, sweat, fever, shortness of breath, orthopnea, PND, chest pain, edema, anasarca, ascites, skin rash, urticaria, fever, arthralgia, coma, seizures, immobility, polyuria, skin rashes, fever, weight loss, epistaxis, hemoptysis, edema, hematuria, proteinuria, sudden onset of flank pain, frequency, urgency, dysuria, dribbling, sudden anuria, alternate episodes of anuria and polyuria, vaginal bleeding or abnormal menstruation, pelvic pain
Acute tubular necrosis	Exposure to IV contrast agent(s), aminoglycosides, NSAIDs
Chronic renal failure	Fatigue, weakness, shortness of breath, dyspnea, orthopnea, PND, anorexia, weight loss, nausea, vomiting, hiccups, bad taste, GI bleeding, bone pain, fractures, amenorrhea, menorrhagia, decreased libido, apathy, confusion, impaired memory, narrowed span of attention, disorientation, irritability, depression, decreased sensation in extremities, burning feet, restless leg syndrome, pruritis, pallor, fever
Glomerulonephritis	Edema, hematuria, proteinuria
Nephrolithiasis	Symptoms of urinary tract infection (UTI), renal colic
Nephrotic syndrome	Shortness of breath, orthopnea, PND, chest pain, edema, anasarca, ascites
Tumor	Flank pain (kidney), fever, weight loss, hematuria, renal colic
Urinary tract infection	Fever, flank pain, hematuria, dysuria, dribbling, frequency, urgency, malodorous urine
Urinary tract obstruction	Urinary frequency, urgency, dysuria, dribbling, sudden anuria, alternating episodes of anuria and polyuria, pelvic pain
Vascular thrombosis, vasculitis	Sudden onset of flank pain or hematuria, shortness of breath, cough, hemoptysis, epistaxis

Table 20-4. NONSPECIFIC SYMPTOMS AND THEIR NEPHROLOGY DISEASE PROCESSES.

SYMPTOM	DISEASE PROCESS
Anasarca	Nephrotic syndrome, ARF
Anuria	Urinary tract obstruction, ARF
Dysuria	UTI, ARF, urinary tract obstruction
Edema	GN, cardiovascular disease, decreased oncotic pressure (liver disease), vascular obstruction
Hematuria	Trauma, vigorous exercise, infection, tumor, genetic kidney disorders, GN, UTI, vascular thrombosis/vasculitis
Polyuria	Urinary obstruction, ARF
Proteinuria	Glomerulonephritis, ARF
Renal colic or flank pain	Nephrolithiasis, renal cell cancer, thrombosis
Pelvic pain	Infection, trauma, transitional cell carcinoma (urothelial carcinoma), prostate/gynecologic (GYN) cancer, acute renal failure

IX. PHYSICAL EXAMINATION

A. Vital Signs: Ensure that vital signs are taken correctly.

1. For all blood pressure measurements:
   - **a.** Patient should have the arm bared.
   - **b.** Refrain from smoking or ingesting caffeine during the 30-minute period before measurement.
   - **c.** Rest for 5 minutes.
   - **d.** Use appropriate cuff size (at least 80% of the arm).
2. To obtain orthostatic vital signs:
   - **a.** Take blood pressure and heart rate measurements in the supine, sitting, and standing positions.
   - **b.** Allow 3-5 minutes between measurements to allow stabilization.
   - **c.** A drop of 10-20 mmHg in the systolic blood pressure or an increase in the pulse rate of more than 15 beats per minute signifies positive orthostatic changes.

B. Nephrology-Focused Physical Examination (Tables 20-5 and 20-6)

X. DIFFERENTIAL DIAGNOSIS (Table 20-7)

XI. INITIAL LABORATORY AND RADIOLOGIC EVALUATION

A. General Studies (Table 20-8)

B. Urinalysis and Assessment of Renal Function by Laboratory Data

1. The urine collected for urinalysis must be fresh because the elements of the urine change with standing.
2. A freshly voided, clean-catch specimen is best.

Table 20-5. NEPHROLOGY-FOCUSED PHYSICAL EXAMINATION.

SYSTEM	ASSESS FOR . . .
Eyes	Conjunctivae, fundi
Ears	Hearing
Nose	Saddle nose deformity, bleeding
Throat	Exudates, erythema
Neck	Jugulovenous distension (JVD), bruits, lymph nodes
Lungs	Decreased breath sounds, crackles
Heart	Murmur, rub, gallops, regularity, distant heart sounds
Breast	Mass, tenderness
Abdomen	Palpable kidneys, masses or tenderness, liver congestion, ascites, distended bladder, bruits
Genitourinary	Pelvic mass or tenderness, prostate enlargement or nodules
Extremities	Edema, skin popping or needle tracks, hemodialysis access
Skin	Color, pallor, excoriations, petechiae, ecchymosis, skin turgor, maculopapular rash, palpable purpura, livido reticularis, Raynaud's phenomenon, "butterfly" rash
Neurologic	Mental status, sensory/motor examination, asterixis

3. If the patient has a Foley catheter in place, withdraw the urine from the proximal port of the catheter tubing. Always do your own urinalysis.

a. Appearance: Check for clarity and color. Normal color (clear to yellow) can be altered by bilirubin, drug metabolites, and presence of blood, crystals, or leukocytes.

b. Specific gravity (dipstick) corresponds roughly to the osmolality. Specific gravity of 1.010 denotes isosthenuria or osmolality equal to the plasma. This is helpful to determine the concentrating ability of the kidneys.

c. Chemical tests (dipstick): The urine dipstick has tabs impregnated with certain chemical reagents that roughly measure the following substances or parameters: pH, protein, glucose, ketones, blood, urobilinogen, bilirubin, nitrites, and leukocyte esterase. Dip the urine specimen and allow the time as listed on the side of the bottle to pass before reading the colorometric changes on each of the tabs.

Text continued on p. 394.

Table 20-6. FINDINGS OF PHYSICAL EXAMINATION AND POSSIBLE DIAGNOSES.

SYSTEM	PHYSICAL EXAMINATION FINDING	POSSIBLE DIAGNOSES
General	Anorexia	ARF
Vitals		
Pulse	Tachycardia	Prerenal fluid loss (dehydration), urosepsis
Blood pressure	Increased (hypertension)	ARF (e.g., acute nephritis [multiple etiologies], CRF etiologies), azotemia, renal arterial obstruction, end-stage renal disease, increased renin production (multiple etiologies), scleroderma renal crisis, Liddle's syndrome
	Decreased (hypotension)	Urosepsis, consider if dehydration if orthostatic
Respiratory rate	Increased	Cardiogenic pulmonary edema (e.g., right-sided heart failure, from renal failure and excess fluid volume)
Weight	Increased	ARF, nephrotic syndrome
	Loss (cachexia)	Malignancy (e.g., renal cancer)
Temperature	Fever	Infections, connective tissue disorders, malignancy (e.g., renal cancer)
	Hypothermia	Azotemia
HEENT		
Eyes	Scleral icterus	Hepatorenal syndrome
	Papilledema	Hypertension associated with renal failure/malignant hypertension
	Corneal opacities	Fabry's disease
	Tortuous retinal veins	Fabry's disease
Ears	Deafness	Alport's syndrome
Nose	Saddle nose deformity	Wegener's granulomatosis
Mouth	Dry mucus membranes	Prerenal fluid loss
	Bad (uriniferous) breath	Uremia
	Mucosal ulceration	Advanced uremia, connective tissue disorders

Face	Edema	ARF (e.g., acute nephritis [multiple etiologies])
Lungs	Rales/rhonchi	Pulmonary edema associated with renal failure (multiple etiologies)
Cardiovascular	Arrest, EKG abnormalities	Hyperkalemia caused by renal failure
	Rub	Pericarditis (uremia)
Abdomen	Suprapubic pain	Urinary tract infection (cystitis, urethritis), urinary tract obstruction
	Upper abdominal pain	Renal infarction (acute arterial occlusion)
	Ascites	Hepatorenal syndrome, fluid overload (dialysis patients)
	Pain	Henoch-Schönlein purpura
	Bruit	Renal artery stenosis
	Palpable kidney(s)	Cancer, polycystic kidney disease
	Lower abdominal pain	Urinary tract obstruction (urinary/renal colic)
Genitourinary		
General	Loin pain	Renal vein thrombosis (nephrotic syndrome), nephrolithiasis
Male	Prostate enlargement	Urinary tract obstruction, prostatitis
	Tender prostate	Prostatitis
	Left varicocele	Renal vein thrombosis (nephrotic syndrome)
Female	Purulent discharge	Urethritis
Skin	Decreased turgor	Prerenal fluid loss
	Petechiae	Hemolytic-uremic syndrome-thrombotic thrombocytopenic purpura (HUS-TTP)
	Jaundice	Hepatorenal syndrome
	Slate-brown color	Hemochromatosis: dialysis patient following multiple transfusions
	Purpura	Henoch-Schönlein purpura, cryoglobulinemia
	Necrotizing skin lesions	Cryoglobulinemia
	Powdery white deposits	Uremic frost (rare in U.S.)

Continued

Table 20-6. FINDINGS OF PHYSICAL EXAMINATION AND POSSIBLE DIAGNOSES—*cont'd*

System	Physical Examination Finding	Possible Diagnoses
Lymphatics	Lymphadenopathy	Lymphoma
Extremities	Edema	ARF (e.g., acute nephritis [multiple etiologies]), CRF (multiple etiologies), nephrotic syndrome (multiple etiologies), DVT (nephrotic syndrome)
	Pain	Pyelonephritis
	Weakness	Hyperkalemia (e.g., rhabdomyolysis with renal failure), renal failure/uremia
	Decreased DTRs	Renal failure/uremia
	Osteodystrophy	Renal insufficiency (encompasses "renal rickets," osteitis fibrosa cystica, and osteosclerosis), renal tubular acidosis, Vitamin D disorder
	Bone pain	Osteomalacia, osteitis fibrosa cystica
	Hip pain	Aseptic necrosis in renal transplant patients
	Dystrophic nails	Nail-Patella syndrome
	Absent patella	Nail-Patella syndrome
Back	Flank pain/tenderness	UTI (pyelonephritis), urinary tract obstruction, renal vein thrombosis (e.g., nephrotic syndrome), renal cancer (primary and metastatic), renal infarction (e.g., acute arterial occlusion), polycystic renal disease, nephrolithiasis
	Bruit	Renal artery stenosis
	Lumbar pain	Renal vein thrombosis (multiple etiologies)
Rectum	Positive guaiac	GI hemorrhage (e.g., associated with acute renal failure, HUS-TTP)
Neurologic	Lethargy/somnolence	ARF, hepatorenal syndrome
	Confusion/dementia	ARF, hepatorenal syndrome, "dialysis dementia"
	Asterixis	ARF, liver failure

Table 20-7. PATHOLOGIC DIAGNOSIS OF KIDNEYS.

Acute renal failure	
Prerenal	Decreased oral intake (elderly), loss of extracellular fluid (true volume depletion), gastrointestinal/skin/respiratory/renal loss of fluid, loss of fluid into body cavity/interstitial space (redistribution of extracellular fluid), compromised cardiac function, nephrotic syndrome, hepatic cirrhosis
Intrinsic	Acute tubular necrosis (ATN), acute interstitial nephritis (AIN), rhabdomyolysis, multisystem disease processes, GN, vascular thrombosis/vasculitis, cholesterol emboli syndrome, pyelonephritis
Postrenal	Nephrolithiasis, urinary tract obstruction
Chronic renal failure	
Glomerulopathies	Allergies, insect bite, accompanies some upper respiratory infections (URIs), associated with some tropical diseases, part of some systemic disease processes (e.g., diabetes mellitus [DM], hypertension, various autoimmune diseases), malignancy, medications
Chronic interstitial nephritis	Medications, heavy metals, connective tissue/immunological disorders, metabolic disorders, hereditary nephritis

Table 20-8. USEFUL TESTS FOR RENAL DISEASE PROCESSES, SIGNS, AND SYMPTOMS.

On Whom	Laboratory or Radiologic Study
All patients with suspected renal disease	Sodium, potassium, chloride, CO_2, blood urea nitrogen (BUN), creatinine, glucose, calcium, phosphorus, magnesium, albumin, complete blood count (CBC) with differential, renal ultrasound, urinalysis performed by the clinician

Continued

Table 20-8. USEFUL TESTS FOR RENAL DISEASE PROCESSES, SIGNS, AND SYMPTOMS—*cont'd*

SELECTED PATIENTS	ADDITIONAL TESTS TO CONSIDER
Patients with proteinuria (depending on history and physical findings)	Hepatitis panel, RPR, serum/urine protein electrophoresis (SPEP/UPEP), antinuclear antibodies (ANA), chest x-ray (CXR), lipid panel, human immunodeficiency virus (HIV), 24-hour urine for creatinine and protein, stool occult × 3, mammogram
Patients with hematuria (depending on history and physical findings)	As above and also cryoglobulins, complement battery, antineutrophil cytoplasmic antibodies (ANCA), antiglomerular basement membrane (GBM), ASO, sickle cell analysis, stone risk assessment
Patients with dysuria, hematuria, pyuria	Urine culture (consider acid-fast bacteria [AFB] or fungal culture if negative)
Patients with sterile pyuria,medications known to cause acute interstitial nephritis, or postvascular procedure	Urine Hansel stain
Patients with acute renal failure	Urine electrolytes to include urine creatinine
Patients with chronic renal failure	Parathyroid hormone (PTH)
Patients with pharyngitis	Throat culture
Patients with fever, IV drug abuse, or new murmur	Blood cultures, echocardiogram
Patients with ascites or abdominal pain	Liver function tests (LFTs), amylase, lipase, acute abdominal series
Patients with renal colic	Kidney-ureter-bladder (KUB) x-ray
History of muscle pain, vigorous physical exertion, heat exposure	Creatine phosphokinase (CPK), urine myoglobin

d. Microscopic examination: Spin the urine in a centrifuge for approximately 5 minutes at 1500 to 2000 rpm. The urine is then poured out, leaving a pellet in the bottom of the tube. Resuspend the pellet in the remaining few drops of urine and place a drop on a microscopic slide with a cover slip.

Scan the slide on low power (100 x), moving to high power (400 x) to examine areas of interest. Table 20-9 lists the elements that may be present.

Table 20-9. ELEMENTS FOUND IN URINE.

ELEMENTS	TYPES
Crystals	Urate, calcium phosphate, oxalate, triple phosphate, cystine
Cells	Erythrocytes (inspect for dysmorphic morphology signifying renal parenchymal origin), leukocytes, renal tubular cells, oval fat bodies, squamous cells
Casts	Hyaline, granular, red blood cells (RBCs), white blood cells (WBCs), tubular cell, degenerating cellular, broad, waxy
Organism	Bacteria, yeast, trichomonas, nematodes
Miscellaneous	Spermatozoa, mucous, fibers

C. Renal Function

1. The glomerular filtration rate (GFR) is the best index of renal function. (There are, however, limitations to this index that are beyond the scope of this text to discuss.)
2. General guidelines are helpful to assess renal function:
   a. The general equation for the renal clearance of any substance, expressed in mL/min:

$$C = UV/P \text{ (then divided by 1440 min/24 hours)}$$

   (1) "U" is the urine concentration (mg/dL).
   (2) "V" is the urine volume in 24 hours (mL).
   (3) "P" is the plasma concentration (mg/dL).

   b. Endogenous creatinine is the substance used most often for the determination of GFR.
   c. This requires the collection of a 24-hour urine for determination of volume and creatinine and a simultaneous determination of plasma creatinine.
   d. Normal range of creatinine clearance for men is 97-137 mL/min/1.73 m^2 and for women 88-128 mL/min/1.73 m^2.
   e. The following equation provides an estimate of creatinine clearance with the age, weight, and serum creatinine without the 24-hour urine:

$$C = (140 - \text{age}) \times \text{lean body weight}) \div (P \times 72).$$
(for women, multiply the above by 0.85)

XII. ACRONYMS AND ABBREVIATIONS (Table 20-10)

Table 20-10. NEPHROLOGY ACRONYMS AND ABBREVIATIONS.

Acronym or Abbreviation	Definition	Acronym or Abbreviation	Definition
ADH	Antidiuretic hormone	**GN**	Glomerulonephritis
AGN	Acute glomerulonephritis	**HUS-TTP**	Hemolytic-uremic syndrome—thrombotic thrombocytopenic purpura
AIN	Acute interstitial nephritis	**IVP**	Intravenous pyelogram
ANA	Antinuclear antibodies	**NS**	Nephrotic syndrome
ANCA	Antineutrophil cytoplasmic antibodies	**PAN**	Polyarteritis nodosum
ARF	Acute renal failure	**PND**	Paroxysmal nocturnal dyspnea
ATN	Acute tubular necrosis	**PSGN**	Post streptococcal glomerulonephritis
BM	Basement membrane	**PTH**	Parathyroid hormone
BUN	Blood urea nitrogen	**RCC**	Renal cell carcinoma
CAPD	Continuous ambulatory peritoneal dialysis	**RPGN**	Rapidly progressive glomerulonephritis
CCPD	Continuous cyclic peritoneal dialysis	**RTA**	Renal tubular acidosis
CGN	Chronic glomerulonephritis	**RTD**	Renal tubular defects
Cr	Creatinine	**RVT**	Renal vein thrombosis
CRF	Chronic renal failure	**UTI**	Urinary tract infection
GBM	Glomerular basement membrane	**VUR**	Vesicoureteral reflux
GFR	Glomerular filtration rate		

XIII. DEFINITIONS (Table 20-11)

Table 20-11. NEPHROLOGY TERMS.

TERMS	DEFINITION
Alleman's syndrome	Association of double kidney and clubbed fingers, sometimes associated with facial asymmetry and degeneration of motor nerves
Alport's syndrome	Hereditary autosomal-dominant disorder characterized by progressive hearing loss, pyelonephritis or glomerulonephritis, and occasional ocular defects
Anasarca	Generalized massive edema
Anuria	Complete suppression/absence of urinary secretion
Azotemia	Excess of urea and other nitrogenous compounds in the blood
Balkan nephropathy	Acquired endemic disorder in the Balkans, characterized by variable renal disease, from focal tubular atrophy, interstitial edema, and mononuclear cell infiltration to diffuse interstitial fibrosis leading to atrophic kidneys
Bartter's syndrome	Hypertrophy and hyperplasia of the juxtaglomerular cells, producing hypokalemic alkalosis and hyperaldosteronism; characterized by absence of hypertension in face of increased plasma renin and insensitivity to pressor effects of angiotensin
Berger's disease	IgA associated GN
Cryoglobulinemia	Presence of immune globulins that precipitate at low temperature, associated with multiple clinical manifestations (e.g., Raynaud's, vascular purpura, urticaria, necrosis of the extremities, bleeding disorders, vasculitis, arthralgia, neurologic changes, glomerulonephritis, hepatosplenomegaly)
Dysuria	Pain with urination
Epstein's syndrome	Nephrotic syndrome
Fabry's syndrome	X-linked lysosomal storage disease, with accumulation or globotriaosylceramide in multiple organs including kidney; patients usually die of kidney failure

Continued

Table 20-11. NEPHROLOGY TERMS—*cont'd*

TERMS	DEFINITION
Fanconi's syndrome	Term for group of diseases characterized by dysfunction of the proximal renal tubules with generalized hyperaminoaciduria, renal glycosuria, hyperphosphaturia, and bicarbonate and water loss; most common cause is cystinosis
Frequency	Need to empty the bladder frequently
Goodpasture's syndrome	Glomerulonephritis associated with pulmonary hemorrhage, association with antibasement membrane antibodies
Hematuria	Blood in the urine
Hemochromatosis	Accumulation of iron in organs (including kidney), eventually leading to failure; may be acquired or inherited
Henoch-Schönlein purpura	Form of nonthrombocytopenic purpura probably caused by a vasculitis; usually see multiorgan involvement including kidneys
Hepatorenal syndrome	Functional renal failure, oliguria, and low urinary sodium without pathologic renal changes; associated with cirrhosis and ascites or with obstructive jaundice
HUS-TTP	Syndrome characterized by renal failure microangiopathic hemolytic anemia, fever, neurologic changes, and thrombocytopenia
Isosthenuria	Urine osmolality equal to the plasma
Liddle's syndrome	Rare inherited disorder characterized by hypertension, hypokalemic alkalosis, and negligible aldosterone secretion
Milk-alkali syndrome	Hypercalcemia without hypercalciuria or hypophosphatemia, with only mild alkalosis, normal serum phosphatase, severe renal insufficiency, with hyperazotemia, and calcinosis
Nephrolithiasis	Kidneys stone(s)
Oliguric	Urine output less than 500 mL in a 24-hour period
Orthostatic	A drop in systolic blood pressure greater than 10 mmHg or increase in pulse of 15 beats per minute with change in position
Osteitis fibrosis cystica	Osteitis with fibrous degeneration and formation of cysts, and with fibrous nodules on the affected bones; caused by hyperfunction of the parathyroid gland and marked osteoclastic activity

Table 20-11—cont'd

Terms	Definition
Osteomalacia	Softening of the bone because of poor mineralization resulting from deficiency of Vitamin D and calcium
Osteosclerosis	Hardening or abnormal density of bone
Nephritic	Urine sediment revealing dysmorphic RBCs and RBC casts
Nephrolithiasis	Renal calculi (stones)
Nephrotic	Greater than 3.5 g of proteinuria in a 24-hour period
Polycystic kidney disease	Inherited disorder characterized by cystic kidneys; infantile form associated with hypertension and high mortality, and adult form associated with progressive renal failure
Polyuria	Passage of a large volume of urine in a short period (e.g., diabetes)
Potter's syndrome	Characteristic facial appearance with renal agenesis or hypoplasia and other defects
Proteinuria	Presence of protein in the urine (greater than 150 mg)
Prune-belly syndrome	Absent lower part rectus abdominis muscle and lower and medial parts of the oblique muscles, associated with greatly dilated ureters and bladder, small and dysplastic kidneys, hydronephrosis, undescended testis, and protruding belly
Pyuria	Presence of WBCs in the urine
Renal colic	Pain that may wax and wane in the flank referred from the kidney
Renal tubular acidosis	Decreased excretion of acid by kidneys with resulting metabolic acidosis; frequently associated with a hyperchloremic acidosis
Restless leg syndrome	Deep discomfort in calves when sitting or lying down, producing an irresistible urge to move legs, especially just before falling asleep
Systemic lupus erythematosus	Multisystem autoimmune disorder of connective tissue within a wide range of clinical manifestations; frequently associated with nephritis
Uremia	Excess of urea, creatinine, and other nitrogenous products in the blood

Continued

Table 20-11. NEPHROLOGY TERMS—*cont'd*

TERMS	DEFINITION
Urgency	Sensation of need to urinate
von Hipple-Lindau	Characterized by congenital angiomatosis of the retina and cerebellum, and cysts of the pancreas, kidneys, and other viscera

XIV. SAMPLE H&P WRITE-UP

Chief Complaint: "My legs have been swelling for a few days, and I fainted this morning."

HPI: T.N. is a single 19-year-old white male who was in his usual state of good health until 5 days ago when he noted swelling in both of his feet. The swelling progressed to where it was noticeable in both of his legs, and it became difficult to put his shoes on. This morning, when the patient stood up from his seat to go to another class, he lost consciousness and collapsed, and was subsequently brought to the emergency room by ambulance. He apparently regained consciousness shortly after falling to the ground. The patient also admits to a decreased ability to walk long distances (more than a block) or up the stairs without getting out of breath, and lightheadedness/dizziness if he stands too quickly from a lying or sitting position. He has recently been quite thirsty and admits to a 15-pound weight gain over the last week. He denies fever, anorexia, nose bleeds, orthopnea, PND, vomiting or change in bowel habits, abdominal pain, depression, chest pain, hemoptysis, flank pain, pruritis, arthralgias, or skin rash.

PMHx: The patient denies any chronic medical problems or recent infections. As far as he knows, all of his social contacts and family are well.

PSHx: History of tonsillectomy and adenoidectomy as a child. No complications.

Emergency and Trauma History: The patient has never been hospitalized, had a blood transfusion, or any trauma-related injuries.

Childhood History: Multiple ear infections as a child. Otherwise, he denies any other childhood illnesses.

Occupational History: Freshman in college. He does not have other employment.

Travel History: No travel since a trip to Hawaii 9 months previously with his family.

Animal and Insect Exposure History: The patient does not have any pets and has not had any unusual reactions to past insect bites or stings.

MEDICATIONS: Aspirin for the past 4 days for foot pain, otherwise none. There are no known drug allergies or history of adverse reactions.

HEALTH MAINTENANCE

Diet: Regular diet with no restrictions. The patient is not a vegetarian. There have been no recent changes.

Exercise: The patient jogs on occasion, but does not exercise regularly.

Sleep Patterns: The patient usually wakes once each night to void, although recently admits to waking 2 to 3 times each night.

Social Habits: The patient denies smoking, tobacco, or illicit drug use.

FAMILY HISTORY

First-Degree Relatives' Medical History: The patient's father has hypertension, otherwise no known medical problems.

Genogram: There is no history of genetic traits or diseases within the patient's family.

PSYCHOSOCIAL HISTORY

Personal and Social History: The patient is white and is a freshman in college. He currently lives in a dormitory and has one roommate. He is not sexually active.

REVIEW OF SYSTEMS

General: 15-pound weight gain in the past week, generalized fatigue, and polydipsia. No fever or chills.

HEENT/Neck: No visual changes or epistaxis.

Respiratory: Mild, nonproductive cough and mild dyspnea on exertion. No hemoptysis.

Cardiovascular: No tachycardia, palpitations, chest pain, or PND.

Gastrointestinal: No abdominal pain, nausea or vomiting, or change in bowel habits.

Genitourinary: Polyuria and frequency. No gross hematuria, urgency, or dribbling.

Hematologic/lymphatic: No easy bruising or bleeding tendencies. No masses in axilla, neck, or groin.

Skin: No rash, pruritis, new lesions, or easy bruising.

Neurologic: Rare mild headaches for the past week as well as dizziness on standing. No history of seizures.

Musculoskeletal: No arthritis or muscle weakness.

Extremities: Significant bilateral peripheral edema over the past week. No paraesthesias, numbness, or tremor.

Psychiatric: No history of depression, mood disorders, or anxiety.

PHYSICAL EXAMINATION

Vital signs: T 98.8°F, P 90, BP 158/94, RR 18, Weight 180 lbs., Height 5′7″

HEENT: Moderate periorbital and facial edema. No scleral icterus. Membranes moist.

Neck: No thyroid enlargement or masses. 4 cm JVD.

Lungs: Bilateral crackles and rales, most notable at the bases.

Cardiovascular: Normal S1 and S2. Regular rate and rhythm. No murmur or rub.

Abdomen: Soft, nontender. No RUQ or epigastric pain. No organomegaly.

Genitourinary: No CVA tenderness. No genital tract lesions or discharge.

Rectal: No masses or BRBPR. Guaiac negative.

Skin: No rash or jaundice. Normal skin turgor.

Extremities: 3+ pitting edema bilateral lower extremities. Strength normal.

Neurologic: Normal reflexes. Oriented to person, place, time, and situation. No focal sensory or musculoskeletal deficits.

ANALYSIS: Probable nephrotic syndrome.

21

NEUROLOGY

Michael S. Jaffee, MD, Gregory Sengstock, MD, PhD, and Eric H. Hanson, MD, MPH

I. CHIEF COMPLAINT

A. Chief Complaint: Common neurology presenting complaints.
1. Vertigo.
2. Visual changes: Diplopia, visual field cut, or unilateral loss of visual acuity.
3. Weakness.
4. Sensory changes: Numbness or paresthesias.
5. Paroxysmal loss of consciousness (LOC).
6. Memory loss.
7. Headaches.

B. Identifying Data: Obtain patient's age, gender, handedness, medical record number, and race/ethnicity.

II. HISTORY OF PRESENT ILLNESS

A. Common Neurologic Symptoms
1. Are you experiencing vertigo?
2. Have you had any visual changes? Diplopia, visual field cut, or unilateral loss of visual acuity?
3. Do you have any weakness?
4. Have you had any sensory changes? Numbness or paresthesias?
5. Have you lost consciousness? Paroxysmal LOC.
6. Are you experiencing memory loss?
7. Do you have headaches?

B. Multiple Complaints: If more than one complaint, obtain history starting sequentially with the first complaint.

C. Onset: For each of the symptoms above, ask whether onset was acute, subacute (within 2 weeks), or gradual.

D. Course: For each symptom, ask the following questions:
1. Has the symptom progressed? Gradual progression, stepwise progression? Had progressed but now stabilized?
2. Has symptom remained unchanged since onset? Or is it paroxysmal (e.g., seizure, migraine)?
3. What occurred before, during, and after the event?

III. PAST MEDICAL AND SURGICAL HISTORY

A. Past Medical History
1. Have you been diagnosed with a chronic medical condition? Obtain date of onset, current status, responses to interventions, complications, or sequelae. Anticipate possible neurologic

complications from certain medical conditions (e.g., hypertension [HTN], heart disease, atrial fibrillation, diabetes, infection).
2. Have you been hospitalized? When? For what reason?
3. Have you had any injuries or accidents? When? Sequelae?

B. Past Surgical History

1. What, if any, surgical procedures have you had? Which procedures? When?
2. Did you have any operative or postoperative complications?
   a. Infection?
   b. Stroke?
   c. Mental status change?
   d. Anoxia? A possible complication of cardiovascular surgery.
   e. Any focal compressive neuropathy from prolonged surgical position (e.g., meralgia paresthetica—numbness of lateral femoral cutaneous nerve caused by prolonged lithotomy position)?
3. What type of anesthesia was used (if known)? Any complications?

C. Emergency and Trauma History

1. Have you made any emergency room visits? When? For what reason?
2. Were you treated for an injury or accident? When? Sequelae? Include history of head trauma and associated LOC.

D. Childhood History

1. What childhood illnesses did you have? Any hereditary or congenital disorders?
2. If known, were there any complications in your delivery or soon after birth?
3. Was your development and growth normal? Were developmental milestones met (similar to other children your age)?
4. Did you have febrile seizures?
5. Did you have meningitis?
6. What immunizations did you receive? Polio, diphtheria, measles?

E. Occupational History

1. What occupations have you had (include military service)? Dates?
2. Have you ever been exposed to hazardous materials (e.g., asbestos, solvents, heavy metals, other chemicals)? Two main patterns of nervous system disease: Peripheral polyneuropathy and cognitive/mental status changes.

F. Travel History

1. Where have you traveled? For what length of time? Prophylaxis taken? Consider areas endemic for arboviruses (e.g., mosquitoes) and certain viral encephalitides.

2. When did the travel occur? Some disease processes such as parasites may not be recognized until decades following the trip.
3. Diet during travel: Did you drink the local water? Were ice cubes used in restaurants made with local water? Did you consume any unwashed fruits or vegetables? Did you consume pork in areas endemic for neurocysticercosis (Mexico)?

IV. MEDICATIONS, ALLERGIES, AND ADVERSE REACTIONS

A. Medications

1. Are you taking any prescription medications? Current dosage and schedule, date initiated, recent changes in dosing?
2. Are you using any over-the-counter (OTC) medicines, herbal preparations, or supplements?
3. What medicines have been tried previously for your condition? Include dose, duration, and tolerability (presence of side effects).

B. Allergies to Medications and Side Effects/Adverse Reactions

1. What, if any, allergic or adverse reactions have you had to medications? What treatments did you receive and with what results?
2. Consider interactions if patient is taking multiple medications.

V. HEALTH MAINTENANCE

A. Prevention: Stroke Risk Factors

1. Do you have hypercholesterolemia?
2. HTN?
3. Do you have diabetes? Is it under control?

B. Diet

1. Have you had any unintentional weight gain or loss?
2. Are your symptoms better or worse with meals?
3. Are your symptoms provoked by certain foods (e.g., migraines triggered by red wine and chocolate, periodic paralysis triggered by carbohydrate load)?
4. What is your usual diet? Having patients keep a food journal may be beneficial.
5. Do you consume any unusual items (e.g., hair, clay, ice)?
6. Are you anorexic? Achieve early satiety? Hyperphagia?
7. When did you have your last meal?

C. Exercise

1. Have you experienced any recent changes?
2. Have you recently started exercising?

D. Sleep Patterns

1. Do you have trouble falling asleep?
2. Is your sleep interrupted?
3. Do you awaken early?
4. Do your legs jerk during sleep (history from bed partner)?

E. Social Habits

1. Do you use tobacco? What type? How much? For how long? Pack-years (packs per day times number of years).
2. Do you use alcohol? Quantity, frequency, physical or legal problems related to use?
3. Do you use illicit drugs? Which ones, frequency, route or administration?
4. Do you use caffeine? Changes in intake (either increase or decrease) can be associated with headaches.

VI. FAMILY HISTORY

A. First-Degree Relatives' Medical History

1. Have first-degree relatives had headaches such as migraines or hemiplegic migraines?
2. Have any first-degree relatives had a movement disorder? Parkinson's disease? Spinocerebellar ataxias (e.g., Friedrich's ataxia)?
3. Are there any hereditary neuropathies (e.g., Charcot-Marie-Tooth)?
4. Dementias (e.g., Alzheimer's, Pick's disease, frontotemporal tauopathy, Huntington's disease)?
5. Hereditary tumors (e.g., neurofibromatosis)?

B. Three-Generation Genogram (see page 341 in Chapter 18)

VII. PSYCHOSOCIAL HISTORY

A. Personal and Social History

1. What is your ethnic background? Ethnicity and race may identify increased risk of disease or variable responses to therapy (e.g., neurosarcoidosis in African-Americans).
2. Socioeconomic status: Are you able to afford medications and therapies?
3. Education: What level of education have you achieved? Assess the patient's ability to understand the disease process and to make lifestyle adjustments.

B. Current Illness Effects on the Patient

1. Gauge the patient's coping skills and support system.
2. Determine whether the patient's expectations of current illness and therapy are realistic.
3. Assess for signs of depression.

C. Interpersonal and Sexual History

1. Are you sexually active?
2. How often do you engage in sexual activity? Some medications (e.g., some hypertensive agents) may affect the ability to achieve erection, decrease libido, or both. This may be intolerable to the patient.

D. Family Support

1. Are family members supportive? Available to assist in an emergency? Family members may need tutoring on neurologic emergencies (e.g., for acute-onset stroke, must present

within 3 hours to be eligible for thrombolysis treatment [IV t-PA]).

2. Do family members know what to expect regarding the course of your disease? They may need to be educated on the expected natural history and course of disease, especially if it is likely to be progressive.

E. Occupational Aspects of the Illness

1. Does your job require you to fulfill physical duties or functions? The patient may need to restrict physical activity at work.
2. Does your job involve driving? Are you responsible for the safety of others? Certain conditions such as seizures may require driving restrictions and inability to work jobs in which a seizure could pose significant risk (e.g., airline pilot, bus driver). The DMV of each state has its own guidelines on driving and seizures.

VIII. REVIEW OF SYSTEMS (Tables 21-1, 21-2, and 21-3)

Table 21-1. GENERAL NEUROLOGY SYMPTOMS BY SYSTEM.

SYSTEM	SYMPTOMS
General and neurovegetative	Transient loss of consciousness, fatigue, fever/shakes/chills
HEENT	Diplopia, dysarthria, dysphagia, vertigo, visual problems, headache
Neck	Stiffness
Cardiovascular	Palpitations
Gastrointestinal	Nausea, abdominal pain
Genitourinary	Urinary incontinence
Obstetrics and gynecologic	Sexual dysfunction (medication induced)
Lymphatic	Lymphadenopathy
Musculoskeletal	Weakness, cramping, back pain, numbness, paresthesias, stiffness, abnormal movement (increased or decreased)
Neuropsychiatric	Depression, cognitive problems (memory)
Anterior (carotid) circulation symptoms	Monocular visual loss, focal numbness or weakness, aphasia, apraxia
Posterior (vertebrobasilar) circulation symptoms	Diplopia, dysarthia, dysphagia, vertigo, visual field cut

Table 21-2. NONSPECIFIC SYMPTOMS AND THEIR NEUROLOGIC DISEASES.

Symptom	Diseases
Transient LOC	Seizure, syncope, TIA, migraine
Weakness	Upper motor neuron (UMN) versus lower motor neuron (LMN): see section III
	Bilateral, proximal: myopathy; bilateral, distal: neuropathy
	One extremity + pain: radiculopathy (nerve root)
	One extremity without pain: stroke, tumor
Numbness	Stroke, neuropathy, radiculopathy
Diplopia	Stroke, myasthenia gravis, multiple sclerosis (MS)
Vertigo	Stroke, multiple sclerosis, peripheral vestibulopathy
Tremor	Parkinson's disease, essential tremor, drug-induced
Headache	Migraine, subarachnoid hemorrhage, temporal arteritis, elevated intracranial pressure (ICP) (mass, pseudotumor, hydrocephalus)

Table 21-3. COMMON NEUROLOGIC DISEASES AND THEIR SYMPTOMS.

Disease	Symptoms
Stroke	Acute onset of focal numbness or weakness, vertigo, or diplopia
Multiple sclerosis	Subacute onset of multifocal lesions separated in space and time
Myopathy	Subacute onset of symmetric weakness
Movement disorders	Hypokinetic-parkinsonism syndrome; hyperkinetic-chorea syndrome

IX. PHYSICAL EXAMINATION (Table 21-4 and Boxes 21-1 and 21-2)

Table 21-4. SELECTED PHYSICAL FINDINGS AND POSSIBLE DIAGNOSIS.

System	Physical Examination Finding	Possible Diagnoses
Vital Signs/ Blood pressure	Orthostatic drop in systolic BP with no increase in pulse	Autonomic dysfunction

Table 21-4—cont'd		
System	**Physical Examination Finding**	**Possible Diagnoses**
HEENT		
Head	Tender temporal areas	Temporal arteritis
Eyes	Marcus-Gunn Pupil	Multiple sclerosis (MS)
	Nystagmus	Vertical nystagmus is a CNS source
	Ptosis	Horner's syndrome or neuromuscular disease (i.e., myasthenia gravis)
Ears	Lesions in external canal	Ramsay-Hunt syndrome
Face	Unilateral droop	Bell's palsy (whole face), central lesion (lower face only)
Neck	Bruit	Possible marker of atherosclerosis (not sensitive or specific)
Posterior neck	Stiffness	Meningitis, cervicalgia
Cardiovascular	Atrial fibrillation or murmur	Cardiac source of embolic stroke
Genitourinary	Saddle anesthesia; loss of anal wink reflex	Lower spinal cord lesion
Skin	Café-au-lait spots	Neurofibromatosis
	Adenoma sebaceum	Tuberous sclerosis
	Heliotropic Rash	Dermatomyositis
Lymphatics	Lymphadenopathy	Cancer, infection
Extremities	Atrophy, fasciculations	Lower motor neuron (LMN) disease
Neurologic	See Box 21-1	

Box 21-1. NEUROLOGIC PHYSICAL EXAMINATION BY SECTION.

I. **Mental Status Examination**
II. **Cranial Nerves:** Optic group (CN II, III, IV, VI), branchiomotor group and tongue (CN V, VII, IX, X, XI, XII), special sensory group (CN I, VIII)
III. **Motor:** Bulk, tone, and strength
IV. **Sensory:** Cutaneous sensory and cortical sensory integration
V. **Reflexes:** Deep, superficial and pathologic reflexes
VI. **Cerebellar**
VII. **Gait and Station**

Box 21-2. NEUROLOGIC PE SEQUENCE OF PATIENT POSITION (ALTERNATE METHOD).

I. **Mental status**

II. **Patient seated on examination table**
Cranial nerve tests (CN I Olfaction), optic group (CN II, III, IV, VI), branchiomotor group and tongue (CN V, VII, IX and X, XII, and XI), special sensory group (CN I, VII, VIII). Sensory examination (superficial sensory modality testing, deep sensory modality testing, dermatomal distribution of sensory loss). Motor: upper extremities strength and coordination. (Optiona)l: lower extremities strength and coordination. Strength testing (grade strength 0 to 5). Coordination and tone. Reflexes (Grade 0 to 4+).

III. **Patient lying down (optional)**
Motor: Lower extremities strength and coordination (strength testing: scale 0-5). Heel-to-shin test, Reflexes to include evaluation for Babinski reflex.

IV. **Patient standing**
Routine gait, toe walking, heel walking, tandem walking, Romberg's test.

V. Special case: Coma Evaluation: Level of consciousness (response to verbal or painful stimuli), pupillary responses, eye movements (doll's eye reflex or cold water calorics), motor posturing, spontaneous movements, or withdrawal of each extremity to pain.

A. Mini-Mental Status Examination (MSE) (Table 21-5)

It is necessary to complete at least part of the mental status examination on every patient. Although most of the information is gathered during the history, specific questions and cognitive function questions need to be asked and introduced. The MSE measures three functions that need to be examined: thinking, feeling, and behavior.

1. Level of consciousness: Estimate the patient's level of consciousness along a continuum: from alert, on the left side of the continuum, to coma, on the right.

Table 21-5. MINI-MENTAL STATUS EXAMINATION

Examination Areas	Questions and Tasks	Score
Orientation	What is the year, season, date, day, and month?	(/ 5)
	Where are we? (state, country, town, hospital, floor).	(/ 5)

Table 21-5—cont'd

EXAMINATION AREAS	QUESTIONS AND TASKS	SCORE
Registration	Name three objects: 1 second to say each. Then ask the patient to repeat all three words after you have said them. Give 1 point for each initial correct answer. Then repeat them until patient learns all three words. Count trials and record. Number of trials ________.	(/ 3)
Attention and Calculation	Serial 7's. 1 point for each correct. Stop after 5 answers. Alternatively spell "world" backwards	(/ 5)
Recall	Ask for the three objects repeated above. Give 1 point for each correct	(/ 3)
Language	Name a pencil and wristwatch (2 points) Repeat the following "No ifs, ands, or buts" (1 point) Follow a three-stage command: 1. "Take a paper in your right hand. 2. Fold it in half. 3. Put it on the floor." (3 points) Read and obey the following: Close your eyes (1 point). Write a sentence (1 point).	(/ 8)
Visuospatial	Copy the design (1 point).	(/ 1)
ASSESS level of consciousness along a continuum:____________ Alert Drowsy Stupor Coma		Total Score (/ 30)

Note that a score <20 is very suggestive of a dementia.
Source: Folstein MF, Folstein SE, McHugh PR. Mini-Mental State: A practical method for grading the state of patients for the clinician. Journal of Psychiatric Research, 12, 189–198.

2. Orientation: Ask patient what the date is (i.e., day of the week, month, year). Then ask specifically for any parts omitted. Ask for additional, related information (e.g., "Can you also tell me what season it is?"). Give one point for each correct answer. Then ask, "Can you tell me the name of this hospital?" "Where

is it located?" (e.g., town, country). Give one point for each correct response.

3. Registration: Ask the patient if you may test his or her memory. Then say the names of three unrelated objects (e.g., "truck, seven, red") clearly and slowly, taking about one second to say each word. After you have said all three words, ask the patient to repeat them. The first repetition determines the score (0-3). Keep saying them, up to six trials, until the patient can repeat all three words. If the patient does not eventually learn all three words, recall cannot be meaningfully tested.
4. Attention and calculation: Ask the patient to count backward by 7, beginning at 100. Stop after 5 subtractions (i.e., 93, 86, 79, 72, 65). Score the total number of correct answers. If the patient cannot or will not perform this task, ask him or her to spell the word "world" backwards. The score is the number of letters given in the correct order (e.g., "dlrow" = 5, "dlorw" = 3).
5. Recall: Ask the patient to recall the three objects that you previously specified in orientation. Score 0-3.
6. Language.
   a. Naming: Show the patient a wristwatch and ask what it is. Repeat for a pencil. Score 0-2.
   b. Repetition: Ask the patient to repeat a sentence after you say it. Allow only one trial. Score 0 or 1.
   c. Three-stage command: "Take a piece of paper in your right hand, fold it in half, and put it on the floor." Give the patient a piece of blank paper and repeat the command. Score 1 point for each part correctly executed.
   d. Reading: On a blank piece of paper, print the sentence "Close your eyes" in letters large enough for the patient to see clearly. Ask the patient to read the sentence and do what it says. Score 1 point if the patient actually closes his or her eyes.
   e. Writing: Give the patient a blank piece of paper and ask him or her to write a sentence for you. Do not dictate the sentence; it is to be written spontaneously. It must contain a subject and verb and be sensible, but correct grammar and punctuation are not important.

B. Cranial Nerves (CN)

1. Olfactory nerve (CN I): Usually not formally tested unless a chief complaint.
   a. Test one nostril at a time with fruit smells, peppermint, and camphor. Do not use noxious substances such as ammonia.
   b. Note whether patient is unable to recognize smells (i.e., anosmia); patient should respond to ammonia. If no smell (including ammonia) is recognized, the patient may not have an organic disease.

2. Optic nerve (CN II).
 a. Visual acuity.
  (1) Check vision with Snellen's chart, near-vision card, newspaper, or magazine.
  (2) Additionally, you can check if viewing an object through a pinhole will correct a patient's refractive problem.
 b. Visual fields.
  (1) Check by confrontation.
  (2) Look for gross abnormalities in both eyes, then carefully assess each eye.
  (3) Test the quadrants: If defect is in only one eye, then a lesion has to be anterior to chiasm. If defect is in both eyes in the same quadrants, the lesion is usually behind the chiasm.
 c. Fundoscopic examination.
  (1) Disc: Assess for color, sharp margins, and flat optic cup. An edematous optic cup can indicate papilledema (increased intracranial pressure, malignant hypertension, or thrombosis of the central retinal vein).
  (2) Blood vessels: Arteriovenous (AV) nicking (hypertension), bright yellow object in artery (cholesterol embolus).
  (3) Retina: Red lesions (hemorrhages), bright yellow object in artery (cholesterol embolus). Note disc, blood vessels, and retinal background.

3. Oculomotor nerve (CN III) is tested with trochlear (CN IV) and abducens (CN VI).
 a. Muscles innervated $(LR_6SO_4)_3$.
  (1) III = Medial rectus, inferior rectus, superior rectus, inferior oblique, palpebral muscle.
  (2) IV = Superior oblique.
  (3) VI = Lateral rectus.
 b. Pupils.
  (1) Parasympathetic (pupilloconstriction) to sympathetic (pupillodilation).
  (2) Pupils of unequal size: Anisocoria of up to 0.5 mm is normal if both pupils react normally.
  (3) Direct and consensual light reflex.
   (a) Direct: Pupil gets smaller when light shines directly on it.
   (b) Consensual: The other pupil constricts to match the opposite eye.
   (c) Swinging flashlight test: Rapidly move the light from the pupil of each eye to the other and hold it for approximately 2-3 seconds. If the pupil dilates when light is swung onto it, the prior consensual response was stronger than the present direct

NEURO

response, indicating afferent pupillary defect or Marcus Gunn pupil (optic nerve lesion).

(d) If no light reflex exists, check accommodation. More fibers do accommodation than do light reflex. Have patient look in the distance and then at your finger, which should be placed 10 cm in front of patient. You should detect pupil constriction.

c. Extraocular muscle testing: Diplopia.

(1) Six positions of cardinal gaze.

(2) Rule: Diplopia is worst in the position of the weak muscle.

(3) Side-by-side diplopia is usually medial or lateral rectus.

(4) Oblique or vertical diplopia: Bielschowsky's head-tilt test.

(a) Determine which eye is higher. If the right eye is higher, then it is a problem with depressors of the right eye or elevators of the left eye.

(b) Have the patient look to both sides. If the diplopia is worse on left lateral gaze, then it is a problem with the right superior oblique (SO) or the left superior rectus (SR) muscle.

(c) Have the patient look up and down on the side that is the worst. If diplopia occurs while looking up, the problem is with the left SR, and if it occurs when looking down, it is the right SO muscle.

d. Nystagmus.

(1) Described by its fast phase, right beating, left beating, up, down, or rotatory.

(2) Etiologies.

(a) Physiologic (e.g., looking out window of moving vehicle).

(b) Retinal (e.g., blind, unable to fixate).

(c) Peripheral (e.g., vestibular system lesion): Vestibular system is a push-push system; a lesion on the left will allow the eyes to slowly deviate to the left and a fast phase to the right (right-beating nystagmus) will be seen.

(d) Central (e.g., brainstem or cerebellum disease). Drugs: Antiepileptics (multidirectional gaze-evoked nystagmus). Pure vertical nystagmus is always central in origin.

4. Trigeminal nerve (CN V).

a. Innervation.

(1) Sensory sensation to the face.

(a) Three divisions: VI = ophthalmic (to vertex of skull), V2 = maxillary, V3 = mandibular.

(b) Subjective test with light touch, pinprick.

(c) Objective test with corneal reflex, touch the cornea with cotton or tissue.

(i) Afferent is CN5, and the efferent is CN7.

(ii) Look for equal bilateral blink; if both slow, either unilateral 5 or bilateral 7. Then test other side; if only one is slow, then it is a 7.

(2) Motor to muscles of mastication: Masseters, temporalis, pterygoids, as well as tensor tympani. Test by having patient resist against open mouth, weakness on side opposite jaw moves.

5. Facial (CN VII).

a. Innervation.

(1) Motor sensation to the face.

(2) Taste to the anterior two thirds of tongue.

(3) Stapedius muscle.

b. Test by raising eyebrow, testing orbicularis oculi, blow out cheeks, pucker lips.

(1) Bell's palsy: Peripheral CN 7 lesion (signs): Weakness of eyebrow, eye closure, pucker lips; may have taste alteration (sweet, sour, salty, bitter); and may have increased sound on the affected side (low frequency common).

6. Acoustic (CN VIII).

a. Assess hearing grossly with ticking watch, rubbing patient's hair between fingers.

b. Weber test.

(1) Hold 516-Hz tuning fork on vertex of head.

(2) Ask which ear it is louder in, the good or deaf ear.

c. Rinne test.

(1) Hold 516-Hz tuning fork on mastoid process (bone conduction [BC]) and alternate with front of ear (air conduction [AC]).

(2) Determine which is heard longer. The normal finding is AC > BC.

7. Mouth CN IX, X, XII and Neck CN XI.

a. Glossopharyngeal (CN IX).

(1) Innervates sensory posterior one third of tongue, motor stylopharyngeus, autonomic parotid gland.

(2) Test by having patient say "ah" and watching movement of uvula, gag reflex (afferent portion).

b. Vagus (CN X).

(1) Innervates sensory tympanic membrane, eternal auditory canal (EAC) and external ear, motor muscles of palate (recurrent laryngeal nerve), autonomic carotid baroreceptors, parasympathetic to thorax and abdomen.

(2) Test by listening to voice for hoarseness, gag reflex (efferent portion), swallow water.

c. Hypoglossal (CN XII).

(1) Innervates motor to intrinsics of the tongue.

(2) Test by having patient push tongue into cheek; protrude tongue; it will deviate toward the weak side.

d. Spinal accessory (CN XI).

(1) Innervates motor to trapezius and sternocleidomastoid (ipsilateral innervation to SCM).

(2) Test by trying to turn the head.

C. **Somatic Motor System**

1. **Muscle Bulk:** Graded as normal, slight, moderate, or severe atrophy.
2. **Muscle Tone:** Use range of motion and relaxation of all extremities for testing of lead pipe and spastic (clasp-knife) reflexes, as well as testing for cogwheel rigidity.
3. **Muscle Strength (Table 21-6).**

a. Scale 0/5 to 5/5.

b. Test strength of movements against resistance. Does the weakness follow a distributional pattern (proximal-distal, right-left, or upper extremity-lower extremity)?

Table 21-6. MRC (MUSCLE RESEARCH COUNCIL) MUSCLE STRENGTH SCALE.

MUSCLE GRADATION	DESCRIPTION
5 / 5 Normal	Complete range of motion against gravity with full resistance. No movement at the joint
4 / 5 Good	Complete range of motion against gravity with some resistance. Movement at the joint with effort
3 / 5 Fair	Complete range of motion against gravity
2 / 5 Poor	Complete range of motion with gravity eliminated. Movement with the arm on a table
1 / 5 Trace	Evidence of slight contractility. No joint motion
0 / 5 Zero	No evidence of contractility

4. **Neck and Upper Extremities**

a. Neck: Flexion and extension, side-to-side movements.

b. Shoulder: Abduction and the "T figure" (resistance against abducted shoulders) for trapezius muscle (CN XI).

(1) Look for scapular winging.

(2) Test infraspinatus muscle (suprascapular nerve C5-6) and teres minor muscle (axillary nerve branch C5) by applying resistance to external rotation of the arm flexed at the elbow.

(3) Test subscapular muscle (upper and lower subscapular muscle C5-6) by applying resistance to internal rotation.

c. Elbow: Flexion by the biceps muscle (musculocutaneous nerve C5) and extension by the triceps muscle (radial nerve C7).

d. Wrist: Dorsiflexion and volar flexion.

e. Fingers.

(1) Thumb abduction (abductor pollicis brevis muscle), adduction, opposition, flexion (all median nerve), and extension (radial nerve).

(2) Finger strength with flexion and extension (grip strength).

(3) Dorsal and palmar interossei muscles abduction and adduction (ulnar nerve).

(4) Mnemonic PADs & DABs (palmar interossei muscle adduction and dorsal interossei muscle abduction).

5. **Lower Extremities.**

a. Hip: Flexion, extension, abduction, and adduction.

b. Knee: Flexion and extension.

c. Ankle.

(1) Dorsiflexion and plantar flexion.

(2) Inversion of plantar flexed foot (tibialis anterior muscle and deep peroneal nerve L4-5).

(3) Walking with foot everted (peroneus longus and brevis muscles and superficial peroneal nerve S1).

d. Toes: Large toe flexion (flexor hallucis longus muscle and tibial nerves L5, S1-2) and extension (extensor hallucis longus muscle and deep peroneal nerves L4-5, S1).

6. **Method of Documenting Motor Strength (Table 21-7).**

7. **Patterns of Muscular Weakness.**

a. Upper Motor Neuron (UMN).

(1) Increased tone, increased reflexes.

(2) Pyramidal pattern of weakness (weak extensions in arms; weak flexors in legs).

(3) Pronator drift in arms when held up for 2 minutes.

b. Lower Motor Neuron (LMN).

(1) Wasting, fasciculation, decreased tone, or decreased reflexes.

(2) Peripheral pattern of weakness (weak flexors in arms; weak extensors in legs).

(a) Muscle disease: Wasting, decreased tone, impaired or absent reflexes.

(b) Neuromuscular junction: Fatigable weakness, normal or decreased tone, normal reflexes.

c. Functional (psychiatric) weakness: Normal tone, normal reflexes, normal bulk, erratic power (give-way weakness).

Table 21-7. MUSCULAR STRENGTH GRADING CHART FOR EXTREMITIES USING THE 5-POINT SCALE.

ARM	SA	EE	EF	IS	WE	WF	FE	FF	IO	APB
R	5	5	5	5	5	5	5	5	5	5
L	5	5	5	5	5	5	5	5	5	5

SA = Shoulder Abductor; EE = Elbow Extenders; EF = Elbow Flexors; IS = Infraspinatus; WE = Wrist Extenders; WF = Wrist Flexors; FE = Finger Extenders; FF = Finger Flexors; IO = Interossei; APB = Abductor Pollicis Brevis.

LEG	HF	HE	HAB	HAD	KF	KE	ADF	APF	AI	AE	EHL
R	5	5	5	5	5	5	5	5	5	5	5
L	5	5	5	5	5	5	5	5	5	5	5

HF = Hip Flexors; HE = Hip Extenders; HAB = Hip Abductors; HAD = Hip Adductors; KF = Knee Flexors; KE = Knee Extenders; ADF = Ankle Dorsiflexion; APF = Ankle Pronator Flexion; AI = Ankle Inversion; AE = Ankle Eversion; EHL = Extensor Hallucis Longus.

D. Sensory System

1. **Five Primary Modalities.**
   a. Spinothalamic tract.
      (1) Pinprick.
      (2) Temperature.
      (3) Light touch.
   b. Posterior column.
      (1) Vibration (128-Hz tuning fork).
      (2) Proprioception.
         (a) Distal extremities such as fingers/toes.
         (b) Trunk (Romberg's test).
      (3) Light touch: Note that light touch is carried by both spinothalomic tract as well as posterior column.
2. **Cortical Sensory Integration Tests (secondary modalities).**
   a. Double simultaneous stimulation.
   b. Graphesthesia: Recognition of written numbers on the back of the hand or the top of the foot.
   c. Stereognosis: Recognition of forms, objects placed into the hand.
   d. Two-point discrimination.
   e. Note: Cannot test for secondary modalities unless primary modalities are intact.
3. **Patterns of Sensory Loss.**
   a. Single nerve: Loss limited to distribution of single nerve.
   b. Root or roots: Common in arm are C5, 6, 7; in the leg are L4, 5, S1.
   c. Peripheral nerve: Glove and stocking, nerves are usually affected distally first.
   d. Spinal cord.
      (1) Complete transverse lesion: Loss of all sensation below level except for some pain sensation a couple of levels below.
      (2) Hemisection of the cord (Brown-Sequard): Loss of proprioception and vibration on the same side and pain and temperature several levels below on the opposite side.
      (3) Central cord: Loss of pain and temperature bilateral at the level of the lesion with sparing of proprioception and vibration. May have a capelike distribution with cervical syringomyelia.
      (4) Posterior column: Loss of proprioception and vibration with intact pain and temperature.
      (5) Anterior spinal syndrome: Loss of pain and temperature below lesion with preserved proprioception and vibration.
   e. Brainstem: Crossed findings of unilateral loss on the face and contralateral loss on the body.

   f. Thalamic: Hemisensory loss of all modalities.
   g. Cortical loss: Intact primary sensations, loss of cortical sensory functions.
   h. Functional loss: Nonanatomical distribution.

E. Reflexes

Assess patient's reflexes, using the reflex grading 4-point scale provided in Box 21-3.

***Box 21-3.* REFLEX GRADING 4-POINT SCALE.**

4	Hyperactive with clonus, indicative of disease.
3	Brisk, spread to involve movement across more than one joint.
2+	More brisk than average, but no spread.
2	Average, normal.
1	Diminished, low normal.
0	No response.

1. **Deep Tendon Reflexes**
   a. Biceps (C5).
   b. Brachioradialis (C6).
   c. Triceps (C7).
   d. Finger flexion (C8).
   e. Knee jerk: Test of quadriceps patellar tendon (L4).
   f. Achilles tendon, ankle jerk, or triceps surae reflex (S1).
2. **Superficial Tendon Reflexes**
   a. Abdominal reflex (T10-12): Stroking abdomen causes umbilicus to move toward area of stimulation; test in four quadrants.
   b. Cremasteric reflex (Afferent L1-Efferent L2): Stroke inner thigh and cause scrotum to rise on stroked side.
   c. Anal wink (S4-S5): Touch areas lightly around the perirectal region and note contraction. Useful for lesions or tumors that present in the sacral regions or cauda equina.
3. **Pathologic Reflexes**
   a. Babinski's sign.
      (1) Positive test is an upgoing large toe when the sole of the foot is scratched in a direction from the heel toward the toes.
      (2) Critical test of upper motor neuron function. Any lesion in the upper motor neuron (UMN) pathway (CNS or spinal cord) may modify this response.
   b. Clonus.
   c. Frontal lobe release reflexes: Rooting, grasping, glabellar, palmomental.

F. **Cerebellar Complex Motor Tests**

1. **Finger-To-Nose Movement**
   a. Evaluate for dysmetria and dystaxia (incoordination) of voluntary movements.
   b. Intention tremors may also be present when a voluntary movement is attempted.
2. **Heel-to-Shin:** Tap heel three times on contralateral patella and move from knee to ankle *slowly* along the shin.
3. **Rapid Alternating Movements (RAMs)**
   a. Hand pronation to supination on the thigh.
   b. Test for the inability to start and control or difficulty in making RAMs (i.e., dysdiadochokinesia) in patients with frontal or cerebellar damage.
4. **Saccades:** Rapid conjugate deviation eye movements regulated by the contralateral cerebral hemisphere through the parapontine reticular formation (PPRF) with a cerebellar component.
   a. Have patient look at your nose then finger . . . nose . . . finger.
   b. Look for dysmetric movements; eyes moving too far (hypermetric) or not far enough (hypometric).
5. **Fisher's Test:** Have patient tap index finger on the interphalangeal joint of thumb.
   a. Test corticospinal system by speed.
   b. Cerebellar system by accuracy.
   c. Basal ganglia system by amplitude.

G. **Gait and Coordination**

1. **Observation**
   a. Tremor at rest or with movement (intention tremor).
   b. Other abnormal movements.
   c. Quantity of movement (hyperactive or bradykinetic).
2. **Gait and Station**
   a. Arm swing.
   b. Width of gait (narrow-based or wide-based).
   c. Toe walking.
   d. Heel walking.
   e. Tandem walking.
   f. Walking with feet inverted or everted.
   g. Deep knee bends.
   h. Romberg's test.
   i. Pronator drift (a motor test).
3. **Abnormal Gaits**
   a. Symmetrical.
      (1) Parkinsonian.
         (a) Flexed posture.
         (b) Festinating (difficult start and stop).
         (c) Small steps (march a petit pas).

(d) En bloc turns (many steps to turn around).
(e) Decreased arm swing bilateral.
(2) Scissoring.
(a) Feet crossing over, toes dragged.
(b) May indicate spastic paraparesis due to multiple sclerosis or cerebral palsy.
(3) Sensory ataxia.
(a) High steppage, wide-based (positive Romberg test).
(b) May indicate posterior column damage or peripheral neuropathy.
(4) Magnetic.
(a) Small steps, feet do not lift off ground.
(b) May indicate frontal lobe process or hydrocephalus.
(5) Astasia-abasia (functional).
(a) Gait is all over the place like the patient is falling, but does not.
(b) Usual cause is psychogenic.

b. Asymmetrical.
(1) Hemiplegic: Usual cause is UMN lesion such as stroke.
(a) Swinging of leg.
(b) Decreased arm swing ipsilateral to the leg swing.
(2) Waddling pelvis—suggestive of a myopathy.
(3) Foot drop: Unable to keep foot up during heel walk.
(a) Can be UMN or LMN.
(b) Usual LMN cause is peroneal palsy or L5 radiculopathy.

H. Additional Information

1. Tremor

a. To test for tremor, have patient place index fingers opposing each other, hands under the nose.
(1) Postural tremor usually indicates benign essential tremor (4-7 Hz).
(2) Resting tremor indicates basal ganglia disease (Parkinson's).

b. Can also have patient do Archimedes spinal.

2. Meningitic Signs

a. Kernig's sign: Patient supine, flex thigh, then straighten leg; patient will experience pain in neck.

b. Brudzinski's sign: Patient supine and lift the patient's head; patient's knees will bend as a response.

3. Postures (in Coma Patients)

a. Decorticate.
(1) Arms both flexed, legs are stiff and extended.
(2) Lesion is usually above the brainstem in thalamus.

b. Decerebrate.
(1) Arms are extended, legs are stiff and extended.
(2) Lesion is usually brainstem lesion (midbrain).

X. DIFFERENTIAL DIAGNOSIS

A. Initial Differential Diagnosis Based on Timing of Onset and Pattern of Examination (Table 21-8)

Table 21-8. INITIAL DIFFERENTIAL DIAGNOSIS BASED ON TIMING OF ONSET AND PATTERN OF EXAMINATION.

TIMING OF ONSET	FOCAL	DIFFUSE
Acute	Vascular	Metabolic
Subacute	Inflammatory	Inflammatory
Chronic	Tumor	Degenerative

B. Classification of Etiologies: A useful mnemonic is "VITAMINS D."

1. **V**ascular.
2. **I**nfectious/inflammatory.
3. **T**rauma.
4. **A**utoimmune.
5. **M**etabolic/toxic.
6. **I**atrogenic.
7. **N**eoplastic.
8. **S**eizure, psychiatric.
9. **D**emyelinating.

XI. LABORATORY STUDIES AND DIAGNOSTIC EVALUATIONS

A. Electromyogram (EMG)/Nerve Conduction Studies (NCS)

1. Electrical studies of nerve and muscle.
2. Can help diagnose and specify diseases of the motor neuron, peripheral nerve, neuromuscular junction, and muscle.

B. Electroencephalogram (EEG)

1. Measurement of electrical activity of the brain cortex.
2. Used in evaluation for seizures and encephalopathy (decreased mental status).

C. Evoked Potentials (EP): Tests cortical pathways of sensory inputs.

1. Visual EP: Used in evaluation of multiple sclerosis or optic neuritis.
2. Brainstem Auditory Evoked Response (BAER): May be used in evaluation of multiple sclerosis or acoustic neuroma.

D. Somatosensory Evoked Potential (SSEP): May be used in evaluation of myelopathy (spinal cord lesion).

E. Neuroimaging

1. Structural: Computed tomography (CT) scan and magnetic resonance imaging (MRI).
2. Functional: Positron emission tomography (PET) scan and single photon emission computed tomography (SPECT).

3. Vascular: Carotid dopplers (ultrasound), magnetic resonance angiography (MRA), and cerebral angiogram.

F. **Cerebrospinal Fluid (CSF)**

1. Opening pressure may be elevated in pseudotumor cerebri.
2. Cell count may be elevated in infection.
3. Protein will be elevated with any form of inflammation.
4. Glucose is decreased in bacterial, fungal, and TB meningitis.

XII. EPONYMS, ACRONYMS, AND ABBREVIATIONS (Table 21-9)

XIII. DEFINITIONS (Table 21-10)

XIV. SAMPLE H&P WRITE-UP

CC: Recurrent transient loss of consciousness (seizure).

ID: J.S. is a right-handed 63-year-old white male with a prior stroke now admitted for new-onset seizures.

HPI: Approximately 10 months ago, the patient presented with the acute onset of right-sided weakness and numbness. This was primarily affecting the lower face and arm and mildly affecting his leg. He had associated expressive aphasia (comprehension intact). Work-up consisted of a head MRI, carotid dopplers, and echocardiogram. He was found to have had an ischemic stroke of the left MCA. His carotids were found to have significant stenosis of the left ICA, and patient underwent a carotid endarterectomy 6 weeks later with no complications.

For the past month, the patient has been having witnessed episodes of generalized tonic-clonic activity. His right arm shakes, and then quickly his body becomes rigid and he has tonic-clonic jerks for 2-3 minutes. He has on two occasions had urinary incontinence associated with these episodes. He has approximately 1 hour of post-episode confusion. The patient has no memory of these events; he does describe a warning of paresthesias on his right side before onset of the jerking.

MHx: Hypertension, peripheral vascular disease, and coronary artery disease.

SHx: Status post three-vessel coronary artery bypass graft (CABG).

Childhood Illnesses: Usual.

Medications: Propanolol 40 mg bid, Aspirin 325 mg po qd, Lisinopril 10 mg po qd.

Allergies: No known drug allergies.

HEALTH MAINTENANCE

Prevention: Blood pressure under good control.

Diet/Nutrition: Gained 10 lbs. over past year due to lack of exercise status post-stroke.

Habits: Tobacco: 22 pack-years, quit 8 months ago after his stroke. Alcohol: Drinks 4 beers approximately 2 nights per week. Caffeine: 2 cups per day.

Family History: Stroke in mother; no family history of seizures.

Social History: No significant travel history or animal exposures. No toxin exposures. Worked as real estate agent; has been on dis-

Table 21-9. NEUROLOGY EPONYMS, ACRONYMS, AND ABBREVIATIONS.

Acronym or Abbreviation	Term	Acronym or Abbreviation	Term
AA	Alcoholics Anonymous	**CT**	Computed tomography
AVM	Arteriovenous malformation	**DTR**	Deep tendon reflex
ALS	Amyotrophic lateral sclerosis	**DPH**	Diphenylhydantoin (Dilantin)
AED	Antiepileptic drug	**ETOH**	Alcohol
APD	Afferent pupillary defect	**EMG**	Electromyogram
ACA	Anterior cerebral artery	**EEG**	Electroencephalogram
ADEM	Acute disseminated encephalomyelitis	**EP**	Evoked potential
BC	Bone conduction	**EAC**	External auditory canal
BAER	Brainstem auditory evoked response	**EOM**	Extraocular movements
CVA	Cerebrovascular accident	**F-N**	Finger-to-nose test of coordination
CN	Cranial nerve	**FSH**	Fascio-scapulo-humeral muscular dystrophy
CNS	Central nervous system	**GBS**	Guillain-Barré syndrome
CSF	Cerebrospinal fluid	**GTC**	Generalized tonic-clonic seizure
CBZ	Carbamazepine	**HNP**	Herniated nucleus pulposus
CIDP	Chronic inflammatory demyelinating neuropathy	**HSMN**	Hereditary sensorimotor neuropathy
CMT	Charcot-Marie tooth (hereditary neuropathy)	**HA**	Headache
CTS	Carpal tunnel syndrome	**HC**	Head circumference
CPS	Complex partial seizure	**HNPP**	Hereditary neuropathy with liability for pressure palsies
CPA	Cerebellopontine angle	**ICP**	Intracranial pressure

Continued

Table 21-9. NEUROLOGY EPONYMS, ACRONYMS, AND ABBREVIATIONS—*cont'd*

Acronym or Abbreviation	Term	Acronym or Abbreviation	Term
ICH	Intracerebral hemorrhage	**PICA**	Posterior inferior cerebellar artery
INO	Intranuclear ophthalmoplegia	**PSP**	Progressive supranuclear palsy
IR	Inferior rectus muscle	**PERRLA**	Pupils equally round and reactive to light and accommodation
IO	Inferior oblique muscle	**PT**	Physical therapy
LOC	Loss of consciousness	**PCS**	Partial complex seizure
LMN	Lower motor neuron	**PET**	Positron emission tomography
LBP	Low back pain	**REM**	Rapid eye movement
LP	Lumbar puncture	**RAMs**	Rapid alternating movements
LE	Lower extremity	**SAH**	Subarachnoid hemorrhage
LR	Lateral rectus muscle	**SO**	Superior oblique muscle
MS	Multiple sclerosis	**SR**	Superior rectus muscle
MSE	Mental status examination	**SCM**	Sternocleidomastoid
MCA	Middle cerebral artery	**SSEP**	Somatosensory evoked potential

MRA	Magnetic resonance angiography	**SPECT**	Single photon emission computed tomography
MD	Muscular dystrophy	**SSPE**	Subacute sclerosing panencephalitis
MLF	Medial longitudinal fasciculus	**TIA**	Transient ischemic attack
MRI	Magnetic resonance imaging	**TLE**	Temporal lobe epilepsy
MR	Mental retardation	**TCA**	Tricyclic antidepressant
MR m.	Medial rectus muscle	**TTE**	Transthoracic echocardiogram
NCV	Nerve conduction velocity	**TEE**	Transesophageal echocardiogram
NPH	Normal pressure hydrocephalus	**UE**	Upper extremity
NMJ	Neuromuscular junction	**UBO**	Unidentified bright object (MRI)
NCSE	Nonconvulsive status epilepticus	**UMN**	Upper motor neuron
OP	Opening pressure	**VDRL**	Venereal disease research laboratory
OPCA	Olivopontocerebellar atrophy	**VEP**	Visual evoked potential
OCB	Oligoclonal bands	**VFFTC**	Visual fields full to confrontation
OT	Occupational therapy	**VPA**	Valproic acid (Depakote)
PPRF	Parapontine reticular formation	**VNS**	Vagal nerve stimulator
PCA	Posterior cerebral artery	**VPS**	Ventriculoperitoneal shunt
PD	Parkinson's disease		

Source: Flaherty AW. The Massachusetts General Hospital Handbook of Neurology. Lippincott Williams & Wilkins, 2000, 50.

Table 21-10. NEUROLOGY-FOCUSED DEFINITIONS.

TERM	DEFINITION
Anosmia	Inability to recognize smells
Agnosia	Inability to process sensory information; not attributable to sensory loss
Alexia	Inability to read
Agraphia	Inability to communicate with writing
Amnesia	Impairment of memory; can be anterograde or retrograde
Anosognosia	Denial of hemiplegia
Aura	Sensory prodrome of seizure or migraine; can involve any of the senses
Automatism	Repetitive movements such as lip-smacking or picking clothes; can be seen in complex partial seizures
Athetosis	Slow, writhing irregular movements, mostly in hands
Asterixis	Flapping jerk of hands when arms extended and palms are facing out; sign of toxic/metabolic problem such as liver disease
Astereognosis	Inability to recognize objects by palpation with intact primary sensory organs (cortical sign)
Apraxia	Inability to perform a motor task with strength and coordination intact (cortical sign)
Aphasia	Disorder of language to include expression or comprehension (cortical sign)
Archimedes spinal	Written test tool used in evaluation of tremor
Ataxia	Difficulty with coordinating ambulation/ walking
Astasia-abasia	Motor incoordination with an inability to stand or walk despite normal ability to move the legs when sitting or lying down; a form of hysterical ataxia
Babinski's reflex	Dorsiflexion of big toe on stimulation of sole of the foot, occurring with lesions of the pyramidal tract
Bradykinesia	Abnormal slowness of movement; sluggishness of physical and mental responses
Bell's palsy	Unifacial paralysis of sudden onset, caused by lesion of the facial nerve

Table 21-10—cont'd	
TERM	**DEFINITION**
Brown-Sequard	Loss or proprioception and vibration on the same side and pain and temperature several levels below on the opposite side with hemisection of the spinal cord
Brudzinski's sign	Flexion of the neck, resulting in flexion of the hip and knee, seen with meningeal irritation
Chorea	Rhythmical movements of a rapid, jerky nature
Coma	Unresponsiveness to external or internal stimuli
Café-au-lait spots	Characteristic skin lesion(s) seen in association with neurofibromatosis
Dermatome	The area of skin supplied by a spinal nerve
Diplopia	The perception of two images of a single object
Dysaphia	Impairment of sense of touch
Dysarthria	Imperfect articulation caused by disturbances in muscular control
Dysdiadochokinesia	Ability to start and control or difficulty in making rapid alternating movements
Dystonia	Co-contraction of agonist and antagonist, which often leads to abnormal posture or position
Encephalopathy	Abnormality of the brain, typically causing altered mental status
Encephalitis	Inflammation of the brain
Glabellar reflex	Blinking when the glabellar area between the eyes is tapped
Graphesthesia	Recognition of written number on back of the hand or the top of the foot
Horner's syndrome	Ptosis, miosis, anhidrosis; indicator of damage to sympathetic fibers l
Hemiballism	Violent and flinging movements affecting one side
Kernig's sign	Sign of meningitis, the patient can completely extend the leg in dorsal decubitus position but not when sitting or with thigh flexed on abdomen
Marcus-Gunn pupil	Afferent pupillary defect: consensual pupil response stronger than direct response, seen best with swinging flashlight test

Continued

Table 21-10. NEUROLOGY-FOCUSED DEFINITIONS—*cont'd*

Term	Definition
Meningitis	Inflammation/infection of the meninges
Myelopathy	Disease of the spinal cord
Myelitis	Inflammation of the spinal cord
Myopathy	Abnormality of muscle
Myositis	Inflammation of muscle
Mononeuropathy	Abnormality of a single nerve
Mononeuritis multiplex	Disorder affecting multiple nerves in an asymmetric pattern
Nystagmus	Involuntary, rapid, rhythmic movement of the eyeball
Palmomental (palm-chin) reflex	Twitching of chin with stimulation of the palm
Plexopathy	Abnormality of a nerve plexus (brachial or lumbar)
Pronator drift	Pronation and flexion of upper extremity with eyes closed
Proprioception	Sense of body position. The mechanism involved in the self-regulation of posture and movement through stimuli originating in the receptors imbedded in the joints, tendons, muscles, and labyrinth
Polyradiculopathy	Abnormality of many nerve roots
Radiculopathy	Abnormality of a nerve root; commonly seen with herniated nucleus pulposus
Ramsey-Hunt syndrome	Herpes zoster involving facial and auditory nerves, associated with ipsilateral facial paralysis and herpetic vesicles of the external ear or tympanic membrane
Saccades	Rapid conjugate deviation eye movements regulated by the contralateral cerebral hemisphere through the parapontine reticular formation with a cerebellar component
Snellen's chart	Common chart used to assess visual acuity during eye examination
Stereognosis	Recognition of forms and objects placed into the hand
Syncope	Loss of consciousness
Vertigo	Sensation of spinning or movement; can be from either central (brain) or peripheral (vestibular nerve) source

	D	T	B	IS	WF	WE	FF	FE	I	HF	KF	KE	DF	PF	EHL
R	4+	3+	4	3+	4+	4	5	3+	5	5	4+	5	4+	5	5
L	5	5	5	5	5	5	5	5	5	5	5	5	5	5	5

	Jaw	Triceps	Biceps	Brachio-radialis	Finger Flex	Patella	Ankle	Plantar
R	—	2+	3	3	1	3	1	Extensor + Babinski
L	—	2	2	2	1	2	1	Flexor

NEURO

ability since his stroke. Lives at home with his wife. Requires ambulation with wheelchair. Since onset of seizures, has been afraid to leave his apartment.

PHYSICAL EXAMINATION

Vital Signs: Blood Pressure 141\87, P 82, T 98.9.

HEENT: Normocephalic, atraumatic, oropharynx is notable for a lateral tongue laceration.

Neck: Supple, no bruits or lymphadenopathy.

Lungs: Clear to auscultation.

Heart: Regular rate and rhythm, no murmurs/gallops/rubs.

Abdomen: Soft, nontender, normal bowel sounds.

NEUROLOGIC EXAMINATION

Mental Status: Patient is alert and oriented × 3. Attention and concentration are normal. Speech is fluent. Comprehension is normal. Patient can repeat. Recall is 3 out of 3 at 5 minutes. Follows three-step commands. Writing: Impaired due to aphasia. Figure reconstruction was intact. Intellect appeared consistent with background. Judgment and insight was normal. Mood was frustrated with dysphoric affect.

Cranial Nerves II-VI: Visual fields are full to confrontation. Discs are sharp. Pupils equal and reactive to light and accommodation, with no APD. No ptosis or Horner's syndrome is present. Extraocular movements are fully intact. There is no nystagmus. VORs were intact. Saccades were intact. **CN V, VII, VIII:** Sensation is normal. Facial strength: Mild lower facial droop. Hearing is intact to voice. **CN IX-XII:** Tongue and palate move in the midline. SCM and trapezius are 5/5 strength.

Motor: (see top Table on page 431) +right fix. +right pronator drift. Muscle bulk: Normal. Muscle tone: Increased in right arm and leg. Right arm in slightly flexed position; right leg slightly extended and externally rotated.

Sensation: Decreased pinprick, temperature, and light touch in right arm; vibration was 10 seconds at the toes and 20 seconds at the fingers. Proprioception intact. Romberg is unable to be tested because of right-sided hemiparesis.

Deep Tendon Reflexes: (see bottom Table on page 431)

Complex motor: Finger-to-nose, heel-to-shin, RAM, and Fisher's tests were limited by weakness, but coordination seemed accurate bilaterally.

Gait/station: Station is normal. Gait is notable for circumduction of right leg with decreased right arm swing. Patient cannot heel/toe/tandem walk.

22

OBSTETRICS

Karrie Francois, MD, and Michael R. Foley, MD

I. CHIEF COMPLAINT

A. **Chief Complaint:** Use the patient's own words for the major complaint or reason for admission.

B. **Identifying Data:** Obtain patient's name, age, race/ethnic background, gravidity/parity (term deliveries, preterm deliveries, abortions, number of living children).

II. HISTORY OF PRESENT ILLNESS

A. What is the estimated date of delivery (EDD) based on the first day of last menstrual period (LMP), ultrasound, or both?

B. When did the onset of symptom(s) occur and what is their duration?

C. Are you having contractions, pelvic cramping, abdominal pain, or back pain?

D. Do you have any vaginal discharge; what is its character and duration? Are there any associated symptoms?

E. Are you experiencing any vaginal bleeding or spotting? If so, what is the amount and duration? Do you have any associated symptoms? Is bleeding associated with any activities?

F. Perform nonstress test or ultrasound assessment of fetal movement if greater than 16 weeks' gestation.

III. PAST MEDICAL AND SURGICAL HISTORY

A. Menstrual History

1. At what age did you undergo menarche?
2. When was the first day of your LMP? Is this date definite or approximate?
3. When was the first day of your last normal menstrual period (LNMP)?
4. Do you menstruate regularly?
5. How frequent are your menstrual periods, using number of days (e.g., menses occurs every ____ days)?
6. How long do your periods last? Does the flow quantity or quality change during your period?
7. Do you have associated pelvic pain, breast tenderness, mood alterations, bloating, or other symptoms before or during your menstrual period?

B. Obstetric History

1. How many times have you been pregnant?
2. Have you had any spontaneous or elective abortions (less than 20 weeks' gestation)? At how many weeks' gestation did these

occur? Did you have any complications or require surgical intervention (e.g., dilatation and curettage [D&C]) with these abortions?

3. Have you had any ectopic (e.g., tubal) pregnancies? If so, how were you treated?
4. How many deliveries (greater than 20 weeks' gestation) have you had? At how many weeks' gestation did you deliver? Where did you deliver? How long was your labor? How much did each infant weigh at delivery? What gender was each infant? What type of delivery did you have with each pregnancy? Did you require any anesthesia during your labor or delivery? Were there any maternal or neonatal complications with a delivery? Were any pregnancies complicated by preterm labor?
5. How many living children do you currently have? If deceased, what caused the child's death?
6. Were you on oral contraceptive pills (OCPs) at the time of conception of this pregnancy?

C. **Gynecologic History**

1. When was your last Papanicolaou (Pap) smear? What was the result?
2. Have you ever had an abnormal Pap smear? Did you require any treatment? If so, what type of treatment did you have?
3. Did your mother take any medications (e.g., hormones) when she was pregnant with you?
4. Have you ever been told that your uterus is abnormally shaped?
5. Do you have a history of uterine fibroids (leiomyomata)?
6. Have you ever had, or been exposed to, any sexually transmitted diseases (STDs)? If so, what type of infections? Were you and/or your partner treated for these infections?
7. Have you ever had any gynecologic surgery?
8. Have you ever had problems with, or treatment for, infertility?

D. **Past Medical History**

1. Have you been diagnosed with any illnesses? What was the date of onset, progression, and response to interventions? Were there any complications or sequelae?
2. Have you ever been exposed to, or immunized against, Hepatitis B?
3. Have you ever been exposed to Hepatitis C?
4. Have you ever been exposed to tuberculosis (TB) or been treated with isoniazid (INH)?
5. Have you had a rash or a viral illness since your LMP?
6. Have you ever been exposed to HIV?

E. **Past Surgical History**

1. Have you undergone surgery? What was the diagnosis?
2. What surgical procedure was performed?
3. What were your responses to interventions?

4. Were there any operative or postoperative complications or sequelae?
5. When and where was the surgery performed (i.e., name of hospital and date of procedure)?
6. Was anesthesia used during the procedure? What type? Were there any complications with its use?

F. **Emergency and Trauma History**

1. Have you ever been hospitalized? What was the date of hospitalization, name of hospital, duration, reason for hospitalization, and diagnosis?
2. Have you ever had a blood transfusion? If yes, for what reason and how many units (if known)?
3. Have you ever had any injuries or trauma-related injuries? What therapy or treatment did you require?

G. **Childhood History:** Have you had any childhood illnesses? If so, what were they?

H. **Occupational History**

1. What is your occupation?
2. Are you exposed to any chemicals, radiation, or other possible teratogens at your workplace?

I. **Travel History**

1. Have you traveled during your pregnancy? If so, where have you traveled?
2. Have you been exposed to any individuals who may have been infected with a disease endemic to a particular area (e.g., tuberculosis)?

J. **Animals and Insects Exposure History**

1. Do you have any cats? If so, do you change the cat litter boxes? Doing so can increase the risk of toxoplasmosis in pregnancy.
2. Have you had any reactions to past bites or stings (i.e., envenomations)?

IV. MEDICATIONS, ALLERGIES, AND ADVERSE REACTIONS

A. Do you currently take any medications? If so, were they prescribed or purchased over-the-counter (OTC)?

B. Have you taken any medications since your LMP?

C. Have you ever had an allergic or adverse reaction to a medication? If so, what type of reaction did you have?

V. HEALTH MAINTENANCE

A. **Prevention**

1. Female preventive screening: Have you had regular Pap smears taken? Do you regularly have your breasts examined? Do you regularly self-examine your breasts? Do you have regular mammograms taken? If applicable, starting at what age or history?
2. Immunizations: Did you receive immunizations during your childhood and adolescence? If so, do you recall for what types of diseases you received immunizations?

B. Diet

1. What type of diet do you follow (e.g., vegetarian, diabetic)?
2. Do you eat raw meat or fish?
3. Approximately how many calories do you consume per day?
4. Do you take any vitamins or supplements? If so, what types and how much?

C. Exercise

1. Do you exercise? If so, how often, what type, how intense, and for what duration?
2. Do you regularly use hot tubs or whirlpools?

D. Sleep Patterns: Do you have any unusual sleep patterns? If so, are they related to your occupation, stress, or medication use?

E. Social Habits

1. Do you use tobacco products? If yes, what type, how much and how often, and for how long?
2. Do you use alcohol? If yes, how often and how much?
3. Do you use illicit drugs? If yes, what types, how much, and how often?

VI. FAMILY HISTORY

A. First-Degree Relatives' Medical History

1. What medical diseases are present within your first-degree relatives?
2. Has anyone in your family had any obstetric complications (e.g., multiple gestations, preeclampsia)?

B. Three-Generation Genogram: Do any of the following medical conditions affect you, the father of the baby, or anyone in either of your families?

1. Advanced maternal age (i.e., 35 years or older at your EDD)?
2. Thalassemia (i.e., Italian, Greek, Mediterranean, African, or Asian backgrounds)?
3. Neural tube defects (e.g., spina bifida, meningomyelocele, or anencephaly)?
4. Congenital heart disease?
5. Down syndrome?
6. Tay-Sachs disease (i.e., Jewish, Cajun, French Canadian backgrounds)?
7. Sickle cell disease or trait (African background)?
8. Hemophilia?
9. Muscular dystrophy?
10. Cystic fibrosis?
11. Huntington chorea?
12. Mental retardation or autism? If yes, has the person been genetically tested for Fragile X syndrome?
13. Other inherited genetic or chromosomal disorders?
14. Maternal metabolic disease such as insulin-dependent diabetes mellitus (IDDM) or phenylketonuria (PKU)?

15. Has the father of the baby had a child with any of the birth defects listed above?
16. Previous child with birth defects not listed above?
17. Recurrent pregnancy loss (3 or more spontaneous abortions) or previous stillbirth?

VII. PSYCHOSOCIAL HISTORY

A. Personal and Social History

1. What is your ethnicity? Certain disease risks are associated with particular ethnicities (e.g., sickle cell disease, Tay-Sachs disease, thalassemias)?
2. Are you able to provide food, car restraints, and care for your infant?
3. What educational level have you attained?

B. Interpersonal History/Family Aspects of Pregnancy

1. What is your marital status?
2. Is the father of the baby involved in the pregnancy?
3. Do you have any religious or cultural preferences that need to be considered during the pregnancy (e.g., refusal of blood products)?
4. Are you, or have you ever been, in a relationship that involves domestic violence?

VIII. REVIEW OF SYMPTOMS (Tables 22-1 to 22-3)

Many symptoms observed during the course of obstetrical care are normal physiologic changes associated with pregnancy, although the symptoms of other medical and surgical conditions may change in quality during pregnancy. Also, some diseases may initially occur during pregnancy, but their diagnoses may be delayed because of the pregnancy. The clinician must differentiate normal physiologic changes of pregnancy from pathologic disease states.

Table 22-1. GENERAL OBSTETRICAL SYMPTOMS BY SYSTEM.

SYSTEM	SYMPTOMS
General	Fatigue, weight changes
HEENT/Neck	Visual changes, scotomata, epistaxis, nasal congestion, thyroid enlargement
Respiratory	Cough, dyspnea, shortness of breath
Chest	Breast enlargement, nipple discharge
Cardiovascular	Tachycardia, palpitations, orthopnea, paroxysmal nocturnal dyspnea, dyspnea with exertion
Gastrointestinal	Nausea, emesis, hematemesis, heartburn, RUQ pain, epigastric pain, constipation, appetite changes

Continued

Table 22-1. GENERAL OBSTETRICAL SYMPTOMS BY SYSTEM—*cont'd*

SYSTEM	SYMPTOMS
Genitourinary	Dysuria, urinary frequency, urinary urgency, vaginal discharge, vaginal bleeding or spotting, vaginal/vulvar discoloration and/or itching, dyspareunia, pelvic pain, uterine cramping, contractions, uterine tenderness (See history section for obstetrical/gynecological review)
Hematologic/ Lymphatic	Easy bruising, bleeding tendencies, lymphadenopathy
Skin	Rash, pigmentary changes and their distribution, spider angiomata, striae, palmar erythema, hirsutism, pruritis
Neurologic	Migraines/headaches, seizures
Musculoskeletal	Arthritis, muscle weakness, back pain
Extremities	Peripheral edema, tremor, paresthesias, numbness
Psychiatric	Mood disorders, substance abuse, depression, anxiety

Table 22-2. NONSPECIFIC SYMPTOMS AND THEIR OBSTETRICAL DISEASES.

SYMPTOM	POSSIBLE DISEASES
Abdominal pain	Uterine contractions, term or preterm labor, placental abruption, chorioamnionitis, preeclampsia/hemolysis, elevated liver enzymes, and low platelets (HELLP) syndrome, ectopic pregnancy, acute fatty liver of pregnancy
Anemia	Dilutional anemia of pregnancy, HELLP syndrome (hemolysis)
Back pain	Term or preterm labor, abruption, hydronephrosis of pregnancy (right kidney more commonly involved than left)
Dyspnea	Dyspnea of pregnancy, underlying disease (e.g., cardiovascular, thromboembolic, pulmonary)
Fever	Chorioamnionitis, septic abortion, underlying disease (infectious, endocrine, connective tissue)
Headache	Preeclampsia

Table 22-2—cont'd

Symptom	Possible Diseases
Nausea/emesis	Nausea and vomiting of pregnancy, hyperemesis gravidarum, HELLP syndrome, acute fatty liver of pregnancy
Skin changes	Normal changes of pregnancy (e.g., hyperpigmentation, spider angiomata, striae, palmar erythema), jaundice (acute fatty liver of pregnancy), rash (e.g., pruritic urticarial papules and plaques of pregnancy [PUPPP] syndrome, herpes gestationis, prurigo gestationis, pruritis (cholestasis of pregnancy)
Tachycardia	Chorioamnionitis, placental abruption, underlying disease (e.g., cardiovascular, thromboembolic, endocrine, infectious)
Thrombocytopenia	Gestational thrombocytopenia, HELLP syndrome, underlying disease (idiopathic thrombocytopenic purpura [ITP], connective tissue disease, thrombotic thrombocytopenic purpura [TTP])
Vaginal discharge	Preterm or term rupture of membranes (ROM), lower genital tract infection, bacterial vaginosis, preterm or term labor, chorioamnionitis
Vaginal bleeding	Spontaneous abortion, threatened abortion, incomplete abortion, subchorionic bleeding, placental abruption, placenta previa, preterm or term labor, ectopic pregnancy, lower genital tract lesion or laceration

Table 22-3. COMMON OBSTETRICAL DISEASES AND THEIR SYMPTOMS.

OB Disease	Symptoms
Preterm labor	Abdominal or pelvic pain, back pain, uterine cramping, vaginal discharge, vaginal bleeding
Preeclampsia	Hypertension, proteinuria, headache, scotomata, peripheral edema (facial and upper extremities), oliguria, rapid weight gain, thrombocytopenia, anemia

Continued

Table 22-3. COMMON OBSTETRICAL DISEASES AND THEIR SYMPTOMS—*cont'd*

OB Disease	Symptoms
Premature rupture of membranes (PROM)	Watery vaginal discharge, sometimes increased uterine cramping, back pain, abdominal pain
Chorioamnionitis	Abdominal pain, uterine tenderness, fever, maternal tachycardia, fetal tachycardia, foul vaginal discharge
Ectopic pregnancy	Early gestation (<12 weeks), abdominal or pelvic pain, vaginal bleeding or spotting, hemodynamic instability if ruptured

IX. PHYSICAL EXAMINATION

The obstetric physical examination must differentiate normal physical changes associated with pregnancy from abnormal obstetric conditions, as well as underlying disease states (Table 22-4).

Table 22-4. PHYSICAL EXAMINATION FINDINGS AND POSSIBLE DIAGNOSES.

Systems	Physical Examination Finding	Possible Diagnoses
Vitals		
Pulse	Tachycardia	Chorioamnionitis, placental abruption, volume contraction, underlying disease state (e.g., cardiovascular, thromboembolic, endocrine, infectious)
Blood pressure	Hypertension	Gestational hypertension, preeclampsia/HELLP syndrome, chronic hypertension, underlying disease state (e.g., endocrine, renal)
	Hypotension	Placental abruption, blood loss, underlying disease state (e.g., infectious/sepsis, endocrine)

Table 22-4—cont'd

Systems	Physical Examination Finding	Possible Diagnoses
Respiratory rate	Tachypnea	Underlying disease state (e.g., thromboembolic, pulmonary, infectious, pain/anxiety)
Weight	Rapid weight gain Weight loss	Preeclampsia Hyperemesis gravidarum
Temperature	Fever	Chorioamnionitis, septic abortion, underlying disease state (e.g., infectious, endocrine, connective tissue)
Heent		
Eyes	Periorbital edema	Preeclampsia
	Retinal hemorrhages, retinal detachment	Preeclampsia/eclampsia
	Icteric sclera	Acute fatty liver of pregnancy, underlying disease state (liver)
Ears	No obstetrical abnormalities	
Nose	Mucosal edema, vascular congestion	Normal changes of pregnancy
Mouth	Gingival edema	Normal changes of pregnancy
	Gingivitis with bleeding	Epulis gravidarum
	Dental caries	Preterm labor risk factor
Face	Facial edema	Pre-eclampsia
	Melasma ("mask of pregnancy")	Normal changes of pregnancy
Neck		
Thyroid	Thyroid enlargement	Normal changes of pregnancy
	Goiter, nodule, tenderness, bruit	Underlying disease state
Lungs	Bilateral diffuse inspiratory crackles, decreased breath sounds in bases	Preeclampsia complicated by pulmonary edema
	Rhonchi, wheezes, focal inspiratory crackles	Underlying disease state (e.g., pulmonary, infectious)

Continued

Table 22-4. PHYSICAL EXAMINATION FINDINGS AND POSSIBLE DIAGNOSES—*cont'd*

Systems	Physical Examination Finding	Possible Diagnoses
Chest	Breast and nipple enlargement, hyperpigmentation of nipples/areolae	Normal changes of pregnancy
	Yellow-white nipple discharge	Colostrum
Cardiovascular	Tachycardia	Chorioamnionitis, placental abruption, volume contraction, underlying disease state (e.g., cardiovascular, thromboembolic, endocrine, infectious)
	Splitting of first and second heart sounds, S3 gallop, systolic ejection murmur	Normal changes of pregnancy
Abdomen	RUQ or epigastric pain	Preeclampsia/HELLP syndrome, liver hematoma, acute fatty liver of pregnancy, underlying disease state state (e.g., gallbladder, infectious, gastrointestinal
	Uterine tenderness	Chorioamnionitis, placental abruption, septic abortion
	Uterine contractions	Term or preterm labor, placental abruption, chorioamnionitis
	Fetal heart tone assessment (if >10 weeks' gestation)	Normal range: 120-160 bpm Tachycardia: fetal hypoxemia, chorioamnionitis Bradycardia: fetal hypoxemia Decelerations: umbilical cord compression, fetal hypoxemia Irregularity: fetal arrhythmia Sinusoidal: fetal anemia

Table 22-4—cont'd

Systems	Physical Examination Finding	Possible Diagnoses
	Fundal height assessment (if >14 weeks' gestation)	Decreased fundal height: intrauterine growth restriction (IUGR), oligohydramnios, size-dates discrepancy Increased fundal height: macrosomia, polyhydramnios, size-dates discrepancy, multiple gestation
Genitourinary	Costovertebral angle (CVA) tenderness	Hydronephrosis of pregnancy (right > left), pyelonephritis
	Lower genital tract lesions (i.e., vulvar, vaginal, cervical)	Condyloma, STD, neoplasm
	Watery vaginal discharge: pooling, nitrazine positive, fern positive	Preterm or term ROM
	Vaginal discharge	Normal physiologic discharge of pregnancy, preterm or term labor (mucus plug), bacterial vaginosis, STD, chorioamnionitis, yeast infection, septic abortion
	Vaginal bleeding	Spontaneous abortion (threatened, incomplete, or complete), subchorionic bleeding, placental abruption, placenta previa, preterm or term labor, ectopic pregnancy, lower genital tract lesion or laceration
	Cervical dilation	Preterm or term labor, cervical incompetence
	Pelvic pain, +/– "fullness"	Ectopic pregnancy, tuboovarian pathology, ovarian torsion

Continued

Table 22-4. PHYSICAL EXAMINATION FINDINGS AND POSSIBLE DIAGNOSES—*cont'd*

Systems	Physical Examination Finding	Possible Diagnoses
Skin	Hyperpigmentation, melasma, spider angiomata, striae, palmar erythema	Normal changes of pregnancy
	Jaundice	Acute fatty liver of pregnancy, cholestasis of pregnancy, underlying disease state (liver)
	Erythematous urticarial papules and plaques	Pruritic urticarial papules and plaques of pregnancy (PUPPP) syndrome
	Erythematous papules, vesicles, and bullae	Herpes gestationalis
	Excoriated papules	Prurigo gestationalis
Extremities	Peripheral edema	Normal changes of pregnancy, preeclampsia, underlying disease state (e.g., renal, cardiovascular)
Neurologic	DTR hyperreflexia, clonus	Preeclampsia/eclampsia, underlying disease state (e.g., endocrine, neurologic)
	Seizures	Eclampsia, underlying disease state (e.g., neurologic, substance abuse)
	Paresthesias, numbness	Carpal tunnel syndrome (hands), underlying disease state (e.g., endocrine, neurologic)

X. DIFFERENTIAL DIAGNOSIS

The differential diagnosis for obstetrics-related diseases varies by the gestational age of the pregnancy. Table 22-5 lists the most common presenting symptoms and their associated differential diagnosis based on gestational age categories.

Table 22-5. OBSTETRIC DIFFERENTIAL DIAGNOSIS.

SYMPTOM	DIAGNOSES
LESS THAN 20 WEEKS' GESTATION	
Cervical dilation	Spontaneous abortion (threatened, incomplete, or complete), cervical incompetence, septic abortion
Hypertension	Chronic hypertension, underlying disease state (endocrine, renal)
Uterine contractions	Spontaneous abortion (threatened, incomplete, or complete), chorioamnionitis/septic abortion
Vaginal bleeding	Spontaneous abortion (threatened, incomplete, or complete), subchorionic bleeding, placenta previa, ectopic pregnancy, lower genital tract lesion or laceration
MORE THAN 20 WEEKS' GESTATION	
Cervical dilation	Preterm or term labor
Hypertension	Gestational hypertension, pre-eclampsia/HELLP syndrome, chronic hypertension +/– superimposed preeclampsia, exacerbation of underlying disease state (endocrine, renal)
Uterine contractions	Preterm or term labor, placental abruption, chorioamnionitis
Vaginal bleeding	Preterm or term labor, subchorionic bleeding, placental abruption, placenta previa, lower genital tract lesion or laceration

OB

XI. LABORATORY STUDIES AND DIAGNOSTIC EVALUATIONS

The recommended laboratory studies and diagnostic evaluations for all pregnant women are listed in Table 22-6. Additional testing may be indicated depending on the patient's past medical history, past obstetric history, family history, and race/ethnicity.

XII. TERMS/ABBREVIATIONS AND DEFINITIONS (TABLE 22-7)

XIII. PRENATAL VISITS: ISSUES TO DISCUSS AND PHYSICAL EXAMINATION FOCUS (Table 22-8)

XIV. SAMPLE H&P WRITE-UP

CC: "I've had a headache for 3 days and my face and legs are swelling."

Table 22-6. OBSTETRICS-FOCUSED LABORATORY EVALUATION.

Initial Visit	8-12 Weeks	15-20 Weeks	24-28 Weeks	35-37 Weeks
Blood type	Consider dating ultrasound with nuchal translucency	Maternal serum alpha-fetoprotein quadruple screen	Antibody screen (if Rh negative or previous positive screen)	Group B streptococcus culture
Antibody screen	Genetic counseling if advanced maternal age or high risk for chromosomal anomalies	Ultrasound for anatomic surveillance, dating confirmation	Rhogam (if indicated)	
Hemoglobin/Hematocrit	Chorionic villus sampling	Genetic amniocentesis	Hemoglobin/Hematocrit	
Rubella titer		Consider bacterial vaginosis screening for high risk patient populations	Diabetes screen (1-hour glucola) 3-hour glucose tolerance test (if abnormal diabetic screen)	

VDRL (RPR)			Consider repeat VDRL if high risk patient population	
Hepatitis B surface antigen	—	—	—	—
HIV counseling/testing	—	—	—	—
TB skin test (PPD)	—	—	—	—
Pap smear	—	—	—	—
Gonorrhea culture	—	—	—	—
Chlamydia culture	—	—	—	—
Hemoglobin electrophoresis (if indicated)	—	—	—	—
Tay-Sachs evaluation (if indicated)	—	—	—	—
Cystic fibrosis evaluation (if desired)	—	—	—	—
Other pending PMHx	—	—	—	—

Table 22-7. OBSTETRICS TERMS/ABBREVIATIONS AND DEFINITIONS.	
TERM/ABBREVIATION	**DEFINITION**
Abortion (AB)	Delivery at less than 20 weeks' gestation; miscarriage
Acute fatty liver of pregnancy (AFLP)	Syndrome related to pregnancy characterized by liver failure
Advanced maternal age (AMA)	Mother 35 years of age or older at time of delivery
Cervical incompetence (CI)	Painless cervical dilation
Cholestasis of pregnancy	Syndrome related to pregnancy characterized by pruritis and bile acid elevation
Chorioamnionitis	Intrauterine infection
Colostrum	Breast secretion of plasma, immunoglobulins, lactoferrin, albumin, electrolytes, and lactose
C/S	Cesarean section
Eclampsia	Syndrome related to pregnancy characterized by hypertension, proteinuria, and seizures
Ectopic pregnancy	Pregnancy outside of the uterine cavity
Estimated date of delivery (EDD)	"Due date" Date obtained from LMP and/or ultrasound for anticipated delivery of infant
Epulis gravidarum	Gingival hypertrophy and edema associated with pregnancy
FAVD	Forceps-assisted vaginal delivery
Gravidity	Number of pregnancies that an individual has had
Gestational hypertension	Hypertension that begins more than 20 weeks' gestation and is not associated with proteinuria
HELLP syndrome	Syndrome related to pregnancy characterized by hemolysis, elevated liver enzymes, and low platelets; usually associated with preeclampsia or eclampsia
Hyperemesis gravidarum (HG)	Nausea and vomiting of pregnancy associated with dehydration and electrolyte disturbances
Intrauterine fetal demise (IUFD)	Death of fetus while in utero; usually refers to death after first trimester

Table 22-7—cont'd

Term/Abbreviation	Definition
Intrauterine growth restriction (IUGR)	Fetal growth less than 10% for gestational age. Now termed FGR (see Chapter 19)
Labor	Uterine contractions associated with cervical change (dilation and/or effacement)
LMP	First day of last menstrual period
LNMP	First day of last normal menstrual period
Macrosomia	Fetal growth more than 90% for gestational age
Menarche	Onset of first menstruation
Oligohydramnios	Low amniotic fluid volume
Parity	Number of deliveries that an individual has had
Placental abruption	Premature separation of placenta from uterine wall
Placenta previa	Placental tissue covering the cervical os
Polyhydramnios	High amniotic fluid volume
Postdates	More than 42 weeks' gestation
PPROM	Preterm premature rupture of membranes
Preeclampsia	Syndrome related to pregnancy characterized by hypertension and proteinuria
Preterm	Less than 37 completed weeks' gestation
PROM	Premature rupture of membranes Rupture of fetal membranes prior to the onset of labor
PUPPP syndrome	Pruritic urticarial papules and plaques of pregnancy
Rupture of fetal membranes (ROM)	Loss of amniotic fluid
SAB	Spontaneous abortion
Septic abortion	Miscarriage complicated by infection
STD	Sexually transmitted disease
SVD	Spontaneous vaginal delivery
Term	37 to 42 weeks' gestation
Teratogen	Substance, organism, or physical agent capable of causing abnormal fetal development
TOL	Trial of labor
VAVD	Vacuum-assisted vaginal delivery
VBAC	Vaginal birth after Cesarean section

OB

Table 22-8. PRENATAL VISITS.

	Discussion Issues	Prenatal Visits	Examination
First trimester	Anticipated prenatal care course Nutrition, anticipated weight gain Indications for ultrasound Discussion of genetic counseling, chorionic villus sampling/amniocentesis Prenatal care classes Toxoplasmosis precautions Environmental/work hazards Physical/sexual activity Warning signs of pregnancy problems (e.g., bleeding, fever with pelvic pain, severe nausea and vomiting)	Every 4 weeks	Initial physical examination Blood pressure, urine for protein/glucose/leukocytes, weight Doppler of fetal heart tones after 10 weeks' gestation
Second trimester	Fetal movement awareness Warning signs of pregnancy problems (e.g., bleeding, preterm labor, loss of fluid)	Every 4 weeks	Blood pressure, urine for protein/glucose/leukocytes, weight Doppler of fetal heart tones Fundal height measurement

Third trimester	Fetal movement charting Warning signs of pregnancy problems (e.g., bleeding, preterm labor, loss of fluid, preeclamptic symptoms [headache, visual disturbances, epigastric/right upper quadrant pain, edema]) Travel limitations Labor instructions, review of hospital facilities Labor medications, anesthesia considerations Possibility of and indications for Cesarean section Review of risks and benefits of VBAC (vaginal birth after Cesarean section) Postdates gestation counseling Counseling regarding feeding options (breast or bottle) Newborn car seat Postpartum birth control options, including consideration of sterilization	Every 4 weeks until 32 weeks Every 2 weeks from 32-36 weeks Every week from 36 weeks until delivery	Blood pressure, urine for protein/glucose/leukocytes, weight Doppler of fetal heart tones Fundal height measurement Assessment of fetal position Baseline vaginal examination at 24 weeks' gestation Vaginal examination per symptoms Evaluation of edema

HPI: M.J. is a single 18-year-old African American G2P0010 female with an EDD of 6/20/02 by LMP of 9/13/01 and second trimester ultrasound confirmation. Patient received full prenatal care and experienced no previous complications with this pregnancy. She presents at 37 4/7 weeks' gestation with a one-week history of intermittent headaches and increasing edema in her extremities and face. The patient presented to her obstetrician today for a routine prenatal visit when her blood pressure was noted to be 155/95 with 3+ proteinuria on a urine dipstick. Prior blood pressures ranged from 100-110/50-60. She denies scotomata or RUQ pain. The patient has noted occasional contractions but denies loss of fluid, vaginal discharge, and vaginal bleeding. The patient has noted good fetal movement.

Menstrual History: The patient underwent menarche at 12 years of age. The first day of her LMP and LNMP was 9/13/02. This date is definite. Her menses are regular, occur every 30 days, and last 5-6 days. The first day of her menses is marked by heavier flow and menstrual cramping. She does have symptoms of breast tenderness and bloating before her menses.

Obstetric History: The patient has had 2 pregnancies. She has had 1 elective abortion at 8 weeks' gestation in 6/01. There were no associated complications. The current pregnancy is her second. She was not taking OCPs at the time of her conception with this pregnancy.

Gynecologic History: The patient's last Pap smear was in 11/01. The result was within normal limits. She has never had an abnormal Pap smear. Her mother did not take any medications during her pregnancy while the patient was in utero, and the patient has never been told that her uterus is abnormally shaped. The patient denies a history of fibroids, past gynecologic surgery, and problems with infertility. The patient was diagnosed with chlamydia at the beginning of her pregnancy and was treated with a negative test of cure culture documented one month after treatment. The patient denies any known exposure to gonorrhea, HSV, or HIV.

PMHx: The patient denies any chronic medical problems. The patient denies any known exposure to hepatitis B, hepatitis C, TB, or HIV. The patient has not had any rashes or viral illnesses during her pregnancy.

PSHx: No prior surgeries.

Emergency and Trauma History: The patient has never been hospitalized, had a blood transfusion, or had any trauma-related injuries.

Childhood History: Chicken pox at age 7. She denies any other childhood illnesses.

Occupational History: Senior in high school and she does not have other employment.

Travel History: No travel during her pregnancy, and she has not been exposed to any individuals from areas with endemic diseases.

Animal and Insect Exposure History: The patient has one cat, and her mother changes the litter box. The patient has not had any unusual reactions to past insect bites or stings.

MEDICATIONS: Tylenol for the past three days for her headaches. She has not taken any other medications since her LMP. The patient reports an allergy to penicillin (rash without respiratory involvement). She has taken prenatal vitamins throughout her pregnancy.

HEALTH MAINTENANCE

Prevention: The patient's last Pap smear was in 11/01. See GYN section. The patient does not practice self-breast examinations. The patient received all of the usual childhood immunizations, including MMR.

Diet: Regular diet with no restrictions. She consumes approximately 2400 calories per day and has gained 32 pounds during her pregnancy. She does not eat raw meat or fish.

Exercise: The patient walks 2-3 times per week. She has not had access to hot tubs or whirlpools.

Sleep Patterns: The patient wakes 1-2 times per night to void since the third trimester began but has had no other unusual sleep patterns during the pregnancy.

Social Habits: The patient denies smoking or tobacco use. The patient used alcohol in the first trimester before knowing that she was pregnant, but stopped once she was diagnosed with pregnancy. The patient denies illicit drug use.

FAMILY HISTORY

First-Degree Relatives' Medical History: The patient's father has hypertension and adult-onset diabetes mellitus. The patient's mother is healthy. The patient's sister had preeclampsia with her first pregnancy.

Three-Generation Genogram: There is no history of genetic traits or diseases within the patient's family or the father of the baby's family.

PSYCHOSOCIAL HISTORY

Personal and Social History: The patient is African American. She is a senior in high school and lives with her parents.

Interpersonal History/Family Aspects of Pregnancy: The patient is single. The father of the baby is involved in the pregnancy. The patient does not have any religious or cultural preferences that would potentially affect the pregnancy. The patient denies a history of domestic violence.

REVIEW OF SYSTEMS

General: 5-pound weight gain in the past week.

HEENT/Neck: No visual changes or scotomata. No epistaxis.

Respiratory: No cough, dyspnea, or shortness of breath.

Cardiovascular: No tachycardia, palpitations, orthopnea, or paroxysmal nocturnal dyspnea.

Gastrointestinal: Nausea and vomiting in the first trimester. Occasional heartburn. No RUQ or epigastric pain. Occasional constipation.

Genitourinary: Urinary frequency for the past 4 weeks. No dysuria, urinary urgency, vaginal discharge, vaginal bleeding, or itching. Occasional cramping over the past 2 weeks but no uterine tenderness.

Hematological/Lymphatic: No easy bruising or bleeding tendencies.

Skin: No rash, pruritis, hirsutism, or pigmentary changes. Abdominal striae.

Neurological: Intermittent headaches for the past week. No history of seizures.

Musculoskeletal: Occasional back discomfort. No arthritis or muscle weakness.

Extremities: Significant peripheral edema over the past week. No paresthesias, numbness, or tremor.

Psychiatric: No history of depression, mood disorders, or anxiety. Alcohol use in the first trimester (3 beers, wine or mixed drinks 1-2 nights per week).

PHYSICAL EXAMINATION

Vital signs: T 98.8°F P 86 BP 158/94 RR 18 Weight 168 lbs.

HEENT: Moderate periorbital and facial edema.

Neck: No thyroid enlargement.

Lungs: Clear to auscultation bilaterally.

Chest: No nipple discharge or masses.

Cardiovascular: Normal S1 and S2. Regular rate and rhythm. Grade I/VI systolic ejection murmur.

Abdomen: Soft, nontender, gravid. No RUQ or epigastric pain. Irregular and mild uterine contractions every 7-10 minutes. Fetal heart tones: 150s and reactive with no decelerations. Fundal height 39 cm. Fetus cephalic by Leopold's maneuvers and ultrasound confirmation.

Genitourinary: No CVA tenderness. No genital tract lesions, vaginal discharge, or vaginal bleeding. Cervix: 1 cm dilated/50% effaced/-2 station/mid-position/soft consistency.

Skin: Striae on abdomen. No rash or jaundice.

Extremities: 3+ pitting edema.

Neurologic: 3+/4 DTR hyperreflexia, 1 beat of clonus. No focal sensory or musculoskeletal deficits.

23

OCCUPATIONAL MEDICINE

Phillip E. Parker, MD, MPH, Katerina M. Neuhauser, MD, PhD, MPH, and Thomas S. Neuhauser, MD

I. OCCUPATIONAL MEDICINE ILLNESS, DISEASE, AND INJURY

A. Occupation-Related Illness and Disease

1. All occupational illnesses and diseases, regardless of severity, are recordable under the Occupational Safety and Health Administration (OSHA).
2. Sometimes it is difficult to determine the work-relatedness of an occupational illness or injury (e.g., dermatitis, cumulative trauma disorders such as carpal tunnel syndrome, and hearing loss).
3. The following statistics establish the significance of occupational illness and disease.
   a. Occupational diseases/illnesses are associated with many workplace hazards: toxic chemicals (e.g., solvents, acids, petroleum fractions, paints, plastics, and resins), dusts, gases, metals, and ergonomic factors (e.g., heavy lifting, repetitive motions, abnormal postures, extremes of temperature, vibration, and noise).
   b. Preexisting diseases in employees that worsen while employed are considered occupationally related.
   c. It is difficult to assess the number of employees with work-related disease, but at least 400,000 new cases of disabling occupational illnesses in the workforce and 100,000 deaths occur annually.
   d. Employees in the manufacturing industry have the highest rates of occupationally related disease and illness, with ergonomic disorders and skin rashes representing most of the cases.

B. Occupational Injury

1. Generally, occupational injuries result from precipitating events (e.g., falls, slips, or electrocutions). Back problems, which are considered injuries even though they usually develop over time, are the exception.
2. Occupational injuries that require first-aid treatment and no medical treatment are not recordable under OSHA regulations.
3. Important injury facts:
   a. Approximately 1 million eye injuries, 1 million back injuries, 400,000 fractures, 21,000 amputations, and 2 million severe lacerations occur annually in the U.S. workforce.

b. At least 2 million employees are permanently or partially disabled each year by occupational injuries.
c. Most occupational injuries involve trauma to the musculoskeletal system.
d. Leading causes of injuries in the workplace involve work-related motor vehicle accidents (MVAs), machines, homicides, falls, electrocutions, and falling objects.
e. Workplaces with high rates of serious nonfatal injuries are manufacturing plants, shipbuilding yards, foundries, sawmills, and meat packing plants.
f. Occupational injuries result in between 20,000 to 75,000 deaths annually.
g. Major causes of occupation-related deaths are work-related MVAs, assaults, falls, trauma, and electric shock.
h. Industries with the highest death rates include mining, construction, transportation, and agriculture.

II. CHIEF COMPLAINT

A. **Occupational Approach to the Chief Complaint:** The occupational medicine chief complaint may represent the most important part of the history and physical. Patients with occupational illnesses and injuries may not attribute their condition to an occupational exposure and present with a variety of multisystem complaints. For this reason, occupational exposures should be considered in each physician-patient encounter.

B. **Frames of Reference:** Consider the following questions:
1. Is some occupational exposure potentially impairing this patient's health?
2. Are health problems potentially affecting the patient's ability to safely perform his or her current job?
3. Will the treatment have potentially iatrogenic effects on safe employment?

III. HISTORY OF PRESENT ILLNESS

A. **Industrial Hygiene (IH) Data**
1. What are your dates of employment?
2. What job positions (titles) have you held?
3. What type of work, including duties, did you perform? Actual job functions must be explored because job titles can be misleading.
4. How often and for how long did you perform each activity?
5. What products were you involved in making? What services were you involved in providing?
6. What is the nature of the agents or substances to which you are exposed in the workplace? How often do you use them? What is the average amount of time you are exposed to them?
7. What relationship, if any, exists between the development of your symptoms and the use of hazardous substances or agents (e.g., the evolution of symptoms in the workplace)? May need

to refer to Material Safety Data Sheets (MSDS) to determine which chemicals the individual was actually exposed to in the workplace.

8. How frequently do you use personnel protective equipment (PPE) in the workplace, for what length of time, and what is the condition of that equipment?
9. What types of chemicals, and for what length of time, are you exposed to at home? Do you use PPE?
10. Where have you traveled? In the United States? To foreign countries? Obtain all geographical and physical details. Inquire about types of water and food consumed, animal and insect exposure, and possible contact with an infectious agent.

B. **Epidemiology:** Care must be taken not to confuse "association" with "causation" (see Table 23-7).

IV. PAST MEDICAL AND SURGICAL HISTORY

A. **Past Medical History:** The occupational medicine consultant is generally not the employee's primary care physician; therefore, obtaining a thorough history is vital.

1. What previous illnesses have you had? Assess previous illnesses (e.g., childhood, physical, psychologic), injuries, surgical procedures, and hospital admissions. Realize that part of the history may be unreliable because there may be no established medical record or the patient may have an incentive to hide specific details of the medical problem for specific secondary gains (e.g., monetary).
2. Have any other co-workers had similar conditions? Assess any co-worker co-morbidity.
3. What other medical conditions do you currently have? Assess ongoing, underlying medical conditions. Realize that the patient may downplay the seriousness of these conditions to continue working.
4. Are you currently involved in any form of litigation, disability claim, or worker's compensation claim?

B. **Past Surgical History:** What surgical procedures have you undergone? Assess prior surgical treatments for potentially work-related conditions (e.g., carpal tunnel release).

V. MEDICATIONS, ALLERGIES, AND ADVERSE REACTIONS

A. Medications

1. What prescription medications are you currently taking? Identify any prescription medications that can have obvious, profound, or even subtle effects on a worker's ability to perform in the workplace (e.g., loss of color vision caused by sildenafil).
2. What over-the-counter (OTC) products do you take? Identify any OTC medications that can affect function.
3. Are you using any herbal preparations or nutritional supplements? Evaluate herbal or nutritional supplements for potential adverse effects.

a. Consider inconsistent potency or product adulteration if the products were purchased outside the United States.
b. Consider whether the substances are resulting in inadequate treatment for serious medical conditions (e.g., depressive symptoms are inadequately treated with use of St. John's Wort).

B. **Allergic Reactions and Adverse Reactions**
1. Have you had an allergic or adverse reaction? Evaluate previous reactions to objects and substances at the workplace (e.g., latex in gloves in the health care setting).
2. Any allergic reactions to medications? What treatment did you receive with what response?
3. Have you had any adverse reactions or side effects to medications?

VI. HEALTH MAINTENANCE

A. **Prevention:** Preventive measures commensurate with age, sex, and occupation should be assessed (e.g., immunizations for health care workers).

B. **Diet:** What is your typical diet? Evaluate any ongoing weight loss plan.

C. **Exercise:** What is your normal exercise activity and schedule? Were any changes made to your regular routine with the onset of symptoms?

D. **Hobbies:** What recreational activities or hobbies do you engage in? Certain recreational activities or hobbies can impair health (e.g., firearm enthusiasts may suffer significant asymmetrical hearing loss).

E. **Sleep Patterns:** What is your normal sleep pattern? Have there been any recent changes? Do you use sleeping aid medications?

F. **Social Habits**
1. Do you drink alcohol? What type, how much, and how often? Alcohol use may influence biologic monitoring for liver toxins.
2. Do you use tobacco? What type, how much, and how often? Tobacco use may have synergistic negative effects with workplace exposures (e.g., asbestosis).
3. Do you use recreational or illicit drugs?
4. Recent travel before onset of illness (see History of Present Illness section).

VII. FAMILY HISTORY

A. **First-Degree Relatives' Medical History:** Obtain age, sex, health status (if deceased, cause of death), and chronic disease.

B. **Delayed Exposures**
1. Obtaining the family medical history can elucidate some clinical patterns of delayed exposures. Some occupations pose a hazard for secondary exposures to spouses and children of employees (e.g., painters may inadvertently bring home significant amounts of lead on their clothing and spouses repeatedly wash their clothes over long periods).

2. What type of chemicals or materials are brought home from work on clothes or tools? A careful history is required to discern risk to family members from workplace exposures.

VIII. PSYCHOSOCIAL HISTORY

A. **Personal and Social History**

1. What is your race/ethnicity background?
2. Do you frequently travel to foreign countries? Which ones and how often? Ethnicity and other disease-associated risks (e.g., glucose-6-phosphate deficiency [G6PD] in a frequent international traveler requiring malaria prophylaxis).

B. **Impact of Current Illness on Patient:** Assess financial, emotional, and family support.

C. **Interpersonal and Sexual History**

1. Are you sexually active?
2. Do you have more than one partner? Do you use protection? Sexual history may reveal risk factors for human immunodeficiency virus (HIV) or hepatitis B or C.

D. **Occupational Aspects of Illness**

1. How many days of work have you missed?
2. How many days have you been late to work? Workplace attendance and tardiness may give clues regarding patient motivation to improve.

IX. REVIEW OF SYMPTOMS (Tables 23-1 and 23-2)

The occupational hazard determines the scope of the examination as well as the potential findings.

OCC

Table 23-1. GENERAL OCCUPATIONAL MEDICINE SYMPTOMS BY SYSTEM.

System	Symptoms
General	Fatigue, weight changes, recurrent febrile illnesses
HEENT/Neck	Visual changes, scotomata, diplopia, tinnitus, vertigo, hearing loss, epistaxis, nasal congestion, thyroid enlargement, headaches, sinusitis, head trauma, mucosal irritation of eyes or nasopharynx, facial flushing when consuming alcohol
Respiratory	Cough, dyspnea, shortness of breath, sputum (color, quantity, duration), hoarseness, hemoptysis, shortness of breath, reactive airway disease, wheezing, bronchitis, pleurisy or pain with breathing

Continued

Table 23-1. GENERAL OCCUPATIONAL MEDICINE SYMPTOMS BY SYSTEM—*cont'd*

System	Symptoms
Chest	Breast enlargement, nipple discharge
Cardiovascular	Tachycardia, palpitations, orthopnea, paroxysmal nocturnal dyspnea, dyspnea with exertion, chest pain, palpitations, murmurs, hypertension, edema, leg pain or cramps, claudication
Gastrointestinal	Nausea, vomiting, hematemesis, dysphagia, appetite changes, heartburn, right upper quadrant pain, jaundice, epigastric pain, abdominal pain, cholecystitis, constipation, diarrhea, melena, hematochezia, steatorrhea
Genitourinary	Dysuria, urinary frequency, urinary urgency, hematuria, nocturia, slowness of stream, vaginal discharge, vaginal bleeding or spotting, amenorrhea, dyspareunia, pelvic pain
Hematologic/ lymphatic	Easy bruising, bleeding tendencies, lymphadenopathy
Skin	Rash, pigmentary changes and their distribution, spider angiomata, striae, palmar erythema, hirsutism, pruritus, defatting dermatitis, chloracne, eczema
Neurologic	Migraines/headaches, seizures, paraesthesia, dysesthesia, tremors, vertigo, dizziness, syncope, memory loss, coordination
Musculoskeletal	Arthritis, back pain, joint pain, stiffness, swelling, soreness, deformity, muscle tenderness, muscle weakness
Extremities	Peripheral edema, tremor, paresthesias, numbness, sensitivity to extremes of temperature
Endocrine	Enlarged lymph nodes, diabetes
Reproductive	Infertility, spontaneous abortions, stillbirths, prematurity and birth defects such as cleft palate, developmental delay in children
Psychiatric	Mood disorders, substance abuse, depression, anxiety

Table 23-2. COMMON OCCUPATIONAL MEDICINE DISEASES AND THEIR SYMPTOMS.

Disease	Symptoms
Carpal tunnel syndrome	Coldness, numbness of hands, frequently dropping or losing grip strength
Chemical hepatitis	Jaundice, icterus, pruritus, encephalopathy, nausea, emesis
Contact dermatitis	Erythema, blistering, cracking, itching of exposed surfaces
De Quervain's syndrome	Tendon tenderness along radial base of thumb
Hypersensitity pneumonitis (e.g., farmer's lung)	Episodic attacks of febrile illness associated with cough, headache, shortness of breath, and malaise resembling recurrent pneumonia
Infertility	Many toxins may result in decreased sperm counts, decreased libido, menstrual irregularities, spontaneous abortions and fetal demise
Metal fume fever	Chills, fevers, malaise, minor respiratory and gastrointestinal complaints
Multiple chemical sensitivities	Multiple ill-defined symptoms related to chemical exposures, including sensitivities to smells. Intensity and pattern of symptoms are often in excess of those expected
Noise-induced hearing loss	Gradual onset of hearing loss in both ears, especially in frequencies higher than 4000 Hz
Occupational asthma	Temporal association with work, although shortness of breath and wheezing often worse at night and early morning hours
Peripheral neuropathy	Numbness, tingling, weakness along nerve distribution and may be due to exposures such as lead, arsenic, mercury, solvents, organophosphates, n-hexane, acrylamide, thallium
Pneumoconiosis	Usually nonspecific symptoms, including dyspnea on exertion. Symptoms may continue to progress despite cessation of exposure because of delayed clearance of inhaled agents such as coal, silica, and asbestos
Respiratory tract malignancies	Hemoptysis, weight loss

Continued

Table 23-2. COMMON OCCUPATIONAL MEDICINE DISEASES AND THEIR SYMPTOMS—*cont'd*

Disease	Symptoms
Trigger finger	Hand flexor tendons swelling, popping, snapping. Fingers may have to be forcibly extended after contraction
White knuckle syndrome	Numbness, blanching, and loss of dexterity at fingertips. Found in those exposed to excessive hand and arm vibration

X. PHYSICAL EXAMINATION (Table 23-3)

XI. DIFFERENTIAL DIAGNOSIS (Table 23-4)

XII. LABORATORY STUDIES

A. **Routine Labs:** Complete blood count (CBC), blood chemistry profile, urinalysis.

B. **Specific Labs:** Dictated by presenting complaints and findings or OSHA requirements.
  1. Direct testing: Tests for a specific agent in a medium (e.g., blood, stool, urine).
  2. Indirect testing: Tests for evidence of an agent's presence (e.g., urinary β2-microglobulin as evidence of cadmium exposure).
     a. Metabolites.
     b. Abnormal enzymatic activity.
     c. Alterations in physiological processes.

C. **Ancillary Testing**
  1. Chest or other x-rays and diagnostic imaging studies.
  2. Liver function tests (LFTs).
  3. Pulmonary function tests (PFTs).
  4. Nerve conduction studies.

XIII. OCCUPATIONAL EXAMINATIONS

A. **Ethical Considerations**
  1. Employers can hire or contract clinicians to provide employee medical examinations. Occupational practitioners serve the needs of the employer and the employee, which can create conflicts of interest. Conflicts of interest also may exist between physicians, employers, worker representatives, the public, and regulatory agencies.
  2. The legal system does not consider the relationship between an occupational medicine physician and an employee a true "physician-patient" relationship. In response, the American College of Occupational and Environmental Medicine (ACOEM) developed a code of ethics to which physicians should adhere.

Table 23-3. FINDINGS OF OCCUPATIONAL MEDICINE PHYSICAL EXAMINATION AND POSSIBLE DIAGNOSES.

System	Physical Examination Finding	Possible Diagnoses
Vitals		
Pulse	Tachycardia	Toxic exposure, underlying disease state (cardiovascular, thromboembolic, endocrine, infectious)
Blood pressure	Hypertension	Toxic exposure such as carbon disulfide, chronic hypertension, underlying disease state (endocrine, renal)
	Hypotension	Dehydration, underlying disease state (infectious/sepsis, endocrine)
Respiratory rate	Tachypnea	Acute or delayed toxic exposure, underlying disease state (thromboembolic, pulmonary, infectious, pain/anxiety)
	Weight loss	Occult malignancy, hyperthyroid, illicit drug use
Temperature	Fever	Toxic exposures, underlying disease state (infectious, endocrine, connective tissue)
Heent		
Head	Visible injuries	Trauma
Eyes	Retinal hemorrhages	Laser exposure
	Icteric sclera	Exposure to liver toxin, underlying disease state (liver)
	Cataracts	RF radiation exposure, trauma, toxic exposures
Ears	Hearing loss	Noise induced loss, otosclerosis, trauma, acoustic neuromas
Nose	Mucosal edema, vascular congestion	Irritant exposure, allergies
	Holes in nasal septum	Chromate exposure, illicit drug use

Continued

Table 23-3. FINDINGS OF OCCUPATIONAL MEDICINE PHYSICAL EXAMINATION AND POSSIBLE DIAGNOSES—*cont'd*

System	Physical Examination Finding	Possible Diagnoses
Mouth	Bluish gingival margin (Burton's lines)	Lead exposure, possible cyanosis
	Bleeding gums	Poor dental hygiene, hematologic disorder caused by benzene or ionizing radiation exposure
Breath	Garlicky smell	Possible exposure to thallium
Face	Facial hair, micrognathia, or disfigurement	Evidence that individual may not be able to get an adequate seal if respirator use is required
Neck		
Thyroid	Thyroid enlargement	Goiter
	Goiter, nodule, tenderness, bruit	Underlying disease state
Lungs	Bilateral diffuse inspiratory crackles, decreased breath sounds in bases	Toxic inhalational exposure, asbestosis, underlying disease state (pulmonary, infectious)
	Rhonchi, wheezes, focal inspiratory crackles	Occupational asthma, underlying disease state (pulmonary, infectious)
Cardiovascular	Tachycardia	Dehydration, underlying disease state (cardiovascular, thromboembolic, endocrine, infectious)
	Arrhythmias	Exposures to solvents, underlying disease state
	Chest pain	Premature arteriosclerosis following carbon disulfide exposure, carbon monoxide exposure, underlying coronary artery disease

Abdomen	Pain	Toxic exposures such as lead, underlying disease state (gallbladder, infectious, gastrointestinal)
	Right upper quadrant (RUQ) or epigastric pain	Toxic exposures such as halogenated hydrocarbons, underlying disease state (gallbladder, infectious, gastrointestinal)
Genitourinary	Costovertebral angle (CVA) tenderness	Kidney disease
	Vaginal bleeding	Spontaneous abortion, underlying disease state
Skin	Acneiform rash	Possible exposure to halogenated aromatic compounds, exposure to grease and lubrication oils
	Jaundice	Acute fatty liver, cholestasis, underlying disease state (liver)
	Eczematous dermatitis	Contact dermatitis (irritant versus allergic)
	Nodular lesions	UV induced skin cancers
	Urticaria	Allergic reactions
	Granuloma	Possible foreign body or beryllium exposure
	Ulcerations	Chromate exposure
	Facial and shoulder flushing	May indicate exposure to TCE if associated with alcohol consumption
	Depigmentation	Toxic exposure such as with phenolic compounds
Extremities	Tendon tenderness along radial base of thumb	De Quervain's syndrome

Continued

Table 23-3. FINDINGS OF OCCUPATIONAL MEDICINE PHYSICAL EXAMINATION AND POSSIBLE DIAGNOSES—*cont'd*

System	Physical Examination Finding	Possible Diagnoses
	Numbness, tingling in first 3 1/2 digits, positive Tinel's and Phalen's signs	Carpal tunnel syndrome
	Numbness, blanching, and loss of dexterity at fingertips	Hand-arm vibration syndrome
	Fingernail transverse white lines (Mees' lines)	Arsenic exposure
	Scleroderma-like changes of distal digits	Vinyl chloride exposure
	Elbow pain	Medial or lateral epicondylitis
Neurologic	Seizures	Toxic exposure, underlying disease state (neurologic, substance abuse)
	Paresthesias, numbness	Carpal tunnel syndrome (hands), underlying disease state (endocrine, neurologic), toxic effect of multiple agents
	Extrapyramidal syndrome	Toxic exposures such as carbon disulfide or manganese
	Peripheral neuropathies	Toxic exposures such as lead or underlying metabolic disorders
Psychiatric	Abnormal mental status examination	Stress, overt psychiatric disease, chronic circadian rhythm disruption, malingering, toxic exposure such as heavy metals

Table 23-4. OCCUPATIONAL DISEASE DIFFERENTIAL DIAGNOSIS.

Symptom	Possible Etiologies
Anemia	Exposure of bone marrow suppressants, preoperative blood loss, surgical blood loss, undiagnosed trauma, hemolysis, overhydration, autologous blood donation, pregnancy-related, sickle cell, thalassemia, intrinsic coagulation defect, high-dose Coumadin or heparin, drug effects
Arrhythmia	Solvent exposure, electrolyte imbalance, intrinsic cardiac rhythm disturbance, acute cardiac event, hypoxia, hypercarbia (respiratory failure), high digitalis level, other drug effects, thyrotoxicosis, anemia, anxiety, hypoglycemia, pheochromocytoma, high caffeine intake
Chest discomfort	Toxic exposure alone or exacerbating underlying acute MI, heartburn, gastroesophageal reflux disease (GERD), surgery-related anxiety, hypoxia, costochondritis, chest trauma, pneumonia, herpes zoster (shingles), pulmonary embolism
Confusion	Toxin-induced encephalopathy such as from mercury, hepatic encephalopathy, other drug effects, hypoxia, hypercarbia, anxiety with hyperventilation, older patient in different environment, electrolyte imbalance, stroke, seizure, hypoglycemia, new head injury, cardiac abnormalities, carotid artery disease, psychiatric illness
Hypertension	Carbon disulfide exposure, inadequate BP medication, pain, anxiety, endocrine abnormality, renal disease, fluid overload, CHF, intracranial pathology
Hypotension	Hypovolemia, blood loss, nothing per os (NPO) status, gastrointestinal (GI) losses, acute cardiac event, status post dialysis for surgery, undiagnosed trauma, vasovagal reaction, pulmonary embolus
Infertility	Possible exposure to toxic agent such as lead versus other physiologic cause
Pain	Cumulative trauma disorder, occupational injury, chronic systemic illness, normal post-surgical pain versus new event, inadequate pain medication ordered (e.g., dose too low, interval too long, drug interaction), ischemia or obstruction of internal organ(s)

Continued

Table 23-4. OCCUPATIONAL DISEASE DIFFERENTIAL DIAGNOSIS—cont'd

Symptom	Possible Etiologies
Shortness of breath	Direct irritant or hypersensitivity reaction, occupational asthma, asthma, pneumoconiosis, airway disease, airway obstruction, cardiac heart failure (CHF), acute arrhythmia or myocardial infarction (MI), severe valvular disease, hypoxia, mild upper respiratory infection (URI) versus pneumonia, chronic obstructive pulmonary disease (COPD), anxiety, anemia, hemoglobin abnormalities, pulmonary embolus, overdose of skeletal muscle relaxants
Somnolence	Chronic circadian disruption, electrolyte imbalance, stroke, COPD with hypercarbia, new head injury, seizures, hypoglycemia

B. **Code of Ethics**

1. Accord the highest priority to the health and safety of individuals in both the workplace and in the environment.
2. Practice on a scientific basis with integrity and strive to acquire and maintain adequate knowledge and expertise upon which to render professional service.
3. Relate honestly and ethically in all professional relationships.
4. Strive to expand and disseminate medical knowledge and participate in ethical research efforts as appropriate.
5. Keep confidential all individual medical information, releasing such information only: when required by law or by overriding public health considerations, to other physicians (according to accepted medical practice), or to others at the request of the individual.
6. Recognize that employers may be entitled to counsel about an individual's medical work fitness, but not to diagnoses or specific details, except in compliance with laws and regulations.
7. Communicate to individuals and/or groups any significant observations and recommendations concerning their health or safety.
8. Recognize those medical impairments in oneself and others, including chemical dependency and abusive personal practices, which interfere with one's ability to follow the above principles, and take appropriate measures.

C. **OSHA Recordkeeping Rules**

1. Providers should be familiar with existing OSHA recordkeeping rules and regulations.

2. For specifics, refer to the OSHA website at www.osha.gov/recordkeeping.

D. **Worker's Compensation**

1. Employees may seek compensation from their employers for sustaining an occupational injury or illness while employed.
2. Physicians may be asked to medically evaluate the individual.
   a. Determine whether an occupationally related injury or illness in fact occurred.
   b. Determine the extent of the injury or illness.
   c. Determine the recuperative potential of the employee and/or rehabilitative needs.
3. Worker's compensation covers all work-related injuries or diseases.
4. Most injuries have an obvious precipitating event that resulted in the injury, but some must be thoroughly investigated before they are considered occupationally related (e.g., hearing loss or repetitive trauma disorders).
5. Providers work with other health care professionals (e.g., public health officials, industrial hygienists, bioenvironmental engineers) to determine whether an occupational injury or illness occurred. These professionals help review workplace practices and hazards, adequacy of control measures, and nonoccupationally related hazards.
6. It is difficult to determine whether a disease is the result of an occupational exposure or whether a previous disease has been aggravated by occupational exposures.
   a. Sometimes it is obvious that a disease was acquired in the workplace (e.g., a needlestick injury before diagnosis of hepatitis B or C, HIV).
   b. More frequently, the association is unclear. Disease may have resulted from aging, poor immunity, predisposition/heredity, excessive use of tobacco or alcohol products, or risky behavior.
7. Before a disease is considered occupationally related, the investigator must weigh the available evidence.
   a. Exposure must have occurred while the individual was employed and working.
   b. Disease cannot be associated with extracurricular activities outside the workplace.
   c. Individual must be demonstrated to have been exposed to hazardous levels of the suspected hazard, in either previous or current jobs. This may involve:
      (1) Reviewing industrial hygiene surveys to evaluate hazardous levels of a particular substance.
      (2) Demonstrating inadequate control measures.
      (3) Identifying failure to use, or improperly using PPE (see Definitions section).

E. Americans with Disabilities Act (ADA)

1. See Definitions section for definitions of impairment, functional limitation, disability, essential functions of a job, and reasonable accommodations. A thorough review of the ADA and associated definitions can be found at www.usdoj.gov/crt/ada/adahom1.htm.
2. Employers must make reasonable accommodations for individuals with disabilities; in other words, the ADA prohibits discrimination based on any disability in a qualified person.
3. The ADA prohibits preemployment medical examinations during the process of hiring an individual with a disability.

F. Conducting Occupational Examinations: Four main types of occupational examinations are provided to employees (current or potential).

1. Preplacement medical examination.
   - **a.** Prospective employees receive physical examinations before employment.
   - **b.** Determinations are made as to whether any significant physical or mental impairment exists that would preclude an individual from performing essential duties related to the job.
2. Occupational periodic examination.
   - **a.** OSHA mandates that certain examinations be offered to workers who have been exposed to specific hazards in the workplace (Table 23-5).
   - **b.** Employers pay for these occupational periodic examinations.
   - **c.** Employees can refuse testing unless specifically required by their employment contract.
   - **d.** Examinations are part of a comprehensive medical surveillance system.
     - **(1)** Early identification of those employees with potentially adverse health consequences caused by occupational hazards.
     - **(2)** Triggering workplace evaluations and investigations to ensure that all available precautions have been taken to ensure the safety of employees.
     - **(3)** Tracking adverse trends to allow for better targeting of prevention efforts.
   - **e.** Biological monitoring (measuring specific agents or metabolites in biological specimens, generally blood or urine) is conducted for specific workplace hazards.
3. Assessment and treatment of occupational injury or illness.
   - **a.** Medical care for injuries or illnesses.
   - **b.** OSHA recordkeeping guidelines must be kept in mind (see Physical Examination section).
4. Return-to-work or fitness-for-duty evaluation ensures that workers are able to safely perform essential functions of their jobs.

Table 23-5. PARTIAL LIST OF WORKPLACE HAZARDS WITH OSHA-MANDATED OCCUPATIONAL EXAMINATIONS.

Acrylonitrile	Bloodborne Pathogens	Lead
Alpha-Naphthylamine	1,2-Butadiene	4,4 Methylenedianiline (MDA)
Arsenic	Cadmium	Methylene Chloride
Asbestos	Carcinogens (specific)	4-Nitrobiphenyl
Benzadine	Coke Oven Emissions	Noise (excessive)
Benzene	Cotton Dust	Silica
Beta-Naphthylamine	Ethyleneimine	Tuberculosis
Bis-Chloromethyl Ether	Formaldehyde	Vinyl Chloride

Note: Refer to the OSHA website for more specific information on mandated medical surveillance for specific occupational hazards (www.osha.gov).

5. Workplace evaluation: Firsthand knowledge of an employee's worksite is critical in the delivery of occupational medicine. There is no substitute for direct observation of industrial operations (refer to occupational medicine texts for further guidance).

XIV. ACRONYMS AND ABBREVIATIONS (Table 23-6)

XV. DEFINITIONS (Table 23-7)

XVI. SAMPLE H&P WRITE-UP

CC: "Hey, Doc. I'm here for my annual checkup. Haven't seen you around the plant much."

HPI: CEV is a divorced 57-year-old white male shop foreman who presents for his annual occupational examination. He recently was hired to his current duties, which are mostly administrative. However, he still assists with routine maintenance procedures at your chemical plant, which produces vinyl monomer. He reports a long history of working in similar plants and relates the "glory days" when he started out cleaning reactors. He states, "In those days, we didn't have all this PPE." He reports his health as "pretty good, but age seems to be taking away my energy."

PMHx: CEV states that he doesn't really have a personal physician because he is rarely ill. He denies any chronic medical problems and reports that he has never had an on-the-job injury or illness before. He has been pretty healthy, unlike some of the guys he started out with years ago. He has never had a worker's compensation or disability claim.

Table 23-6. OCCUPATIONAL MEDICINE ACRONYMS AND ABBREVIATIONS.

Acronym or Abbreviation	Term	Acronym or Abbreviation	Term
ACGIH	American Conference of Governmental Industrial Hygienists	**IME**	Independent medical examiner
ACOEM	American College of Occupational and Environmental Medicine	**MCS**	Multiple chemical sensitivities
ADA	Americans with Disabilities Act	**MRO**	Medical Review Officer
AL	Action limit	**MSDS**	Material Safety Data Sheet
ATSDR	Agency for Toxic Substances Disease Registry	**MSHA**	Mine Safety and Health Administration
BLS	Bureau of Labor Statistics	**NFPA**	National Fire Protection Association
CERCLA	Comprehensive Environmental Response, Compensation, and Liability Act	**NIHL**	Noise-induced hearing loss
CTD	Cumulative trauma disorder	**NIOSH**	National Institute of Occupational Safety and Health

CWP	Coal worker's pneumoconiosis	NOEL	No observed effect level
DOD	Department of Defense	NRC	Nuclear Regulatory Commission
DOE	Department of Energy	OSHA	Occupational Safety and Health Administration
DOT	Department of Transportation	OWC	Office of Worker's Compensation
EAP	Employee Assistance Program	PEL	Permissible exposure limit
EPA	Environmental Protection Agency	PPE	Personal protective equipment
FAA	Federal Aviation Administration	RCRA	Resource Conservation and Recovery Act
FHA	Federal Highway Administration	SARA	Superfund Amendments and Reauthorization Act
FIFRA	Federal Insecticide, Fungicide and Rodenticide Act	STEL	Short-term exposure limit
FRA	Federal Railroad Administration	STS	Significant threshold shift
HAZMAT	Hazardous materials	TLV	Threshold limit value
HIPAA	Health Insurance Portability and Accountability Act	TSCA	Toxic Substances Control Act
IH	Industrial hygiene		

Table 23-7. DEFINITIONS OF OCCUPATIONAL MEDICINE TERMS.

TERM	DEFINITION
Administrative controls	Administrative method to minimize hazard exposure in the workplace, such as rotating shifts
Association versus causation	Key tenet of occupational medicine that comes up in "work-relatedness" determinations, liability cases, epidemiologic studies, etc. An association must be present but is only one of several principles required to prove causality (see epidemiology texts)
Biological hazards	Infectious or immunologically active agents in the workplace (e.g., molds, fungi, bacteria)
Case management	Team approach toward minimizing lost productivity as a result of occupational injury or illness
Chemical hazards	Chemicals in the form of mists, vapors, gases, or airborne particles (i.e., dust and fumes) that can be inadvertently inhaled, ingested, or absorbed through the skin
Disability	Limitation in ability to perform an activity. This is a managerial determination. Specific definitions may vary among regulatory agencies
Engineering controls	Methods of physically separating hazards and employees to minimize potential exposure such as using enclosed automated processes
Ergonomic factors	Elements of a workstation that place an employee at risk for repetitive or cumulative motion disorders (e.g., vibrating tools, chronic repetitive use of instruments in awkward positions, excessive bending and reaching)
Essential functions of the job	The specific duties for which an offer of employment is extended
Functional impairment	Restriction resulting in less than normal ability or range of performance

Table 23-7—cont'd

TERM	DEFINITION
Hazard control	Controlling hazards in the workplace through (1) substitution or elimination of known hazardous materials or processes, (2) modifying industrial processes to limit exposure, (3) modifying the workplace to isolate the worker from the hazard, (4) removing the hazard through ventilation, (5) modifying work practices to reduce exposure, and (6) using personal protective equipment when other methods are ineffective
Health hazards	Chemical and biologic materials capable of producing adverse acute or chronic health effects
Impairment	Loss of function at the physiologic level. This is a medical determination
Industrial hygiene	Health profession responsible for recognizing, evaluating, and controlling hazards in the work environment
Occupational hazards	Physical, chemical, and biologic hazards or ergonomic factors in the work environment that cause or contribute to injury, disease, impaired function, or discomfort
Occupational injuries	Injuries resulting from a specific event in the workplace (e.g., motor vehicle accidents [MVAs], homicides, falling, slipping)
Occupational illnesses and diseases	Disease processes resulting from occupational exposures (e.g., hepatitis B and C, dermatitis, asbestosis, cumulative motion disorders, hearing loss) or preexisting diseases exacerbated by current working conditions (e.g., asthmatic attacks, worsened allergies)
OSHA "general duty" clause	Section 5(a)(1) of the OSHA Act states that "employer shall furnish to each of his employees employment and a place of employment which are free from recognized hazards that are causing or are likely to cause death or serious physical harm to his employees." This clause covers any hazard not specifically addressed in the Act elsewhere

Continued

Table 23-7. DEFINITIONS OF OCCUPATIONAL MEDICINE TERMS—*cont'd*

Term	Definition
Personal protective equipment (PPE)	Devices that provide a barrier between worker and the occupational hazard that protect the eyes (safety glasses, goggles, face shields), skin (gloves, aprons, full body suits), and respiratory tract (respiratory protection devices)
Physical hazards	Hazardous elements of the work environment, including explosives, flammable and/or combustible liquids, oxidizers, compressed gases, reactive chemicals, excessive noise, ionizing and nonionizing radiation, and temperature extremes
Reasonable accommodation	Efforts required of employers by the ADA to enable an employee with a disability to perform the essential function of a position
Risk assessment	Characterization of a hazard and its risks
Risk communication	Conveyance of actual risk in the appropriate perspective to the patient, public, or decision makers
Risk management	Efforts to mitigate risk
Work hardening	Rehabilitative therapy designed for early return to work and minimization of future injury and lost duty time

PSHx: Right inguinal hernia repair approximately 20 years prior.

MEDICATIONS: Tylenol for the past three days for some generalized body aches. Had been prescribed Benadryl in the past for mild seasonal allergies, but made him too drowsy. The patient reports no known drug allergies and doesn't take any nutritional supplements.

HEALTH MAINTENANCE

Prevention: The patient received all of the usual childhood immunizations, including MMR. He has never had a screening colon study or fecal occult blood test. He does not recall when his cholesterol was last checked, but he is sure it must have been looked at during prior occupational health examinations.

Diet: Regular diet with no restrictions. Lately he hasn't had as much of an appetite and reports losing a few pounds.

Exercise and Hobbies: The patient walks extensively on the job. He used to enjoy model building but has lost dexterity in his hands over the years.

Sleep Patterns: The patient has had no other unusual sleep patterns except some difficulty adjusting after working rotating shifts.

Social Habits: The patient denies smoking or tobacco use. He used to consume alcohol socially, but recently just hasn't had much desire. The patient denies illicit drug use.

Travel: He denies any recent travel. He was assigned overseas during one tour in the Vietnam conflict. He denies any known unusual exposures during that time.

FAMILY HISTORY

First-Degree Relatives' Medical History: The patient's father died in a coal mine accident and had hypertension. The patient's mother is alive and well. He has no siblings or children.

Three-Generation Genogram: There is no history of genetic traits or diseases within the patient's family.

PSYCHOSOCIAL HISTORY

Personal and Social History: The patient is a Caucasian born in Pennsylvania before moving to Texas. He currently lives alone.

Current Illness Effects on the Patient: The patient denies current illness.

Interpersonal and Sexual History: The patient is single, but "always looking." He reports a few regular female friends and has been treated for "the clap" several times in the past.

Family Support: He occasionally visits his mother, who lives in a skilled nursing center. He has several cousins with whom he doesn't keep in close contact.

Occupational Aspects of Illness: The patient denies any ongoing illness and has not missed a day since hiring into his current job.

REVIEW OF SYSTEMS

General: 15-pound weight loss over the past few weeks.

HEENT/Neck: No visual changes or scotomata. No epistaxis.

Respiratory: No cough, dyspnea, or shortness of breath.

Cardiovascular: No tachycardia, palpitations, orthopnea, or paroxysmal nocturnal dyspnea.

Gastrointestinal: Some slight nausea without vomiting. Occasional heartburn and decreased appetite. No RUQ or epigastric pain. Occasional constipation and "hemorrhoidal" bleeding.

Genitourinary: No dysuria, urinary urgency, penile lesions, or discharge.

Hematologic/Lymphatic: Some increased bruising tendencies.

Skin: No rash, pruritis, hirsutism, or pigmentary changes except for chronic cracking of skin around his distal fingertips.

Neurologic: No history of seizures, headaches, or dizziness.

Musculoskeletal: Occasional back discomfort. No arthritis or muscle weakness.

Extremities: Some peripheral edema over the past few weeks. No paresthesias, numbness, or tremor. Has some decreased dexterity of distal fingertips, which are also sensitive to cold air.

Endocrine: No polydipsia, polyphagia, or nocturia.

Reproductive: Not applicable.

Psychiatric: No history of depression, mood disorders, or anxiety.

PHYSICAL EXAMINATION

Vitals: T 98.8°F P 86 BP 155/96 RR 18 Weight 153 lbs.

HEENT: Slight facial edema. Sclera icteric and fundoscopic examination normal. Bilateral high-frequency hearing loss on audiogram. Poor oral hygiene with some evidence of friable gums.

Neck: No thyroid enlargement. Slight jugular venous distension.

Lungs: Clear to auscultation bilaterally.

Chest: No nipple discharge or masses.

Cardiovascular: Normal S1 and S2. Regular rate and rhythm. Grade I/VI systolic ejection murmur.

Abdomen: Soft and slightly distended. Some evidence of hepatosplenomegaly. RUQ discomfort to direct palpation. No rebound or peritoneal signs.

Genitourinary: No CVA tenderness. No genital tract lesions.

Rectal: Large external hemorrhoids. Prostate slightly enlarged but symmetrical. Stool guaiac positive.

Skin: No obvious jaundice. Extensive sun damage with scattered salmon-colored plaques over forearms and face. Small 1- to 2-cm lesion on posterior left ear with raised pearly borders and central ulceration.

Extremities: 1-2+ pitting pretibial edema. Scleroderma-like lesion over distal fingertips.

Neurologic: 2+ deep tendon reflexes, symmetrically. No focal sensory or musculoskeletal deficits.

Psychiatric: Mini-mental status examination normal.

24

ONCOLOGY

Thomas S. Neuhauser, MD, Michael Osswald, MD,
and Nina J. Karlin, MD

I. CHIEF COMPLAINT: What brings the patient in to be evaluated?

A. Cardinal Symptoms of Cancer

1. **New mass**: Have you noticed a new breast mass, neck mass, or bony mass?
2. **Bleeding:** Epistaxis, hemoptysis, hematemesis, rectal bleeding, irregular menstrual patterns or vaginal bleeding, blood in urine, or easy bruising could indicate the presence of cancer or cancer-associated thrombocytopenia.
3. **Hoarse voice**: Do you have a hoarse voice? A hoarse voice is a sign of cancer of the head and neck region or a mediastinal mass that paralyzes the recurrent laryngeal nerve.
4. **Cough:** Have you recently developed a chronic cough? This could suggest a lung mass.
5. **Weight loss:** Have you lost weight? Weight loss is a sign of generalized illness, but in the absence of another etiology, metastatic cancer needs to be considered.
6. **Pain:** Do you have any new pain that does not go away? New pain that does not resolve could suggest a primary or metastatic cancer; it is especially common in metastases to bone but also could be caused by a mass in any location.
7. **Change in bowel habits**: Has there been a change in your bowel habits? Such a change specifically suggests gastrointestinal cancers.
8. **Swollen glands:** Are any of your glands swollen? Lymphadenopathy often has an infectious source, but when generalized, it suggests lymphoma. If the lymphoma is localized, it could suggest a local organ cancer (e.g., axillary nodes suggest breast cancer and neck nodes suggest head and neck cancer).

B. Identifying Data

1. Age: Incidence of many cancers vary with the age of the patient (e.g., Hodgkin's lymphoma in young adults, chronic lymphocytic leukemia [CLL] in older adults, Wilm's tumor in children).
2. Gender: Incidence of malignancy varies with or unique to sex of patient (e.g., much higher incidence of breast cancer in women, prostate cancer in men).
3. Race: Certain races may be predisposed to certain malignancies (e.g., increased incidence of gastric cancer in Asian, African, and Hispanic patients).

4. Country of origin or residence: Incidence of many cancers vary with country (e.g., natural killer [NK] cell malignancies in Thailand, gastric cancer in the Orient).

II. HISTORY OF PRESENT ILLNESS

A. **Duration:** How long have you had these symptoms? A symptom that has been present for many years is more likely to be benign.

B. **Relievers:** What have you already tried to help resolve symptoms? Did it help?

C. **Evaluations:** What work-ups, if any, have been done?

D. **Performance Status:** What is your performance of daily activities? Has it changed?

E. **Quality of Life:** How do these symptoms affect your daily life, if at all?

F. **Treatment:** Have you been able to tolerate past treatments for this disorder? Do you think you'll be able to tolerate recommended treatment(s)?

G. **Oncology-Specific History for Cancers (Table 24-1)**

Table 24-1. SPECIFIC REGIONS AND ONCOLOGY-FOCUSED HISTORY TOPICS.

REGION	HISTORY TOPICS
Bladder	Exposure to aniline dye, leather/paint/rubber occupational exposure, history of travel to Middle East or Africa (exposure to *Schistosomiasis haematobium*), tobacco use, pelvic irradiation, history of use of cyclophosphamide, history of spinal cord compression (chronic urinary retention), chronic low fluid intake, caffeine intake
Breast	Diet, patient age, oral contraceptive use, family or previous history of breast cancer, early menarche/late menopause, history of other malignancies, diabetes mellitus (DM), alcohol use, dermatomyositis, obesity, late first pregnancy or nulliparity, history of ductal carcinoma in situ (DCIS), lobular carcinoma in situ (LCIS), or atypical ductal hyperplasia (ADH), BRCA/Her-2-neu status, ethnicity, prior biopsies

Table 24-1—cont'd

REGION	HISTORY TOPICS
Colorectal	Polyps (especially if greater than 3 cm and villous subtype), high-grade dysplasia, poor diet (increased dietary fat/oil), inflammatory bowel disease (IBD) (e.g., ulcerative colitis or Crohn's disease), family history of polyps/colorectal carcinoma (e.g., familial adenomatous polyposis syndrome, Gardner's syndrome, Turcot's syndrome), smoking, asbestos exposure, history of ureterosigmoidostomy
Esophageal	Tobacco and alcohol use (each one is a risk, but synergistic in combination), race, history of esophagitis (with or without intestinal metaplasia/Barrett's), Plummer-Vinson syndrome, achalasia, esophageal web/diverticula, short esophagus, thermal/caustic injury, history of strictures, tylosis
Gastric	*Helicobacter pylori* infection, achlorhydria, atrophic gastritis, pernicious anemia, previous resection, mucosal dysplasia, increased consumption of smoked/pickled foods (e.g., nitrates), tobacco use
Gynecologic (cervical, endometrial, ovarian, vulvar)	Abnormal Pap smears, history of human papilloma virus (HPV) (types 16, 18, 31, 33, 35), young age at first intercourse, low socioeconomic group, multiple sexual partners, pelvic inflammatory disease (PID)/history of sexually transmitted diseases (STDs), palpable pelvic mass(es), history of human immunodeficiency virus (HIV), exogenous estrogen use, polycystic ovary disease, anovulatory cycles, obesity, hypertension (HTN), family history of cancer, DM, infertility, hereditary nonpolyposis colon cancer syndrome, ovarian cancer, change in or abnormal vaginal bleeding, late menopause, prior pelvic radiation therapy, history of diethylstilbestrol (DES) use/vaginal adenosis, vulvar lump/mass, bleeding, pain, infection, pruritis, rash, toxin/drug exposure, history of colon/breast/endometrial cancer, nulliparity, urinary frequency, constipation, abdominal discomfort/distention, high animal fat diet, BRCA status

Continued

ONC

Table 24-1. SPECIFIC REGIONS AND ONCOLOGY FOCUSED HISTORY TOPICS—*cont'd*

Region	History Topics
Head and neck	Tobacco (smoking or chewing), long-standing hyperkeratosis, chronic inflammatory conditions, xeroderma pigmentosa, prior history of head and neck disease, occupational history (nickel-refining, hardwood dust), MEN II syndrome (Sipple's)
Hematopoietic	Social class, family size, history of immunosuppression (HIV status), prior history of malignancy/lymphoma, history of radiation therapy, inherited or acquired immunodeficiency states, chronic inflammatory disorder, collagen-vascular diseases, travel history
Kidney	Tobacco use, family history, thorotrast exposure, von Hippel-Lindau syndrome, polycystic kidney disease, DM, chronic dialysis, industrial dye exposure, history of chronic analgesic nephropathy
Neurologic	Ionizing radiation, exposure to vinyl chloride, history of: neurofibromatosis, tuberous sclerosis, von Hippel-Lindau, Turcot syndrome, nevoid basal-cell syndrome, Li-Fraumeni syndrome; immune suppression (e.g., HIV, transplant), family history of brain cancer
Pancreas	Tobacco use, diet, partial gastrectomy, glucose intolerance/diabetes mellitus, chronic pancreatitis, toxin exposure, idiopathic deep venous thrombosis (DVT, think Trousseau's), dermatomyositis/polymyositis, family history, MEN I syndrome (Wermer's syndrome)
Prostate	Race, age, occupational exposure: chemists, loggers, cadmium industrial workers, farmers, painters, rubber tire workers, textile workers; family history of prostate cancer; cirrhosis (associated with increased estrogen level); diet (increased animal fats/decreased fibers); history of vasectomy
Pulmonary	Smoking (pack-years), asbestos/radon/chemical exposure, occupational exposures, prior history of lung disease, performance status, cardiac history, history of solitary pulmonary nodule, history of other malignancies

Table 24-1—cont'd

REGION	HISTORY TOPICS
Sarcoma	History of mass, neurofibromatosis, chronic lymphedema, radiation injury, prior radiation (especially for breast cancer and lymphoma), chemical carcinogen exposure, family history of sarcoma
Skin	Sun exposure, race, history of previous skin malignancies, arsenic/sun exposure, irradiation, coal tar/quinacrine exposure, chronic draining osteomyelitis, fistulae, stasis dermatitis, thermal/electric burns, chronic heat exposure, atrophic skin lesions, xeroderma pigmentosum, basal cell nevus syndrome, HPV infection, immunosuppression, poor tanning capacity, level of education, presence of large number of moles (especially atypical), family history of melanoma/dysplastic nevus syndrome, propensity to sunburn, history of severe sunburn as a child
Testicular	Cryptorchidism (undescended testes), infertility, genitourinary anomalies, history of atypical melanocytic nevi

III. PAST MEDICAL AND SURGICAL HISTORY

A. Past Medical History

1. Have you previously been diagnosed with cancer? Is your current cancer a relapse or a new primary? Have you received chemotherapy or radiation therapy treatments in the past that could have been carcinogenic?
2. Do you have any major illnesses? If so, what are they? A patient's ability to receive cancer therapy may be hindered by the presence of other major illness. For example, chemotherapy dosing may be limited in a patient with hepatic or renal disease. Cardiopulmonary disease may limit a patient's ability to tolerate a curative surgical resection of a cancer.
3. Do you have any of the following illnesses (that can predispose to cancer)?
   - **a.** Chronic liver disease (e.g., cirrhosis or iron overload) may lead to hepatocellular cancer.
   - **b.** Human immunodeficiency virus (HIV) predisposes patients to a host of hematopoietic malignancies and Kaposi's sarcoma.

c. Xeroderma pigmentosum predisposes to multiple malignancies, esophageal cancer in patients with Barrett's esophagus, gastric lymphoma in patients with *Helicobacter pylori,* colon cancer in patients with inflammatory bowel disease, penile squamous cell carcinoma in patient's with history of erythroplasia of Queyrat.

d. History of dysplasia or carcinoma-in-situ (CIS).

4. Have you been hospitalized? When? Where? For what reason?
5. Have you had blood transfusions? Multiple transfusions predispose to formation of alloantibodies. Important for oncology patients who frequently utilize numerous blood products.
6. Have you had irradiation? For what reason? How much? Radiation is associated with numerous malignancies.

B. **Past Surgical History:** Have you undergone any surgical procedures? If so, what were they and when did you have them? Were there any complications or sequelae?

C. **Childhood History**

1. Was your childhood development normal? Undescended testis predispose to testicular cancer.
2. Did you have radiation treatments? Radiation was used in the past to treat acne; increased risk for thyroid cancer.
3. Where did you grow up?
4. What immunizations did you have?
5. Have you had prior cancers?

D. **Occupational History**

1. Are you exposed to any potential carcinogens at your workplace? Aromatic amines, arsenic, asbestos, benzene, chromium, ionizing radiation, nickel, vinyl chloride, polycyclic hydrocarbons, industrial dyes, or hazardous wastes?
2. Do any co-workers have similar problems or malignancies? Some malignancies can be traced to a common source (e.g., hematopoietic malignancy following nuclear plant accident and mesothelioma in shipyard workers).
3. Do you use appropriate safety equipment or attire?

IV. **MEDICATIONS, ALLERGIES, AND ADVERSE REACTIONS**

1. Are you currently taking any medications? Some drugs may interfere with chemotherapy or surgery (e.g., anticoagulants) or potentiate the effects of others.
2. Are you taking any drugs that have been associated with an increased risk of cancer? Estrogens may increase risk of breast cancer; Tamoxifen may increase the risk of uterine cancer.
3. Have you had any allergic reactions to prior medicines (e.g., classic example is penicillin and cross-reactivity with penicillin derivatives/cephalosporins)?
4. Have you had previous reactions to transfusions? Anaphylaxis?

5. Have you ever experienced any intolerable side effects to medications (e.g., impotence, intractable itching, coughing, headaches)?

V. HEALTH MAINTENANCE

A. Prevention

1. Do you use tobacco? Have you tried to quit? Have you taken any smoking cessation classes?
2. Do you use or abuse alcohol? If so, do you have a desire to quit? Have you made any attempts?
3. Are you sexually active? Do you have more than one partner? Do you use protective measures?
4. Are you exposed to toxins or chemicals at work? Do you use appropriate personal protective equipment (PPE), safety equipment, and attire?
5. Are your immunizations up to date? This is important if the patient is currently or is soon to be immunocompromised or undergo a splenectomy.
6. Do you avoid sun damage and sunburn? Do you use sunscreen? What SPF?

B. Screening Tests

1. Pulmonary: Large-scale screening of smoking population for lung cancer is not justified at this time because early detection does not appear to alter long-term mortality.
2. Colorectal: Annual hemoccult starting at age 50 and flexible sigmoidoscopy starting at age 50 and every 3 to 5 years thereafter.
3. Esophageal cancer: If documented history of Barrett's, then annual esophagogastric duodenoscopy (EGD) with biopsy, to assess for dysplasia/neoplasia.
4. Breast cancer: Annual mammogram starting at age 40. Breast self-examination 5 days after each menses in women over 20 years of age.
5. Gynecologic
   a. Cervical cancer: Annual Pap smear for 3 years for women who are older than 18 years or who are sexually active, and if consecutively negative, every 2-3 years thereafter.
   b. Ovarian cancer: Use of vaginal ultrasound and serial CA 125 measurements have not shown any survival benefit (currently investigational).
6. Prostate: Controversial because no studies have proved beneficial. Currently done in patients with life expectancy of more than 10 years.
   a. Men age 40-50: Annual digital rectal examination (DRE).
   b. Men over 50: Annual DRE and serum prostatic specific antigen (PSA) (age 40 if positive family history).
7. Melanoma: In high-risk patients, annual full-body examination of melanocytic nevi (moles)/lesions by a dermatologist.

8. Testis: Monthly testis self-examination. Correct undescended/cryptorchid testis.

C. **Diet:** Is associated with cancers of the gastrointestinal (GI) tract and cancers affected by hormones (e.g., breast, endometrial, ovary, prostate).

1. Excess caloric intake should be avoided. Intake of fat (<30% of calories), salt-cured, nitrate-cured, smoked, and pickled foods should be decreased or moderated.
2. Intake of foods containing fiber, vitamin C, and beta-carotene should be increased.
3. Intake of salty or smoked foods, red meats, and alcohol should be limited.

D. **Exercise**

1. Do you engage in regular exercise? Lack of exercise is a risk factor for certain cancers.
2. Have you experienced any recent changes in your exercise regimen or in your endurance?

E. **Sleep Patterns**: Has your sleep pattern recently changed? Have you had night sweats? Chills? Nocturia?

F. **Social Habits**

1. Do you use tobacco products? How many packs per day for how many years (pack-years)? Clearly related to cancer of lung, head and neck, esophageal, bladder, and other malignancies.
2. Do you consume alcohol? How much? How long? Clearly related to liver and head and neck cancers.
3. Are you sexually active? Have you had an STD? Are your partners healthy?
4. How would you describe your personal hygiene? Failure to bathe and poor oral hygiene can cause chronic irritation that may predispose to malignancy.

VI. FAMILY HISTORY

A. **First-Degree Relatives' Medical History:** Assess for familial cancer syndromes. Breast, ovary, and colon cancers have strong familial components, although true hereditary cancers probably make up the minority of cases.

B. **Three-Generation Genogram**

1. Diagram may be best method for organizing information.
2. Also query patient's children, parents, and spouse or partner (as available and appropriate).

VII. PSYCHOSOCIAL HISTORY

A. **Personal and Social History**

1. What is your place of birth (country and city), religious and race/ethnicity background?
2. Are you married? Any children?
3. What level of education have you attained (e.g., years of schooling, college and advanced degrees)?

4. Where do you currently reside? Determine proximity to treatment center. Some cancer treatments require long stays at the hospital and frequent follow-up.

B. **Current Illness Effects on the Patient**
1. Assess patient's understanding of why he or she is here. Discuss possible illness, treatment options, potential consequences, and complications. Some patients may want a second opinion.
2. Can you afford treatments and medications? Long hospital stays, frequent clinical follow-ups, and expensive medications may be necessary (e.g., bone marrow transplantation [BMT], surgery).
3. Genetic counseling may be necessary (e.g., familial syndromes, predisposition to certain cancers/additional malignancies).
4. How will your illness affect your employment?
5. Any emotional/psychiatric problems? May expect psychiatric difficulties with some illnesses and treatments (e.g., depression, guilt, change in self-image, anxiety, fear).
6. With some patients, will need to discuss issues related to dying.
7. May need to address fertility concerns with patient, including the effect of chemotherapy on germ cells (testis/ovaries) and the effect of radical surgery on sexual function (impotence, loss of libido, dyspareunia, vaginal fibrosis). For some patients, sperm banking/egg banking may be an option or concern. For pregnant women, will have to address effect of therapy and malignancy on fetus.

C. **Interpersonal and Sexual History:** Obtain detailed sexual history, including health of partners (if known).

D. **Family/Friend Support**
1. What social support and resources do you have (e.g., family, friends, church, employer)?
2. What family stressors (e.g., young children, poor support systems) do you have?
3. Do you have concerns or fears regarding the effect of your cancer on your family? Cancer and its treatment can place an incredible social, financial, and time burden on patients and their families.
4. Will you need referrals for home health care or assistance or transportation?
5. Consider whether family as well as patient needs genetic counseling.

E. **Occupation Aspects of Illness**
1. How will the illness/treatment affect your employment?
2. Will special arrangements be necessary during or following treatment? Do you have a flexible work schedule? It is easier to deal with problems that come up if they are discussed and anticipated.

VIII. REVIEW OF SYSTEMS (Tables 24-2, 24-3, and 24-4)

Note: Many malignancies are accompanied by weight loss/cachexia, fatigue, fever, bone pain (with metastases). Lung metastases will result in pleural effusions/rubs. Dentition should be examined because this may affect therapy decisions or propensity to infection. Good neurologic examination should be performed to assess for metastasis, paraneoplastic syndromes/chemotherapy effects (peripheral neuropathies). A good skin survey is important to assess for metastasis, rashes associated with drugs. Assess for hydration.

Table 24-2. GENERAL SYMPTOMS BY SYSTEM.

System	Symptoms
General	Performance status, weakness, fevers, malaise
HEENT	Headache, tinnitus, hearing loss, visual changes, conjunctivitis, epistaxis, mouth ulcers, dental pain, loss of taste, neck masses/enlarged lymph nodes, sore throat, decreased hearing (unilateral), hoarseness, nasal obstruction, change in fitting of dentures
Respiratory	Shortness of breath, pleurisy, hemoptysis, hoarseness, anorexia, weight loss, dyspnea, paresthesias (e.g., Pancoast's tumor), jaundice, abdominal distention/discomfort (metastasis, advanced disease)
Cardiovascular	Chest pain, palpitations
Gastrointestinal	Nausea, vomiting, abdominal distention, dyspepsia, hiccups, diarrhea, constipation, rectal bleeding, dysphagia, early satiety, distaste for meat, weakness, hematemesis, jaundice
Genitourinary	Dysuria, frequency, color of urine, odor, hematuria
Obstetric/ gynecologic	Menstruation or cessation thereof, pregnancy, vaginal discharge
Hematopoietic	Fatigue, infections, easy bruising
Lymphatic	Lymphadenopathy, extremity swelling/edema
Musculoskeletal	Muscle weakness or pain, bony pain or swelling, lymphedema
Dermatologic	Rashes, sun sensitivity
Central nervous system	Headache, photophobia, nausea, weakness
Psychiatric	Depression, insomnia, mania, restlessness, mood changes

Table 24-3. NONSPECIFIC SYMPTOMS AND ASSOCIATED DISEASE PROCESSES.

SYMPTOM	DISEASE PROCESS
Bony pain/swelling	Trauma, osteomyelitis, tumor/metastasis
Cough	New chronic cough could suggest infection, irritation, aspiration, a lung mass
Dysphonia (hoarse voice)	Cancer of the head and neck region/ mediastinal mass paralyzing recurrent laryngeal nerve, infection, trauma, irritation
Hematuria	Infection, trauma, mass lesion
Hemoptysis	Pneumonia, associated with chronic cough, tumor/metastases
Lymphedema	Obstruction/poor drainage (mass lesion, clot), decreased oncotic pressure, infection
Rectal bleeding	Trauma/hemorrhoids, liver disease/ cirrhosis, GI bleeding (mass, coagulopathy, trauma, vascular abnormalities, infarction)
Swollen glands	Lymphadenopathy is often from an infectious source; generalized suggests lymphoma, localized could suggest a local organ cancer

Table 24-4. COMMON MALIGNANT DISEASE PROCESSES AND THEIR SYMPTOMS.

CANCER TYPE AND ORGAN SYSTEM(S) AFFECTED	SYMPTOMS
Bladder	Hematuria, hesitancy, frequency, dysuria, post-voiding discomfort, pelvic/flank pain, constipation, nocturia, urinary obstruction
Breast	Mass, pain, bloody nipple discharge, skin changes (dimpling/erythema/induration), axillary mass (lymphadenopathy), breast pain, eczema
Colorectal	Abdominal pain/distension, palpable mass, hematochezia, changes in bowel habits, organomegaly (liver/spleen metastases, biliary obstruction, portal hypertension), ascites, consistent gas pain, decrease in stool caliber, severe pain (anal)

Continued

Table 24-4. COMMON MALIGNANT DISEASE PROCESSES AND THEIR SYMPTOMS—cont'd

Cancer Type and Organ System(s) Affected	Symptoms
Esophageal	Throat/chest pain, hematemesis, dysphagia, pain radiating to back, odynophagia
Gastric	Abdominal distension/fullness, early satiety, hematemesis, loss of appetite, distaste for meat, dysphagia, melena, dyspnea, ovarian mass (Krukenberg tumor)
Gynecologic	Change in/abnormal vaginal bleeding, bleeding during pregnancy (trophoblastic malignancies), abdominal fullness, infertility, mass(es), recurrent infections, urinary frequency, constipation, abdominal pain/distension, dysuria, dyspareunia, ulceration, pruritis, vaginal discharge, pelvic pain
Head and neck	Mass lesion(s), head and neck pain, mucosal ulcers, pain, recurrent unilateral sinusitis/nasal obstruction, odynophagia, dysphagia, cough, aspiration pneumonia, visual disturbances, hearing loss, erythroplakia, loosening teeth, poorly fitting dentures, epistaxis, ptosis, cranial nerve neuralgia(s), weakness of muscles (e.g., tongue, sternocleidomastoid), hoarseness, otalgia
Hematopoietic	Lymphadenopathy (palpable masses), night sweats, bone pain, lymph node pain with alcohol ingestion, symptoms related to site of involvement (e.g., kidney, mediastinum), anergy
Kidney	Flank pain, mass/organomegaly, hematuria, features of paraneoplastic syndromes (erythrocytosis, hypercalcemia, fever, hepatomegaly, hypertension, amyloidosis), left-sided varicocele, lower extremity edema, plethora, polyuria, constipation, anemia
Neurologic	Headache, seizures, hemiparesis, aphasia, hemineglect, hemianopsia, diabetes insipidus, hyperphagia, visual field defects, extremity weakness, hearing loss, dysmetria, ataxia, vertigo, nystagmus, nausea/emesis, mental status changes
Liver	Pain in right subcostal area, pain radiating to shoulder, fatigue, anorexia, fever, ascites (advanced disease)

Table 24-4—cont'd

Cancer Type and Organ System(s) Affected	Symptoms
Pancreas	Abdominal mass, jaundice, pancreatitis, vague/intermittent abdominal pain, migratory thrombophlebitis, weight loss, early satiety, fatigability, nausea, constipation, depression, vomiting, bloating, dyspepsia
Prostate	Hematochezia, changes in bowel habits, bone pain, urinary obstruction, hesitancy, urgency, nocturia, poor urinary stream, dribbling, terminal hematuria, sudden-onset paraplegia/incontinence/encopresis, nodular prostate/seminal vesicles, groin mass (lymphadenopathy), hematospermia
Pulmonary	Chest pain, hemoptysis, clubbing, pleural effusions, rubs, stridor, new/changing/persistent cough, hoarseness, dyspnea, nonresolving/recurrent pneumonia, chest pain, paraesthesia/weakness of upper extremities (Pancoast's tumor), ptosis/miosis/anhidrosis (Horner's syndrome), erythema/edema upper extremity/facial plethora/dyspnea (superior vena cava/SVC syndrome), abdominal symptoms (pain, distention, organomegaly)/jaundice (liver metastasis), adenopathy
Sarcoma	Abdominal fullness and/or pain, early satiety, back pain, soft/painless mass in soft tissue or extremity
Skin	Lesion, ulceration, regional lymphadenopathy, change in shape/color/border of nevus, bleeding of nevus (melanoma)
Testicular	Orchitis, mass, abdominal pain, gynecomastia, infertility, dysuria, back pain

IX. PHYSICAL EXAMINATION (Tables 24-5 and 24-6)

To document suspicious findings, delineate possible stage of disease, and determine what further studies may need to be done. Vitals and full examination are required for all cancer patients. There are common sites of cancer involvement/metastasis for many malignancies (see general H&P section).

Table 24-5. CANCER SITES AND ORGAN SYSTEMS AFFECTED AND PHYSICAL EXAMINATION FOCUS AREAS.

ORGAN OR REGION	PHYSICAL EXAMINATION
Bladder	Abdominal/pelvic/rectal examination: Note flank pain, lower extremity or genital edema
Breast	Breast/axillary examination: Palpate for breast/axillary masses/painful areas, skin changes (erythema/induration/dimpling), nipple retraction/discharge, bone pain
Colorectal	Abdominal/rectal examination: Check for ascites, masses, changes in abdominal girth, hepatomegaly, pain, blood in stool (guaiac)
Esophageal	Chest/abdominal examination: Hepatomegaly, cachexia, pulmonary examination
Gastric	Abdominal/pelvic examination: Abdominal masses/distension/ascites, ovarian mass(es), blood in stool (guaiac)
Gynecologic	Pelvic/abdominal/breast/rectal examination: Perform Pap (if not recent), note discharge, mass(es), asymmetric ovaries, lymphadenopathy, vulvar lesions/pain/erythema/rash/ulceration, abdominal distension/increased girth
Head and neck	Head/neck/cranial nerve examination: Mass lesions, lymphadenopathy, asymmetry (including tonsils/salivary glands), vision/hearing, erythroleukoplakia, loosening teeth, trismus
Hematopoietic	Lymph node examination: Lymphadenopathy, hepatosplenomegaly, signs related to site of involvement (e.g., mediastinum, lung, liver, kidney, brain, bone marrow)
Kidney	Abdominal/neural examination: Organomegaly (amyloidosis), flank mass/pain, left sided varicocele, lower extremity edema, plethora, hypotonia, mental status changes
Neurologic	Neurologic examination: Hemianopsia, visual field defects, weakness, cranial nerve defects, hearing loss, dysmetria, ataxia, nystagmus, mental status changes, changes in reflexes

Table 24-5—cont'd

ORGAN OR REGION	PHYSICAL EXAMINATION
Pancreas	Abdominal/skin examination: Mass, distension, pain, ascites, skin rash(es), peripheral vessels (migratory thrombophlebitis)
Prostate	Rectal/abdominal examination: Masses/irregularities (prostate), bone pain, blood in stool (guaiac)
Pulmonary	Chest examination: Signs of Cushing's disease, paresthesias, upper extremity weakness/edema, neck/supraclavicular mass(es), ptosis, miosis, facial plethora, dyspnea, rubs, dullness to percussion
Sarcoma	Abdominal/peripheral examination: Soft tissue mass(es), back discomfort
Skin	Skin/lymph node examination: Color/size of lesions, irregularities, distribution, change in color/border (pigmented lesions), lymphadenopathy
Testicular	Scrotal/abdominal/neurologic examination: Note mass(es), gynecomastia, neural deficiencies (metastasis), hydrocele, varicocele, features of epididymitis

X. DIFFERENTIAL DIAGNOSIS (Table 24-7)

XI. LABORATORY STUDIES AND DIAGNOSTIC EVALUATIONS

A. Laboratory Studies

1. New cancer patients.
   a. Complete blood count (CBC).
   b. Basic chemistries.
   c. Liver function tests (LFTs).
   d. Lactate dehydrogenase (LDH).
   e. Calcium.
   f. Urinalysis.
2. Tumor markers.
   a. Measured in body fluids (most commonly serum).
   b. Assist in determination of tumor type as well as serving as markers of treatment effect and recurrent disease.
   c. Some markers by organ system include the following:
      (1) Pulmonary: CA 125, CA 15-3.
      (2) Gastric: Carcinoembryonic antigen (CEA).
      (3) Colorectal: CEA.

Table 24-6. FINDINGS ON PHYSICAL EXAMINATION AND POSSIBLE DIAGNOSES.

System	Physical Examination Finding	Possible Diagnoses
General and systemic	Cachexia	Advanced malignancy (e.g., poor nutrition resulting from loss of appetite/dysphagia/emesis, widespread disease)
	Pallor	Anemia resulting from chronic blood loss (colon cancer, renal cancer), bone marrow involvement (pulmonary, prostate, breast cancer)
Vital signs		
Temperature	Fever	Frequently associated with malignancy
Pulse	Tachycardia	Paraneoplastic hyperthyroidism, dehydration, pheochromocytoma, paraganglioma, hypoglycemia
Blood pressure	Hypertension	Renal cancer (increased renin production), pheochromocytoma (90%), adrenal tumor, Wilm's tumor (children), paraganglioma
	Hypotension	VIPoma, adrenal gland metastasis (orthostatic), systemic mastocytosis, tumor lysis syndrome
Respiratory rate	Increased respirations	Right heart failure (e.g., carcinoid syndrome)
Weight	Unintentional loss	See cachexia above
Height posture	Decrease from previous	Pathologic fracture of spine caused by primary of metastatic malignancy, Paget's disease of bone
HEENT		
Head	Bulging fontanelles (young children)	Brain tumor

Eyes	Ptosis	Nasopharyngeal cancer, pulmonary cancer (e.g., Horner's syndrome), thymoma (associated with myasthenia gravis)
	Proptosis	Rhabdomyosarcoma (children), olfactory esthesioneuroblastoma
	Papilledema	Increased intracranial pressure (brain tumor)
	Visual field defect	Tumor of hypothalamus
	Nystagmus	Cerebellar tumor
	White pupil (leukocoria)	Retinoblastoma
	Fluffy calcifications of retina	Retinoblastoma
	Venous dilation	Hyperviscosity (e.g., Waldenstrom's macroglobulinemia)
Ears	Decreased hearing	Nasopharyngeal cancer, acoustic neuroma
Nasal cavity and sinuses	Pain/tenderness	Tumor
	Bloody discharge	Nasal mass, DIC
Mouth	Ulceration	Carcinoma, glucagonoma
	Tumors floor of mouth (oral tongue, buccal mucosa, gingiva, retromolar, hard palate)	Cancer
	Hyperpigmentation (mouth, gums)	Adrenal gland metastasis
	Enlargement or asymmetric hypertrophy of Waldeyer's ring (tonsils, adenoids)	Lymphoma

Continued

Table 24-6. FINDINGS ON PHYSICAL EXAMINATION AND POSSIBLE DIAGNOSES—*cont'd*

System	Physical Examination Finding	Possible Diagnoses
	Macroglossia	Amyloidosis
	Gingival hypertrophy	Acute myelogenous leukemia (AML)
	Brown-black spots around vermilion border	Peutz-Jeghers syndrome
Face	Massive facial edema	End-stage/advanced cancer with lymphovascular obstruction of neck/mediastinum (superior vena cava [SVC] syndrome)
	Painless swelling	Tumor (e.g., salivary gland)
	Plethora	Renal cancer (erythrocytosis with increased erythropoietin production), polycythemia vera (PVC), SVC syndrome
	Numbness/weakness	Involvement of facial nerve (e.g., acoustic neuroma)
	Flushing	Carcinoid tumor (syndrome), systemic mastocytosis
	Thickening facial features	Carcinoid tumor
	Acromegaly	Pituitary tumor, carcinoid tumor
	Sinus pain	Tumor (e.g., olfactory esthesioneuroblastoma)
Neck	Thyroid nodule/mass	Adenoma, carcinoma (primary and metastatic)
	Lymphadenopathy	Metastatic malignancy (e.g., nasopharynx), lymphoma
	Persistent induration of skin	Radiation effect, persistent tumor
Lungs	Airway obstruction	Head and neck cancer
	Dullness to percussion	Effusion (primary and metastatic malignancy, e.g., lung, breast, GI, GU, lymphoma), post-obstructive pneumonia, lymphatic obstruction
	Hoarseness	Laryngeal carcinoma, thyroid cancer, posterior mediastinal tumors

Chest	Gynecomastia (males)	Pulmonary carcinoma, testicular cancer, adrenal carcinoma, melanoma
	Breast mass	Cancer, fibroadenoma
	Skin changes (induration, erythema)	Breast cancer
	Unilateral nipple eczema	Paget's disease
	Pain	Mediastinal tumor, acute leukemia
Cardiovascular	Thrombosis	Hypercoagulable state (e.g., pulmonary carcinoma, myeloproliferative disorder [MPD])
	Thrombophlebitis	Pancreatic, ovarian, breast cancer
	Rub/decreased heart sounds	Pericardial effusion (tumor related; e.g., breast, lung, melanoma, lymphoma)
	Murmur/thrombus cardiac chamber	Hypereosinophilic syndrome
	Arrhythmia	Cardiac involvement by malignancy, tumor lysis syndrome
Abdomen	Increasing abdominal girth/ascites	Metastatic carcinoma or primary carcinoma (e.g., ovary, stomach, colon, pancreas); Wilm's tumor, neuroblastoma, or rhabdomyosarcoma in children
	Right upper quadrant mass, hepatomegaly	Liver cancer (primary or metastatic, e.g., pancreatic, gastric, colonic, pulmonary, leukemia), gallbladder malignancy, bile duct cancer, carcinoid tumor, amyloidosis
	Right lower quadrant pain	Torsion of mass involving cryptorchid testis
	Lower midline abdominal wall mass	Urachal cancer

Continued

Table 24-6. FINDINGS ON PHYSICAL EXAMINATION AND POSSIBLE DIAGNOSES—*cont'd*

System	Physical Examination Finding	Possible Diagnoses
	Left upper quadrant pain/mass	Splenomegaly (e.g., primary and metastatic malignancy, portal hypertension caused by liver disease, storage disease), extramedullary hematopoiesis caused by bone marrow replacement, amyloidosis
Back	Pain	Renal cancer, testicular cancer, bladder cancer, prostate cancer, retroperitoneal tumors
	Mass	Renal cancer, retroperitoneal tumor
Genitourinary		
General	Pelvic pain	Bladder cancer
	Precocious puberty	Adrenal tumor
Male	Painless testicular enlargement	Testicular cancer
	Varicocele	Testicular cancer, renal cancer (left sided, 3%)
	Hydrocele	Testicular cancer (10%)
	Epididymitis	Testicular cancer
	Edema of genitalia	Bladder cancer
	Erythematous rash of penis	Erythroplasia of Queyrat: a lesion predisposing to penile squamous cell carcinoma
	Leukoplakia of penis	Associated with squamous cell carcinoma
	Exophytic mass of penis	Squamous cell carcinoma
	Multiple penile papules	Bowenoid papulosis

Female	Cervical mass	Cervical cancer
	Vulvar lump/mass	Vulvar cancer
	Velvety red skin rash	Paget's disease
	Lower abdominal mass	Ovarian cancer, colon cancer
	Abnormally large uterus	Trophoblastic malignancy
	Virilization	Adrenal carcinoma
	"Cluster of grapes" protruding from vagina	Sarcoma botryoides
Skin	Jaundice	Biliary obstruction (whatever etiology, including malignancy or liver/bile ducts)
	Multiple masses	Metastatic malignancy (e.g., choriocarcinoma)
	Hirsutism	Adrenal cancer
	Eczematous plaque	Bowen's disease (carcinoma in situ)
	Painful wheals	Gastric carcinoid
	Photosensitivity/atrophy	Carcinoid tumor
	Telangiectasias	Carcinoid tumor, liver disease
	Migratory erythematous rash	Glucagonoma
	Hyperpigmentation	Adrenal gland metastasis
	Pearly white papule(s) (some with ulceration)	Basal cell carcinoma
	Vitiligo	Melanoma
	Ulcerated, firm (hyperkeratotic) lesion	Squamous cell carcinoma

Continued

Table 24-6. FINDINGS ON PHYSICAL EXAMINATION AND POSSIBLE DIAGNOSES—*cont'd*

System	Physical Examination Finding	Possible Diagnoses
	Variable-colored lesion with irregular borders with or without bleeding	Melanoma
	Bluish nodules/blotches	Kaposi's sarcoma
	Ulcerating lesions/nodules distal extremities	Epithelioid sarcoma
	Cyanosis	Tumor thromboemboli (e.g., cardiac tumor), myeloproliferative disorder
	Brownish skin lesion/dermographia	Mastocytosis
	Herpes zoster	May see reactive with malignancy (e.g., lymphoma)
	Diffuse, exfoliative erythroderma/plaques	Mycosis fungoides
	Purpura	Thrombocytopenia: Multiple etiologies (e.g., bone marrow replacement, splenomegaly, hyperviscosity syndrome), periorbital associated with amyloidosis
	Petechiae	Thrombocytopenia: Multiple etiologies (e.g., splenomegaly, bone marrow replacement)
	Erythema gyratum repens	Associated with underlying malignancy (e.g., rectal, esophageal, head and neck, pulmonary, breast, uterine cervical)
	Ichthyosis	Hodgkin's lymphoma
	Pyoderma gangrenosum	Acute myelogenous leukemia (AML), myeloma, lymphoma, myeloproliferative disorders, solid tumors

Lymphatics	Lymphadenopathy	Regional metastatic tumor, lymphoma
	Arm edema (post mastectomy)	Lymphangiosarcoma
Extremities and spine	Hypertrophic osteoarthropathy	Pulmonary carcinoma, primary mediastinal malignancy, thymoma
	Upper extremity weakness	Pulmonary carcinoma (Pancoast's tumor)
	Bone pain	Metastatic tumor, osteosarcoma, chondrosarcoma, Ewing's sarcoma
	Upper extremity edema	SVC syndrome, status post-mastectomy
	Generalized weakness	Brain tumor, advanced stage malignancy, VIPoma
	Dermatomyositis, polymyositis	Paraneoplastic syndrome, multiple cancers (e.g., pancreatic cancer, breast cancer, melanoma, thymoma, lymphoma, lung, stomach, bowel, colon)
	Arthritis	Pancreatic cancer, amyloidosis
	Lower extremity edema	Tumor obstruction of lymphatics (e.g., renal cell carcinoma, prostate cancer, bladder cancer), retroperitoneal tumors, primary intravascular sarcomas, heart failure caused by amyloidosis
	Firm, spherical mass tendon sheath	Clear cell sarcoma
	Deep thigh/buttock mass	Liposarcoma, malignant fibrous histiocytoma
	Firm mass near joint/tendon	Synovial sarcoma
	Deep seated bony mass	Chondrosarcoma, osteosarcoma
	Pathologic fracture	Primary and metastatic malignancies
	Arthritic pain	Heart tumor

Continued

Table 24-6. FINDINGS ON PHYSICAL EXAMINATION AND POSSIBLE DIAGNOSES—*cont'd*

System	Physical Examination Finding	Possible Diagnoses
Neurologic	Cranial nerve palsy	Nasopharyngeal cancer
	Mental status changes/dementia	Primary tumor, carcinomatous meningitis, metastatic tumor (e.g., lung, breast, GI), paraneoplastic syndrome, VIPoma, parathyroid carcinoma, hypereosinophilic syndrome, hyperviscosity syndrome
	Cerebellar ataxia	Paraneoplastic syndrome, brain tumor, hypereosinophilic syndrome, hyperviscosity syndrome
	Personality change	Tumor, glucagonoma
	Peripheral neuropathy	Paraneoplastic syndrome, Waldenstrom's macroglobulinemia, hypereosinophilic syndrome
	Headache	Primary tumor, carcinomatous meningitis, metastatic tumor, bleeding, hyperviscosity syndrome
	Seizure	Primary or secondary CNS tumor, hyperviscosity syndrome
	Cranial nerve abnormalities	Brain tumor
	Hemiparesis	Supratentorial tumor
	Aphasia	Left frontal, posterior temporal lobe tumor
	Hemineglect	Parietal lobe tumor
	Hemianopsia	Occipital lobe tumor, pituitary adenoma
	Spastic paraparesis	Spinal cord tumor/compression (e.g., pulmonary, breast, prostate, renal, GI, lymphoma, myeloma, sarcoma)
Rectal	Mass	Anal cancer, prostate cancer/nodule
	Bright red blood per rectum (positive guaiac)	Hollow viscous malignancy (esophageal, small intestine, large intestine, stomach), portal hypertension resulting from liver disease

Table 24-7. AREAS OF LYMPHADENOPATHY AND POSSIBLE CAUSES.

LYMPH NODE	POSSIBLE DIAGNOSES
Upper and middle cervical	Head and neck malignancy, lymphoma, infectious disease
Lower cervical and supraclavicular	Right: Lung and breast malignancy, lymphoma, infectious disease Left: GI, breast, pulmonary malignancies, lymphoma, infectious disease
Axillary	Breast, upper extremity malignancies, lymphoma, infectious disease
Inguinal	Lower extremity, vulvar, anal/rectal, bladder, and prostate malignancies, lymphoma, infectious disease

(4) Endocrine: Thyrocalcitonin (medullary cancer).

(5) Gynecologic: CA-125, β-human chorionic gonadotropin (β-HCG), and alpha fetoprotein (AFP) (ovary), CA 15-3 (ovary).

(6) Genitourinary: PSA (prostate).

(7) Gastroenterology: CA 15-3 (liver), CA19-9 (biliary, hepatic, gastric, colon), CA 72-4 (gastric, colon).

(8) Hematopoietic: LDH (leukemia), β2-microglobulin (myeloma, lymphoma).

(9) Testicular: β-HCG, AFP, placental alkaline phosphatase (PLAP), LDH.

(10) Dermatology: LDH (melanoma).

3. Some laboratory studies have prognostic and treatment significance (e.g., estrogen/progesterone receptors [ER/PR], Ki-67, c-erb-2 [HER-2/neu] status in breast malignancies).
4. Chemistries.
   a. Endocrine studies may be useful if electrolyte imbalance, to assess for a paraneoplastic syndrome (e.g., pulmonary, breast).
   b. LFTs are useful for assessment of liver dysfunction/involvement by malignancy.
   c. Renal function tests are useful for assessment of renal function/involvement by malignancy (may be abnormal in both direct involvement by malignancy and urinary tract obstruction).
   d. Serum protein electrophoresis (SPEP) is useful for assessment for hematopoietic malignancies (e.g., lymphoma, myeloma).

e. Serum hyperviscosity (e.g., Waldenstrom's macroglobulinemia).

5. Alkaline phosphatase and calcium may be useful if concerned about primary bone malignancy or bony metastasis (e.g., myeloma, lymphoma, genitourinary malignancy).
6. Cytogenetic/molecular studies may be useful to assess for oncogenes/translocations associated with specific malignancies.
7. Flow cytometry may be useful for detection and subclassification of hematopoietic malignancies.
8. Cytologic examination of body fluids may provide relatively easy for obtaining/confirming diagnosis (e.g., examine cerebrospinal fluid [CSF] for central nervous system [CNS] disease, ascitic fluid for peritoneal disease, sputum/bronchial lavage for pulmonary disease, urine for bladder malignancy, fine needle aspirate [FNA] for regional malignancies).

B. Diagnostic Studies

1. Endoscopic studies with biopsy are useful for head and neck, lung (transbronchial), GI, pancreatic, endometrium (hysteroscopy), cervix (culposcopy), bladder (cystoscopy), mediastinum (mediastinoscopy), colon (colonoscopy), pancreas (endoscopic retrograde cholangiography [ERCP]), peritoneum (laparoscopy).
2. Biopsy allows for histologic proof of malignancy, determination of type of malignancy, and assists in staging. Bone marrow biopsy is useful for staging (metastasis) and diagnosis (hematopoietic malignancies).
3. Lumbar puncture obtains CSF to examine for malignancy.
4. Radiologic studies: Patients with newly diagnosed malignancies usually have chest x-ray, computed tomography/magnetic resonance imaging (CT/MRI) of affected areas, as well as symptom directed scans.
   a. Positron emission tomography (PET) scan is useful for assessment of deep-seated lesions.
   b. Bone scan is useful for determination of presence and extent of primary and metastatic malignancies (e.g., myeloma).
   c. Gallium imaging is useful for evaluating response to therapy of lymphoma.
   d. Cardiac function studies are useful for assessing cardiac failure and for monitoring changes following treatment by potentially cardiotoxic drugs.
   e. Lymphoscintigraphy may be used to determine direction of lymph node drainage from tumors.
   f. Radioisotopes are used for treatment of some malignancies (e.g., iodine 131 for thyroid cancer).
   g. Angiography may be used for measuring major vascular involvement.

h. Inferior vena cavography may be used to locate thrombi in patients with large tumor masses.
i. Intravenous pyelogram (IVP) is useful to assess kidneys in patients suspected to have renal tumors or prostate cancer.

XII. EPONYMS, ACRONYMS, AND ABBREVIATIONS (Table 24-8)

XIII. DEFINITIONS (Table 24-9)

XIV. SAMPLE H&P WRITE-UP

Chief Complaint: "I started coughing up blood a couple of months ago."

History of Present Illness: J.B. is a 54-year-old Caucasian male with a 40-year history of smoking (3 packs per day; 120 pack-years). He was in his usual state of health until 3 months prior, when he started to experience hemoptysis. At first this occurred one time every third to fourth day, but it has gradually increased to 1 to 2 times per day. J.B. additionally admits to an unintentional 30-pound weight loss over the last 6 months. He has had a long history of emphysema associated with a nonproductive cough, and a history of stable angina for 5 years. He can walk approximately six blocks before developing chest pain, although he sometimes has trouble "catching his breath" after one block.

Past Medical History: Medical history is notable for a 10-year history of hypertension (HTN) and stable angina for 5 years, both well controlled by medication. A stress test two years previously showed "EKG changes" after 5 minutes. The patient has no history of malignancy.

Past Surgical History: History of tonsillectomy and adenoidectomy as a child.

Emergency and Trauma History: Patient has never been hospitalized.

Childhood History: Chicken pox at age 6. He denies any other childhood illnesses. He had all of the appropriate childhood immunizations and cannot remember the time of his last tetanus diphtheria toxoid.

Occupational History: Electrician for 36 years following graduation from high school. He denies exposure to toxins or hazardous materials.

Travel History: Occasionally visits grown kids, who live within a couple hundred miles. No history of travel overseas.

Pets: One dog, that lives at home with the patient.

Medications and Allergies: Aspirin (ECASA) 1 po qd, Atenolol 50 mg qd. No known allergies to foods or medications.

HEALTH MAINTENANCE

Prevention: Patient has tried to quit smoking several times without success. His last checkup was approximately one year ago for his heart. He cannot remember when his last chest x-ray was taken.

Table 24-8. ONCOLOGY-FOCUSED EPONYMS, ACRONYMS, AND ABBREVIATIONS.

Acronym or Abbreviation	Definition	Acronym or Abbreviation	Definition
AFP	Alpha fetoprotein	**IEF**	Immunofixation
AML	Acute myelogenous leukemia	**Ig**	Immunoglobulin
APR	Abdominoperineal resection	**IL-2**	Interleukin-2
CD	Cluster of differentiation	**IVC**	Inferior vena cava
CEA	Carcinoembryonic antigen	**LAR**	Low anterior resection
CHOP	Cyclophosphamide, adriamycin, vincristine, prednisone	**LCIS**	Lobular carcinoma in situ
CLL	Chronic lymphocytic leukemia	**MEN**	Multiple endocrine neoplasia (syndrome)
CPT-11	Irenotecan	**MPUS**	Monoclonal protein of undetermined significance
CTCL	Cutaneous T-cell lymphoma	**MRM**	Modified radical mastectomy
CTX	Cyclophosphamide	**MTX**	Methotrexate
DCIS	Ductal carcinoma in situ	**NHL**	Non-Hodgkin's lymphoma
DES	Diethylstilbestrol	**NSHD**	Nodular sclerosing Hodgkin's disease
DVT	Deep venous thrombosis	**PLAP**	Placental alkaline phosphatase
ERCP	Endoscopic retrograde cholangiography	**PSA**	Prostate specific antigen
FAC	5-Fluorouricil, adriamycin, cyclophosphamide	**SLL**	Small lymphocytic lymphoma
FOBT	Fecal occult blood testing	**SPEP**	Serum protein electrophoresis
HCG	Human chorionic gonadotropin	**SVC**	Superior vena cava
HPV	Human papilloma virus	**VAD**	Vincristine, adriamycin, decadron
IBD	Inflammatory bowel disease	**VIP**	Vasoactive intestinal peptide
IDDM	Insulin-dependent diabetes mellitus	**WM**	Waldenstrom's macroglobulinemia

Table 24-9. DEFINITIONS OF ONCOLOGIC TERMS.

TERM	DEFINITION
Acanthosis nigricans	Diffuse, velvety rash (gray, brown, black), mostly in skin folds, often associated with internal carcinoma
Achalasia	Failure to relax smooth muscle of gastrointestinal tract, especially the gastroesophageal sphincter, resulting in esophageal dilation
Beckwith-Wiedemann syndrome	Associated with Wilm's tumor, GU anomalies, aniridia, and hemihypertrophy
Blumer's shelf	Rectal shelf in men
Cryptorchid testis	Undescended testis
Cushing's disease	Hypercortisolism secondary to excessive anterior pituitary secretion of adrenocorticotropic hormone, with or without an adenoma
Dysplastic nevus syndrome	Acquired atypical appearing nevi that are associated with melanoma; autosomal dominant with incomplete expression and penetration
Eaton-Lambert syndrome	Myasthenia-like syndrome, in which the weakness usually affects the limbs, and ocular and bulbar muscles are spared; often associated with small cell carcinoma of lung
Erythroleukoplakia	Erythema or white discoloration of oral mucosa
Erythema gyratum repens	Rare condition characterized by undulating bands of urticarial eruptions over the entire body, associated with underlying malignancy
Familial adenomatous polyposis syndrome	Autosomal-dominant disorders, including Peutz-Jeghers syndrome (modest increased risk of carcinoma) and familial adenomatous polyposis (markedly increased risk of carcinoma)
Gardner's syndrome	Familial polyposis of large bowel, fibrous dysplasia of skull, osteomas, fibromas, epithelial cysts, supernumerary teeth
Hematochezia	Passage of bloody stools
Grawitz tumor	Renal cell carcinoma (all types)
Hemianopsia	Defective vision or blindness in half of visual field of one or both eyes

Continued

Table 24-9. DEFINITIONS OF ONCOLOGIC TERMS—*cont'd*

TERM	DEFINITION
Horner's syndrome	Combination of miosis, ptosis, and anhidrosis
Hypernephroma	Renal cell carcinoma (all types)
Hyperviscosity syndrome	Associated with Waldenstrom's macroglobulinemia (WM), characterized by bleeding, neurologic dysfunction, visual disturbances, and congestive heart failure
Ichthyosis	Fish scale-like patches of the skin, associated with Hodgkin's lymphoma
Krukenberg's tumor	Metastasis to the ovary in women
Li-Fraumeni syndrome	Fragile chromosomes, predisposing to numerous malignancies, related to p53 gene mutation
Meig's syndrome	Ascites and hydrothorax associated with ovarian fibroma or other pelvic tumor
Mondor's disease	Superficial thrombophlebitis associated with breast cancer
Multiple endocrine (MEN) neoplasia syndrome	Autonomous function of one or more endocrine glands, usually associated with tumors (e.g., type I/Wermer's syndrome, type II, Sipple's syndrome, type III, mucosal neuroma syndrome)
Neurofibromatosis	Syndrome associated with neurofibromas, optic gliomas, intracranial tumors, embryonal tumors, and leukemia. Type II associated with multiple schwannomas (especially acoustic), meningiomas, and ependymomas
Nevoid basal cell syndrome	Predisposition to numerous basal cell carcinomas
Nevus	Hamartoma. There are many types of nevi in addition to the melanocytic types
Odynophagia	Pain on swallowing
Pancoast's tumor	Supraclavicular tumor resulting in paraesthesia/weakness of upper extremities
Otalgia	Pain in the ear
Paget's disease	Intraductal carcinoma of the breast, with involvement of the nipple or areola causing an eczematous-like rash; also a neoplasm of the vulva and perianal region with similar appearance, but less strong association with underlying invasive malignancy

Table 24-9—cont'd

Term	Definition
Paraneoplastic syndrome	Symptom complex arising in cancer-bearing patient that cannot be explained by local or distant spread of tumor
Pernicious anemia	Megaloblastic anemia secondary to failure of absorption of vitamin B_{12}; may be associated with achlorhydria
Plummer-Vinson syndrome	Usually occurring in middle-aged women with hypochromic anemia, chiefly characterized by cracks or fissures at the corners of the mouth, painful tongue with atrophy of papillae, and dysphagia caused by esophageal stenosis/webs
Pyoderma gangrenosum	Painful skin ulcers with necrotic base and purplish border, associated with solid tumors and lymphoreticular disorders
Sister Joseph nodule	Nodule deep in the subcutis in the periumbilical area, associated with metastasizing intra-abdominal cancer
SVC syndrome	Obstruction of superior vena cava, resulting in progressive unilateral erythema/edema of upper extremity, facial plethora, and dyspnea
Trousseau's sign	Spontaneous venous thrombosis of extremities occurring in association with visceral malignancies
Tylosis	Formation of callous (keratosis)
Tumor lysis syndrome	Sign/symptoms following chemotherapy, resulting from massive release of electrolytes and other breakdown products from dying tumor cells
Turcot's syndrome	Familial polyposis in association with malignant CNS tumors
Virchow's node	Supraclavicular node, involved by metastatic malignancy
Von Hippel-Lindau syndrome	Constellation of vascular malformations throughout body (including CNS), polycythemia, renal/epididymal tumors, cysts of liver, kidney, pancreas, hemangioblastoma of cerebellum, pheochromocytoma

Continued

Table 24-9. DEFINITIONS OF ONCOLOGIC TERMS—*cont'd*

TERM	DEFINITION
Xeroderma pigmentosum	Autosomal recessive disease characterized by extreme dermal photosensitivity to UV light, with predisposition to numerous skin lesions and malignancies, and severe ophthalmologic abnormalities; neurologic abnormalities may also be observed

Diet: Unmodified since being diagnosed with angina 5 years ago. His meals are rich in red meats and starch ("I am a meat and potatoes man."). Eats approximately 3 times each day. Drinks five cups of coffee per day and denies consumption of tea or sodas.

Exercise: Patient does not currently exercise.

Sleep Patterns: Rarely wakes up to void at night. Recently has woken up "sweating."

Interpersonal and Sexual History: Patient has been married to his second wife for 15 years. He has two adult children by his first wife, and one child by his second. His youngest child is currently in his last year at a four-year college. There have been no other sexual contacts other than his wife.

Social Habits: Patient admits to smoking 3 packs per day for 40 years. The patient does not drink and denies illicit drug use.

FAMILY HISTORY

First-Degree Relatives' Medical History: Patient's father died of myocardial infarction at 50 years of age and had high blood pressure for "many years." The patient's mother is alive and healthy at 78. She had breast cancer in her 50s, but to his knowledge she has had no recurrence. Both sets of grandparents died of "old age," although the patient recalls his paternal grandfather had "heart problems."

Three-Generation Genogram: No known history of genetic traits within the patient's family.

PSYCHOSOCIAL HISTORY

Personal and Social History: Patient is Caucasian and lives with his second wife. He completed high school at 18 and apprenticed to become an electrician. The couple have a child going to college approximately 40 miles from their home. His wife is a homemaker. The patient is the sole source of income for the family.

Interpersonal History and Sexual History: Patient is in a monogamous relationship. His wife had a hysterectomy for "bleeding problems" but is otherwise healthy.

Understanding of Potential Illness: Patient is worried about lung cancer, given his long history of smoking. He wants to know how long "he has left."

REVIEW OF SYSTEMS

General: Patient can walk up to 5 blocks without developing chest pain. He admits to night sweats and general malaise.

HEENT/Neck: Denies headache, tinnitus, hearing loss/changes, epistaxis, loss of taste, and neck masses.

Respiratory: Admits to shortness of breath (SOB) that has become worse over last half year. Sputum sometimes tinged with blood. He admits to a dry hacking cough over last "decade" that has gradually grown worse. He also admits to hemoptysis over last 3 months that has gradually increased in frequency. Denies pleurisy.

Cardiovascular: Admits to chest pain when he "walks too far" approximately once every other week. The pain is quickly relieved by rest and a nitroglycerin capsule. Denies palpitations or claudication.

Gastrointestinal: Denies nausea, vomiting, diarrhea, abdominal distension, bright red blood per rectum (BRBPR), dysphagia, hematemesis, constipation, or recent changes in bowel habits.

Genitourinary: No dysuria, urinary urgency, or hematuria.

Hematologic/Lymphatic: No easy bruising or spontaneous epistaxis. Denies masses in neck, axilla, or groin.

Skin: No rashes, pigmentary changes, or lesions.

Neurologic: No history of seizures or muscular weakness.

Musculoskeletal: No arthritis.

Extremities: No joint pain.

Psychiatric: No history of mental status changes.

PHYSICAL EXAMINATION

Vitals: T 99.0°F P 89 BP 144/85 RR 18 Weight 155 lbs.

General: Thin, anxious Caucasian male, approximately 5′11″. He has a harsh "smokers' voice." The patient's lips are pursed upon inspiration.

HEENT: No sinus tenderness or facial plethora. Neck with normal range of motion and supple. An approximately 1 cm supraclavicular lymph node detected on the right. Sclerae normal, pupils equally round and reactive to light (PERRLA). Normal fundoscopic examination without retinal lesions; no miosis or ptosis noted. Nares patent without discharge or blood. Gums not inflamed.

Lungs: Clear to auscultation with the exception of a rub noted on the right. Dullness to percussion noted at the right base.

Cardiovascular: Regular rate and rhythm and without extra heart sounds. Pulses 2 to 3+ all extremities.

Abdomen: Soft, nontender, without organomegaly.

Genitourinary: No CVA tenderness. Normal circumcised male.

Skin: No rash, petechiae, unexplained bruises, or jaundice.

Extremities: Slight weakness detected on right upper extremity with flexion and extension, otherwise normal strength and range of motion without joint swelling or tenderness. Clubbing noted on upper extremity digits with detectable cyanosis of nail beds.

Neurologic: Normal reflexes, gait, and station.

25

OPHTHALMOLOGY

Patrick S. Kelley, MD

I. CHIEF COMPLAINT

A. Chief Complaint: Use the patient's own words.

B. Identifying Data: Listing the patient's age, sex, and race/ethnicity may seem insignificant, but several illnesses run along these lines.

II. HISTORY OF PRESENT ILLNESS

At the medical student, intern, and early resident level, a good ophthalmologic history focuses on three basic problems: the patient doesn't see as well as he or she used to; the patient's eye(s) feels different or painful; or the patient's eye(s) looks different.

A. Decreased Vision or Change in Vision

1. How long have you had these symptoms?
2. Do they affect one or both eyes (monocular or binocular)?
3. Are the symptoms always present or just for a certain time period?
4. Describe any changes in your vision (or specific visual field).
5. If patient describes flashes (photopsias) or floaters, are they new?
6. Did you see a veil or curtain come across your vision?
7. If patient reports having double vision, ask if it is monocular, binocular, horizontal, vertical, or oblique.
8. Do you wear glasses? Are these glasses your most current prescription? This is a frequent source of confusion.

B. Foreign Body Sensations or Painful Eye

1. How long have you had this sensation?
2. Were you wearing eye protection at the time?
3. What were you doing at the time when you felt something go into your eye?
4. What type of pain are you experiencing (sharp or dull)?
5. Does the pain get worse in light or when I shine the penlight in it?
6. Does the pain occur with eye movement? If so, which direction does it occur in?
7. Have you had any recent trauma?

C. My Eye Looks Different!

1. What specifically looks different to you?
2. How long has it looked this way? Can you show me pictures of yourself before the eye looked different?
3. Is this symptom getting worse, better, or staying the same?

III. PAST MEDICAL AND SURGICAL HISTORY

A. Ocular History

1. Have your current symptoms occurred previously?
2. Have you had previous eye pathologies or surgeries?
3. Have you had amblyopia?
4. History of patching as a child or a lazy eye?
5. What different types of glasses and contact lenses have you worn, and for how long? How have you cared for your contact lenses?
6. Have you been infected with herpes virus?

B. Past Medical History

1. Do you have diabetes mellitus? If so, for how many years? Do you require insulin? Do you have your fasting blood sugar levels tested regularly (diabetic retinopathy)?
2. Do you have hypertension? If so, how well is your blood pressure (BP) controlled (hypertensive retinopathy, branch vein occlusion [BRVO])?
3. Have you had, or do you currently have, thyroid disease, tuberculosis (TB), sarcoidosis, or syphilis (uveitis)?
4. Have you been diagnosed with a rheumatologic disease? Ankylosing spondylitis, rheumatoid arthritis, inflammatory bowel disease (IBD), Reiter's syndrome, juvenile rheumatoid arthritis (uveitis)?
5. Have you been diagnosed with any type of vasculitis (Behçet's, Wegener's, polyarteritis nodosum, Vogt-Koyanagi-Harada)?

C. Past Surgical History:
Diagnosis, procedures, responses to interventions, operative and postoperative sequelae, anesthesia used.

D. Emergency and Trauma History

1. Have you had any head or neck surgeries?
2. Have you had any hypoperfusion or ischemic events (e.g., stroke, shock)?
3. Any traumatic blows to your head?

E. Childhood History

1. Have you undergone surgery for strabismus?
2. Any patching of your eyes during childhood?
3. Did you have any inflammatory diseases?

F. Occupational History

1. What is your work environment?
2. Do you have adequate eye protection against any flying debris?
3. Are you exposed to toxic fumes (epithelial damage)?
4. Do you engage in occupational activities or hobbies that require eye protection (e.g., woodworking, chemical exposure)?

G. Travel History

1. Have you traveled to foreign countries (onchocerciasis)?
2. Have you been camping (giardiasis)?

H. Animal and Insects Exposure History

1. Have you been exposed to any dogs or cats (toxocariasis, toxoplasmosis)?

2. Have you been exposed to a tarantula? The fine hairs on the abdomen of tarantulas can be particularly irritating to mucosal membranes and to the conjunctiva.
3. Have you been exposed to snakes?

IV. MEDICATIONS, ALLERGIES, AND ADVERSE REACTIONS

A. **Medications:** What prescribed and over-the-counter (OTC) eye medications are you currently taking?

B. **Allergies and Adverse Reactions**: Have you had any reaction to systemic medications and eye drops? What type of reaction? Include the type of reaction to the systemic medication(s) and eye drops.

V. HEALTH MAINTENANCE

A. Prevention

1. Visual acuity assessment recommendations. If any concerns, refer to an ophthalmologist.
   a. Children: Ages child should be screened by trained technician, nurse, or pediatrician (at least once).
      (1) Between newborn and age 3 months.
      (2) Between age 6 months and 1 year.
      (3) Once at approximately age 3.
      (4) Once at approximately age 5.
   b. Adult: Comprehensive eye examination by an ophthalmologist.
      (1) Once between ages 20 to 39.
      (2) Every two to four years between age 40 to 64.
      (3) Every one to two years for ages 65 and older.
2. Glaucoma screening recommendations are usually included as part of a complete optometric/ophthalmologic eye examination.

B. **Diet:** Does your regular diet include meals rich in vitamins? Look for Vitamin A deficiency.

C. **Exercise/Recreation:** Do any symptoms occur after you exercise? Eye complaint following exercise suggests possible pigment dispersion syndrome.

D. **Sleep Patterns:** Do you experience vision loss following sleep? Suggests possible hypotensive event.

E. Social Habits

1. Do you use tobacco? What type, how much, and for how long?
2. Do you use illicit or intravenous (IV) drugs (embolic/infectious events)?

VI. FAMILY HISTORY

A. First-Degree Relatives' Medical History

1. Do your parents or siblings have glaucoma, a history of retinoblastoma, or corneal disorders?
2. Does anyone in your family have night blindness or color blindness?
3. Is anyone in your family blind?

4. Did anyone in your family ever have a lazy eye or crossed eyes, or wear a patch over one eye?

B. **Three-Generation Genogram:** Family history of diabetes, hypertension, heart disease, asthma, and cancers.

VII. PSYCHOSOCIAL HISTORY

A. **Personal and Social History**

1. Can you afford drops or medications?
2. Does Social Services need to be involved?

B. **Current Illness Effects on the Patient:** Has your illness affected your mood or relationships with others? Decreased vision or blindness may cause significant depression or interpersonal problems.

C. **Interpersonal and Sexual History**

1. Do you have a sexually transmitted disease (e.g., chlamydia, syphilis, herpes [HSV], HIV)?
2. Do you use protection during intercourse?

D. **Family Support:** Do you have family or friends to support you during your illness?

E. **Occupational Aspects of Illness:** Will you still be able to function at your current place of employment?

VIII. REVIEW OF SYSTEMS (Tables 25-1 to 25-3)

Table 25-1. GENERAL OPHTHALMOLOGIC SYMPTOMS BY SYSTEM.

System	Symptoms
General	Fatigue, malaise, nausea, fever, headache, weakness
HEENT	Tinnitis, vertigo, epistaxis, mouth ulcers, preauricular or neck masses
Respiratory	Hemoptysis, shortness of breath, orthopnea
Cardiovascular	Palpitations, bradycardia, tachycardia
Gastrointestinal	Diarrhea, constipation, rectal bleeding, steatorrhea, abdominal pain
Genitourinary	Hematuria, dysuria, discharge, flank pain
Endocrine	Change in menstrual pattern, abnormal lactation, weight loss/gain, infertility, growth retardation
Musculoskeletal	Arthritis, joint swelling, myalgia, cramping/contractures, pathologic fractures
Skin	Rashes, bruising, itching, scaling, hypo/hyperpigmented lesions, "growing or changing bump"
Neurologic	Headache, cranial nerve functions, depression, ataxia, paraesthesia, tremor

Table 25-2. NONSPECIFIC OCULAR SYMPTOMS AND THEIR ASSOCIATED DISEASES.

SYMPTOM	DISEASES
Burning or itching	Blepharitis, conjunctivitis, contact lens overwear, contact dermatitis, dry eye, episcleritis, pterygium, topical ocular solution/medication allergy
Decreased vision	Less than 24 hours: Migraine, transient ischemic attack, vertebrobasilar insufficiency, hypoperfusion event, papilledema, ischemic optic neuropathy/giant cell arteritis, acute angle-closure glaucoma, functional. More than 24 hours: Retinal detachment, vitreous hemorrhage, optic neuritis, giant cell arteritis, retinal vascular occlusive event, cataract, corneal scarring, uveitis, glaucoma, age-related macular degeneration, diabetic retinopathy, open/closed-angle glaucoma, refractive error, functional
Distorted vision	Dry-eye syndrome, corneal irregularity, cataract, refractive error/astigmatism, macular disease
Double vision	Monocular: Cataract, corneal opacity, lens dislocation, multiple pupils. Binocular: Isolated or multiple third-, fourth-, or sixth-nerve palsy, thyroid disease, orbital inflammatory pseudotumor, myasthenia gravis, displacement/entrapment from trauma/surgery/orbital disease
Flashes	Posterior vitreous detachment, retinal tear or detachment, migraine
Floaters	Posterior vitreous detachment, uveitis, vitreous hemorrhage, migraine
Halos	Angle-closure glaucoma, corneal edema, cataract
Pain	Ocular: Blepharitis, conjunctivitis, corneal surface disease, dry eye, episcleritis, inflamed pterygium, scleritis. Orbital: Orbital inflammatory pseudotumor, optic neuritis, sinusitis
Photophobia	Corneal abrasion/edema, conjunctivitis, uveitis, albinism, aniridia, migraine, optic neuritis
Red eye	Conjunctivitis (allergic, bacterial, chemical, viral), blepharitis, canaliculitis, dacryocystitis, inflamed pingueculum/pterygium, episcleritis, scleritis, acute angle- closure glaucoma, carotid-cavernous sinus fistula, subconjunctival hemorrhage, conjunctival tumor
Tearing	Conjunctival/corneal irritation (foreign body, trichiasis, laceration, erosion), conjunctivitis, dry eye, ectropion, nasal lacrimal duct obstruction

Table 25-3. COMMON OPHTHALMOLOGIC DISEASES ASSOCIATED WITH COMPONENTS OF THE EYE (SEE DIFFERENTIAL DIAGNOSIS SECTION).

Component	Diseases
Lids	Xanthalasma and hyperlipidemia
Conjunctiva	Argyrosis (silver-containing compounds), adrenochrome deposition
Cornea	Arcus senilis (especially if younger than 50 years of age, hyperlipidemia), clouding (mucopolysaccaridoses), band keratopathy (chronic ocular disease), Kayser-Fleischer ring (copper deposition in Wilson's disease), verticillata (amiodarone, chloroquine, chlorpromazine, indomethacin, Fabry disease)
Lens	Cataracts (diabetes, galactosemia), dislocation (Marfan's, homocysteinuria, trauma, simple ectopia lentis)
Retina	Diabetic retinopathy, Roth spots (septic chorioretinitis, leukemia)

IX. PHYSICAL EXAMINATION

The eight-part eye examination is the basis for the ophthalmologist's examination. Most clinic offices will have an eye chart for distance vision, penlight, near card, and direct ophthalmoscope for a very basic examination. If these items are unavailable, improvise with available resources (flashlight, magazine, etc.) to obtain what information you can.

A. Visual Acuity: Ask the patient to wear his or her most current prescription. Make sure the lenses are clean and that the vision in each eye is tested individually and together.

1. Distance vision.
   - **a.** Place the patient at the designated testing distance from a well-illuminated chart or projection screen.
   - **b.** Occlude each eye individually, asking the patient to say each character on the lines of steadily smaller optotypes until the patient misses half of the characters on that line.
   - **c.** Record each eye individually and together.
   - **d.** To test an infant's visual ability, use a small toy or colorful object that will attract the child's attention by sight, not sound.
   - **e.** Hold the object a couple of feet from the child's face and move it from side to side. Infants up to about 6 months old will usually fix on and follow the moving object.

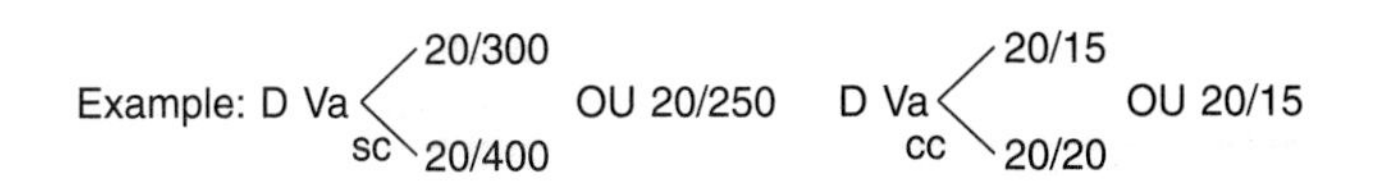

2. Near vision.
   a. With the patient wearing corrective lenses used for near reading or a +3.00 spherical lens over the testing eye, have the patient hold the well-illuminated near card at the distance indicated on the card.
   b. Test each eye individually similar to distance vision above and record appropriately.

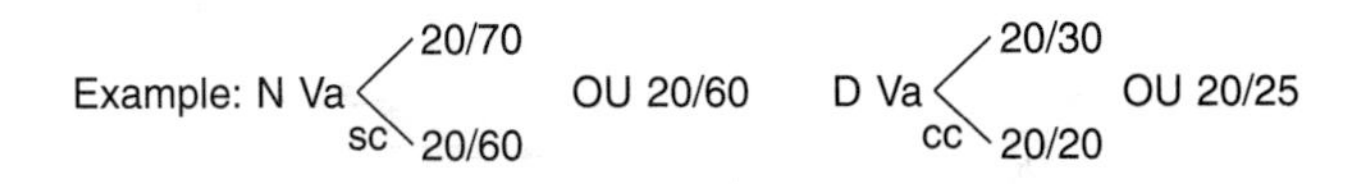

3. Special situations: If you are presented with a patient with decreased vision or in the emergency room with someone with significant trauma, use what is available to obtain a vision determination. For example, documenting the ability to count fingers at whatever distance, the ability to perceive light (no light perception [NLP]) is useful.

B. **Visual Fields**
   1. Place yourself about 3 feet across from the patient, closing the eye directly across from the patient's occluded eye.
   2. Have the patient fixate on your open eye and hold your hand halfway between the patient and yourself.
   3. Move your hand from the periphery toward the center, asking the patient to count your fingers or tell you when he or she sees your fingers wiggling.
   4. Perform this assessment in all quadrants of each eye individually.
   5. For more sensitive testing of the visual fields, a red cap may be used to identify smaller or more central field defects.

Example: Visual fields (Vf)- Full to confrontation (FTC) OU or Vf-

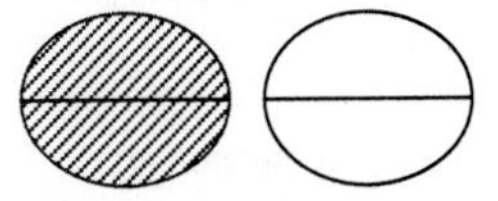

C. **External (Adnexal) Examination**
   1. The adnexal examination is an observation of the patient's face, scalp, and surrounding structures.
   2. You should note any lacerations, scars, or lesions (e.g., herpes zoster [HZV]) and their location in relation to the eyes.

OPHTHO

3. Also note any brow or facial ptosis, preauricular nodes, scalp tenderness, or decreased skin sensitivity here.

D. **Extraocular Motility**
   1. Six extraocular muscles combine to provide movement for the eye.
   2. Each of these extraocular muscles can be isolated by having the patient look in the "six cardinal positions."
   3. Have the patient follow your finger or a small object in the six cardinal positions and up and down along the midline.
   4. Make sure to elevate both lids when in downgaze to note any restriction or overaction.
   5. Compare each eye against the other in all fields of gaze, using normal motility as zero and rating overactions or underactions accordingly.
   6. Use the number 4 as the maximum level of over or underaction.
   7. Note any nystagmus according to its direction and amplitude if present.

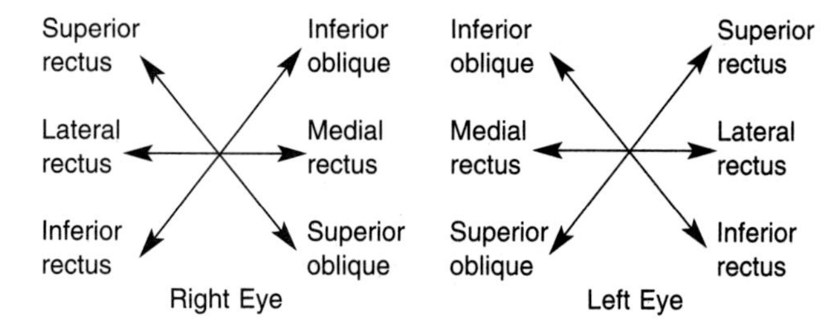

Example: Right CN VI Palsy

– 1/2 0 0 0
– 1 0 0 0
– 1/2 0 0 0

E. **Pupil Response:** A good pupil examination can give you a lot of information regarding the patient's status.
   1. First look at the shape of the pupil; normal pupils are round.
   2. A peaked or oval pupil may indicate previous surgery or trauma. This peak or teardrop will usually point toward the problem, such as synechiae, prolapsed vitreous, or open globe.
   3. Another important piece of information is the presence or absence of a relative afferent pupillary defect (RAPD).

a. Presence of an RAPD indicates asymmetric damage to the afferent visual pathway (afferent nerve fibers from the retinal surface to the pretectal nucleus).
b. An RAPD is not present in symmetric damage to the anterior visual pathway or patients with cataracts, refractive errors, cortical lesions, or malingering.
c. Checking for an RAPD can be performed with the swinging light test:
   (1) Have the patient fixate on a distant object in a dimly lit room. Shine a bright light into the patient's right eye and note the pupillary constriction in both eyes.
   (2) Quickly move the light to the patient's left eye, noting the pupillary response in that eye. In a normal eye, the pupil will constrict slightly or remain the same size. If the pupil dilates when the light is shown into it, there is an afferent pupillary defect, indicating a probable disorder of the retina or optic nerve.
   (3) Move the light back to the patient's right eye and evaluate the pupil's response. If the eye is normal, the pupil will remain the same or constrict minimally; an abnormal response would be either moderate constriction or dilation.
   (4) Repeat illumination of each eye until it is clear that the pupil responds normally or one pupil dilates consistently.
d. Grading of the RAPD is +1 (mild afferent defect) to +4 indicating a severe defect with no afferent light response.

Example

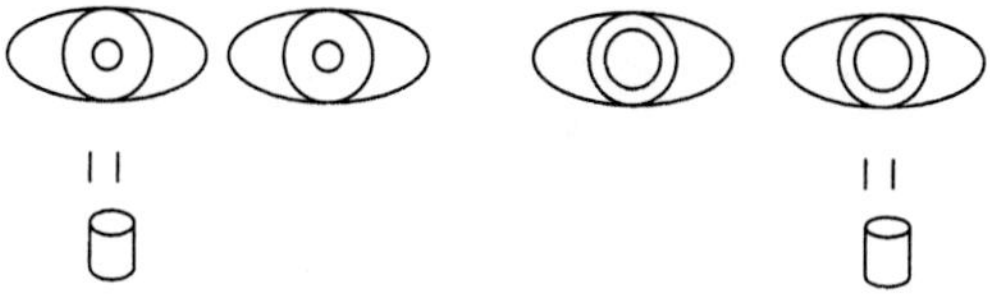

e. With an afferent pathway problem in the left eye, both eyes constrict fully with the light shown in the right eye; however, if the left eye constricts less fully with the light stimulus when compared to the right eye, an RAPD is identified.

F. Ocular Pressure

1. Intraocular pressure (IOP) is measured in millimeters of mercury (mmHg).
2. Along with age, family history, and race, IOP is one of the main risk factors for glaucoma.
3. Normal IOP ranges between 10 and 21 mmHg and is variable throughout the day.

4. Instruction on performing IOP measurements is beyond the scope of this text; however, measurement of IOP is generally performed by two methods.
   a. Applanation tonometry measures the force required to flatten a certain known area of cornea (Goldman tonometer, Tonopen air-puff tonometer).
   b. Indentation tonometry measures the depth of indentation of part of the cornea by a known weight (Schiotz tonometer).

G. Slit Lamp Examination

1. Lids, Lashes, Lacrimals (LLL).
   a. Compare one eye with the other, noting any ptosis, growths or deformities, ectropion, entropion, and loss or discoloration of lashes.
   b. Press on the lacrimal sac, noting any mass or discharge from the puncta.
   c. Be sure to flip the lids if there is concern for a foreign body.
2. Conjunctiva and Sclera (C/S): The conjunctiva is divided into palpebral and bulbar portions.
   a. Look for papillae, follicles, granulomas, scarring, symblepharon, or trapped foreign bodies on the palpebral conjunctiva.
   b. Observe any chemosis, hyperemia or telangiectasia, discharge or secretions, and limbal flush or follicles.
   c. Note any sectoral hyperemia, discoloration, and conjunctival or subconjunctival masses.
3. Cornea (K).
   a. The cornea is best observed with a slit lamp, but gross lesions can be identified with a direct ophthalmoscope and some fluorescein.
   b. Corneal abrasions, epithelial defects, elevations, and filaments are brought out well with fluorescein.
   c. Stromal opacifications and defects should be noted, along with their location on the cornea.
4. Anterior Chamber (A/C).
   a. The anterior chamber is the area between the corneal endothelium and the iris and anterior lens capsule.
   b. Evaluate the depth of the anterior chamber, comparing it with the fellow eye.
   c. Note any cell or flare (dust in a movie theater), hyphema, hypopyon, lens material, vitreous stranding, or foreign bodies and their location.
   d. Make a drawing of any hyphema or hypopyon in relation to the pupil (e.g., 50% filling of the anterior chamber).
5. Iris (I).
   a. The normal iris is completely opaque, with the only light being transmitted through the pupil.
   b. Transillumination may reveal partial- or full-thickness iris defects.

c. Draw these defects or any abnormality in the pupil shape or corectopia.
d. Note any cysts, masses, pigmented lesions, or nodules and their location on the iris.

6. Lens (L).
   a. The lens is a laminated structure enclosed within the lens capsule.
   b. With an undilated pupil, obtaining a good view of the lens is very difficult.
   c. One lens may be compared against the fellow eye by looking at the red reflex.
   d. Indicate if one red reflex is greater in one eye or the other by shining a light source into each eye from about 4 feet in a dimly lit room.
   e. If possible, note the color of the lens.

H. **Fundoscopic Examination or Dilated Fundoscopic Examination (DFE):** This examination is usually performed with the patient's eye dilated, but a limited view of the fundus, optic nerve, and major vessels may be seen with the direct ophthalmoscope.

1. Set the focusing lens at zero on the direct ophthalmoscope, and then place the light beam on the tip of one finger, adjusting the focusing lenses to bring your fingerprint in focus.
2. Have the patient focus at a distant object, and approach the eye at about 15 degrees temporal to the patient's fixation.
3. As the patient's retina comes into focus, adjust the focusing lenses accordingly.
4. If the optic disc isn't in view, follow one of the large vessels back to the disc.
5. Note the size of the disc, sharpness of the edge, approximate cup-to-disc ratio, and presence of hemorrhage, swelling, or venous pulsations.
6. In a normal adult, the size of the optic nerve should be about the size of the small circle on the direct ophthalmoscope.
7. View the vessels, leaving the disc to look for arteriovenous (AV) crossing changes, sheathing of the vessels, or tortuosity.
8. Have the patient slowly look directly at the light, and note any abnormalities in the fundus.
9. Remember that at the medical student/intern level, if you get a good view of the disc and vessels, you are doing well.

X. DIFFERENTIAL DIAGNOSIS

A. Lids

1. Lid crusting: Blepharitis, meibomian gland dysfunction, *phthirus pubis* infestation.
2. Inflammatory lid lesions: Chalazion, hordeolum, pyogenic granuloma, acne, psoriasis, chlamydia, impetigo, erysipelas, herpes, varicella.
3. Malposition of lids: Entropion, ectropion, euryblepharon, coloboma, epiblepharon, thyroid lid retraction, dermatochalasis.

4. Lid masses: Xalanthalasma, milia, retention cysts, nevus, molluscum contagiosum, capillary hemangioma, keratoacanthoma, neurofibromatosis, basal cell carcinoma, squamous cell carcinoma, melanoma.

B. Conjunctiva

1. Acute conjunctivitis.
   - **a.** Noninfectious: Allergic, chemical, foreign body, ultraviolet (UV) radiation.
   - **b.** Infectious.
     - **(1)** Bacterial: Ophthalmia neonatorum: hyperacute purulent conjunctivitis caused by *Neisseria gonorrhea* (medical emergency), streptococcus, Haemophilus influenza, staphylococcus, chlamydia.
     - **(2)** Viral: Epidemic keratoconjunctivitis, pharyngoconjunctival fever, herpes, varicella.
     - **(3)** Fungal.
   - **c.** Autoimmune/vasculitis: Benign ocular pemphigoid, oculomucocutaneous syndrome (Stevens-Johnson syndrome), ligneous conjunctivitis, Wegener's granulomatosis.
2. Chronic conjunctivitis.
   - **a.** Noninfectious: Allergic, chemical, keratoconjunctivitis sicca, giant papillary conjunctivitis.
   - **b.** Infectious: Trachoma, angular blepharoconjunctivitis, Parinaud's oculoglandular syndrome.
3. Conjunctival tumors/masses: Conjunctival cysts, pinguecula, Bitôt spots, leukoplakia, dermoid, nevi, hemangioma, lymphangioma, prolapsed lacrimal gland, melanoma, Bowen's disease, conjunctival carcinoma.

C. Cornea

1. Corneal edema.
   - **a.** Congenital: Birth trauma, glaucoma, congenital hereditary endothelial dystrophy, posterior polymorphous dystrophy.
   - **b.** Acquired: Epithelial defect, iatrogenic/postsurgical, acute closed-angle glaucoma, Fuch's endothelial dystrophy, posterior polymorphous dystrophy, acute hydrops, herpes/varicella keratitis, iridocorneal endothelial syndrome, failed corneal graft.
2. Corneal opacification.
   - **a.** Congenital/early childhood: Birth trauma, congenital hereditary endothelial dystrophy, congenital hereditary stromal dystrophy, Peter's anomaly, herpes/varicella keratitis, corneal ulcer, sclerocornea, metabolic disorders (e.g., Mucopolysaccharidoses), dermoid.
   - **b.** Acquired: Trauma, corneal ulcer, band keratopathy, stromal dystrophies, herpes/varicella keratitis, arcus senilis.

D. Anterior chamber

1. Hyphema.

   a. Children: Trauma, juvenile xanthogranuloma, leukemia, retinoblastoma, herpes/varicella.
   b. Adults: Trauma, postsurgical, herpes/varicella, blood dyscrasia, intraocular tumor, neovascularization.
2. Hypopyon: Corneal ulcer, endophthalmitis, iritis/uveitis, Behçet's disease, intraocular tumor.

E. **Iris**

1. Heterochromia.
   a. Lighter-colored iris: Congenital Horner's syndrome, Fuch's heterochromic iridocyclitis, juvenile xanthogranuloma, chronic iritis, albinism.
   b. Darker-colored iris: Iridocorneal endothelial syndrome, oculodermal melanocytosis, malignant melanoma.
2. Corectopia/polycoria: Surgical/laser peripheral iridotomy, herpes/varicella, trauma, iridocorneal endothelial syndrome, posterior polymorphous dystrophy, aniridia, congenital coloboma, Axenfeld-Rieger syndrome.
3. Neovascularization: Proliferative diabetic retinopathy, vascular occlusive disease (central retinal artery/vein, branch vein occlusion), ocular ischemic syndrome.

F. **Lens**

1. Dislocation: Marfan's, homocysteinuria, Weil-Marchesani, simple ectopia lentis, trauma, Ehlers-Danlos.
2. Cataract.
   a. Congenital: Hereditary, galactosemia, viral (mumps, measles, herpes/varicella, mononucleosis, hepatitis), syphilis, toxoplasmosis, gestational diabetes, thalidomide, Lowe's syndrome, Alport syndrome, Ehlers-Danlos syndrome, Albright's syndrome.
   b. Acquired: Senile, traumatic, myotonic dystrophy (Christmas tree cataract), sunflower cataract (copper foreign body or Wilson's disease), brown subcapsular discoloration (siderosis).

XI. LABORATORY STUDIES AND DIAGNOSTIC EVALUATIONS

A. **Cornea:** Corneal cultures should generally be taken with supervision of an ophthalmologist/ophthalmology resident. Following are common culture media and stains available:

1. Blood agar: Aerobic, anaerobic, mycobacteria, acanthamoeba, fungi.
2. Chocolate agar: Aerobic, *N. gonorrhea,* and Haemophilus species (increased CO_2 environment).
3. Thioglycolate broth: Aerobic and anaerobic bacteria.
4. Sabouraud agar: Fungi.
5. Lowenstein-Jensen agar: Mycobacteria, Nocardia.
6. Gram stain: Bacteria, fungi.
7. Giemsa stain: Bacteria, fungi, acanthamoeba.
8. Calcofluor white: Fungi, acanthamoeba.

B. **Systemic Conditions:** Ophthalmic manifestations should be correlated with a complete physical examination. Following are a few systemic conditions and labs:
   1. Giant cell arteritis: Complete blood count (CBC), C-reactive protein (CRP), erythrocyte sedimentation rate (ESR).
   2. Sarcoidosis: Angiotensin-converting enzyme (ACE), serum lysozyme, biopsy (of highly suspicious tissue).
   3. Syphilis: Reactive plasma reagin (RPR), microhemagglutination assay for *T. pallidum* (MHA-TP).

C. **Uveitis:** The differential for etiologies of uveitis is extensive and beyond the scope of this text. Following are some baseline tests that could be considered with correlation of other historical or physical findings:
   1. Anterior uveitis: Human leukocyte antigen (HLA)-B27, ESR, chest x-ray (CXR), purified protein derivative (PPD), urinalysis (UA), ACE, lysozyme, sacroiliac/spine films, MHA-TP, rapid plasma reagin (RPR), antineutrophil cytoplasmic antibody (ANCA).
   2. Intermediate uveitis: CXR, lysozyme, ACE, MHA-TP, RPR, enzyme-linked immunosorbent assay (ELISA) for toxocara, toxoplasmosis, and Lyme disease, consider magnetic resonance imaging (MRI) if history of multiple sclerosis-like symptoms.
   3. Posterior uveitis: ANCA, MHA-TP, RPR, human immunodeficiency virus (HIV), cytomegalovirus (CMV) titers, ACE, lysozyme, HLA-B5, PPD, ESR, titers for herpes simplex, varicella-zoster, or rubella, antinuclear antibody (ANA).

XII. EPONYMS, ACRONYMS, AND ABBREVIATIONS (Table 25-4)

XIII. DEFINITIONS

One of the big fears of confronting a patient with an eye problem is understanding the terminology that ophthalmologists use. The following is an example of a standard eight-part eye examination.

A. **Visual Acuity:** Often abbreviated as DVA (distance) or NVA (near). A short abbreviation of cc or sc will be written nearby, indicating with or without corrective lenses, respectively. When writing the vision of each eye, the right eye (OD) is always written above the left eye (OS).

B. **Visual Fields:** Again written OD over OS, often as full to confrontation (FTC) or as a drawing with the specific defect indicated (always as if you were looking at the patient).

C. **Pupils:** The first number indicates the size of the pupil before a direct light stimulus. The second number indicates the pupil size with a direct light stimulus.

D. **Pressure** is often denoted as Ta (applanation tonometry) or Tp (tonopen).

E. **Extraocular Motility (EOM)** can be denoted in several ways. Examples include lines indicating the eight areas of gaze or "+" or "–" signs in the patient's direction of gaze, indicating overaction, underaction, or restriction.

Table 25-4. OPHTHALMOLOGY EPONYMS, ACRONYMS, AND ABBREVIATIONS.

Acronym or Abbreviation	Definition	Acronym or Abbreviation	Definition
A/C	Anterior chamber	**EKC**	Epidemic keratoconjunctivitis
ARMD	Age-related macular degeneration	**ERM**	Epiretinal membrane
A.Vx	Anterior vitrectomy	**ET**	Esotropia
BC	Base curve	**FA**	Fluorescein angiogram
BRVO	Branch vein occlusion	**FTC**	Full to confrontation
BSCL	Bandage soft contact lens	**GVF**	Goldman visual field
CA	Corneal abrasion	**HSV**	Herpes simplex virus
CAI	Carbonic anhydrase inhibitor	**HT**	Hypertropia
cc	With correction	**HVF**	Humphrey visual field
c/d	Cup-to-disc ratio	**HZO**	Herpes zoster ophthalmia
CE	Cataract extraction	**IO**	Inferior oblique
CF	Count fingers	**IOFB**	Intraocular foreign body
CME	Cystoid macular edema	**IOL**	Intraocular lens
CNVM	Choroidal neovascular membrane	**IOP**	Intraocular pressure
CRx	Cycloplegic refraction	**J**	Jager
CSME	Clinically significant macular edema	**KP**	Keratic precipitate
DM	Diabetes mellitus	**LLL**	Left lower lid
D&Q	Deep and quiet	**LR**	Lateral rectus
DR	Diabetic retinopathy	**LUL**	Left upper lid
DVD	Dissociated vertical deviation	**MDF**	Map-dot-fingerprint
ECCE	Extracapsular cataract extraction	**MGD**	Meibomian gland dysfunction

Continued

Table 25-4. OPHTHALMOLOGY EPONYMS, ACRONYMS, AND ABBREVIATIONS—*cont'd*

Acronym or Abbreviation	Definition	Acronym or Abbreviation	Definition
MR	Medial rectus	**RAPD**	Relative afferent pupillary defect
MRx	Manifest refraction	**RD**	Retinal detachment
NLP	No light perception	**RGP**	Rigid gas-permeable contact lens
NPDR	Nonproliferative diabetic retinopathy	**RK**	Radial keratotomy
NS	Nuclear sclerosis	**RLL**	Right lower lid
NVD	Neovascularization of the disc	**RP**	Retinitis pigmentosa
NVE	Neovascularization elsewhere	**ROP**	Retinopathy of prematurity
OD	Right eye	**RUL**	Right upper lid
OHTN	Ocular hypertension	**sc**	Without correction
ON	Optic nerve	**SCL**	Soft contact lens
OS	Left eye	**SO**	Superior oblique
OU	Both eyes	**SR**	Superior rectus
PCIOL	Posterior chamber intraocular lens	**SRNVM**	Subretinal neovascular membrane
PDR	Proliferative diabetic retinopathy	**TID**	Transillumination defect of the iris
PEK	Punctate epithelial keratopathy	**TM**	Trabecular meshwork
PK	Penetrating keratoplasty	**Va**	Visual acuity
POAG	Primary open-angle glaucoma	**VH**	Vitreous hemorrhage
PRK	Photorefractive keratectomy	**WWP**	White without pressure
PRP	Panretinal photocoagulation	**XT**	Exotropia
PSC	Posterior subcapsular cataract	**YAG**	Neodymium yttrium-aluminum-garnet laser
PVD	Posterior vitreous detachment		

F. **External (Adnexal) Examination:** Description of the rest of the face and head structures.

G. **Slit Lamp Examination:** Includes all of the structures of the eye from the lids to the anterior vitreous chamber.

H. **Dilated Fundus Examination:** Includes the vitreous chamber, optic nerve and disc, retinal blood vessels, macula and fovea, and peripheral retinal surface.

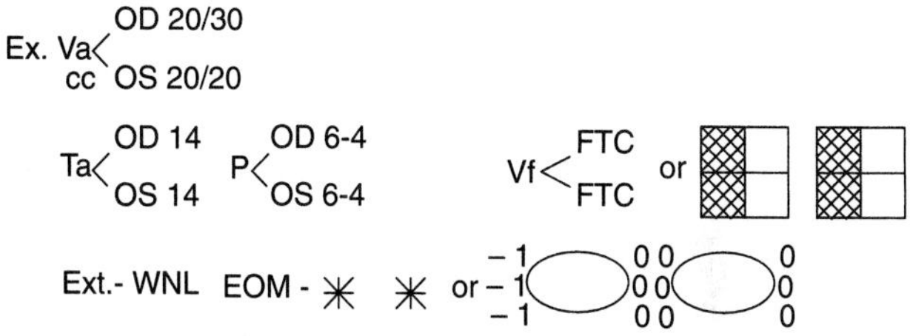

Ex. Va cc < OD 20/30, OS 20/20

Ta < OD 14, OS 14   P < OD 6-4, OS 6-4   Vf < FTC, FTC or [visual field diagrams]

Ext.- WNL   EOM - ✳ ✳ or −1 −1 −1 (OD) 0 0 0 0 0 0 ; 0 0 0 (OS)

SLE (slit lamp exam)

LLL (lids, lashes, lacrimals)
C/S (conjunctiva and sclera)
K (cornea)
A/C (anterior chamber)
I (iris)
L (lens)
Ant. Vit. (anterior vitreous)
DFE (dilated fundus exam)
C/D (cup-to-disc ratio)
M/V/P (macula, vessels, periphery)

XIV. SAMPLE H&P WRITE-UP

CC: M.K. is a 65-year-old male complaining of decreased vision and glare in his right eye.

HPI: Vision loss has been gradual over the past year, and glare symptoms are worse at night with oncoming headlights while driving. He has no complaints of pain or other ocular symptoms.

PMHx: Unremarkable.

Ophthalmologic History: Cataract surgery OS, cataract OD.

PSHx: T&A as child, appendectomy 1989.

Family History: Coronary artery disease (CAD), hypertension (HTN).

Social History: No tobacco or alcohol use.

Physical (Eye) Examination:

Va < 20/70 ph 20/60 -2, 20/20   WRx < −3.50 sphere, −0.50 sphere   Add + 2.50   MRx < −3.75 sphere 20/60, −0.50 sphere 20/20

VF—FTC OU. EOM—Full. Pupils 5—2.5 mm OU.   Ta < 18, 17.

Slit Lamp Examination:
External exam: WNL OU
LLL: Dermatochalasis OU
C/S: White and Quiet OU
K: Clear OU
A/C: Deep and Quiet OU
I: Flat, Round and Reactive
L: 3 + NS OD, PCIOL OS
Dilated Fundus Examination:
C/D ratio: 0.3 OU
N: MVP OU

26

ORTHOPEDICS

Theodore W. Parsons III, MD, FACS, and Eric H. Hanson, MD, MPH

I. CHIEF COMPLAINT

A. **Chief Complaint**—patient's reason for seeking medical attention, including onset of symptoms, location, duration, and any associated problems.

B. **Identifying Data**

1. Name, age (and date of birth), handedness (right or left), vocation, location of injury or problem, and inciting event.
2. For example, Mr. David Smith is a 45-year-old right-hand dominant professional pianist with a left thumb laceration from a table saw accident.

II. HISTORY OF PRESENT ILLNESS

The following outline represents an in-depth patient evaluation and interview. Generally, with musculoskeletal patients, the history is concise and should be modified to the situation, as appropriate. A typical clinic visit would include part but certainly not all of the following information. Hospital admissions or preoperative evaluations are generally more in-depth and might require most or all of this information. Most operative orthopedic patients with any significant medical history require preoperative clearance by their internist or treating physician. Don't forget to avail yourself of that additional, important source of information. It will save you both time and potential perioperative problems.

A. **Area Involved**

1. Can you show me where it hurts? Try to determine whether the pain and symptoms are bone, joint, or muscular in nature, while recognizing that considerable overlapping of symptoms may occur.
2. Is the pain generally a deep ache, frequently localized, or associated with loading or weight-bearing activities? A "yes" answer suggests bone involvement. Fractures are associated with severe, sharp pain, which is exacerbated with movement or loading.
3. Do you have any joint pain, stiffness, tightness, or pain with motion? Joint pain is often associated with crepitance and becomes worse with loading of the joint. Beware of referred pain from hip to knee, knee to thigh, back to buttock, etc.
4. Do you have any muscular pain? Muscular soreness, diffuse ache, or spasm are generally associated with activity and occasionally associated with fatigue or atrophy.

B. Nature of Symptoms and Chronology

1. When did the pain begin (onset)? It is important to note the circumstances associated with the onset of symptoms.
   a. Did the pain begin suddenly or acutely (traumatic)? Did it result from a direct blow? Sudden burst of energy? Did you feel a pop, snap, or tear? Was there immediate swelling (acute vascular) or delayed swelling (edema)?
   b. Subacute: Presentation to care within six weeks of onset. Is the pain improving? Is the pain still present and worsening? Is the pain recurrent? Many joint or ligamentous injuries present in this fashion.
   c. Did the pain begin gradually (overuse, inflammatory, neoplastic)? Is the frequency or intensity of the pain worsening? Was the presentation of symptoms slow without an inciting event?
2. How long have you had the symptoms (duration)?
3. Is the pain progressive? Intermittent? Waxing and waning in nature?
4. Has the pain increased in severity?

C. Characterization of Pain

1. Type of pain.
   a. Is the pain dull and aching? (bone or muscle).
   b. Is it sharp, lancinating or shooting, radicular pain? (neurogenic).
   c. Burning, crushing, or aching pain? (neurogenic, possibly sympathetic).
   d. Throbbing, diffuse, poorly localized pain? (vascular).
   e. Throbbing, intense, well-localized pain? (infection).
   f. Aching, stiffness, tightness character of pain? (arthritic or other joint involvement).
   g. Severe, sharp, intolerable pain, often with deformity (fracture).
2. Intensity of pain.
   a. How severe is the pain (on a scale from 1 to 10)?
   b. Is the pain constant, occasional, or sporadic? Is it increasing or decreasing in intensity?
   c. Is the pain worse at night? Beware of neoplastic or infectious process.
   d. Does the pain awaken you from sleep? Beware of neoplastic, infectious, or possibly arthritic process.
3. Associated factors.
   a. What makes the pain worse? Activity? Certain positions or movements? Symptoms associated with movement or loading are often associated with joint abnormalities. Temperature? Cold exacerbation is common in arthritic conditions. Is the pain worse in the morning or at the end of the day?

b. What makes the pain better? Rest? Medications? Beware of pain that requires narcotics for control. Frequent change of positions? Common in arthritic and inflammatory conditions.

c. Do you trust the joint? Does it give way (either from pain or instability)?

d. Is there locking, catching, or grinding present with motion? Suggests mechanical or arthritic etiology.

e. Is there weakness or clumsiness present? Suggests muscular or neurogenic source.

f. Is there numbness or tingling? If so, where specifically? True neurogenic pain is dermatomal, whereas vascular pain is more diffuse.

g. Was pain present in the joint before injury?

h. Do you have pain when you walk? How far are you able to walk? Throughout your community, within your residence, or only from your bed to a chair? How ambulatory the patient is has a great impact on the type of treatment selected.

i. What makes the pain subside? Standing still for relief suggests vascular claudication; the need to lean over or sit down suggests neurogenic claudication.

D. Medical History Pertinent to the HPI

1. Have you had any similar problems in the past? If so, how long did the symptoms last? What treatments were required?
2. Have you had any history of trauma to the area? Do you engage in any unusual or aggressive activities (e.g., skydiving, playing football, marathon running)?
3. Are any other joints painful? If so, which ones?
4. Do you regularly take anti-inflammatory medications for pain? Do you regularly take narcotics for pain control?

E. Lifestyle Effects Pertinent to the HPI

1. How is the current problem affecting your activity level?
2. Are you able to pursue customary recreational activities? What would you like to be able to do that you are unable to do now?
3. Are the current symptoms severe enough that you would consider surgical intervention?
4. Have you modified your activities in an attempt to alleviate the symptoms?
5. Are you able to continuing working in your current position? If not, why not? If not working, how long has it been since you last worked?
6. Is there a lawsuit pending with this situation? Is this a worker's compensation claim? Be cautious of cases associated with litigation or worker's compensation, which generally are very poor predictive factors for a good outcome.

III. PAST MEDICAL AND SURGICAL HISTORY

A. Past Medical History

1. Have you had any prior musculoskeletal problems, injuries, and treatments?
2. Have you had any back or extremity injuries? Any consequent hospitalizations or transfusions? List any pertinent information regarding such injuries (e.g., sports, vocational)?
3. How would you describe your overall health? Obtain a general assessment of the patient's overall health, including any other major medical problems.

B. Past Surgical History

1. Have you undergone previous surgical procedures? Which procedures and when? Did you have any associated complications (e.g., infection, deep venous thrombosis [DVT])?
2. Have you ever had a problem with anesthetics?
3. Have you ever experienced excessive bleeding after an injury or tooth extraction? Do you bruise easily?

C. Childhood History

1. Did you have any growth abnormalities during childhood development?
2. Did you wear braces or use special appliances?
3. Did you fracture any bones during childhood?

D. Occupational History

1. Has your condition affected your ability to perform your job?
2. Does your occupation involve activities that affect your illness?
3. Do you expect to continue your job functions?

E. Travel History: Have you traveled in the United States? To foreign countries? If so, where? This is typically only important if considering unusual exposure as an etiology for diffuse arthralgias (e.g., Lyme disease) or a possible source of atypical infection (e.g., tuberculosis).

F. Animal and Insect Exposure History: Are you currently exposed, or have you recently been exposed, to animals or insects? This is important information when considering unusual infections or exposures.

IV. MEDICATIONS, ALLERGIES, AND ADVERSE REACTIONS

A. Medications

1. Are you currently taking any prescription medications? Which ones? List current medications.
2. Are you currently using, or have you recently used, steroids for any condition. If steroids have been taken during the past year, may need perioperative stress coverage.
3. Are you taking any over-the-counter (OTC) medications, including herbal preparation and supplements (common in young athletes)?

B. Allergies to Medications and the Side Effects: Have you had any allergic reactions to medications? If so, which ones and when?

C. **Adverse Reactions to Medications:** Have you had any adverse reactions to medications? If the answer is yes, these reactions should be clearly noted in the record, and anesthesiologists should be made aware of these reactions before any surgical intervention.

V. **HEALTH MAINTENANCE**

A. **Prevention**

1. How active are you? Understand the current activity level of the patient *and* ascertain that he or she understands the importance of personal fitness.
2. What type of activities? This must be individualized for each patient depending on age, health status, and capabilities. Typically, the clinic nurse or physical therapist is a good resource for patient teaching beyond interaction of the H&P.

B. **Diet**

1. What is your usual diet?
2. How many calories do you consume daily? Importance here is generally limited to ensuring that caloric intake (in an appropriately balanced diet) is adequate for healing in the perioperative period or during fracture healing. Particular attention should be given to elderly patients, whose diet may be suboptimal.

C. **Exercise/Recreation:** Do you exercise? What type and how much? It is extremely important to understand what activity expectations any patient may have and to assess whether the expectations are realistic. Unrealistic activity expectations are a major source of patient dissatisfaction and potentially a source of litigation.

D. **Sleep Patterns:** Does pain disturb your sleep? Any patient seeking medical attention for a painful condition should be queried regarding pain that awakens them from sleep. Such nocturnal pain is worrisome for underlying malignancy.

E. **Social Habits**

1. Do you use tobacco (current or previous)? What type? Years smoked, packs per day? Tobacco use may significantly alter the healing potential of fusions and certain wounds.
2. Do you drink alcohol (current or previous)? How much consumed daily? How many days per week?
3. Do you use any illicit drugs? Which ones? How often? For how long? Any complications? (Knowing about IV drug use is helpful, particularly in trauma cases, for the surgeon's own protection.)

VI. **FAMILY HISTORY**

A. **First-Degree Relatives' Medical History:** Do any family members have musculoskeletal conditions, such as neurofibromatosis or muscular dystrophies, which have a hereditary component.

B. **Three-Generation Genogram** where appropriate. Some musculoskeletal disorders may be genetic in origin and/or be part of a syndrome.

VII. PSYCHOSOCIAL HISTORY

A. Personal and Social History

1. Ascertain any socioeconomic factors that may affect treatment or prognosis. High school graduate, worker's compensation case, litigation?
2. Briefly determine, as appropriate, the patient's living situation, environment, location, etc. for rehabilitation purposes. Especially appropriate for elderly patients after joint arthroplasty or patients who may require a wheelchair or prolonged use of assistive devices.

B. Current Illness Effects on the Patient

1. How is your condition affecting your life?
2. What limitations has it imposed on your normal functioning? Understand the patient's perceived limitations of the current problem. Allowing patients to express their concerns will help clarify their expectations of care and will facilitate rehabilitation.
3. How do you feel about your condition? Do you feel depressed? Beware that depression is a common finding associated with low-back pain, and may complicate recovery and rehabilitation.

C. Interpersonal and Sexual History

1. Are you sexually active? Information here is typically limited to difficulties with positioning during sexual activity secondary to musculoskeletal pain or joint stiffness (e.g., low-back pain, hip arthritis). Information can be provided to patients educating them on alternatives that may be less painful. Reassurance and educational materials can be therapeutic and are generally well received.
2. Have you had an arthoplasty? Patients with previous arthoplasties may need education regarding methods of protecting the reconstructed joints.

D. Family Support

1. Are family members available to provide support? A support system is important to any patient who will require rehabilitation or may simply be in a cast or wheelchair.
2. Helping clarify with the patient what he or she will need and ascertaining what resources are available is important. The social worker can be invaluable here.

E. Occupational Aspects of Illness

1. What physical demands are placed on you in your job? In your nonwork life? Understanding the physical demands placed on patients by virtue of their occupations is important, as well as their expectations regarding physical performance, both in and out of the work environment. Treatment offered must realistically fit in with any physical demands on patients.

2. How will your condition and time off work (needed for recovery) affect your job? The effect of the illness on occupation, the time for recovery after any treatment, the length of incapacitation, and the projected return-to-work date are important to delineate. Beware of the worker's compensation claimant who is seeking prolonged "off-duty" status.

VIII. REVIEW OF SYMPTOMS (Tables 26-1, 26-2, and 26-3)

Table 26-1. GENERAL ORTHOPEDIC SYMPTOMS BY SYSTEM.

SYSTEM	SYMPTOMS
General	Fatigue, weight loss, night pain, AM stiffness, PM stiffness, pain with activity, history of cancer, fevers, chills, sweats/night sweats, loss of appetite, history of congenital abnormalities
HEENT/neck	Neck stiffness or pain, spasms, radiating pain
Respiratory	Cough, dyspnea, shortness of breath
Chest	Pain, restriction of expansion, costrochondral or sternochondral symptoms
Cardiovascular	Tachycardia, palpitations, orthopnea, paroxysmal nocturnal dyspnea, dyspnea with exertion
Gastrointestinal	Nausea, emesis, hematemesis, heartburn, right upper quadrant pain, epigastric pain, constipation, appetite changes
Genitourinary	Dysuria, urinary frequency, urinary urgency, nocturia
Hematologic/ lymphatic	Easy bruising, bleeding tendencies, lymphadenopathy
Skin	Rash, pigmentary lesions (café au lait), angiomata, masses
Neurologic	Headaches, seizures, numbness or tingling, weakness, any focal abnormalities
Musculoskeletal	Covered in pertinent history: Focus on other extremities not covered in depth. History of rheumatoid arthritis (obtain cervical spine films before any surgery)
Extremities	Dependent edema, lymphedema, peripheral pulses, hair on extremities
Psychiatric	Mood disorders, substance abuse, depression, anxiety

Table 26-2. NONSPECIFIC SYMPTOMS AND THEIR ORTHOPEDIC DISEASES.

SYMPTOM	DISEASES
Neck or back pain	Arthritic changes, disk herniation, internal derangement or desiccation, muscular strain; chronic pain syndromes
Joint pain/ stiffness	Arthritis (degenerative and inflammatory), trauma, instability, infection
Fever	Osteomyelitis, indolent septic arthritis
Night pain	Infection or malignancy
Joint swelling	Sympathetic effusion from extra-articular pathology *or* internal derangement of joint
Weakness/ numbness	Disk herniation or peripheral nerve entrapment
Limp	Painful joint, weakness, mechanical symptoms

Table 26-3. COMMON ORTHOPEDIC DISEASES AND THEIR SYMPTOMS.

DISEASE	SYMPTOMS
Disk herniation	Limb pain (radiating), weakness or numbness, associated neck or back pain
Rotator cuff tear	Weakness in shoulder elevation, pain, decreased range of motion (ROM)
Shoulder impingement	Pain with overhead activities, crepitance of motion, similar to rotator cuff tear
Carpal tunnel syndrome	Pain in hand (thumb, index, middle), night pain and numbness, weakness and clumsiness of grip
Hip arthritis	Groin pain with ambulation, pain with internal rotation, stiffness
Knee arthritis	Gradual stiffness, pain with ambulation, swelling
Anterior knee pain	Peripatellar pain, pain with stairs, slopes, squatting, kneeling, stiffness with prolonged sitting
Knee meniscal tear	Acute or subacute knee pain, swelling, history of twisting trauma
Anterior cruciate ligament tear (knee)	Acute history of twisting or hyperextension trauma to knee. "Pop," inability to ambulate, acute swelling, instability
Posterior tibial tendon dysfunction	Progressive flat foot deformity, arch pain with weight bearing, weakness in plantar flexion, "too many toes" sign with toe rise

IX. PHYSICAL EXAMINATION (Table 26-4)

For the musculoskeletal portion of the general physical examination, patients should put on a gown for uninhibited evaluation of the area involved and surrounding joints (rolling up the pant leg is not sufficient for an examination of the knee, for example). The contralateral limb is also examined for comparison's sake. Observation of patients moving (e.g., walking, dressing) while they are not aware of the observation may provide valuable information, particularly compared to activity and movement observed during formal examination.

Table 26-4. PHYSICAL EXAMINATION FINDINGS AND POSSIBLE DIAGNOSES.

System	Physical Examination Finding	Possible Diagnoses
Vital signs		
Pulse	Tachycardia	Pain
Blood pressure	Hypertension	Pain
Respiratory rate	Tachypnea	Underlying disease state (thromboembolic, pulmonary, infectious pain/anxiety)
Weight	Rapid loss	Underlying malignancy
Weight	Obesity	Arthritic condition in LEs and back
Neck	Stiffness, loss of lordosis	Arthritis, trauma, congenital anomaly
Lungs	Rhonchi, wheezes, focal inspiratory crackles	Underlying disease state (pulmonary, infectious)
Cardiovascular	Murmur, rub	Underlying cardiovascular disease
Abdomen	Masses	Musculoskeletal neoplasm
Genitourinary		
Male	Presence of posterior rectal mass	Consider chordoma
Female	Presence of posterior rectal mass	Consider chordoma
Skin	Multiple café-au-lait lesions	Neurofibromatosis, tibial pseudoarthrosis (kids)

Continued

Table 26-4. PHYSICAL EXAMINATION FINDINGS AND POSSIBLE DIAGNOSES—*cont'd*

System	Physical Examination Finding	Possible Diagnoses
Lymphatics	Persistent lymphedema	Mass, chronic infection
Extremities	See specific examinations	
Neurologic	Focal findings of weakness or sensory loss	Correlate with spinal nerve root or with peripheral nerve root

1. **General.**
   - **a.** Height/weight.
   - **b.** Overall appearance (e.g., slender, muscular, obese).
   - **c.** Gait (e.g., normal, antalgic, stooped, steppage, gluteal lurch).
   - **d.** Any assistive or therapeutic devices used (e.g., brace, cane, TENS unit, wrap). Remove these devices for the examination.
   - **e.** Any obvious deformity (e.g., amputation, altered limb appearance, scoliosis, kyphosis). This observation should include any asymmetry present (e.g., structural or muscular abnormality, possibly neoplastic).
   - **f.** Muscle atrophy (e.g., generalized to the limb, focal area). Measure and record limb circumference of both extremities.
   - **g.** Diffuse ligamentous laxity (e.g., hyperextension of the knees, elbows, digits). This is important in evaluation of ligamentous problems and in shoulder instabilities.
   - **h.** Scars, skin markings (e.g., café-au-lait spots, hair patch).
2. **Extremity:** In general, visually inspect each area before any palpation. Look for scars, abnormal-appearing skin or lesions, joint contracture(s), etc.
   - **a.** Gentle palpation to ascertain focal tenderness *before* any manipulation.
     - **(1)** Start away from the suspected area of pathology and work toward the painful area.
     - **(2)** Palpate *all* areas (bone, soft tissue, joint) of the painful limb and associated proximal and distal joints.
   - **b.** Range of motion (ROM).

(1) Record active *and* passive ROM and any pain and/or crepitance associated with movement. Notice any apprehension (patient anxiety) with certain movements.
(2) Use a goniometer and avoid guessing at degrees of motion.

c. Motor examination.
(1) Examine strength, function, and appearance of associated muscle groups. Compare to contralateral extremity.
(2) Grade strength on a scale of 0 to 5.
5 = Full active range of motion and strength against resistance.
4 = Full active range of motion with some weakness against resistance.
3 = Full active range of motion against gravity only.
2 = Full active range of motion with gravity eliminated.
1 = Palpable or visible contracture of the muscle with minimal to no motion of joint.
0 = No contracture.

d. Sensory examination.
(1) Determine the presence/absence of light-touch, pinprick, and proprioception.
(2) Determine whether any sensory changes follow a specific dermatomal pattern (nerve root pathology), a peripheral nerve pattern (entrapment neuropathy such as carpal tunnel syndrome, or focal pathology), or a "stocking/glove" pattern (e.g., diabetes, peripheral neuropathy, symptom exaggeration).

e. Ligamentous examination.
(1) Test the ligamentous structures (including collateral and secondary stabilizing ligaments) for stability.
(2) Note any laxity, rupture, and the quality of the "endpoint" (i.e., good endpoint = firm resistance when stressed; soft endpoint = mushy resistance when stressed; no endpoint = joint continues to gap open when stressed).

f. Reflexes (Table 26-5).
(1) Examine as appropriate the deep tendon reflexes (DTRs) of the knee, ankle, triceps, biceps, and brachioradialis.
(2) Grade as absent, trace, normal, or hyperactive.
(3) Examine both limbs. Unilateral absence may suggest lower motor neuron lesion; hyperactivity may suggest upper motor neuron lesion.
(4) Note presence of Hoffman's, Babinski, or Oppenheimer pathologic reflexes.

Table 26-5. MUSCULAR INNERVATION AND REFLEXES OF UPPER AND LOWER LIMBS.

Root	Muscles	Reflexes
C5	Deltoid	N/A
C6	Biceps, wrist extensors	Biceps, brachioradialis
C7	Triceps, wrist flexors, finger extensors	Triceps
C8	Finger flexors	N/A
T1	Interossei	N/A
L1-2	Iliopsoas	N/A
L3	Quadriceps, hip adductors	Patellar tendon
L4	Quadriceps, tibialis anterior	Patellar tendon
L5	Tibialis posterior, extensor hallucis longus	Posterior tibial tendon
S1	Gastroc-soleus, flexor hallucis longus	Achilles tendon

g. Peripheral circulation.
   (1) Look for skin changes associated with venous insufficiency (e.g., edema, discoloration, ulcerations).
   (2) Evaluate bilateral pulses. Look for pallor of elevation/dependent rubor associated with arterial disease.

h. Lymphatics: Look for any lymphangetic streaking (infection), regional adenopathy (+/– tenderness) that may be present.

i. Limb length.
   (1) More important in lower extremity (LE) than in upper extremity (UE) because of gait and stance.
   (2) Measure in LE from anterior superior iliac spine (ASIS) to the medial malleolus, or in UE from C7 to the tip of the middle finger.

3. Regional specific examination: Following are some of the basic aspects of site-specific examination:

a. Spine: Back pain, a common complaint, is often referred into the buttock or into the posterior thigh. Patients often complain of hip pain and point to the buttock area. Remember to consider neurogenic claudication from stenosis in patients with otherwise normal examination.
   (1) Patients should wear a gown, open to the back (and disrobed to undergarments), to expose the entire spine for evaluation.
   (2) Assess for palpable spasm in the musculature and any tenderness to palpation (e.g., focal tenderness in muscle as compared to diffuse, nondescript tenderness

of symptom magnification). Feel for any palpable gap or step-off, suggesting displacement of elements.

(3) Assess and record motion in all directions (i.e., flexion, extension, lateral bend, rotation), and look for pain reproduction or exacerbation with certain movements.

(4) Look for deformity, loss of normal position (lordosis for cervical and lumbar spine, kyphosis for thoracic spine). Evaluate for any scoliosis or imbalance and any rigidity or abnormal posture.

(5) Look for rib hump and increased or decreased kyphosis in forward flexion.

(6) Evaluate DTRs in upper and lower extremities. Look for any absent or pathologic reflexes.

(7) Carefully assess the motor and sensory examination, looking for nerve root involvement.

(8) Tension signs (e.g., straight leg raise, lasegue, bowstring) suggest nerve root irritation.

(9) Perform a vascular examination to rule out a vascular source of lower extremity pain.

(10) Check hip motion to rule out arthritic pain as the etiology of lower extremity symptoms.

(11) Palpate the sacroiliac joint (SIJ) for tenderness. Perform Flexion, ABduction, and External Rotation of the hip (FABER) test or Gaenslen maneuver to assess SIJ involvement.

(12) Look for presence of Waddell signs, suggesting nonorganic or functional overlay elements to the examination. The presence of three or more signs suggests symptom exaggeration.

(a) Diffuse, superficial tenderness to palpation of the lumbar area.

(b) Simulation: Rotating the hips or light pressure on the apex of the head causes back pain.

(c) Distraction: While distracted, patient can do a seated straight-leg raise to 90 degrees, but while supine patient resists straight-leg raise and gives pain response.

(d) Overreaction: Patient gives exaggerated responses, grabs examiner's hands, cries out or grimaces with pain.

(e) Regional abnormality: Pain or numbness in the limb is distinctly nonphysiologic and not associated with a specific dermatomal pattern.

b. Hip.

(1) Patient wears a gown to expose hip, buttock, groin, and knee. It is important to examine the knee as well as to look for referred pain.

(2) Observe the gait. Look for any gluteal lurch (e.g., patient leans over weak abductors during gait).

(3) Palpate over the greater trochanter for pain (bursitis).

(4) Test ROM in supine position. Normal: 120 degrees flexion, 45 degrees abduction, 20 degrees adduction. Compare motion with contralateral hip. Note any limitation of motion or crepitance present.

(5) Passive flexion/internal rotation is sensitive for intra-articular hip pathology (causes pain). Resisted straight-leg raise (Stinchfield test) also reproduces pain with joint pathology.

c. **Knee**

(1) Observe gait and position of knee (valgus = knock-kneed, varus = bow-legged).

(2) Look and palpate for fluid in joint, indicating inflammation. Palpate for synovitic fullness.

(3) Palpate the patella and perform patellar grind and entrapment tests against the trochlear groove (pain and crepitance suggests patello-femoral arthralgia).

(4) Look for hypermobility or poor tracking (usually lateral) of the patella. Apprehension with lateral pressure suggests chronic subluxation.

(5) Palpate the inferior pole of the patella/tibial tubercle for pain, suggesting tendonitis.

(6) Fullness and pain at tubercle in adolescent suggests Osgood-Schlatter disease.

(7) Test and record ROM. Normal = 0 to 135 degrees. Look and feel for catching, grinding, etc. Note any pain present.

(8) Stress the medial and lateral collateral ligaments at 30 degrees of flexion to determine stability. Palpate the origin and insertion of each for presence of pain.

(9) Palpate the joint lines (medial and lateral) for pain (meniscal tear, synovitis, arthritis). Perform McMurray test for meniscal pathology.

(10) Test the anterior cruciate ligament (ACL) with Lachman test and anterior drawer. Perform pivot shift, looking for rotatory instability.

(11) Test posterior cruciate ligament (PCL) with posterior drawer, posterior sag, and extension recurvatum tests.

(12) Test posterolateral corner with reverse pivot shift and external rotation drawer.

(13) Palpate the pez anserine for pain, swelling, and synovitis.

(14) Look for any atrophy in the quadricep mechanism. Compare with contralateral thigh. Measure thigh circumference and record differences.

d. Ankle.

(1) Observe gait and weight-bearing position.

(2) Palpate malleoli and syndesmosis for pain or deformity.

(3) Palpate the anterior talofibular ligament (ATFL), calcaneofibular ligament (CFL), Achilles tendon, deltoid ligament, peroneal tendons, and medial flexors for pain, synovitis, etc. Ensure that the posterior tibial tendon is functioning (e.g., look for heel varus with toe rise).

(4) Palpate the joint line for pain, synovitis, etc. Persistent pain in the anterolateral jointline after injury may suggest a meniscoid lesion.

(5) Test for any anterior-posterior, lateral, inversion, or eversion instability (e.g., anterior drawer, cotton, dorsiflexion internal rotation).

(6) Test the ATFL, CFL, deltoid ligament, and syndesmotic ligament.

(7) Test and record ROM (dorsiflexion 15 degrees, plantarflexion 45 degrees, inversion and eversion are variable). Stabilize talus in dorsiflexion and evaluate subtalar motion.

e. Shoulder.

(1) Palpate acromion, coracoid, tuberosities, and scapular spine for tenderness.

(2) Observe for any atrophy of the shoulder girdle.

(3) Palpate the acromioclavicular joint for pain, prominence, and deformity. Perform cross-arm or hyperadduction test and assess for pain.

(4) Palpate biceps. Observe for rupture (trauma or chronic impingement). Palpate the long head tendon for pain.

(5) Test and record ROM. Normal is forward flexion 170 degrees, abduction 170 degrees, external rotation 50 degrees, and internal rotation reach to T7. Feel for any crepitance with motion; check for weakness in external rotation or with scapular lift-off (rotator cuff pathology).

(6) Look for impingement pain with forward flexion or with flexion, adduction, or internal rotation movement. Pain with resisted abduction in the thumb down position (supraspinatous test) suggests impingement.

Tenderness in the subacromial bursa is common in impingement.

(7) Test for anterior or posterior apprehension, suggesting instability. Hawkins relocation test is helpful in determining antero-inferior instability.

(8) Pain with resisted abduction or with sudden giving way while lowering an abducted arm (drop arm sign) may suggest a rotator cuff tear.

f. **Elbow.**

(1) Palpate the condyles, olecranon, and radial head for tenderness or deformity.

(2) Test and record ROM. Normal is 0 to 140 degrees and pronation/supination arc of 160 degrees.

(3) Palpate for fullness in joint, especially at lateral joint line.

(4) Palpate for pain (especially with resisted wrist extension or flexion) over the epicondyles, suggestive of overuse syndromes (e.g., tennis elbow).

(5) Note any crepitance with motion.

(6) Test for medial and lateral stability.

(7) Palpate the cubital tunnel for tenderness. Feel for any subluxation of the ulnar nerve with motion.

g. **Wrist.**

(1) Palpate the distal radioulnar joint, radial and ulnar styloids, and the carpus for tenderness, deformity, or fullness.

(2) Palpate the "snuff box" for pain (scaphoid pathology).

(3) Palpate the wrist extensors and flexors for pain, fullness, etc. Test against resisted motion.

(4) Perform provocative tests of the carpal tunnel to evaluate for carpal tunnel syndrome (CTS).

(a) Conduct Tinel, Phalen's, and median nerve compression tests. Check sensation of thumb, index, and middle fingers.

(b) Look for any thenar atrophy.

(5) Palpate the first dorsal compartment for fullness, tenderness. Perform Finklestein test, looking for DeQuervain disease.

(6) Palpate the triangulofibrocartilagenous complex (TFCC) at the ulnar wrist for pain and crepitance. Pain with pressure and ulnar deviation of the wrist suggests TFCC pathology.

(7) Test and record ROM. Normal is extension of 60 degrees, flexion of 75 degrees, ulnar deviation of 30 degrees, and radial deviation of 20 degrees.

(8) Palpate for masses (often ganglia) on dorsal and volar aspects of wrist.

X. DIFFERENTIAL DIAGNOSIS (Table 26-6)

The differential diagnosis for orthopedic diseases is typically associated with a particular joint or region. Table 26-6 lists the more common symptoms and the appropriate differential.

Table 26-6. PATHOLOGICAL DIFFERENTIAL DIAGNOSIS OF PAIN.

Location	Possible Diagnoses
Neck/back	Arthritis (inflammatory, degenerative, posttraumatic), disc desiccation or herniation, instability, congenital anomaly, stenosis, chronic pain syndrome
Shoulder	Rotator cuff tear, AC joint arthritis, glenohumeral arthritis, impingement syndrome, labral tear, instability, referred neck pain, fracture
Elbow	Arthritis, osteochondral lesion, instability, mass, fracture
Forearm	Entrapment neuropathy, trauma, muscular overuse
Hand/wrist	Arthritis, carpal instability, tenosynovitis, peripheral nerve entrapment, trauma, osteonecrosis, fracture
Hip	Arthritis, trauma, osteonecrosis, tumor, referred back pain, greater trochanteric bursitis, labral tear, fracture
Knee	Arthritis, osteonecrosis, osteochondral defect, meniscal tear, fracture, patellofemoral arthralgia malalignment, plica impingement, tendonitis, instability, ligament sprain, referred hip pain
Leg	Stress fracture or syndrome, referred back pain
Ankle/foot	Arthritis, tendonitis or tendonopathy, osteochondral defect, instability, ligamentous laxity, fracture, meniscoid impingement, sprain

XI. LABORATORY STUDIES AND DIAGNOSTIC EVALUATIONS

A. Imaging Studies

1. Obtain radiographs of any anatomic area being examined in at least two planes.
2. Examine the patient before evaluation of the radiograph to avoid focusing on any obvious problems and missing other, more subtle findings on the examination.
3. Examine the radiographs for fractures, deformity, joint changes, destructive lesions, soft tissue mineralization, swelling, etc. Remember that straight lines in bone density, even if subtle, generally reflect pathology.

4. In the trauma setting, radiographs of the joint above and below the area of obvious trauma should be obtained.
5. Always image both the hips and the knees when evaluating children and adolescents with hip or knee pain.
6. Special studies such as bone scans, computed tomography (CT) scans, and magnetic resonance imaging (MRI) may be obtained, when appropriate, for additional diagnostic information.

B. Laboratory Studies

1. Standard: Complete blood count (CBC), erythrocyte sedimentation rate (ESR), C-reactive protein (CRP), and cultures of aspirates or open wounds as appropriate.
2. Urinalysis (UA), CBC, and coagulation studies preoperatively in appropriate age group.
3. Type and screen/cross for matched blood as appropriate preoperatively. Consider donation of autologous blood for joint replacement surgery.

XII. ACRONYMS AND ABBREVIATIONS (Table 26-7)

XIII. DEFINITIONS (Table 26-8)

XIV. SAMPLE H&P WRITE-UP

Chief Complaint: Right knee pain.

History of Present Illness: Mr. Jones is a 23-year-old white male construction worker who suffered the acute onset of right medial knee pain following a twisting injury while playing basketball 5 days ago. The patient did not fall at the time of injury. He denies any acute swelling or audible pop, but he did have to stop playing and was able to walk unassisted to the bench. The following morning, he noted significant swelling and pain with ambulation. The swelling has decreased somewhat over the last 2 or 3 days, but the pain and stiffness persist. He denies locking but does have a catching sensation in the joint. The pain is characterized as a sharp pain localized to the medial knee, exacerbated with weight-bearing activities and improved somewhat with rest. Currently, Mr. Jones is able to ambulate only minimal distances secondary to pain. He has not returned to work since the injury. He admits to a previous left knee injury (also basketball related) last year, resulting in a meniscal tear and requiring surgical intervention.

Medical History: Mr. Jones is an otherwise healthy 23-year-old male.

Surgical History: Left knee arthroscopy last year with partial medial menisectomy. Patient denies subsequent problems with the left knee.

Childhood History: Unremarkable.

Occupational History: Construction worker, involved in heavy manual labor six days per week.

Medications: Takes Motrin rarely for muscular aches and pains (800 mg TID prn).

Drug Allergies: NKDA.

Table 26-7. ORTHOPEDIC ACRONYMS AND ABBREVIATIONS.

ACRONYM OR ABBREVIATION	DEFINITION	ACRONYM OR ABBREVIATION	DEFINITION
ABC	Aneurysmal bone cyst	CFL	Calcaneofibular ligament
ABI	Ankle-brachial index	CMC	Carpal-metacarpal/metatarsal joint
ACL	Anterior cruciate ligament	CR	Closed reduction
AD	Anterior drawer	CS	Cervical spine
AEA	Above-elbow amputation	CT	Computed tomography scan
AFO	Ankle-foot orthosis	CTR	Carpal tunnel release
AIIS	Anterior inferior iliac spine	CTS	Carpal tunnel syndrome
AKA	Above-knee amputation	DBM	Demineralized bone matrix
APB	Abductor policis brevis	DDD	Degenerative disc disease
APL	Abductor policis longus	DF	Dorsoflexion
ASIS	Anterior superior iliac spine	DIP	Distal interphalangeal joint
AT	Anterior tibialis	DJD	Degenerative joint disease
ATFL	Anterior talofibular ligament	DRF	Distal radius fracture
BEA	Below-elbow amputation	DRUJ	Distal radioulnar joint
BKA	Below-knee amputation	ECRB	Extensor carpi radialis brevis
BMP	Bone morphogenic protein	ECRL	Extensor carpi radialis longus
BS	Bone scan	ECU	Extensor carpi ulnaris

Continued

ORTHO

Table 26-7. ORTHOPEDIC ACRONYMS AND ABBREVIATIONS—*cont'd*

Acronym or Abbreviation	Definition	Acronym or Abbreviation	Definition
EDC	Extensor digitorum comminus	**MPJ**	Metatarsal/metacarpal phalangeal joint
EDL	Extensor digitorum longus	**MTP**	Medial tibial plateau
EDQ	Extensor digiti quinti	**MUA**	Manipulation under anesthesia
EHL	Extensor halicis longus	**OCD**	Osteochondral defect
EIP	Extensor indicis proprius	**OCE**	Osteochondroma
EPB	Extensor policis brevis	**ORIF**	Open-reduction internal fixation
EPL	Extensor policis longus	**OSA**	Osteogenic sarcoma
FPL	Flexor policis longus	**PCL**	Posterior cruciate ligament
EIP	Extensor indicis proprius	**PD**	Posterior drawer
EUA	Exam under anesthesia	**PF**	Plantar/palmar flexion
Ex-fix	External fixation device	**PFA**	Patellofemoral arthralgia (anterior knee pain)
FCU	Flexor carpi ulnaris	**PIP**	Proximal interphalangeal joint
FDP	Flexor digitorum profundus	**PSIS**	Posterior superior iliac spine
FDS	Flexor digitorum superficialis	**PT**	Posterior tibialis
FHL	Flexor halicis longus	**PTFL**	Posterior talofibular ligament

FX	Fracture	**RCR**	Rotator cuff repair
FOOSH	Fall on outstretched hand	**ROM**	Range of motion (A = Active, P = Passive)
GCT	Giant cell tumor	**RTHA**	Revision total hip arthroplasty
IPJ	Interphalangeal joint	**RTKA**	Revision total knee arthroplasty
KAFO	Knee-ankle-foot orthosis	**RTC**	Rotator cuff tear
HNP	Herniated nucleus pulposis	**RCR**	Rotator cuff repair
LBP	Low-back pain	**SAD**	Subacromial decompression
LCL	Lateral collateral ligament	**SCI**	Spinal cord injury
LE	Lower extremity (R = right, L = left)	**SCIWORA**	Spinal cord injury without radiographic abnormality
LFC	Lateral femoral condyle	**SIJ**	Sacroiliac joint
LJL	Lateral joint line	**TFCC**	Triangular fibrocartilagenous complex (ulnar wrist)
LMT	Lateral meniscal tear	**THA**	Total hip arthroplasty
LSO	Lumbosacral orthosis	**TKA**	Total knee arthroplasty
LSS	Lumbosacral spine	**TLJ**	Thoracolumbar junction
LTP	Lateral tibial plateau	**TLSO**	Thoracolumbosacral orthosis
MCL	Medial collateral ligament	**TS**	Thoracic spine
MFC	Medial femoral condyle	**TSA**	Total shoulder arthoplasty
MFH	Malignant fibrous histiocytoma	**UBC**	Unicameral bone cyst
MJL	Medial joint line	**UE**	Upper extremity (R = right, L = left)
MMT	Medial meniscal tear	**V/V**	Varus/valgus

Table 26-8. ORTHOPEDIC-FOCUSED DEFINITIONS.

TERM	DEFINITION
Abduction	Movement away from midline
Adduction	Movement toward midline
Ankylosis	Stiffness of a joint (e.g., trauma, arthritis, scarring)
Antalgic	As applied to gait, refers to short stance phase secondary to painful weight bearing
Anteversion	Usually applied to femur or humerus, describes internal torsion
Arthrodesis	Fusion of a joint
Arthroplasty	Operation on joint, typically to gain mobility
Babinski reflex	Flexor plantar response: Stroking of plantar foot with great toe extension and fanning of the lesser toes. Denotes long-tract spinal cord involvement
Bowstring	Supine patient with hips and knees flexed; passive extension of knee and compression into popliteal space causes radiating leg pain in presence of nerve root compression
Calcaneus	Dorsiflexed position of ankle
Carpal tunnel syndrome	Compressive neuropathy of the medial nerve in the wrist, associated with pain, weakness, and numbness
Cavus	Exaggerated longitudinal arch of foot
Comminuted	More than two fragments in fracture
Contracture	Pathologic condition of joint, loss of full extension
Contralateral	Pertaining to the other side of the body
Coxa	Hip
Dislocation	Complete separation of a joint (no contact of articular surfaces)
Equinus	Plantarflexed position of ankle
FABER test	Flexion ABduction and External Rotation (FABER) of the hip joint, pushing on the flexed ipsilateral knee and contralateral pelvis. Pain indicates sacroiliac joint pathology
Finkelstein test	With thumb inside of flexed fingers making a fist, passive ulnar deviation of the wrist causes radial-sided wrist pain. Positive in stenosing tenosynovitis of the first dorsal compartment of the wrist (De Quervain's disease)
Genu	Knee

Table 26-8—cont'd

TERM	DEFINITION
Girdlestone	Resection arthroplasty of the hip
Greenstick	Incomplete fracture in children; cortex on tension side only appears to be involved
Hallux	Great toe
Hoffman's reflex	In relaxed hand, flicking the middle fingernail causes index and thumb flexion. Denotes long-tract spinal cord involvement in neck
Impacted	Fracture where one fragment is driven into another
Ipsilateral	Pertaining to the same side of the body
Kyphosis	Posterior curvature of spine
Lachman's test	With knee flexed 20 degrees, gentle forward translation of the tibia and posterior translation of the femur. Lack of endpoint suggests injury to anterior cruciate ligament
Lasegue	Forced dorsiflexion of foot during passive straight-leg raise that causes leg pain, indicative of nerve root compression
Lordosis	Anterior curvature to spine
McMurray test	Valgus of varus stress on the fully flexed knee with the tibia internally or externally rotated, "pinching" the meniscus. Bringing the knee into full extension may elicit a painful click on the medial/lateral joint line. Test may imply meniscal pathology, but is nonspecific
Malunion	Fracture healed with deformity
Mumford	Resection of distal clavicle
Nonunion	Failure of fracture of osteotomy to heal
Olisthy	Slippage of one vertebra on another in any direction
Open	Fracture that has penetrated the skin, deep laceration exposing joint
Osteotomy	Operative separation/cut of bone
Pathologic fracture	Fracture through abnormal bone (e.g., tumor, osteopenia)
Pes	Foot
Planus	Flattening of longitudinal arch of foot
Pronation	Rotational movement of forearm turning palm down

Continued

Table 26-8. ORTHOPEDIC-FOCUSED DEFINITIONS—*cont'd*

Term	Definition
Recurvatum	Extension of knee beyond 0 degrees
Retrolisthesis	Posterior slippage of one vertebra on another
Retroversion	Usually applied to femur or humerus, describes external torsion
Scoliosis	Abnormal curvature of the spine
Segmental	Two or more fractures involving the entire width of the bone, producing full-thickness segments of bone
Spondylolisthesis	Anterior slippage of one vertebra on another
Spondylolysis	Defect in the pars interarticularis, may be associated with olisthy
Spondylosis	Degenerative disease of the spine
Sprain	Incomplete tear of a ligament
Stinchfield test	Pain with resisted straight-leg raise, nonspecific for hip joint pathology
Strain	Incomplete tear of a muscle
Stress fracture	Fracture from repetitive trauma
Subluxation	Partial displacement of a joint, articular surfaces retain some contact
Supination	Rotational movement of forearm turning palm up
Tenodesis	Fixation of tendon to bone
Tenolysis	Freeing of tendon, usually removing adhesions
Tenotomy	Operative division of a tendon
Torus	Incomplete fracture in children, where the concave cortex buckles (also know as a buckle fracture)
Valgus	Angulation of a limb where distal part is directed away from the midline (normal knee is valgus)
Varus	Angulation of a limb where distal part is directed toward the midline
Waddell signs	Five described signs suggestive of nonorganic findings: 1. Superficial tenderness 2. Overreaction 3. Distraction 4. Simulation 5. Regional (nonanatomic) sensory changes

Family History: Unremarkable.

Social History: Married male with 2 young children. Wife is not employed outside the home. Patient plays basketball every weekend.

Review of Symptoms: Reveals periodic low-back pain at the end of the day when involved in heavy lifting. Otherwise unremarkable.

Physical Examination: Well-developed, well-nourished, 6′5″, 205-lb., fit-appearing white male in no acute distress, who ambulates with an antalgic gait.

Examination of the left knee reveals well-healed, nontender arthroscopic portal sites. ROM is 0-135 degrees without pain. There is no joint line tenderness, no effusion, no crepitance, no instability, and no atrophy. The patella tracks well with no pain.

Examination of the right knee reveals obvious swelling with a 2+ effusion in the joint. There is diffuse tenderness over the medial knee, particularly at the medial joint line. Range of motion is limited to 5-95 degrees and is painful at the extremes of motion. There is moderate tenderness to valgus stress with a solid endpoint and no significant laxity, and mild tenderness over the femoral insertion of the MCL. Attempts at McMurray's test are met with resistance and marked pain response. Lachman's test shows a 1+ excursion with a good endpoint, symmetric with the contralateral knee. The patella tracks well, with no medial facet tenderness and no patellar tendon or quad tendon tenderness to palpation.

There are no skin changes over the knee. The motor sensory examination in the RLE is unremarkable.

Right hip ROM is full without pain. The right ankle examination is unremarkable.

Imaging Studies: Plain radiographs of the knee reveal evidence of an effusion but show no bony abnormality.

Diagnosis: Medial right knee pain, presumed medial meniscal tear.

27

OTOLARYNGOLOGY AND EAR, NOSE, AND THROAT SURGERY

William Clark, MD, DDS, FACS

I. CHIEF COMPLAINT

A. **Chief Complaint:** Why is the patient here to see you? Use the patient's or parent's own words (open-ended questioning).

B. **Chronology of Events:** Onset (acute, subacute, or chronic), duration (minutes, hours, days, weeks, months, or years), and frequency of symptom(s).

C. **Identifying Data:** Name, age, gender, race/ethnicity; admission date, time, and site.

II. HISTORY OF PRESENT ILLNESS

A. **Ear:** The ear has only a few functions and can manifest only a handful of signs and symptoms.

1. Hearing.
   - **a.** Have you had any hearing loss?
     - **(1)** If yes, when did it begin and how long has it lasted (onset and duration)?
     - **(2)** Is your hearing loss continuous or intermittent?
     - **(3)** Is it symmetrical?
   - **b.** Do you have any distortions in hearing?
2. Balance and vertigo.
   - **a.** Have you experienced vertigo (i.e., the illusion of motion)? If so, do you sense that the environment is moving about you (objective vertigo) or do you feel that you are moving in relation to your environment (subjective vertigo)? Lightheadedness, "swimming-headed" feelings, and similar symptoms are rarely associated with ear pathology and suggest a nonotologic etiology.
   - **b.** When did any of these symptoms begin (onset)?
   - **c.** How long does it typically last (duration)?
   - **d.** How often does it occur (frequency)?
   - **e.** Is the symptom associated with a positional change? For example, does it occur when you turn your head or when you roll over in bed? Is it associated with hearing loss or tinnitus? Is it accompanied by nausea or vomiting? Nausea with or without vomiting may accompany severe vertigo of otologic origin.
3. Pain.
   - **a.** Do you have any ear pain?

b. If so, do you have any tenderness? Ear pain with a tender ear canal suggests otitis externa but may also occur with carcinoma of the ear canal.
c. Is your pain accompanied by any hearing loss? Hearing loss may accompany either otitis externa or carcinoma because of ear canal obstruction. Ear pain with hearing loss and no tenderness suggests otitis media.
d. The ear is often the recipient of pain referred from other areas. Common sites of such pain are the temporomandibular joint (TMJ), pharynx, larynx, oral cavity, tooth pathology, and inflammation in a neck structure. The setting of a painful ear with a normal ear examination suggests the need to look elsewhere for the etiology of the pain.

4. Drainage.
   a. Have you had any drainage from the ear? Ask this question of all patients who are being evaluated for chronic ear problems.
   b. Is the ear drainage recurrent and associated with a tender ear canal (otitis externa)? Has your ear been exposed to water recently? In the absence of associated water exposure, consider carcinoma of the ear canal. Recurrent ear drainage without canal tenderness suggests chronic otitis media with tympanic membrane perforation or cholesteatoma.
5. Tinnitus.
   a. How loud is your tinnitus?
      (1) Is it keeping you awake?
      (2) Does it impair conversations?
   b. When does it bother you? Most continuous tinnitus will be more bothersome at night.
   c. Is it accompanied by vertigo? Tinnitus that precedes the onset of severe vertigo suggests endolymphatic hydrops as the etiology (Ménière's disease is idiopathic endolymphatic hydrops).
   d. What is its pitch or quality? High-pitched ringing is common and has many causes; high-frequency hearing loss is the most common. Low-pitched tinnitus (often described as roaring or buzzing) is classical for endolymphatic hydrops.
   e. Is it continuous or pulsatile? Pulsatile tinnitus suggests a vascular etiology, and the patient should be referred for an otolaryngology consultation. Continuous tinnitus is nonspecific. All tinnitus will be made more noticeable by impairment of the ear's conduction system, including impaction of the ear canal by cerumen.

B. Nose

1. Nasal obstruction.
   a. Do you use any prescription medications or over-the-counter (OTC) products?

b. When did the symptom begin (onset)?
c. Which side is involved?
d. Does it occur seasonally or year-round?
e. Any associated symptoms?
   (1) Do you have any sneezing?
   (2) Any discharge?
   (3) Postnasal discharge?
   (4) Do you have eye or conjunctival itching or erythema?
   (5) Do you have facial pain or headaches?

2. Olfactory disturbance.
   a. When was your sense of smell affected (onset)?
   b. Did it occur after a head trauma?
   c. Is the symptom intermittent or continuous?
   d. Is it associated with nasal obstruction? Absence of such association suggests possibility of non-nasal etiology (e.g., olfactory system, brain).
3. Epistaxis.
   a. Have you taken anticoagulant medications?
   b. When did the symptom begin (onset)?
   c. How often does it occur (frequency)?
   d. How long does it last (duration)?
   e. What is the typical amount of blood lost (volume)? How much blood have you lost in the last 24 hours?
   f. When blood is flowing and your head is upright, where does most of the blood go? Most blood flowing down the pharynx in a middle-aged or older patient suggests a posterior epistaxis, a potentially life-threatening condition. Emergent referral is in order, even if no bleeding is present on examination.

C. Throat

1. Pain.
   a. When did the pain begin (onset)?
   b. Where is it located?
   c. Is the pain symmetrically located?
   d. Have you had any recent weight loss? If answer is yes, promptly refer patient to an oncologist.
   e. Do you have any associated symptoms?
2. Dysphagia.
   a. When did the symptom begin (onset)?
   b. Is it continuous or intermittent?
   c. Any apparent level of obstruction? Have patient point it out.
   d. Is it associated with pain?
   e. Associated with weight loss?
   f. Associated with any types of foods?
   g. Do you have a tendency for rancid foods to come back up? This would suggest a Zenker's diverticulum.

h. Do you have any signs or symptoms of gastrointestinal reflux?

3. Snoring: Much of this information is best obtained from the observations of the bed partner of an adult or of a child's parent.
   a. When did the snoring begin (onset)?
   b. When does snoring begin after the initiation of sleep?
   c. Is the snoring associated with the use of alcohol or other central nervous system (CNS) depressant?
   d. How loud is the snoring?
   e. Does changing position in bed alter the effects of snoring?
   f. Any signs of obstruction or apnea?
4. Vocal complaints.
   a. When did the symptom begin (onset)?
   b. Is it intermittent or continuous?
   c. Is it worse in the morning or at the end of the day? When the symptom is worse in early morning, it suggests gastroesophageal (GE) reflux as an etiologic factor, although daytime gastroesophagopharyngeal reflux is also a common cause of vocal complaints. When worse at the end of the day, it is nonspecific and probably worsened by use of the voice.
   d. How do you use your voice? Do you regularly experience problems from overuse (e.g., professional singer, announcer, teacher)? Are any other signs or symptoms associated with the symptom? Dysphagia? Weight loss? Throat or neck pain? All of these are signs of possible malignancy and signal the need for referral.
   e. Any stridor? Suggests serious problem such as malignancy in the adult. Suggests serious airway obstruction such as epiglottitis or laryngeal papillomatosis in the child.
   f. Do you have GE reflux? This is the etiology of, or a complicating factor in, many if not most vocal complaints.

D. Face and Neck Masses

1. When did the mass become noticeable and how long has it been present (onset and duration)?
2. Has it changed in size (growth, fluctuations)?
3. Do you currently drink alcohol or use tobacco? Have you in the past?
4. Are there masses in other locations? Axillae? Inguinal region?
5. Do you have any systemic signs or symptoms? Fever? Chills? Malaise? Weight loss? Pruritis? These suggest the possibility of lymphoma.

III. PAST MEDICAL AND SURGICAL HISTORY

A. Past Medical History

1. Have you had any head or neck radiation? Radiation therapy in the 1950s and 1960s for acne or thymus or thyroid

conditions increased the risk for papillary carcinoma of the thyroid.

2. Have you had any trauma?
3. Have you had cancer?

B. Past Surgical History

1. Have you had any surgical procedures? Patients with chronic middle ear problems have often had one or more prior surgical procedures, and the details of these operations can be critical to understanding and treating the present condition.
2. Have you had a malignancy of the head and neck region? If so, have you had prior surgery on the area, prior radiation, or prior chemotherapy to treat it?
3. Have you had recent surgery that involved endotracheal intubation? This may be related to pharyngeal or laryngeal complaints.

C. Childhood History

1. What type of sun exposure did you have as a child? Did you have episodes of sunburn?
2. Were you intubated as an infant? Children who were intubated as infants are at risk for developing acquired subglottic stenosis.

D. Occupational History

1. Do you work with wood? Woodworkers, especially those who work with softwood without filtration masks, have an increased incidence of adenocarcinoma of the sinuses.
2. Are you exposed to radium at work? Individuals who painted watch dials with radium would sometimes lick the paintbrush on their tongue for a fine point, which increased their risk for tongue carcinomas.
3. Are you exposed to nickel? Nickel exposure has been correlated with carcinoma of the sinuses.

E. Travel History: Have you traveled within the United States? Have you traveled to foreign countries? Some inflammatory processes are endemic to certain regions. Examples of endemic diseases, which might present in the head and neck region are Hansen's disease (leprosy), *Leishmaniasis* exposure area, Rhinosporidiosis, and Rhinoscleroma.

F. Animal and Insect Exposure History: Are you exposed to cats and other companion animals? Such exposure is associated with the transfer of "cat scratch disease," which often presents with impressive cervical lymphadenopathy.

IV. MEDICATIONS, ALLERGIES, AND ADVERSE REACTIONS

A. Medications

1. Are you currently taking any prescription medications? Indications, last dose, duration of use, and possible drug interactions? Annotate date started and regimen changes.

2. Do you use OTC medications such as analgesics, sleeping medications, vitamins, supplements, herbal preparations, or diet pills?
3. Alternative medicine therapies?

B. Allergies and Adverse Reactions: Differentiate between allergic manifestations and adverse reactions. Often an adverse effect does not represent a true IgE-mediated allergy, but rather intolerance to the medication (e.g., gastrointestinal upset with codeine).

1. Have you had an allergic reaction to medication?
   a. What was the allergic reaction (e.g., respiratory or neurologic manifestations)?
   b. How was the allergic reaction treated?
   c. What was the route of medication administration when the allergy occurred (oral, intravenous, subcutaneous)?
2. Have you had any environmental allergies? Have you had reactive airways disease (RAD), hay fevers or allergic rhinitis, food allergies, or dermatologic reactions (e.g., nickel in earrings)?

V. HEALTH MAINTENANCE

A. Prevention: The immunization for invasive *Haemophilus influenza* B is effective for prevention of epiglottitis.

B. Sleep Patterns

1. Do you have difficulty rising in the morning? This may be a sign of disturbed sleep.
2. Do you sleep or feel sleepy during the day? Daytime somnolence suggests sleep disturbance.

C. Social Habits

1. Do you use tobacco? What form? How much and for how long?
2. Do you drink alcohol? What type? How much and for how long?

VI. FAMILY HISTORY

A. First-Degree Relatives' Medical History

1. Have any family members had cancer?
2. Have any family members had multiple endocrine neoplasia (MEN) syndrome? A patient with a medullary carcinoma may have a MEN syndrome.
3. Have family members had allergic rhinitis/atopy?

B. Three-Generation Genogram: Expand family history to create a three-generation family genogram if increased susceptibility (genetic predisposition) is known to occur with the disease or syndrome (e.g., basal cell nevus syndrome, Sturge-Weber syndrome, Gardner's syndrome, cherubism, white sponge nevus syndrome).

VII. PSYCHOSOCIAL HISTORY

A. Personal and Social History

1. What is your country of birth and ethnicity? This information may help identify increased risk for certain conditions (e.g., recently emigrated from China, particularly the region of Canton, would place that individual at higher risk for nasopharyngeal carcinoma).

B. **Current Illness Effects on the Patient:** How have you been affected by your symptom(s)? Loss of senses (e.g., taste and/or smell, hearing) can be a severe emotional stressor. Assess prognosis early on with your patients.

C. **Interpersonal and Sexual History:** Are you sexually active? How many partners do you have and of what gender? What protective measures do you use? Assess for HIV risk factors.

D. **Occupational Aspects of Illness or Condition:** How has your illness affected your physical functioning and job (i.e., adaptation)?

VIII. REVIEW OF SYSTEMS (Tables 27-1, 27-2, and 27-3)

Table 27-1. GENERAL OTOLARYNGOLOGY SYMPTOMS BY SYSTEM.

System	Symptoms
Ear	Pain, tenderness, vertigo, drainage, hearing loss
Nose	Obstruction, odor perception, discharge, post nasal drip, bleeding
Mouth/ oropharynx	Pain, tenderness, masses, bleeding, odors, dysphagia, snoring, apnea
Larynx	Vocal quality, vocal endurance, airway, pain, effectiveness of cough
Neck	Masses, pain, tenderness

Table 27-2. NONSPECIFIC SYMPTOMS AND ENT DISEASES.

Symptom	Possible Diseases
Pulsatile tinnitus	Venus hum, arteriovenous malformation, globus tumor of ear, neck, or skull base
Low-pitched tinnitus	Endolymphatic hydrops (especially when accompanied by fluctuating hearing loss and ear fullness)
Ear canal tenderness	Otitis externa, carcinoma of ear canal
Unilateral hearing loss	One-sided noise trauma, cerumen impaction, otosclerosis, tympanic membrane perforation, cholesteatoma (especially when accompanied by chronic, malodorous drainage), neoplasm of cerebellar pontine angle or internal auditory canal (so-called acoustic neuroma or vestibular schwannoma)

Table 27-2—cont'd

SYMPTOM	POSSIBLE DISEASES
Hoarseness	Gastrolaryngopharyngeal reflux, laryngeal mass (malignant neoplasm, vocal polyp, vocal nodule), acute laryngitis, vocal cord paralysis (unilateral has ineffective cough but good airway, bilateral usually has stridor)
Dysphagia	Gastroesophagopharyngeal reflux, neoplasm, stricture
Snoring	Obstructive sleep apnea syndrome
Morning headache	Obstructive sleep apnea syndrome
Daytime somnolence	Obstructive sleep apnea syndrome
Postnasal drip	Gastro-pharyngeal reflux, sinusitis
Unilateral ear pain	Malignant neoplasm with referred pain must be considered if the ear examination is normal; otitis media (accompanying hearing loss and no tenderness), otitis externa (accompanying tenderness)

Table 27-3. FIVE MOST COMMON ENT DISEASES AND THEIR SYMPTOMS.

DISEASE	SYMPTOMS
Recurrent otitis media	Ear pain, hearing loss
Recurrent tonsillitis	Throat pain, fever, odynophagia
Obstructive sleep apnea syndrome	Snoring, disturbed sleep, morning headache, difficult morning awakening, daytime somnolence
Laryngopharyngeal reflux (related to GERD)	Postnasal drip, hoarseness, dysphagia, recurrent sinusitis, recurrent middle ear problems
Hearing loss	Decreased hearing (often with tinnitus), difficulty understanding conversations in noisy environment

IX. PHYSICAL EXAMINATION (Table 27-4)

Table 27-4. PHYSICAL EXAMINATION FINDINGS AND POSSIBLE DIAGNOSES.

System	Physical Examination Finding	Possible Diagnoses
Ears		
External canal	Canal occluded with cerumen	Cerumen impaction (a sign of canal instrumentation by patient or parent)
	Tender, swollen ear canal	Otitis externa, carcinoma
	Multiple rounded protuberances of bony portion of canal	Exostoses of bone of ear canal (often associated with frequent cold water exposure; "surfer's ear")
Tympanic membrane	Immobile tympanic membrane	Middle ear effusion (may be sign of nasopharyngeal mass in the adult), unseen perforation
	Inflamed, bulging tympanic membrane	Otitis media
	Retraction of TM	Eustachian tube dysfunction, developing cholesteatoma, cholesteatoma
	Perforation	Sharp angles and fresh blood indicate acute TM perforation, rounded edges and no blood indicate chronic perforation
	Perforation and/or deep retraction with epithelial debris	Acquired cholesteatoma. The superior tympanic membrane (pars flaccida) and the posterior-superior quadrant of the TM are the high-risk areas for acquired cholesteatoma formation
Nose		
External	Asymmetrical external nose	External nasal deformity, possible nasal trauma
Nasal cavities	Pale mucous membranes with copious, clear secretions	Allergic rhinitis

Table 27-4—cont'd

System	Physical Examination Finding	Possible Diagnoses
	Nasal septum not in midline	Deviated nasal septum
	Smooth, firm, mucus-covered masses of lateral nasal walls, symmetrically distributed	Nasal turbinates (normal structures often mistaken for nasal polyps)
	Smooth, soft mucus-covered masses of nasal cavities	Nasal polyps, neoplasm, encephalocele, manifestation of cystic fibrosis (CF) when seen in children
	Erythema of mucous membranes with purulent discharge	Infectious rhinitis and/or sinusitis
	Mass lesion other than those above	Possible neoplasm
Mouth	Tender, erythematous mass	Squamous cell carcinoma
	Bony-hard mass midline of palate	Torus palatinus (benign bony outgrowth)
	Bony-hard globular masses, lingual surface of mandible	Torus mandibularis (benign bony outgrowth)
Face	Mass, region of parotid gland	Neoplasm requiring treatment until proven otherwise
	Swelling over anterior surface of maxilla	Inflammatory mass of dental etiology
Neck	Abnormal mass in adult's neck	Serious neoplasm until proven otherwise
	Cystic mass, midline, between larynx and hyoid bone	Thyroglossal duct cyst
	Cystic mass deep and just anterior to lower one third of SCM muscle	Branchial arch cyst (second arch)
	Sinus tract opening just anterior to lower one third of SCM muscle	Branchial cleft sinus (second arch)

Continued

Table 27-1. PHYSICAL EXAMINATION FINDINGS AND POSSIBLE DIAGNOSES—*cont'd*

System	Physical Examination Finding	Possible Diagnoses
	Cystic mass posterior to SCM muscle	Lymphatic malformation (so-called cystic hygroma or lymphangioma)
Thyroid	Mass	Cyst, benign neoplasm, malignant neoplasm
	Mass in supraclavicular region of adult	Metastatic lesion from below the clavicle
Posterior neck	Firm, unilateral mass(es) in adult	Metastatic carcinoma from nasopharynx

A. Examination of the Ears

1. Pinna (auricle).
   - **a.** Note presence of lesions.
   - **b.** Record tenderness to palpation.
2. Ear canal.
   - **a.** Inspect lateral canal without speculum to avoid looking past pathology.
   - **b.** Pull pinna posteriorly and superiorly to help straighten the lateral portion of the cartilaginous portion of the canal while placing the largest ear speculum that will fit in the canal.
   - **c.** Note presence of any lesions, foreign bodies, and excessive cerumen.
     - **(1)** Obstructing cerumen will need to be removed to facilitate the examination.
     - **(2)** The presence of cerumen suggests that the skin of the ear canal is healthy.
     - **(3)** The presence of cerumen deep in the bony portion of the canal suggests self-instrumentation of the canal because cerumen is secreted only in the cartilaginous portion.
   - **d.** A swollen, wet, and tender ear canal suggests otitis externa but, in long-standing cases, may represent carcinoma.
   - **e.** The most common mass lesions of the ear canal are benign bony growths (e.g., osteomas and exostoses).
     - **(1)** Exostoses are thought to be related to frequent exposure to cold water.
     - **(2)** The term "surfer's ear" has been applied to ears affected with these lesions.
3. Tympanic membrane (TM) and middle ear.

a. Much information about the health of the middle ear may be obtained by careful and skillful otoscopy.

b. In general, the largest possible ear speculum is used. This gives a broad view of the ear, prevents the speculum from contacting the sensitive bony portion of the canal, and makes pneumatic otoscopy easier.

c. Posterior-superior pulling of the pinna facilitates placement of the speculum.

d. The otoscope is angled to permit visualization of as much of the TM as possible.

(1) If you attempt to visualize the annulus of the TM, you will only see as much as the patient's anatomy permits. This varies among patients.

(2) It is usual for the curvature of the bony ear canal to block visualization of the anterior-most portion of the TM.

(3) Two areas that should receive special attention are the pars flaccida (superior-most portion of the TM) and the posterior-superior quadrant of the TM.

(a) The pars flaccida should be inspected for signs of retraction, apparent perforation, and epithelial debris. Any of these findings suggests the presence or development of a cholesteatoma.

(b) The posterior-superior quadrant of the TM overlies the ossicles. Retractions are common in this area. The ossicles are at risk of damage by retractions.

(i) Cholesteatomas may develop from retractions in this area.

(ii) Moisture, granulation tissue, and squamous debris all suggest the possibility of cholesteatoma formation.

e. Pneumatic otoscopy.

(1) Otoscope in place with large speculum sealing the canal.

(2) Puffs of air delivered by bulb.

(3) With a normal middle ear, the TM should move freely in and out.

(4) An open TM perforation or PE tube will result in no motion because the hole prevents a pressure differential.

(5) A middle ear filled with an effusion will show diminished motion.

(6) Air bubbles in an effusion will move separately from the TM.

(7) TM changes simulating bubbles will move with it.

(8) TM changes simulating a perforation (dimeric membrane) will move with the TM while a "real" TM perforation will prevent motion.

4. Special examinations with hearing loss, vertigo, and tinnitus.
   a. Test function and symmetry of the trigeminal nerves (CN V).
      (1) Light touch to skin of face.
      (2) Corneal reflex is more sensitive and also tests facial nerve function.
   b. Test function and symmetry of facial nerve (CN VII).
      (1) Raising eyebrows.
      (2) Grimacing.
   c. Audiogram.
   d. Positional testing.
   e. Romberg test.
   f. Evaluation of gait.

B. Examination of the Nose

1. Inspect external nose for lesions and symmetry.
2. Anterior rhinoscopy may be performed by using an otoscope with a large speculum.
   a. The nasal septum medially and the inferior turbinates laterally are the most prominent landmarks seen.
   b. Note the position of the septum: Should be near midline.
   c. Note color of mucous membranes: Medium pink is the usual; redness suggests inflammation; pale gray to light blue suggest allergy.
   d. Note presence or absence of masses.
   e. Observe quantity and quality of secretions.
   f. A variation in the size of inferior turbinates is common because they fluctuate with the nasal cycle.
   g. Polyps are pale and movable, whereas turbinates are pink and fixed.

C. Examination of the Throat

1. Inspect lips for lesions.
2. Inspect buccal and labial cavities for lesions.
3. Inspect teeth and their supporting tissues.
4. Inspect hard and soft palates.
5. Inspect the tongue for masses, ulcerations, and tenderness.
6. Have the patient lift his or her tongue to the palate to facilitate inspection of its ventral surface and the floor of the mouth.
7. Inspect the lateral and posterior walls of the oropharynx for lesions.
   a. The tonsils occupy the lateral wall.
      (1) Note their presence, size, and symmetry.
      (2) Epithelial debris in tonsillar crypts is normal.
   b. The posterior wall of the oropharynx may reveal the presence of drainage from the nasal cavities or nasopharynx above.
8. Without the special mirrors or scopes of the specialist, the base of the tongue is best examined by palpation.

9. Examination of the hypopharynx and larynx are likewise limited in the primary care setting.
   a. Note the quality of the voice.
   b. Have the patient cough to evaluate the strength of glottic closure.
   c. Listen for stertor, stridor, and wheezes.
      (1) Stertor is the low-pitched, inspiratory, snorelike sound characteristic of obstructing lesions above the larynx.
      (2) Stridor is the higher-pitched, inspiratory or expiratory airway sound associated with narrowing of the airway at the laryngeal or tracheal level.
      (3) Wheezes are musical airway sounds associated with obstructive pathology below the tracheal level. They are typical of asthma. Wheezes may be present with an airway foreign body.

D. Examination of the Face and Neck

1. Observe for symmetry.
2. Palpate the parotid regions.
   a. A mass in this region is usually a parotid neoplasm.
   b. A referral to an otolaryngologist is in order without further evaluation.
3. Palpate the entire neck; normal structures that are often palpable are listed as follows:
   a. Hyoid bone.
   b. Larynx.
      (1) Thyroid cartilage.
      (2) Cricoid cartilage.
   c. Trachea.
   d. Thyroid gland: All masses deserve specialty referral.
   e. Submandibular glands: Often ptotic in the senior citizen. Any mass is a neoplasm until proven otherwise.
   f. Sternocleidomastoid (SCM) muscles.
   g. Carotid arteries.
   h. Transverse process of atlas (posterior to mandible, near the mastoid tip).
4. Many solid masses in an adult's neck will represent a neoplastic process, and the patient should be referred without additional evaluation or trials of treatment.
5. Congenital masses occur in predictable locations and may present in adulthood.
   a. Thyroglossal duct cyst.
      (1) Occur midline from submental area to larynx.
      (2) Cystic feel on palpation.
      (3) Often have history of past infection.
      (4) May transilluminate.
      (5) May move upward on extrusion of tongue.
   b. Branchial cleft abnormality.

(1) Second arch cysts will present at the anterior border of the SCM muscle.
(2) Second arch fistulae will present at the same location.
(3) First, fourth, and sixth arch abnormalities are rare and often offer a diagnostic challenge to the specialist.

6. The face and neck region contains many lymph nodes. Lymph node groups are recognized and are detailed as follows:
   a. Facial group.
      (1) Parotid region is the most important. The gland contains several lymph nodes, which may receive metastases from the auriculotemporal region and elsewhere. Lymph nodes near the parotid also drain the auriculotemporal area.
      (2) Other facial lymph nodes may react to inflammatory processes of the face and scalp.
   b. Submental region.
      (1) Drains the lower lip and anterior oral cavity and is a frequent site for inflammatory lymphadenopathy. Carcinoma of the lower lip, labial cavity, and anterior floor of mouth/tip of tongue may metastasize to this area.
      (2) Referred to as a part of "Level I" by those who treat head and neck malignancies.
   c. Submandibular triangle.
      (1) Makes up the rest of "Level I."
      (2) Contains the submandibular (submaxillary) salivary gland and associated lymph nodes.
      (3) Drains the submandibular and sublingual salivary glands, buccal and labial cavities, the floor of the mouth, the mandibular alveolus, and the tongue.
      (4) A common site for nodal enlargement by both inflammatory and neoplastic processes.
      (5) Any mass in the region demands specialty referral.
   d. Deep jugular chain of lymph nodes.
      (1) Centered around the carotid sheath contents (deep jugular vein, carotid artery, vagus nerve) just anterior to the anterior border of the SCM muscle.
      (2) The upper one third is called "Level II."
         (a) Drains the oral cavity, oropharynx, hypopharynx, and larynx.
         (b) Masses here are often inflammatory in the child but usually represent metastases in the adult.
      (3) The middle third is called "Level III."
         (a) Drains the same areas as Level II plus the thyroid gland, trachea, and cervical esophagus.
         (b) A common site for metastases in the adult.
      (4) The lower third is called "Level IV."

(a) Drains the same areas as Levels II and III and may be the site of distant metastases from below the clavicle.

(b) Any mass in this region without an obvious inflammatory explanation requires specialty consultation, as do similar masses in Levels II and III.

e. Posterior triangle lymph nodes.

(1) Called "Level V."

(2) Primarily drains the nasopharynx and posterior scalp.

(3) Masses without obvious inflammatory etiologies suggest nasopharyngeal carcinoma.

X. DIFFERENTIAL DIAGNOSIS (Table 27-5)

Table 27-5. ENT DIFFERENTIAL DIAGNOSIS.

Signs and Symptoms	Possible Diagnoses
Conductive hearing loss	Ear canal impaction (cerumen, foreign body), tympanic membrane perforation, otosclerosis, cholesteatoma, congenital ossicular fixation, middle ear effusion
Sensorineural hearing loss	Presbycusis, noise exposure, acoustic trauma, endolymphatic hydrops, congenital malformation, ototoxicity to drug, otosclerosis
Vertigo	Benign paroxysmal positional vertigo, vestibular neuronitis ("bacterial labyrinthitis"), endolymphatic hydrops
Ear pain	Otitis media, otitis externa, carcinoma of ear canal, referred pain (pharynx, larynx, neck, teeth, temporomandibular joint)
Nasal obstruction	Allergic rhinitis, nonallergic rhinitis, deviated nasal septum, nasal polyps, neoplasm of nose or nasopharynx, adenoid hypertrophy (child), choanal atresia (child), nasal crusting, chronic sinusitis, laryngopharyngeal reflux
Snoring	Uncomplicated snoring, obstructive sleep-apnea syndrome, hypertrophy of adenoids and/or tonsils (child)
Parotid gland mass	Benign neoplasm, malignant neoplasm, cystic lesion (HIV association), benign lymphoepithelial lesions (collagen-vascular association), definitive diagnosis important
Stridor in the neonate	Laryngomalacia, vocal cord paralysis, laryngeal cleft, subglottic stenosis

XI. LABORATORY STUDIES AND DIAGNOSTIC EVALUATIONS

A. Cultures

1. A throat culture is of some value in differentiating a viral from a bacterial pharyngitis.
2. Nasal cultures are of limited value in the treatment of sinusitis because there is poor correlation between organisms in the nose versus the sinuses.
3. Cultures of the ear canal for otitis externa are of limited value because the common organisms are well known (e.g., *Pseudomonas, Proteus, Staphylococcus),* and topical agents are usually the treatment of choice.
4. Cultures of middle ear drainage via a perforation are of limited value because they are often contaminated by the time the patient presents for treatment. Cultures obtained by tympanocentesis or myringotomy are reliable.

B. Blood Tests: Complete blood count (CBC) with differential with or without a Mono Spot test is useful in differentiating between bacterial tonsillitis and mononuclear tonsillitis.

C. Audiometric Testing

1. Impedance audiometry is useful for evaluating the middle ear. Using this technology to evaluate a sensorineural hearing test may help differentiate between problems of the inner ear versus the auditory nerve. Some aspects of facial nerve function may also be measured by this testing.
2. Pure-tone audiometry tests the perception thresholds for a series of tones, usually 250 through 8000 Hz. The results are recorded in decibels on a scale from −20 to 110, with −20 to +20 being the range of normal.
   a. Air conduction is tested using headsets or ear canal inserts and tests the conduction system, the inner ear, and the acoustic nerve.
   b. Bone conduction is tested with bone vibrators. The sound signal bypasses the conduction system. The difference, if any, between air and bone conduction is called the air-bone gap and defines the conductive portion of a hearing impairment.
   c. Speech audiometry uses the spoken word to test the speech reception threshold (SRT, reported in decibels) and speech discrimination (reported as percentage correct).

D. Radiologic Imaging

1. Computed tomography (CT) scans are used to evaluate the temporal bone and paranasal sinuses for infection or tumor masses. They are also useful for evaluating neck masses and helping define the extent of primary neoplasms and their metastases. This technology is also used extensively in evaluating facial trauma.

2. Magnetic resonance imaging (MRI) with gadolinium enhancement is the gold standard for evaluation of the internal auditory canal and/or the cerebellar-pontine angle for neoplasms. MRI is also used to evaluate soft tissues of the face and neck and is a complement to CT studies of these same areas.

XII. ACRONYMS AND ABBREVIATIONS (Table 27-6)

XIII. DEFINITIONS (Table 27-7)

XIV. SAMPLE H&P WRITE-UP

CC: "My child has had many ear infections and doesn't seem to hear well much of the time."

HPI: E.C. is a 28-month-old female with a history of six episodes of acute otitis media. She has also been noted to have middle ear fluid on several of her examinations. Her first episode of acute otitis media occurred at 15 months of age. Over the last 13 months, she has had six such episodes, with the most recent being about 2 weeks ago. She finished taking a course of oral amoxicillin a few days ago. Mom states that her daughter's hearing is decreased.

PMHx: Has had frequent URIs, often leading to AOM. Immunizations are all up to date.

PSHx: Unremarkable.

Emergency and Trauma History: Unremarkable.

Childhood History: Prenatal history of full-term product of an uncomplicated pregnancy. Perinatal history of spontaneous vaginal delivery at 42 weeks' gestation. Left the hospital at 48 hours.

Prevention: All immunizations are up to date. Several were delayed for a week or two when acutely ill with AOM.

Diet: Breast milk, cow's milk, and prepared baby foods (fruits, vegetables, and meats). Takes nighttime and nap bottles of milk in the flat and supine position.

Exercise: Usual for age.

Social Habits: Her father smokes, but not in the home.

Family History: Mom is 32 years old. The patient's father is 36. Both are in excellent health. The mother had mild asthma as a child and is allergic to several pollens. The father also has inhalant allergies.

REVIEW OF SYSTEMS

General: Near 50th percentile for weight and height.

HEENT: Question of hearing loss. AOM as per HPI above. Frequent rhinorrhea, clear to yellow-green. Frequent nasal congestion. Sneezes a lot, especially in the spring and fall.

Respiratory: Often has mild cough when manifesting a URI and/or episode of AOM. No history of wheezing.

Gastrointestinal: No feeding problems. Occasional mild diarrhea with AOM.

Genitourinary: Unremarkable.

Hematologic/lymphatic: Unremarkable.

Skin: Unremarkable.

Neurologic: Unremarkable.

Table 27-6. OTOLARYNGOLOGY ACRONYMS AND ABBREVIATIONS.

Acronym or Abbreviation	Definition	Acronym or Abbreviation	Definition
AD	Right ear	**JV**	Jugular vein
AOM	Acute otitis media	**LM**	Lymphatic malformation
AS	Left ear	**LPR**	Laryngopharyngeal reflux
AU	Both ears	**M-RND**	Modified radical neck dissection
BMT	Bilateral myringotomy with tubes	**OM**	Otitis media
BOM	Bilateral otitis media	**PET**	Pressure-equalizing tubes
BPV	Benign positional vertigo	**RND**	Radical neck dissection
CA	Carotid artery	**RRP**	Recurrent respiratory papillomatosis
CHL	Congenital hearing loss; Conductive hearing loss	**SCC**	Squamous cell carcinoma
CN	Cranial nerve	**SNHL**	Sensorineural hearing loss
COM	Chronic otitis media	**T&A**	Tonsillectomy and adenoidectomy
CPA	Cerebellopontine angle	**TC**	Throat culture
EAC	External auditory canal	**TGDC**	Thyroglossal duct cyst
EOM	External otitis media	**TMJ**	Temporomandibular joint
GERD	Gastroesophageal reflux disease	**TT**	Tympanostomy tube (same as PET)
HA	Headache	**UPP (or UP2)**	Uvulo-palatoplasty
HEENT	Head, eyes, ears, nose, throat	**UPPP (or UP3)**	Uvulo-pharyngo-palatoplasty
HL	Hearing loss	**VM**	Vascular malformation; Venus malformation
IAC	Internal auditory canal	**ZMC**	Zygomatico-maxillary complex

Table 27-7. OTOLARYNGOLOGY TERMS.

TERM	DEFINITION
Benign positional paroxysmal vertigo	Sudden, unexpected episode of vertigo induced by body position. Thought to be caused by accumulation of debris in the posterior semicircular canal and potentially relieved by positional maneuvers that move the debris out of the canal
Branchial cleft cyst (second arch)	Congenital cyst extending from the region of the tonsillar fossa to the anterior border of the sternocleidomastoid muscle and thought to be a remnant of the primitive branchial apparatus
Branchial cleft sinus (second arch)	Congenital sinus extending from the anterior neck to the tonsillar fossa and thought to be a remnant of the primitive branchial apparatus
Cholesteatoma	A poorly named pathologic process of the middle ear. Usually results from retraction of the tympanic membrane into the middle ear space and perhaps into the mastoid. Histopathologically represented by keratinizing squamous epithelium lining a cystlike sac filled with epithelial debris. These lesions are surprisingly destructive of middle ear and mastoid structures and may damage the facial nerve, erode through the dense bone of the inner ear, and even enter the cranial cavity
Congenital cholesteatoma	Rare congenital cyst of the middle ear or temporal bone with the same histologic findings as an acquired cholesteatoma. These lesions are of uncertain origin. Some are seen through the anterior-superior quadrant of the tympanic membrane as a white middle ear mass. Others form deep in the temporal bone and are often quite large before discovery
Endolymphatic hydrops	A condition in which the endolymph of the inner ear develops an abnormally high pressure, producing aural fullness, low-pitched tinnitus, hearing loss, and vertigo. Ménière's disease is idiopathic endolymphatic hydrops

Continued

Table 27-7. OTOLARYNGOLOGY TERMS—cont'd

TERM	DEFINITION
Epistaxis (anterior)	Responsible for 90% of all epistaxis cases and almost 100% before middle age. Occurs from relatively small vessels of the anterior nasal septum (Little's area, Kiesselbach's plexus). Probably occurs as a result of dryness of thin mucous membranes, which offer limited protection form the harsh environment of the nasal cavity. Rarely dangerous but a source of inconvenience and worry to the patient and the family
Epistaxis (posterior)	Bleeding from a vessel in the posterior portion of the nasal cavities. Rare before middle age and possibly associated with atherosclerotic changes in the posterior nasal arteries. The patient will often report a series of starts and stops before a potentially exsanguinating bleed
Nasal turbinate	A sidewall structure of the lateral wall of the nasal cavity made of bone covered by a respiratory mucous membrane. The inferior turbinate contains erectile tissue, which functions to produce the respiratory cycle
Odynophagia	Painful swallowing
Positional vertigo	Vertigo precipitated by body motion
Respiratory cycle	Alternating congestion/decongestion of the nasal cavities caused by changes in the blood supply to the erectile tissue of the inferior turbinate. The relative congestion of the inferior turbinates is affected by head position and is responsible for the congestion of the downside of the nose when lying on the side during sleep
Surfer's ear	Condition of the ear canal characterized by numerous bony exostoses of the medial portion of the bony ear canal. Thought to be caused by chronic exposure to cold water
Thyroglossal duct cyst	Congenital neck lesion from a remnant of the thyroglossal duct, the embryonic precursor of the thyroid gland that extends from the foramen caecum of the base of the tongue to the lower neck

Table 27-7—cont'd

TERM	DEFINITION
Vertigo	The illusion of motion
Zenker's diverticulum	A pulsion diverticulum of the lower hypopharynx or upper esophagus. Tends to collect food, resulting in dysphagia and later regurgitation of rancid materials
Laryngopharyngeal reflux	Reflux of gastric contents to the pharynx and larynx. Soft tissue damage thought to be from pepsin, which is activated by the lowered pH

Extremities: Unremarkable.

Psychiatric: Unremarkable.

PHYSICAL EXAMINATION

Vital signs: T 98.4°F (tympanic) P 104 BP 109/72 R 28.

Ears: Tympanic membranes slightly retracted, opaque, pink, and poorly mobile with pneumatic otoscopy.

Nose: Mucous membranes pink with coating of clear to white mucous. No masses.

Mouth/oropharynx: Tonsils 2+ in size, no inflammation. Hard and soft palates normal to inspection and palpation (no evidence of submucosal cleft palate).

Neck: Scattered palpable lymph nodes from .5 to 1 cm in anterior and posterior triangles.

Chest: Clear to percussion and auscultation.

28

PATHOLOGY (AUTOPSY AND LAB UTILIZATION)

Thomas S. Neuhauser, MD, and Stephen J. Cina, MD

PATHOLOGY (FOCUS ON AUTOPSY AND LAB UTILIZATION)

I. IDENTIFYING DATA

Patient demographics (e.g., age, sex, race, place of residence) and medical and surgical history may be invaluable in the assessment of patient-generated material. This information helps the pathologist or laboratory personnel in guiding the clinician as to the best utilization of laboratory studies and construction of a differential diagnosis.

A. Medical and Surgical History

1. Autopsy and postmortem examination may provide the following information:
   a. Guidance to the prosector on what areas to pay special attention to (e.g., history of cardiovascular disease [CVD], malignancy, infectious disease).
   b. Explanation of anatomic abnormalities (e.g., history of splenectomy, appendectomy, bypass surgery, situs inversus, cardiac conduction abnormalities).

c. Recommendation of additional laboratory studies (e.g., alcohol level in a victim of a motor vehicle accident (MVA), cytogenetic studies for possible congenital disease or suspected hematopoietic disease).
d. Need for more detailed examination of specific areas (e.g., if suspect foul play, look under nails for biologic material, perform careful neck dissection to assess for strangulation).

2. Anatomic pathology (histologic examination of lesions/tumors and body fluids, exfoliative specimens, aspirates [cytology]) requires the following information:
   a. Patient's age: For example, renal tumors in children (Wilm's tumor, sarcoma) versus renal tumors in adults (renal cell carcinoma).
   b. Sex: Incidence of many tumors vary with patient's sex.
   c. Race/ethnicity: Many disease processes are associated with the patient's race (e.g., medullary carcinoma of the renal pelvis more common in African-American patients with sickle trait).
   d. Previous evaluations and surgeries (e.g., patient with bone metastasis with history of prostate cancer).
   e. Location of lesion or biopsy: Different tumors and cells may have an identical histologic appearance (e.g., chondrosarcoma of pelvis and enchondroma of finger, mesothelial cells in pleura, and malignant cells in cerebrospinal fluid [CSF]).
   f. Length of time lesion(s) present: Tumors present for long periods and unchanging in size are more likely to be benign.
   g. Radiologic or diagnostic imaging studies are critical (e.g., in assessment of bony lesions).
   h. Syndromes: For example, angiomyolipoma of the kidney more common in patients with tuberous sclerosis.
   i. Exposure to toxins: For example, patients exposed to thorotrast have an increased incidence of hepatic angiosarcoma.
3. Clinical pathology.
   a. Age.
      (1) Normal components of blood vary depending on age of patient (e.g., 60% lymphocytes is normal for children but abnormal for adults, not uncommon to see nucleated red blood cells [NRBCs] in newborn infants, but always abnormal for adults).
      (2) Incidence of disease processes vary with age (e.g., acute lymphoblastic leukemia [ALL] more common in children and myelodysplastic syndrome [MDS] more common in adults).
   b. Sex: For example, identify potential alloantibodies in women of child-bearing age; normal components in blood vary with sex of patient (e.g., hematocrit higher in men than women).

c. Race/ethnicity: For example, cells of different racial groups share common surface antigens; some abnormalities and antigen profiles more common in specific racial groups (e.g., sickle cell anemia in African-American patients, human leukocyte antigen [HLA] haplotype).
d. Past medical history: For example, important for screening of donors (see blood components section), history of immunodeficiency (e.g., cytomegalovirus [CMV] negative/irradiated products in bone marrow transplant patients), history of infection (may explain coagulation abnormality such as disseminated intravascular coagulation [DIC] or prompt specific studies such as examination of a peripheral smear in patient with possible malaria).
e. Past surgical history: For example, consider pneumococcal sepsis in asplenic patient.
f. Prior transfusions/use of blood products: Assessment for alloantibodies, selection of appropriate products (e.g., IgA-free products in patients with IgA deficiency).
g. Previous evaluations: For example, radiologic studies showing lytic bone lesion may prompt work-up for multiple myeloma.
h. Syndromes may explain findings in blood (e.g., anemia in Fanconi's anemia and congenital dyserythropoietic anemia [CDA]).
i. Exposure to toxins: For example, explain abnormalities/dyspoiesis of red cell precursors in bone marrow examination.
j. Travel history: Travel to foreign country or specific area of the continental United States may prompt investigation for infectious disease processes and assessment for specific organisms (e.g., babesiosis in New England).

B. Medications

1. History of medications may be necessary to interpret laboratory studies (e.g., increased bleeding time may be explained by nonsteroidal antiinflammatory drug [NSAID] use, increased partial thromboplastin time [PTT] may be explained by heparin use, skin lesion/rash may be explained by exposure to certain medications [fixed drug eruption, erythema multiforme]).
2. Therapeutic drug monitoring: For example, drug level will vary depending on how many doses, time from administration to blood draw, peak versus trough concentrations.

C. Health Maintenance

1. Diet: For example, failure to fast before blood draw may affect lipid profile.
2. Exercise: For example, creatine kinase (CK) may increase following rigorous physical activity.

3. Social habits: For example, history of alcohol use may help distinguish alcoholic liver disease from nonalcoholic steatohepatitis, which may have an identical histologic appearance.

D. **Family History:** Many disease processes have a definite inheritance pattern/familial predisposition.

E. **Psychosocial History:** For example, history of promiscuity or sexually transmitted diseases (STDs) may prompt microbiologist to use specific culture media.

II. AUTOPSY OR POSTMORTEM EXAMINATION

A. Uses of Autopsies

1. Cause of death determination and for documenting the presence of concurrent disease.
2. Quality assurance of medical care (e.g., useful for assessing accuracy of clinical diagnosis), medical education, diagnosis of new/rare diseases, detection of environmental hazards, and for assessing adequacy of new imaging techniques and treatment protocols.
3. Can provide useful information to surviving family members (e.g., detection of undiagnosed familial hypercholesterolemia) or to society in general (e.g., identifying a hantavirus, Sin nombre virus outbreak).

B. **Types of Autopsies:** Roughly divided into medical autopsies and forensic (medicolegal) autopsies. Key difference is who can authorize an autopsy.

1. In many jurisdictions, all suspicious deaths, unnatural deaths, child deaths, therapeutic misadventures, and deaths within 24 hours of arrival to an ED must be reported to the local medical examiner, coroner, or justice of the peace.
2. Official may order a forensic autopsy or release the body to the next of kin.
3. A medical autopsy is usually performed at the request of the family or treating physician and requires a written permit for the procedure signed by the legal next of kin (usually the spouse of an adult or parent of a child).
4. Both types of autopsies include a review of all pertinent data (e.g., medical records, investigative report), an external examination, a detailed internal dissection, and adjunctive studies as needed (e.g., cultures, toxicology).
5. The forensic autopsy also seeks to determine the manner of death (natural, accident, suicide, homicide, or undetermined), the mechanism of injury, possible weapons, possible time of death, and positive identification of the decedent (often involves scene investigation and consultation with investigating agencies) (Table 28-1).

Table 28-1. MECHANISMS OF DEATH AND CLASSIC LESIONS.

Mechanism of Death	Classic Lesions	Things To Note
Firearms	Entrance and exit wounds	Soot and powder deposition, lacerated hard-contact entrance wounds mimic exit wounds
Sharp force	Stabs and cuts	Defense wounds, hesitation marks
Blunt force	Abrasions, contusions, lacerations, fractures	Patterned injuries, "bumper fractures" in hit and runs
Asphyxiation	Hanging, strangulation, choking, smothering, carbon monoxide (CO)	Ligature furrow, fingernail scratches on throat, no physical signs in smothering
Sudden infant death syndrome (SIDS)	No anatomic, microscopic, or toxicologic cause of death; found face down in bedding	Thymic petechiae, must have a negative scene investigation and complete autopsy
"Shaken baby" syndrome	Subdural hemorrhage, retinal hemorrhages, diffuse axonal injury, parent reports "a fall"	Many will have an impact site on the back of the head, although not necessary
Child abuse	Multiple fractures of various ages, burns, "failure to thrive"	Rule out osteogenesis imperfecta, metabolic conditions
Intravenous drug abuse (IVDA) overdose	Needle tracks, fresh needle punctures, pulmonary edema	Toxicologic analysis, consider AIDS and hepatitis
Thermal	"Pugilistic attitude," soot in airways if alive during fire	Carbon monoxide (CO) levels, artifactual epidural hematoma common
Rape-homicide	Vaginal/rectal trauma, especially in very young and old victims	Oral, rectal, vaginal swabs for semen, nail clippings, hair samples to police
Decomposition	Bloating of soft tissues, purging of body fluids, green-black discoloration	Do not confuse these postmortem artifacts with premortem trauma

C. Death Certificate (for Additional Guidance, See Death Certification, Chapter 6)

1. The immediate cause of death goes on line 1 of the death certificate.
2. The most important line on the death certificate is the lowest line, where the proximate or underlying cause of death is indicated.
3. Common death certificate errors include nonspecific causes of death (e.g., cardiac arrest) or confusion as to the order of the immediate and proximate cause of death (e.g., coronary artery disease [CAD] due to acute myocardial infarct [AMI]).
4. The manner of death will usually be related to the proximate cause of death (e.g., with "Pulmonary embolus (PE) due to deep venous thrombosis (DVT) due to hip fracture due to unwitnessed fall," the manner of death is accident).
5. If an autopsy is to be performed, it is acceptable to call the cause of death "pending autopsy" and issue an addendum when the final diagnoses have been rendered.

III. LABORATORIES AND STUDIES

A. Histology

1. Fixation: Most tissue received in the anatomic lab is placed in fixative (e.g., formaldehyde) and subsequently processed for examination on glass slides.
2. A myriad of histochemical stains are available for use; however, most cases start with examination of hematoxylin-eosin (H&E) stained sections (Table 28-2).
3. The final diagnosis is based both on what is observed on the slides and on the clinical context of the case (e.g., site of origin/organ system involved, concomitant disease, symptoms, presence/absence of distinct tumor).

Table 28-2. USEFUL HISTOCHEMICAL STAINS.

Stain	Target	Common Uses
Luxol fast blue	Myelin	Highlight deficient nerves (demyelinating diseases)
ATPase (variable pH)	Muscle fibers	Evaluation of muscle disease/weakness
Chloracetate esterase	Myeloid cells	Highlight myeloid precursors (granulocytic sarcoma)
PAS-Alcian blue	Mucins	Highlight acidic mucins (Barrett's metaplasia)
Mucicarmine	Mucins	Highlight mucin (adenocarcinoma)

Continued

Table 28-2. USEFUL HISTOCHEMICAL STAINS—*cont'd*

STAIN	TARGET	COMMON USES
Periodic acid schiff (PAS)	Multiple	Highlight fungal organisms, storage disease processes, glycogen (diastase sensitive), Whipple's disease, α-1-antitrypsin inclusions in liver, basement membrane thickening, some mucins
Trichrome stain	Collagen (blue)	Demonstrate extracellular collagen, muscle
Acetylcholinesterase	Ganglion cells	Hirschprung's disease (frozen tissue)
Reticulin	Reticulin framework and basement membrane material	Highlight fibrosis in liver and bone marrow, basement membrane patterns characteristic of specific tumors, determination if neoplasm is invasive
Perls iron	Iron	Iron stores in liver
Congo red	Amyloid	Highlight amyloid
Fontana-Masson	Melanin	Identify melanin pigment
PTAH	Fibrin	Highlight fibrin, demonstrate cross-striations of skeletal muscle
Warthin-Starry	Organisms	Demonstrate *Spirochetes* and *Rochalimaea* species
Grocott's methenamine silver (GMS)	Organisms	Pneumocystis carinii, fungal elements
Dieterle's	Organisms	Highlight Legionella species
Rhodamine-Auramine	Organisms	Highlight mycobacteria in tissue
Van den Bergh	Bilirubin	Highlight bilirubin
Giemsa	Granules mast cells, certain organisms	Highlight mast cells and some microorganisms in tissue

Table 28-2—cont'd

STAIN	TARGET	COMMON USES
Brown and Brenn	Bacteria	Determination if Gram-positive or Gram-negative organisms in tissue
Ziehl-Neelsen	Acid-fast organisms	Highlight mycobacteria
Von Kossa	Calcium	Demonstrate extracellular calcium
Oil Red O (fresh tissue only)	Lipid	Demonstration of lipid in certain neoplasms
Fite	Mycobacteria	Demonstrate mycobacteria in tissue
Cresyl violet	Helicobacter	Demonstrate organisms on gastric mucosa (usually found in mucin)

4. Histologic examination of neoplastic processes allows for the determination of benignancy versus malignancy, the cell type of origin (e.g., sarcoma, lymphoma, carcinoma, melanoma), and may facilitate a specific diagnosis.
5. Pathologic assessment provides information necessary for staging and treatment (tumor size, status of surgical margins, identification of involved lymph nodes, presence/absence of lymphovascular invasion, assessment for proliferative indices).
6. Use of immunohistochemical stains (labeled antibodies applied against specific cell antigens) may be helpful in identification of tumor type if small biopsy or poorly differentiated (Table 28-3).

Table 28-3. USEFUL IMMUNOHISTOCHEMICAL STAINS.

GENERAL TISSUE CATEGORY	IMMUNOHISTOCHEMICAL STAIN
Epithelial tumors	Cytokeratins, epithelial membrane antigen (EMA), B72.3, carcinoembryonic antigen (CEA), Ber-EP4, calretinin
Neuroendocrine differentiation	Neuron-specific enolase (NSE), CD57 (leu-7), chromogranin, synaptophysin, glial fibrillary acidic protein (GFAP)

Continued

Table 28-3. USEFUL IMMUNOHISTOCHEMICAL STAINS—*cont'd*

General Tissue Category	Immunohistochemical Stain
Mesenchymal tumors (sarcomas)	Vimentin, desmin, CD34, CD31, Factor VIII, actin, muscle specific actin (MSA), smooth muscle actin (SMA), S-100, myoglobin, CD68, lysozyme
Melanoma	S-100, Mart-1, HMB-45
Germ cell tumors	Pancytokeratin, vimentin, alpha fetoprotein (AFP), placental alkaline phosphatase (PLAP), β-human chorionic gonadotropin (β-HCG)
Non-Hodgkin's lymphoma	Pan-B and T-cell markers, kappa and lambda light chains, CD5, CD23, cyclin-D1, bcl-2
Hodgkin lymphoma	CD45RB (leukocyte common antigen), CD15, CD30, latent membrane protein (LMP-1) of Epstein-Barr virus (EBV)
Prognostic markers	Estrogen receptors (ER), progesterone receptors (PR), HER2-neu, p53

7. For a poorly differentiated tumor, initial markers ordered may include pancytokeratin, vimentin, leukocyte common antigen (LCA/CD45RB), and S-100.
8. Intraoperative consultation.
   a. Requested in some cases where information gleaned from immediate pathologic examination of frozen tissue can have immediate management consequences.
   b. Indications generally include determining specimen adequacy (for diagnosis and/or excision), staging malignant neoplasms, and rendering a diagnosis that may change intraoperative management.
   c. Frozen section of tissue allows for immediate microscopic examination, but artifacts created during the freezing can make interpretation difficult and can alter subsequent routine histologic analysis.
   d. Frozen section is discouraged or refused when requested "for interest only."

B. Cytology

1. Cytology is roughly defined as the study of cellular morphology.
2. Specimens are generally obtained by exfoliation (e.g., Papanicolaou [Pap] smear, bronchial wash, bladder wash, brushings) or through fine-needle aspiration (FNA).

3. Specimens are examined for cellular morphology (e.g., cell size and shape, shape and size of nuclei compared to cytoplasm, presence of nucleoli, state of chromatin) as well as cellular relationships (e.g., clusters, papillary formation, presence of blood vessels).
4. Cytology may be used to screen for disease (e.g., yearly Pap smear or assessment of bladder wash in a patient with a history of transitional cell carcinoma), for primary diagnosis of a tumor (e.g., assessment of a thyroid nodule), and in some cases for therapy (e.g., aspiration of a benign fluid-filled cyst of the breast).
5. Although these techniques are minimally invasive and can often provide useful information, biopsy remains the gold standard and may still be necessary.

C. **Electron Microscopy**

1. Electron microscopy (EM) allows for the ultrastructural study of tissue and is used to assess unclassifiable neoplasms (by light microscopy/immunohistochemistry); to clarify poorly differentiated (similar) neoplasms, kidney disease (assessment of glomeruli), metabolic storage diseases, and some infectious disorders (progressive multifocal leukoencephalopathy [PML], herpes simplex virus [HSV], Michaelis-Gutman bodies, and Nocardia); and to identify foreign materials (in tissue).
2. Ideal tissue fixatives are gluteraldehyde and Karnovsky's solution; tissue is subsequently embedded in plastic (epoxy resin).
3. Formalin-fixed tissue can be used; however, the results are suboptimal.

D. **Blood Bank**

1. Blood donation.
   a. Require full name, permanent address, date of birth (age), date of last donation (longer than 8 weeks for whole blood and longer than 48 hours for apheresis).
   b. Permanent deferrals: Viral hepatitis following 11th birthday, high-risk behavior for human immunodeficiency virus (HIV) (or HIV positive), positive for hepatitis B virus (HBV), hepatitis C virus (HCV), and human T lymphotropic virus (HTLV), history of babesiosis, Chaga's disease, tegison ingestion, receive money or drugs for sex.
   c. Three-year deferral: History of malaria or immigrant from endemic country.
   d. Twelve-month deferral: Needle stick, transfusion, travel to country endemic for malaria, receiving hepatitis B immunoglobulin (HBIG), incarcerated more than 72 hours, rabies vaccination.
   e. Six-week deferral: Pregnancy.
   f. Four-week deferral: Rubella/chickenpox vaccine.
   g. Thirty-day deferral: Use of Accutane or Proscar.

PATH

h. Two-week deferral: Measles, mumps, oral polio (MMP) vaccines.
i. Three-day deferral: Nonroutine dental work.
j. Donor must possess the following criteria: Weight 110 lbs. or more, temperature 99.58°F or lower, pulse 50-100 bpm, BP 180/100 or lower, hemoglobin 12.5 (homologous donation) or 11 (autologous donation) or higher, and minimum age 17 years (homologous).

2. Apheresis indications.
   a. Therapeutic hemapheresis (removal of a specific blood component) is useful for hyperviscosity syndromes, hyperleukocytosis (fractional volume >20%, symptomatic patients with white cell count >100,000/uL, blasts >50,000/uL), thrombocythemia (platelet count >1,500,000/uL), hemolytic uremic syndrome/thrombotic thrombocytopenic purpura (HUS/TTP), complications of sickle cell disease (SSDx), post-transfusion purpura, myasthenia gravis, acute Guillain-Barré syndrome, and chronic inflammatory demyelinating polyneuropathy.
   b. Replacement of the product removed depends on the disease process and frequency of the procedure.
   c. Stem cell collection (hematopoietic precursors) and granulocyte collection (infected neutropenic patients).
3. Blood components.
   a. Transfusion of blood products (Table 28-4): Give only what is clinically indicated. Do not "treat numbers" from the lab.
   b. Dosage.
      (1) Dosage will vary depending on clinical situation and response to infusion(s).
      (2) Apheresis product may be better choice if worried about alloimmunization or refractory to transfusion.
      (3) RBCs: *Do not* infuse with lactated Ringer's, 0.45 normal saline, antibiotics, or total parenteral nutrition (TPN). Cells will *lyse*. Use normal saline, ABO-compatible plasma, or 5% albumin.
      (4) Fourth-generation filters remove 99.99% aggregates/white blood cells (WBCs).
      (5) Donor red blood cells (RBCs) should be compatible with recipient plasma.
4. Transfusion reactions.
   a. Transfusion ABO incompatibility results in severe hemolytic transfusion reaction (most cases result from clerical error).
   b. Reactions may manifest as fever, chills, hypotension/shock, disseminated intravascular coagulation (DIC), and pain in infusion site, back, and chest. May also see bleeding, oozing from wounds, hemoglobinuria, and oliguria.

Table 28-4. INDICATIONS AND CONTRAINDICATIONS FOR TRANSFUSIONS OF BLOOD COMPONENTS.

PRODUCT	INDICATIONS	CONTRAINDICATIONS	EXPECTED RESULT
Whole blood	Rapid hemorrhage >30% volume, exchange transfusion in neonates, autologous transfusion	Volume-sensitive patients, chronic anemia (volume), hemorrhage <30%	
Platelets	Thrombocytopenia if <10-20,000 or <50,000 with bleeding thrombocytopathy	TTP, HIT, ITP (relative)	↑ platelet count 5-10,000/mm^3 in 70 kg adult
Leukocyte-reduced platelets	Prevent HLA alloimmunization, febrile transfusion reaction, prevent CMV, prevent immunomodulatory effects of transfusion		
Washed platelets	Same as washed RBCs, repeated febrile reactions	Time consuming; only use if necessary	
Irradiated platelets	Prevention of transfusion associated-graft versus host disease (TA-GVHD)		
RBCs	Volume loss >30%, decreased RBC survival/ production	Hemorrhage <20%, when crystalloid, will serve nutritional deficiency (replace)	↑ Hematocrit 3%/unit, ↑ Hemoglobin 1 gm/dL

Continued

Table 28-4. INDICATIONS AND CONTRAINDICATIONS FOR TRANSFUSIONS OF BLOOD COMPONENTS—*cont'd*

Product	Indications	Contraindications	Expected Result
Apheresis platelets	Limit exposure to donors, refractory to platelet transfusion		Same as a "six-pack" of platelets
Washed RBCs	IgA-deficient patients, anaphylactic-like reactions to plasma proteins, repeated febrile transfusion reactions, out of ABO-group transfusion, infants	Does not prevent GVHD	
Frozen RBCs	Storage rare RBC units, hypersensitivity to plasma proteins, repeated febrile transfusion reactions		
Leukocyte-reduced RBCs	Same as leukocyte-reduced platelets	Does not prevent GVHD, prevention of transfusion-related acute lung injury (TRALI)	
Irradiated RBCs	Transfusion associated GVHD, bone marrow failure, immunosuppression, neonatal transfusion, transfusion from 1st degree relative	Stem cell infusion, prevention of CMV (use CMV-negative products or filter)	

Granulocytes	Neutropenia, fever, *and* reversible bone marrow hypoplasia	Prophylaxis, nonbacterial infection, advanced malignancy	
Fresh frozen plasma (FFP)	Coagulopathy caused by multiple factor decrease, reverse warfarin effect, dilutional coagulopathy, replacement apheresis for TTP, antithrombin III deficiency	Volume expansion (use crystalloids), factor ↓ when specific product available	Each unit ↑ factor level 20-30%, see ↓ PT/PTT
Cryoprecipitate	Low fibrinogen, treatment von Willebrand's disease/hemophilia A, bleeding uremic patients, factor XIII deficiency, topical glue		
Factor concentrates	FVIII/severe hemophilia A, FIX/hemophilia B		
DDAVP (synthetic ADH)	Release FVIII:vWF, uremic thrombocytopathy, mild hemophilia A, von Willebrand's except IIb/III, hepatic failure	Decreased effectiveness with repeated use	Increase vWF and FVIII

TTP = thrombotic thrombocytopenic purpura; ITP = idiopathic thrombocytopenia; HIT = heparin-induced thrombocytopenia; TA = transfusion associated; GVHD = graft versus host disease; F = factor; vWF = von Willebrand's factor; TRALI = transfusion-related acute lung injury (noncardiogenic pulmonary edema); Neg = negative.

c. Need to stop transfusion and check all paperwork. If concerned about hemolytic transfusion reaction, examine serum for hemolysis (pink color), do complete blood count (CBC), direct antiglobulin test (DAT), bilirubin, urinalysis, disseminated intravascular coagulation DIC panel, and examine peripheral smear for red cell fragments (schistocytes).

d. Unused blood should be returned to the blood bank. Culture of product bags should be performed if there is a concern of infection/bacterial contamination.

e. Delayed hemolytic reactions with fever may occur with Kidd, Duffy, and Kell blood groups and may be apparent only by laboratory studies (increased bilirubin). Blood bank should be alerted to work up blood for alloantibodies.

f. Febrile nonhemolytic reaction (most common) is a diagnosis of exclusion. Need to exclude hemolytic reaction. Transfusion should be suspended pending evaluation.

g. Additional transfusion reactions.
   (1) Urticarial reaction: Sensitivity to plasma proteins.
   (2) Anaphylactic reaction: IgA deficiency.
   (3) TRALI (transfusion-associated lung injury): Likely secondary interaction of patient WBCs and donor antibodies or vice versa.
   (4) Post-transfusion purpura (delayed, anti-PL^{A1} antibodies).

h. Other considerations of transfusion include iron overload (repeated transfusions), potassium overload (renal patients), citrate toxicity/hypocalcemia (patients with renal/liver disease), and air embolism.

5. Transfusion of products (Table 28-5).

Table 28-5. TRANSFUSION OF RED BLOOD CELLS (RBCS).

	Donor ABO Type			
Recipient ABO Type	A	B	AB	O
A	X			X
B		X		X
AB	X	X	X	X
O				X

a. Fresh frozen plasma (FFP): Infuse 2 units at a time in adult, 10-15 mL/kg neonate.

b. Donor FFP should be compatible with recipient RBCs (Table 28-6).

Table 28-6. TRANSFUSION OF FRESH FROZEN PLASMA (FFP).

	Donor ABO Type			
Recipient ABO Type	**A**	**B**	**AB**	**O**
A	X		X	
B		X	X	
AB			X	
O	X	X	X	X

c. Calculations (ex: FVIII) plasma volume = (Patient kg × 70 mL/kg)(1-hematocrit).
   (1) Calculate VIII needed by multiplying plasma volume × % desired activity increase (usually want 50 %).
   (2) Answer: 80 units FVIII/bag gives number of bags.
d. Calculate other factors the same way, except use amount on bag rather than 80.

6. Hemolytic disease of the newborn (HDN).
   a. Most common cause in the United States is ABO^- related and is generally mild.
   b. May occur with first as well as later pregnancy, and most commonly occurs in type O mothers with type A or B babies.
   c. DAT may be positive or negative, and antibody screen negative.
   d. Most severe form of HDN is Rh incompatibility, with Rh-negative moms and Rh-positive babies. DAT positive, antibody screen positive with anti-D, indirect bilirubin positive.
      (1) One full dose (300 mg/vial) Rhogam given to mother protects against 30 mL Rh-positive blood. Kleihauer-Betke determines amount of Rh-positive contamination.
      (2) Calculation: KB % × blood volume = baby volume.
      (3) Baby volume/30 = vials needed. Round up to whole number (example, if determine 2.5 vials are needed, give 3).
   e. HDN may also be seen with Kidd (mild), Duffy (severe), and Kell (severe) blood groups.
7. Parentage testing.
   a. Direct exclusion if child has antigen that could not have come from either parent.
   b. Indirect exclusion if child does not have antigen that he or she should have inherited from a parent.
8. Testing recipient blood.
   a. Specimen required every 3 days if transfusion/pregnancy in last 3 months.

b. Type and screen (T&S) includes records check, ABO/Rh testing, antibody screen (need to antibody identify if a positive screen).
c. Type and cross (T&C) includes everything in T&S plus cross-match between recipient specimen and donor unit.

9. Testing donor blood type (ABO/Rh), HbsAg, anti-HCV, reactive plasma reagin (RPR), anti-HTLV I/II, HIV I/II.

E. Molecular Diagnostics

1. Neoplasia: Hematopoietic disorders.
   a. Examine for immunoglobulin heavy chain (IgH) and light chain (kappa and lambda) rearrangements for B-cell malignancies and T-cell receptors (TCRs) for T-cell malignancies.
   b. Sensitivity and specificity varies between labs as well as between tumors.
   c. Specificity is not 100%. Occasional B-cell neoplasms show rearrangement of TCRs, and rare T-cell neoplasms show rearrangement of IgH.
   d. Rearrangement may rarely be identified in reactive processes. Correlation with clinical history and findings and laboratory studies is mandatory.
   e. It is possible to assess solid-tissue tumors for chromosomal abnormalities associated with those disease processes. This is of invaluable assistance in those cases with a similar clinical history and appearance.
      (1) Breast cancer: Can assess for HER-2/*neu* gene amplification and presence for BRCA-1 and 2 genes.
      (2) Cervical cancer: Can confirm the presence of human papilloma virus (HPV) and determine the type(s).
      (3) Colon cancer: Can assess for the presence of K-*ras*, MCC, DCC, p53.
      (4) Neuroblastoma: n-*myc* amplification helps define the stage of disease.
2. Assessment for microorganisms: Viruses, bacteria, pathogenic fungi, and protozoa.
3. Evaluation for genetic disorders.
4. Transplantation can be used for DNA matching for organ transplant and may play a role in bone marrow transplantation.
5. DNA fingerprinting.
6. Paternity testing and forensics.

F. Chemistry

1. Plasma proteins.
   a. Many plasma proteins increase or decrease during inflammatory conditions. Some increase (positive acute phase reactants [APRs]) and some decrease (negative APRs).
      (1) Positive APRs: α1-chymotrypsin, α1-antichymotrypsin, haptoglobin, ceruloplasmin, fibrinogen, C3, C-reactive protein (CRP), hemopexin.
      (2) Negative APRs: Prealbumin, albumin, retinol-binding protein (RBP), transferrin (initially decreases; later increases).

   b. Plasma proteins migrate to distinct areas when placed in a solid medium (agarose gel); an electric current is applied, and subsequent densiometry scan of the gel yields a curve with five distinct regions.
   c. A monoclonal protein (M-spike) may be seen with various hematopoietic disease processes and appears as a distinct peak in the β or γ region.
2. Liver disease, cardiac disease, hematologic disease, renal disease, endocrinology (see Gastrointestinal, Cardiac, Hematology, Nephrology, and Endocrinology Chapters, respectively).
3. Pancreatic disease.
   a. Amylase and lipase are useful in evaluation of patients with pancreatic diseases.
   b. Clinical sensitivity for both is approximately 90%.
   c. False-negative results occur in patients with recurrent attacks and with little pancreatic tissue.
4. Tumor markers: Substances found in the serum associated with malignancy.
   a. Markers may be used for screening, confirmation, monitoring response to therapy, predicting disease course (prognosis), and detecting recurrence (Table 28-7).
   b. Measuring multiple markers for some disease processes may yield increased specificity.
   c. Markers other than those found in serum (e.g., molecular markers BRAC-1 and 2 genes for breast cancer, and urine markers VMA/HVA, 5-HIAA, and calcitonin for neuroendocrine tumors, carcinoid of the GI tract, and medullary thyroid carcinoma, respectively) are also useful.
5. Lipids.
   a. Specimens should be collected following 12 to 14 hours fasting. Patient should be in a sitting position, and a tourniquet should be used less than 2 minutes.
   b. Finger sticks are used in some situations; however, they may underestimate true levels.
   c. Cholesterol may be broken down into high-density lipoproteins (HDLs), chylomicrons, low-density lipoproteins (LDLs), and very low-density lipoproteins (VLDLs).
   d. Levels of these components comprise the Fredrickson-Levy classification of hyperlipidemias. Total cholesterol = VLDL (Triglycerides/5) + LDL + HDL.
   e. Cholesterol is increased with familial hypercholesterolemias, diabetes mellitus (DM), pancreatitis, hypothyroidism, biliary obstruction, liver disease, high-cholesterol diet, nephrotic syndrome, alcohol use, pregnancy (secondary to estrogen effect), and gout.
6. Electrolytes and acid-base balance (Table 28-8).
   a. Acid-base (intake/output of hydrogen ions) is regulated by plasma (bicarbonate, proteins, inorganic phosphorous),

Table 28-7. SELECTED CLINICALLY USEFUL SERUM TUMOR MARKERS (ALSO SEE ONCOLOGY).

Marker	Normal Expression	Association	Sensitivity	Limitations
CA 125	Body cavity epithelium	Ovarian cancer	>35 U 80% Cases	↑ 66% patients with nonneoplastic disease
CEA	GI Tract	GI, liver, pancreatic, malignancies	>3.0 ng/mL 41-59% cases	Also ↑ 14-21% benign diseases of GI tract
CA27.29		Breast cancer		
CA15.3		Breast cancer		
CA19-9	Lewis^{ab} Blood Group Antigen	Pancreatic cancer	>37 U/mL 72-100% cases	↑ Liver malignancies (76%), GI tract malignancy (19%), and some cases of pancreatitis
βHCG	Placenta	Persistent elevation GTD, nonseminomatous GCT (70%)	>8000 ng/mL GTD >21 days after delivery	↑ Normal pregnancies, assessment for possible tubal pregnancy
AFP	Fetal liver, yolk sac, and GI tract	Hepatocellular cancer (72%), pancreatic cancer (23%), testes teratocarcinoma (75%)	>40 ng/mL	↑ in some benign liver diseases
PSA	Prostate	Prostate cancer	Variable; % free PSA when total 4-10 ng/mL	Found normally in serum and level varies with age

CEA = carcinoembryonic antigen; GI = gastrointestinal; HCG = human chorionic gonadotropin; GTD = gestational trophoblastic disease; GCT = germ cell tumor; AFP = alpha-fetoprotein; PSA = prostate-specific antigen.

Table 28-8. LABORATORY FINDINGS IN ACIDOSIS AND ALKALOSIS.

CONDITION	PH	PCO_2	HCO_3	COMPENSATORY RESPONSE
Metabolic acidosis	↓		↓	pCO_2 ↓ 1.2 mmHg for each ↓ 1.0 mEq/L HCO_3
Respiratory acidosis	↓	↑		HCO_3 ↑ 1 mEq/L each ↑ 10 mmHg pCO_2
Metabolic alkalosis	↑		↑	pCO_2 ↑ 0.4-0.7 mmHg for each ↑ 1.0 mEq/l HCO_3
Respiratory alkalosis	↑	↓		HCO_3 ↓ 5 mEq/L each ↓ 10 mmHg pCO_2

mmHg = millimeters of mercury; mEq = milliequivalents.

RBCs (bicarbonate, proteins, inorganic phosphates, hemoglobin), renal hydrogen excretion (weak acids), and renal reabsorption of bicarbonate.

b. pH = pK + log (base/acid) or 6.1 + log (HCO_3/pCO_2).

c. Acidosis is defined as pH < 7.35 and alkalosis as pH > 7.45.

7. Therapeutic drug monitoring.

a. Ideal candidates for monitoring are those with narrow therapeutic index ranges.

b. Levels may be ordered for subtherapeutic response, suspected toxicity, concomitant use of interacting drug, high-risk patients, and "routine" level.

c. Ideal to assess compliance.

d. V_d = amount of drug in body/C_p = $V_p + V_t \times f_p/f_t$, where V_d = volume distribution, C_p = plasma drug concentration, V_p = plasma volume, V_t = tissue volume, f_p/f_t = fraction unbound drug in plasma/tissue.

e. Rate of elimination = Cl × C_p, where Cl = clearance.

f. $t_{1/2}$ (time for drug to decrease to 1/2 its level) = 0.693/k_1 where k_1 = Cl/V_d. This assumes first-order kinetics, where plasma concentration proportional to dose.

g. Dose = ($C_p \times V_d$)/f, where f = bioavailability.

h. Levels of drugs are influenced by changes in physiology (e.g., poor clearance, changes in rate of metabolism, hepatic/renal disease), drug-drug interactions, and very high doses.

i. Approximately five half-lives is necessary to reach steady state; samples collected too soon will give misleading information. Ideally, lab reports should include dose, date, and time specimen submitted for meaningful interpretation.

j. Drugs with known therapeutic levels include antiarrhythmics (lidocaine, procainamide, quinidine, disopyramide, tocainide, mexiletine, propafenone, amiodarone, digoxin, verapamil), antibiotics (aminoglycosides, vancomycin, chloramphenicol, sulfonamides), antidepressants (amitriptyline, nortriptyline, imipramine, desipramine, trazodone, fluoxetine, lithium), antiepileptics (phenobarbitol, phenytoin, carbamazepine, primidone, valproic acid, ethosuximide, benzodiazapines, diazepam, clonazepam), bronchodilators (theophylline, caffeine), and immunosuppressants (e.g., cyclosporine, FK 506).

k. Quantitative levels are most commonly performed for acetominophen, alcohols, salicylates, barbiturates, phenytoin, theophylline, lithium, digoxin, cyclosporine, FK506, and aminoglycosides.

l. The dosage of some drugs depends on renal function (such as aminoglycosides). Both peak and trough levels may be ordered; troughs are generally drawn just before the next dose.

8. Toxicology testing assists in the diagnosis and treatment of poisonings and documentation and management of drug dependency.
   a. Tests may be qualitative or quantitative.
   b. A basic toxicology service characteristically includes ethanol, salicylates, acetominophen, barbiturates, ethanol, tricyclics, serum iron, total iron-binding capacity (TIBC), carboxyhemoglobin, methemoglobin; additional drugs reflect local prevalence (e.g., cocaine, marijuana, opiates, benzodiazapines, phenothyazine, sedative-hypnotics).
   c. Nomograms have been developed for salicylates and acetominophen.
   d. Specimens frequently submitted include urine, serum (blood), and gastric fluid.
   e. Screens are most frequently performed on urine; however, they may be complicated by metabolites.
   f. Quantitative tests require more time to perform and should not be done unless the level is important for patient management.
   g. Positive results trigger performance of confirmatory tests, and serum quantitation for alcohol is required. For tests with legal consequences, a strict chain of custody must be followed (must be able to answer what, who, and when).
9. Immunology (also see Chapter 7, Allergy and Immunology).
   a. Human leukocyte antigen (HLA) system.
      (1) Class I: HLA-A, B, and C on all nucleated cells and platelets. Certain haplotypes associated with certain autoimmune diseases.
      (2) Class II: HLA-DR, DP, and DQ on antigen-presenting cells (monocytes, macrophages, interdigitating/dendritic reticulum cells, activated T and B-cells). Autosomal codominant: Siblings have a 1 in 4 chance of being HLA identical.
      (3) Class III: Certain complement proteins and some cytokines.
      (4) HLA matching improves survival of transplanted kidneys, hearts, and lungs. ABO (blood group) and HLA compatibility of the donor and results of lymphocytotoxicity crossmatch between patient serum and donor cells are used to assess suitability of potential candidate for donation, when organs become available.
   b. Autoimmune diseases: Many autoimmune disease processes are associated with antibodies directed against "self" antigens/antinuclear antibodies (ANAs) because of break down in self-tolerance. ANAs should not be ordered for random screening because they are associated with a large number of disease processes and are found in a significant number of healthy people.

c. Cryoglobulins: Serum immunoglobulins that precipitate in cold conditions and are categorized into three types:
   (1) Type I: Single monoclonal immunoglobulin, associated with lymphoid malignancies.
   (2) Type II: Monoclonal immunoglobulin with activity against a polyclonal immunoglobulin with rheumatoid factor activity (present as circulating immune complexes), associated with lymphoid malignancies, macroglobulinemia, rheumatoid arthritis, Sjogren's, and hepatitis C.
   (3) Type III: Mixed polyclonal immunoglobulins with rheumatoid factor activity (present as circulating immune complexes), associated with autoimmune disease, infectious mononucleosis (IM), CMV, viral and chronic hepatitis, primary biliary cirrhosis (PBC), post-streptococcal glomerulonephritis, infective endocarditis, leprosy, kala-azar, and tropical splenomegaly syndrome. Blood must be collected in warm syringe and kept at 37°C until it clots (see directions for each individual lab).

d. Flow cytometry studies the antigenic composition of cells.
   (1) Most frequently utilized in the assessment of hematopoietic disease processes.
   (2) Additional uses include assessment of CD4+ (helper T) cells (HIV patients), progenitor cell counts in stem cell collections, reticulocyte counts in anemias, and assessment of CD4/CD8 ratios.
   (3) DNA may also be examined for ploidy (DNA content), which has prognostic significance for some tumors, and is essential for assessment of molar pregnancies.

e. Erythrocyte sedimentation rate (ESR) is increased in most chronic inflammatory disease processes, including temporal arteritis.

G. Specimen and Venipuncture Tube Collection (Tables 28-9 and 28-10)

Table 28-9. SPECIMEN COLLECTION.

SPECIMEN	INDICATIONS	LOCATION/METHOD
Arterial blood	Oxygen, carbon dioxide (P_{CO_2}), pH	Brachial, radial, femoral arteries
Venous blood	Serum analytes, culture	Extremity veins
Skin puncture	Pediatric patients (infants), some geriatric patients with poor access	Finger, ear lobe

Table 28-9—cont'd

SPECIMEN	INDICATIONS	LOCATION/METHOD
Urine	Chemical analysis, bacteriologic culture, microscopic examination	Clean catch, catheter collection
Body fluids (e.g., CSF, thoracentesis)	Assess for neoplasia, transudate vs. exudate, bacteriologic culture	Collect sterile; method dependent on body site
Pap smear	Screening study for cervical neoplasia/ viral cytopathic effect	Dependent on system used
Tissue	Tumor type, disease status, staging, assess neoplasia/infection (culture)	Bring fresh to lab; send portion sterile to microbiology if considering infection
Semen	Counts, morphology, directional movement (infertility work-up)	Ejaculate

Note, many urine studies require 24-hour collection and may require specific preservatives.

Table 28-10. VENIPUNCTURE TUBE COLLECTION.

TUBE	LABORATORY STUDIES
Red top	Blood bank studies, most chemistries/ immunologic studies, haptoglobin, LE preparation, serum viscosity
Green top (Na Heparin)	Ammonia (ice), carboxyhemoglobin, cholinesterase, erythrocyte K^+, methemoglobin, pH, plasma hemoglobin
Gray top (NaF Oxalate)	Glucose tolerance, lactate (on ice), lactose intolerance
Lavender top (EDTA)	CBC, CEA, PB, renin (on ice), ESR, reticulocyte count, sickle cell preparation, eosinophil count, flow cytometric studies
Blue top (Na Citrate)	Coagulation studies, G-6-PD assay
Green top (Na Heparin)	Nitroblue tetrazolium, phagocytosis

LE = lupus erythematosis; CBC = complete blood count; CEA = carcinoembryonic antigen; ESR = erythrocyte sedimentation rate; G-6-PD = glucose-6-phosphate deficiency.

IV. ACRONYMS AND ABBREVIATIONS (TABLE 28-11)

Table 28-11. PATHOLOGY ACRONYMS AND ABBREVIATIONS.

Acronym or Abbreviation	Term	Acronym or Abbreviation	Term
ACA	Anticardiolipin antibody	HPV	Human papilloma virus
ACTH	Adrenocorticotropic hormone	HTLV	Human T-cell leukemia virus
AFP	Alpha-fetoprotein	HUS	Hemolytic uremic syndrome
ALL	Acute lymphocytic leukemia	Ig	Immunoglobulin
ALT	Alanine aminotransferase	IgH	Immunoglobulin heavy chain
AML	Acute myelogenous leukemia	ITP	Idiopathic thrombocytopenic purpura
APR	Acute phase reactant	IVDA	Intravenous drug abuse
AST	Aspartate aminotransferase	LA	Lupus anticoagulant
BUN	Blood urea nitrogen	LDH	Lactate dehydrogenase
CBC	Complete blood count	LDL	Low density lipoprotein
CD	Cluster of differentiation	LH	Leutinizing hormone
CGD	Chronic granulomatous disease	LMP	Latent membrane protein
CGL	Chronic granulocytic leukemia	MCH	Mean corpuscular hemoglobin
CK	Creatine kinase	MCHC	Mean corpuscular hemoglobin concentration
CML	Chronic myelogenous leukemia	MCV	Mean corpuscular volume
CMV	Cytomegalovirus	MDS	Myelodysplastic syndrome
CO	Carbon monoxide	MSA	Muscle specific antigen
CRP	C-reactive protein	NRBC	Nucleated red blood cell
CSF	Cerebrospinal fluid	NSE	Neuron specific enolase

DAT	Direct antiglobulin test	**PDW**	Platelet distribution width
DIC	Disseminated intravascular coagulation	**PLAP**	Placental alkaline phosphatase
dRVVT	Dilute Russell viper venom time	**PNH**	Paroxysmal nocturnal hemoglobinuria
DVT	Deep venous thrombosis	**PRBCs**	Packed red blood cells
EBL	Estimated blood loss	**PSA**	Prostate specific antigen
EM	Electron microscopy	**PT**	Prothrombin time
EMA	Epithelial membrane antigen	**PTH**	Parathyroid hormone
ESR	Erythrocyte sedimentation rate	**PTT**	Partial thromboplastin time
FFP	Fresh frozen plasma	**RBCs**	Red blood cells
FNA	Fine needle aspiration	**RDW**	Red (cell) distribution width
FSH	Follicle stimulating hormone	**SPEP**	Serum protein electrophoresis
GFAP	Glial fibrillary acidic protein	**TA**	Transfusion associated
GVHD	Graft versus host disease	**T&C**	Type and cross
HAV	Hepatitis A virus	**TCR**	T-cell receptor
HBV	Hepatitis B virus	**T&H**	Type and hold
HCG	Human chorionic gonadotropin	**TRALI**	Transfusion-related acute lung injury
HCL	Hairy cell leukemia	**TRAP**	Tartrate resistant alkaline phosphatase
HCT	Hematocrit	**T&S**	Type and screen
HCV	Hepatitis C virus	**TSH**	Thyroid stimulating hormone
HDL	High density lipoprotein	**TT**	Thrombin time
HDN	Hemolytic disease of the newborn	**TTP**	Thrombotic thrombocytopenic purpura
Hgb	Hemoglobin	**VLDL**	Very low density lipoprotein
HIT	Heparin induced thrombocytopenia	**vWF**	von Willebrand's factor
HIV	Human immunodeficiency virus	**WBCs**	White blood cells
HLA	Human leukocyte antigen		

V. DEFINITIONS (TABLE 28-12)

Table 28-12. PATHOLOGY TERMS.

Term	Definition
Allogenic	In bone marrow transplantation, denotes tissues of the same species
Apheresis	Procedure in which blood is removed and then returned to the patient, and a component is removed in the process
Autologous	Relating to self; used in context of blood bank (return packed cells drawn from patient in preparation for surgery) and bone marrow transplant (return stem cells collected from patient following chemotherapy)
Carcinoma	Malignancy originating from epithelial tissue
Cluster of differentiation (CD)	Refers to antigens of surface of blood cells; used to differentiate normal white cells and subclassify hematopoietic malignancies
Dysplasia	Abnormality of development; in pathology refers to alteration in cellular size, shape, and organization and may represent a precursor to invasive malignancy
Dyspoiesis	Abnormal development of hematopoietic precursors; may be reactive or a manifestation of neoplasia
Forensic	Pertaining to legal proceeding (e.g., forensic postmortem examination of a murder victim)
Immunohistochemical	Special stains or studies used to determine cellular characteristics and origin
Kleihauer-Betke	Test used to assess for fetal hemoglobin in red cells; used in pathology to assess presence of fetal blood in pregnant patients (e.g., status postmotor vehicle accident [MVA], following delivery of a child with mismatched Rh antigen)
Oncogene	Gene found in chromosomes of tumor cells, associated with development of malignancy

Table 28-12—cont'd

Term	Definition
Plasma	Fluid portion of blood in which particulate components are suspended
Poorly differentiated tumor	The cell of origin/type of malignancy is not obvious based solely on morphologic assessment; frequently need assistance of additional studies
Rearrangement	In pathology, refers to realignment of chromosomes of heavy and light chains during development of lymphocytes; demonstration of a single rearrangement of B or T-cells in a lymphoid tumor suggests neoplasia
Sarcoma	Malignancy originating from mesenchymal tissue
Serum	The clear liquid that separates from blood upon clotting
Therapeutic misadventure	Death or injury occurring as a direct result of a medical intervention

29

PEDIATRICS

Christine Johnson, MD, Woodson Scott Jones, MD, and Eric H. Hanson, MD, MPH

I. CHIEF COMPLAINT

A. Chief Complaint

1. Succinctly determine the reason for the visit (in patient's or parents' own words, if possible) and the source of referral, if applicable.
2. Age, sex, and underlying conditions.

B. Identifying Data/Source

1. The history should be obtained from the parent or primary caregiver, and from the child when possible. Regardless of who gives the history, the informant should be identified and the reliability of the information should be documented.
2. Adolescents should be interviewed in private, if acceptable to the parent and the child.

II. HISTORY OF PRESENT ILLNESS

A. History of Present Illness

1. Delineate pertinent signs and symptoms in chronologic order.
2. Include any associated signs and symptoms, including pertinent positives and negatives.
3. Include pertinent past history and therapies.

B. Complaint Details: For each complaint, include onset, severity, duration, frequency, location, distribution, radiation, alleviating and exacerbating factors, current treatments/medications, and remedies.

III. PAST MEDICAL AND SURGICAL HISTORY

A. Past Medical History

1. Hospitalizations: Record reason for admission, age at admission or date of admission, findings, length of stay, and disposition.
2. Ask about any frequent or recurring infections (e.g., otitis media, sinusitis, pneumonia, urinary tract infections).
3. Inquire about chronic illnesses (e.g., asthma, eczema, neoplastic disease, genetic disorder, behavioral disorder).

B. Birth History

1. Prenatal: Mother's health during pregnancy, age at delivery, diet, use of tobacco, ethanol, or illicit drugs, infectious disease (e.g., hepatitis B virus [HBV], HIV, group B streptococcus [GBS] status) or other illnesses, pregnancy-associated complications (e.g., preeclampsia), maternal medications.

2. Birth history: Duration of pregnancy and labor, presentation, type of delivery (e.g., spontaneous, forceps-assisted, or Cesarean section), complications with delivery, APGAR scores, and birth weight.
3. Neonatal.
    a. Inquire about illnesses or congenital abnormalities noted at birth, especially cardiopulmonary and neurologic abnormalities, jaundice, and infections.
    b. Note the level of care provided to the neonate (i.e., term nursery versus Neonatal Intensive Care Unit [NICU], any resuscitation provided, procedures or interventions needed).
    c. Note the length of hospital stay and discharge weight.

C. **Growth and Development**

1. Review growth charts for weight, height, and head circumference (if 3 years or younger), and note any deviation from expected. Compare growth with that of family members (see Figs. 29-1, 29-2, and 29-3 for National Center for Health Statistics [NCHS] Growth Charts).
2. Use a standardized developmental screening test (e.g., DENVER II; see Box 29-1) to assess achievement of developmental milestones. Note age of achievement of major milestones (e.g., "rolled-over," "walking").
3. Describe urinary and bowel habits.
4. Address school performance and any issues brought to the parent's attention by teachers.
5. Address social skills and behavior.

D. **Surgical History:** Record type of surgery and reason, age at time of operation, any complications, and occurrence of excessive bleeding. Include minor surgical procedures such as circumcision and/or dental extractions.

E. **Emergency and Trauma History**

1. Obtain information about any accidents and/or injuries (e.g., burns, fractures, toxic ingestions, head injuries).
2. Be cognizant of any unusual injuries, not explained by the HPI that might suggest nonaccidental trauma or child abuse/neglect.

F. **Travel History:** Inquire about any recent travel (e.g., camping, out of the country).

G. **Human, Animal, and Insect Exposure History:** Inquire about day care, other care providers' health, pets, and infestations in house, yard, or school.

IV. **MEDICATIONS, ALLERGIES, AND ADVERSE REACTIONS**

A. **Medications**

1. Document the use of prescription drugs, indications for usage, type and duration of use, and specific dosing.
2. Document the use of over-the-counter (OTC) medications and home remedies or alternative therapies. Include specifics

Box 29-1. DENVER DEVELOPMENTAL SCREENING TEST.

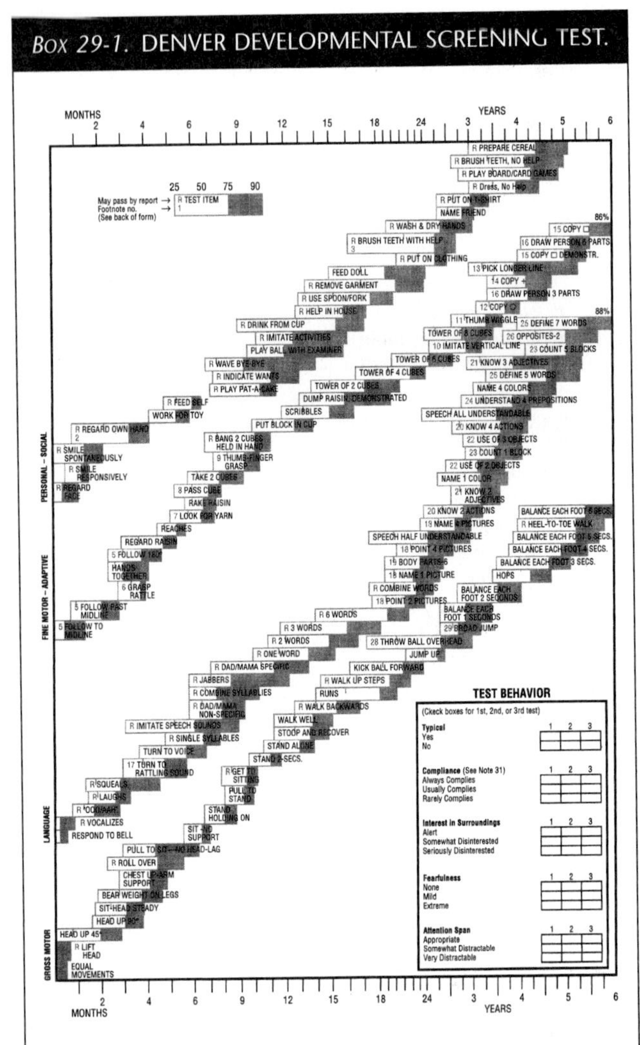

The Denver II is a standardized screen for children 0-6 years of age. Social, fine-motor, language, and gross-motor development are all assessed with the screen. To interpret the results appropriately, preestablished, specific methods for administering the test must be followed. This screening tool helps identify children who may have developmental delays. Re-screen in one to two weeks to

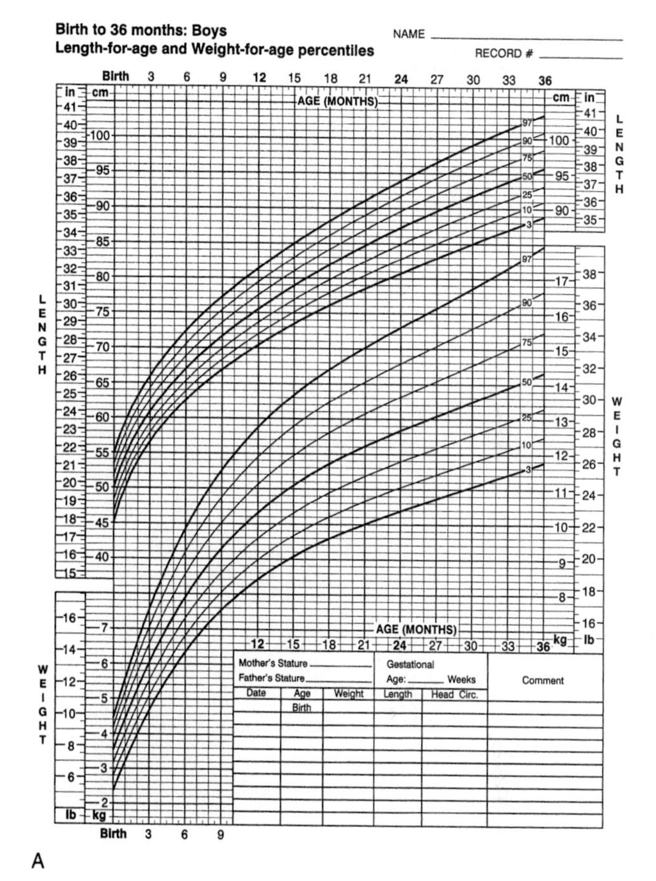

A

Figure 29-1. Growth Charts for Males 0 to 36 months of age. **A.** Boys' length-for-age and weight-for-age percentiles.

Continued

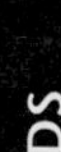

rule out temporary factors such as fatigue, fear or illness is recommended. Subsequent referral for more definitive developmental testing should follow for children with "suspect" Denver II screens. The screening test reports the percentage (25-90%) of children who successfully perform a specific task.

Reproduced with permission from Frankenburg WK, et al. Denver Developmental Screening Test (Denver II), Denver Developmental Materials, Inc. Denver, 1992.

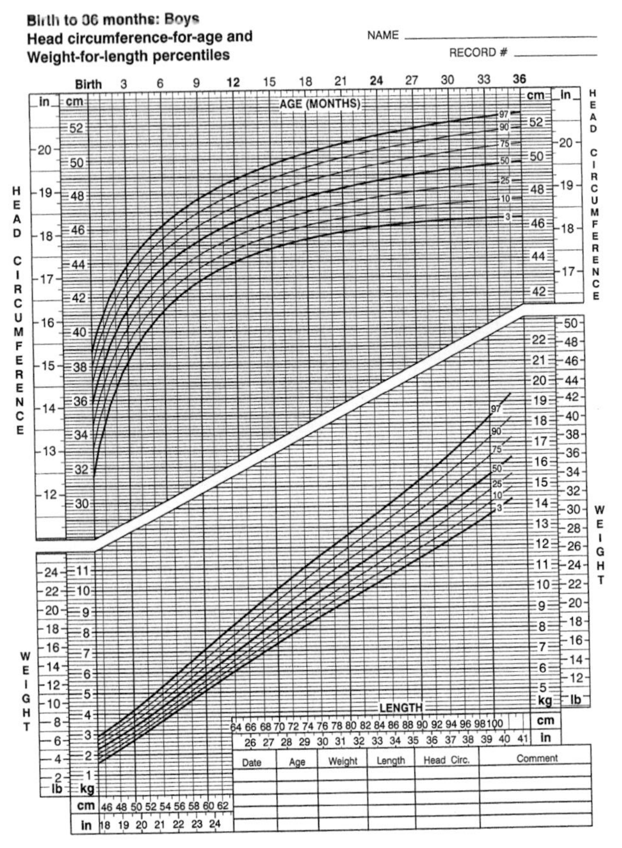

B

Figure 29-1. *cont'd.* **B.** Boys' head circumference-for-age and weight-for-length percentiles. (Source: Centers for Disease Control and Prevention. National Center for Health Statistics. Hyatsville, MD, 2002.)

regarding dosing, indications for usage, type and duration of use, specific dosing, effectiveness, and side effects).

B. Allergies

1. Document any previous reactions to medications or foods, elucidating allergic versus adverse reactions.
2. Document any environmental allergies (e.g., venomous insects, animals, grass, pollen, dust).

V. HEALTH MAINTAINANCE

A. Prevention

1. Immunizations (Figure 29-4): The Recommended Childhood Immunization Schedule is updated yearly by the Centers of

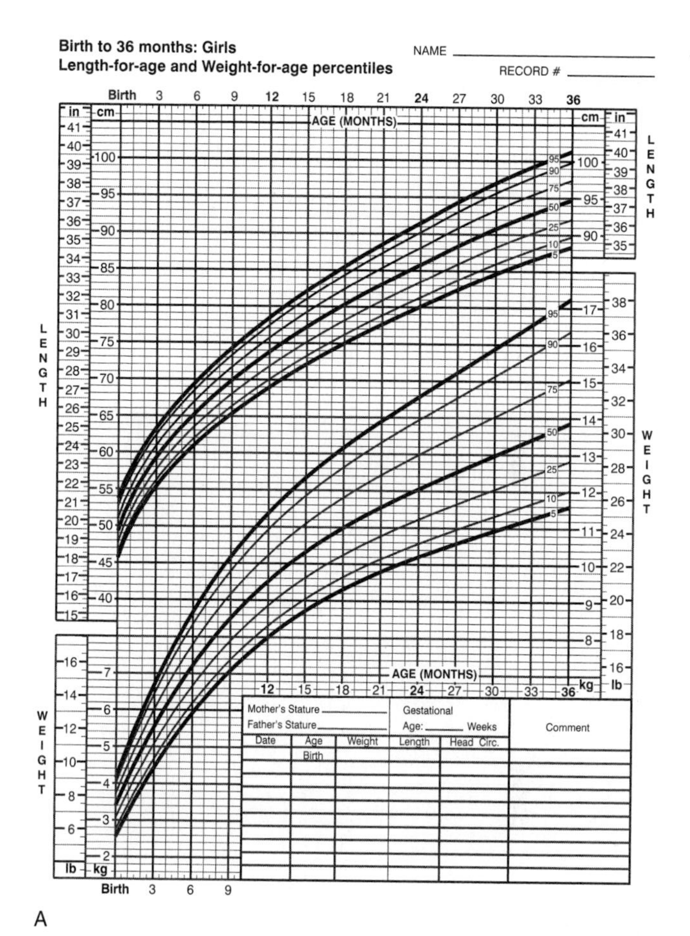

A

Figure 29-2. Growth charts for females 0 to 36 months of age. **A.** Girls' length-for-age and weight-for-age percentiles.

Continued

Disease Control and Prevention (CDC), along with input and approval of other professional organizations.

2. Injury prevention and safety counseling. Include age-appropriate discussion of:
   a. Travel: Car seat appropriate for age/weight. Note: Car seat legislation may vary from state to state. See National Highway Traffic Safety Administration Site for general guidelines (www.nhtsa.dot.gov/people/injury/childps/).
   b. Childproof home: Inquire about and discuss exposure to poisons, electric outlets, stairs, small objects, stove, and

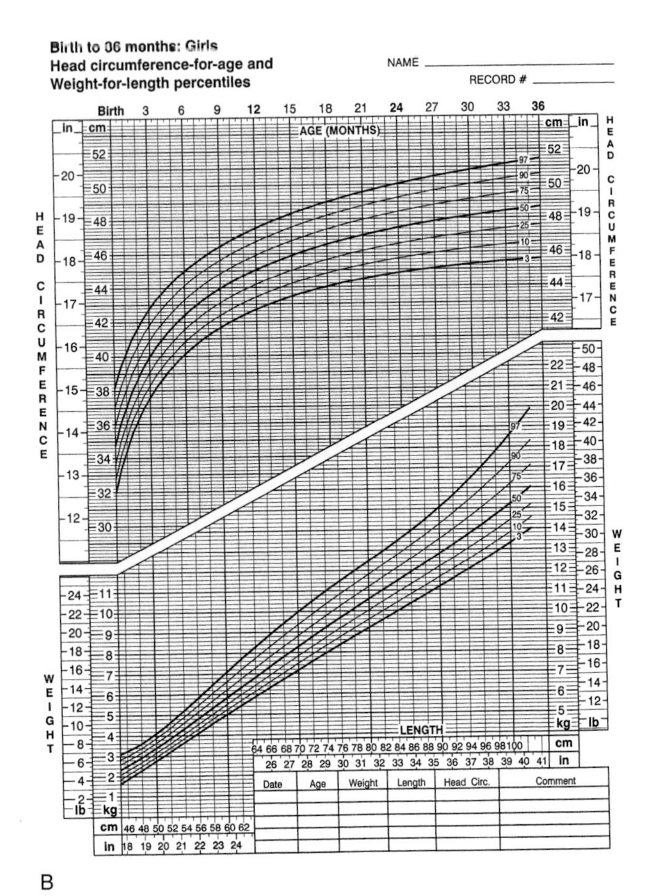

B

Figure 29-2. *cont'd.* **B.** Girls' head circumference-for-age and weight-for-length percentiles. (Source: Centers for Disease Control and Prevention. National Center for Health Statistics. Hyatsville, MD, 2002.)

firearms; access to pools; availability of smoke detectors/carbon monoxide (CO) detectors; hot water setting of water heater; bicycle helmets and use of seatbelts.

c. Sun protection: Sunscreen with 15 SPF or higher, use of hats, clothing, and umbrellas for protection.

d. Insect repellant if high exposure to insects or spends a great deal of time outside.

e. Tobacco use by patient or family members, and exposure to second-hand smoke in other settings. Discuss smoking cessation.

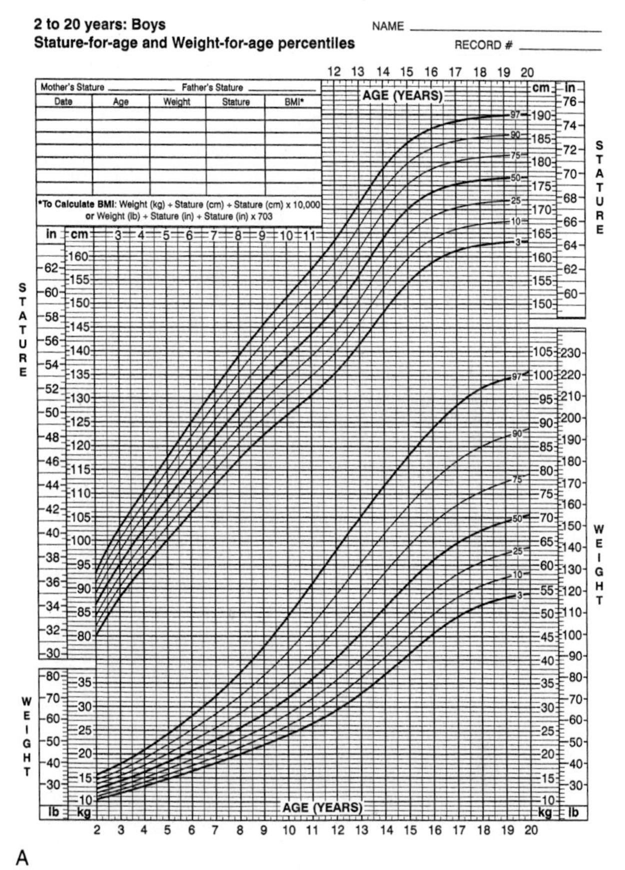

A

Figure 29-3. Growth Charts for Males **(A)** and Females **(B)** 2 to 20 years of age. (Source: Centers for Disease Control and Prevention. National Center for Health Statistics. Hyatsville, MD, 2002.)

Continued

f. Media exposure: Discuss American Academy of Pediatrics (AAP) recommendations for avoiding television viewing in children younger than 2 years and keeping total television viewing time to less than 2 hours per day for others.

B. Nutrition/Diet

1. Ask about specifics of diet: Breast milk or formula, type of formula, amount of intake and interval, formula changes, type of solid foods if any and time of introduction into diet, appetite in general, unconventional dietary habits, food allergies.

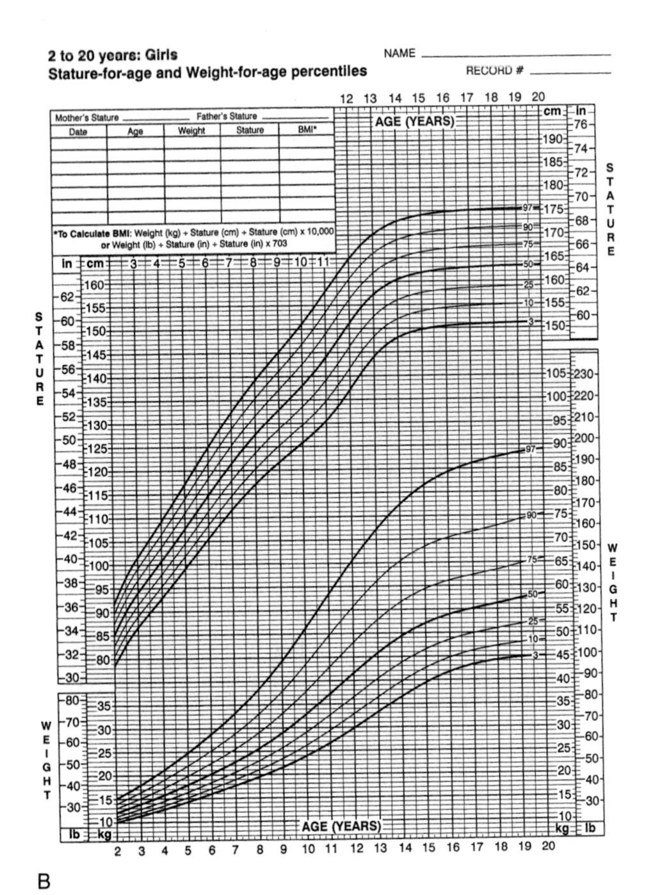

B

Figure 29-3. *cont'd.*

2. In older children, ask about volume of milk, juice, and soda intake, appetite or dietary concerns, and family's response to them.
3. Document use of vitamins and fluoride (inquire whether fluoride is in water source).
4. Note any unusual eating habits or cravings (e.g., pica).

C. **Sleep Patterns**

1. Ask about child's routine sleep pattern, bed sharing, history of nightmares and night terrors, sleepwalking, and bedwetting.
2. Document any recent changes to the routine pattern.

D. **Exercise/Recreation/Physical Activity:** Inquire about daily involvement in physical activity (e.g., chores, sports).

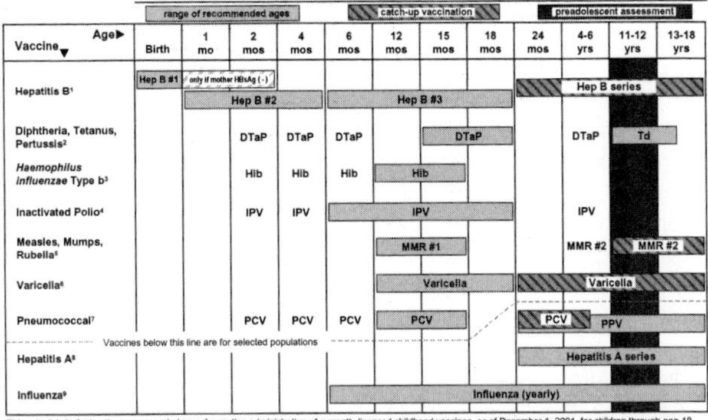

Recommended Childhood Immunization Schedule
United States, 2002

range of recommended ages | catch-up vaccination | preadolescent assessment

Vaccine ▼ / Age ▶	Birth	1 mo	2 mos	4 mos	6 mos	12 mos	15 mos	18 mos	24 mos	4-6 yrs	11-12 yrs	13-18 yrs
Hepatitis B[1]	Hep B #1	only if mother HBsAg (-)							Hep B series			
		Hep B #2			Hep B #3							
Diphtheria, Tetanus, Pertussis[2]			DTaP	DTaP	DTaP		DTaP			DTaP	Td	
Haemophilus influenzae Type b[3]			Hib	Hib	Hib	Hib						
Inactivated Polio[4]			IPV	IPV	IPV					IPV		
Measles, Mumps, Rubella[5]						MMR #1				MMR #2	MMR #2	
Varicella[6]						Varicella			Varicella			
Pneumococcal[7]			PCV	PCV	PCV	PCV			PCV	PPV		
Vaccines below this line are for selected populations												
Hepatitis A[8]									Hepatitis A series			
Influenza[9]					Influenza (yearly)							

This schedule indicates the recommended ages for routine administration of currently licensed childhood vaccines, as of December 1, 2001, for children through age 18 years. Any dose not given at the recommended age should be given at any subsequent visit when indicated and feasible. ▨ Indicates age groups that warrant special effort to administer those vaccines not previously given. Additional vaccines may be licensed and recommended during the year. Licensed combination vaccines may be used whenever any components of the combination are indicated and the vaccine's other components are not contraindicated. Providers should consult the manufacturers' package inserts for detailed recommendations.

1. Hepatitis B vaccine (Hep B). All infants should receive the first dose of hepatitis B vaccine soon after birth and before hospital discharge; the first dose may also be given by age 2 months if the infant's mother is HBsAg-negative. Only monovalent hepatitis B vaccine can be used for the birth dose. Monovalent or combination vaccine containing Hep B may be used to complete the series; four doses of vaccine may be administered if combination vaccine is used. The second dose should be given at least 4 weeks after the first dose, except for Hib-containing vaccine which cannot be administered before age 6 weeks. The third dose should be given at least 16 weeks after the first dose and at least 8 weeks after the second dose. The last dose in the vaccination series (third or fourth dose) should not be administered before age 6 months.

Infants born to HBsAg-positive mothers should receive hepatitis B vaccine and 0.5 mL hepatitis B immune globulin (HBIG) within 12 hours of birth at separate sites. The second dose is recommended at age 1-2 months and the vaccination series should be completed (third or fourth dose) at age 6 months.

Infants born to mothers whose HBsAg status is unknown should receive the first dose of the hepatitis B vaccine series within 12 hours of birth. Maternal blood should be drawn at the time of delivery to determine the mother's HBsAg status; if the HBsAg test is positive, the infant should receive HBIG as soon as possible (no later than age 1 week).

2. Diphtheria and tetanus toxoids and acellular pertussis vaccine (DTaP). The fourth dose of DTaP may be administered as early as age 12 months, provided 6 months have elapsed since the third dose and the child is unlikely to return at age 15-18 months. **Tetanus and diphtheria toxoids (Td)** is recommended at age 11-12 years if at least 5 years have elapsed since the last dose of tetanus and diphtheria toxoid-containing vaccine. Subsequent routine Td boosters are recommended every 10 years.

3. *Haemophilus influenzae* type b (Hib) conjugate vaccine. Three Hib conjugate vaccines are licensed for infant use. If PRP-OMP (PedvaxHIB® or ComVax® [Merck]) is administered at ages 2 and 4 months, a dose at age 6 months is not required. DTaP/Hib combination products should not be used for primary immunization in infants at age 2, 4 or 6 months, but can be used as boosters following any Hib vaccine.

4. Inactivated poliovirus vaccine (IPV). An all-IPV schedule is recommended for routine childhood poliovirus vaccination in the United States. All children should receive four doses of IPV at age 2 months, 4 months, 6-18 months, and 4-6 years.

5. Measles, mumps, and rubella vaccine (MMR). The second dose of MMR is recommended routinely at age 4-6 years but may be administered during any visit, provided at least 4 weeks have elapsed since the first dose and that both doses are administered beginning at or after age 12 months. Those who have not previously received the second dose should complete the schedule by the visit at 11-12 years.

6. Varicella vaccine. Varicella vaccine is recommended at any visit at or after age 12 months for susceptible children (i.e. those who lack a reliable history of chickenpox). Susceptible persons aged $\geq$13 years should receive two doses, given at least 4 weeks apart.

7. Pneumococcal vaccine. The heptavalent **pneumococcal conjugate vaccine (PCV)** is recommended for all children aged 2-23 months and for certain children aged 24-59 months. **Pneumococcal polysaccharide vaccine (PPV)** is recommended in addition to PCV for certain high-risk groups. See *MMWR* 2000;49(RR-9);1-37.

8. Hepatitis A vaccine. Hepatitis A vaccine is recommended for use in selected states and regions, and for certain high-risk groups; consult your local public health authority. See *MMWR* 1999;48(RR-12);1-37.

9. Influenza vaccine. Influenza vaccine is recommended annually for children age $\geq$ 6 months with certain risk factors (including but not limited to asthma, cardiac disease, sickle cell disease, HIV, and diabetes; see *MMWR* 2001;50(RR-4);1-44), and can be administered to all others wishing to obtain immunity. Children aged $\leq$12 years should receive vaccine in a dosage appropriate for their age (0.25 mL if age 6-35 months or 0.5 mL if aged $\geq$ 3 years). Children aged $\leq$ 8 years who are receiving influenza vaccine for the first time should receive two doses separated by at least 4 weeks.

For additional information about vaccines, vaccine supply, and contraindications for immunization, please visit the National Immunization Program Website at www.cdc.gov/nip or call the National Immunization Hotline at 800-232-2522 (English) or 800-232-0233 (Spanish).

Approved by the Advisory Committee on Immunization Practices (www.cdc.gov/nip/acip), the American Academy of Pediatrics (www.aap.org), and the American Academy of Family Physicians (www.aafp.org).

Figure 29-4. Recommended Childhood Immunizations Schedule. For the most up-to-date schedules, go to the CDC website: www.cdc.gov/nip/recs/child-schedule.pdf (Source: Centers for Disease Control and Prevention. Division of Epidemiology and Surveillance. National Immunization Program. Atlanta, 2002.) (Figure 29-4 does not include catch-up vaccination schedule or vaccines indicated for certain risk groups.)

VI. FAMILY HISTORY

A. Parents

1. Note general health and pertinent diseases/diagnoses on both sides of the family.
2. Describe family living arrangements (e.g., single-parent family, parent involvement if being raised by individual other than parent).

3. Document educational levels of the primary caregivers.

B. **Family Health Habits:** Document smoking, dietary habits, physical activity, or substance abuse.

C. **Sibling Health:** Describe any chronic, recurrent, or current medical concerns.

D. **Predispositions/Exposures:** Depending on the chief complaint, consider asking more specific questions about family history of mental conditions, seizure disorders, learning disorders, hearing or vision deficits, infectious diseases, metabolic diseases, renal diseases, cardiovascular or pulmonary diseases, neoplastic diseases, syndromes, and congenital anomalies.

VII. PSYCHOSOCIAL, BEHAVIORAL, AND EDUCATIONAL HISTORY

Obtain basic information about the child's social behavior.

A. **Personality:** Is the child extroverted or introverted?

B. **Social Skills:** Does the child have many playmates? Do they play well together?

C. **Behavior:** Does the child have any troublesome behavior problems (e.g., temper tantrums, breath holding spells, tics, enuresis, poor attention span)?

D. **Hobbies:** Favorite activities? toys? games/sports? Any recent/sudden changes?

E. **School:** Obtain information about school/academic performance and recent changes.

F. **Learning Disorders:** Are there any recognized learning or perceptual disorders (e.g., dyslexia, color blindness)?

G. **Adolescents:** The approach to the psychosocial assessment of the adolescent is typically referred to by the mnemonic HEADSS. This history is optimally taken with the teen alone, accom-panied with counseling regarding confidentiality issues (review individual state laws regarding confidentiality and age at which an adolescent can consent to medical procedures or therapies).

1. **H**ome: Who lives at home? How do you get along? Do you feel safe?
2. **E**ducation/Employment: What school, level, and grades? Ever failed? Do you have a job?
3. **A**ctivities: What do you do for fun? Best friend? Trouble with police?
4. **D**rugs: Do your friends smoke or drink alcohol? Have you ever tried smoking? Have you ever tried drinking alcohol? Any other drugs (pattern, frequency, amount)?
5. **S**exuality: Questions regarding sexual development? Have you ever had sex? (If affirmative, question further the age of first encounter, age of partner, number of partners, if consensual, birth control, and pregnancy).
6. **S**uicide: Do you ever feel down or depressed? Weight loss? Have you ever thought about hurting yourself?

H. **Effects of Illness on Child/Family and Family Support**

1. Assess how well the child and family understand the illness.

2. Consider genetic counseling, as appropriate.
3. Note any special arrangements or needs at home or school (e.g., special bed, wheelchair, home health care).
4. Note specific family strengths (e.g., cohesiveness, resilience).

VIII. REVIEW OF SYSTEMS (Tables 29-1, 29-2, and 29-3)

IX. PHYSICAL EXAMINATION (Table 29-4)

The American Academy of Pediatrics Recommendations for Preventive Pediatric Health Care contains timing of routine health care, appropriate measurements, screening tests, procedures, and anticipatory guidance for children and can be found at the following website: www.aap.org/policy/periodicity.pdf.

A. Vital signs should be recorded at each visit: Temperature, respirations, pulse; blood pressure recording is recommended starting at three years of age (Tables 29-5 and 29-6).

Table 29-1. GENERAL PEDIATRIC SIGNS AND SYMPTOMS BY SYSTEM.

System	Signs and Symptoms
General review	Stability of weight, dietary habits, fatigue, growth, behavioral problems
Skin	Rashes, bumps, bruising
Eyes	Record date of last eye examination, any perceived visual difficulty or change in vision, use of corrective lenses or contact lenses, diplopia
Ears	Hearing concerns, frequency of ear infections
Nose/sinuses	Frequency of nasal discharge, cold symptoms
Throat	Frequency of throat infections
Dental	Quality of dental hygiene
Cardiovascular	Disturbances in rate or rhythm, history of murmur, hypertension, chest pain
Respiratory	Frequent cough, wheezing, history of lower respiratory infections
Gastrointestinal system	Heartburn, abdominal pain, vomiting, diarrhea, change in bowel habits
Genitourinary system	Irritative voiding symptoms, vaginal or urethral discharge, menstrual history
Neuromuscular system	Seizures, headaches, dizziness, unsteady gait, weakness
Skeletal system	Scoliosis, limp, swollen and/or painful joints, back pain
Endocrine	Linear growth, weight, pubertal changes, thyroid enlargement, food and fluid intake

Table 29-2. NONSPECIFIC SYMPTOMS AND ASSOCIATED PEDIATRIC DISEASE PROCESSES.

Symptom	Disease Process
Abdominal pain (Acute, <2 yrs)	Incarcerated inguinal hernia, intussusception, colic, gastroenteritis
Abdominal pain (Acute, >2 yrs)	Gastroenteritis, constipation, appendicitis, peptic ulcer disease, pelvic inflammatory disease (PID), ectopic pregnancy, ovarian or testicular torsion, pancreatitis, inflammatory bowel disease (IBD), pyelonephritis/UTI, Henoch-Schönlein purpura (HSP), gastritis, lead toxicity
Abdominal pain, chronic	Distinguish organic (5%) versus nonorganic (95%)
Acute ear pain	Acute otitis media/externa, mastoiditis, trauma, foreign body, temporomandibular joint (TMJ), caries
Bruising (petechiae/ purpura)	Trauma, viral infections, streptococcal infections, vasculitis, cough and vomiting, idiopathic thrombocytopenic purpura (ITP), coagulopathies, systemic bacterial infection (e.g., meningococcemia, sepsis, disseminated intravascular coagulation [DIC]), nonaccidental trauma (NAT)
Bone pain	Trauma, infection (osteomyelitis), tumor (solid or leukemia), "growing pains"
Constipation	Mechanical obstruction (imperforate anus, intestinal obstruction), abnormal motility (Hirschsprung's disease/colonic aganglionosis), drugs, dehydration, anal fissure, perirectal abscess, behavioral
Cough	Upper respiratory infection (common cold, sinusitis, croup [barking cough]), lower respiratory infection (bronchiolitis, viral or bacterial pneumonia), asthma, aspiration, gastroesophageal reflux, allergic rhinitis, cystic fibrosis, interstitial lung disease, pertussis (whooping cough), tuberculosis, habit cough
Diarrhea	Gastroenteritis (viral, parasitic, bacterial), inflammatory bowel disease, urinary tract infection (UTI), carbohydrate or protein intolerance, celiac disease, malabsorption, pancreatic disease, toddler's diarrhea

Table 29-2—cont'd

SYMPTOM	DISEASE PROCESS
Fever (rectal >100.4°F or 38°C)	Viral illnesses, UTI, occult bacteremia, bacteremia/sepsis, meningitis, osteomyelitis, septic arthritis, cellulitis, Kawasaki disease, systemic onset juvenile rheumatoid arthritis (JRA), malignancy, acute rheumatic fever, Lyme disease (Remember, even a well-appearing infant younger than 3 months of age with any fever may have a serious bacterial illness.)
Headache	Migraine, tension headache, meningitis, tumor, hydrocephalus, increased intracranial pressure (ICP), sinusitis, systemic illness
Joint pain/limp	Trauma/fracture, infection (septic arthritis), transient "toxic" synovitis, avascular necrosis of the proximal femur (Legg-Calve-Perthes disease), epiphysiolysis: slipped capital femoral epiphysis, bone tumor, osteomyelitis, juvenile rheumatoid arthritis (JRA), Lyme arthritis, rheumatic fever, SLE, Nursemaid's elbow (subluxation of the radial head), sickle cell crisis, Osgood Schlatter disease, arthralgia
Ocular erythema, pain, and/or discharge	Conjunctivitis-allergic, bacteria (chlamydia/gonorrhea in neonate), viral, trauma or foreign body, chemical (toxic), orbital and periorbital cellulitis, hordeolum (stye), chalazion, glaucoma, obstructed nasolacrimal ducts
Rash	Bacterial infection: Impetigo (Staphylococcus, Streptococcus), fungal infection (cutaneous dermatophytes, Tinea versicolor, Candida), viral infection (herpes, varicella, Roseola/human herpes virus 6 [HHV6], erythema infectiosum/parvovirus), insect bites or infestation (scabies), dermatitis (eczema, contact dermatitis, dry skin, psoriasis, pityriasis rosea, seborrhea), drug reaction (Stevens-Johnson Syndrome, erythema multiforme), urticaria

Continued

Table 29-2. NONSPECIFIC SYMPTOMS AND ASSOCIATED PEDIATRIC DISEASE PROCESSES—*cont'd*

SYMPTOM	DISEASE PROCESS
Rhinorrhea	Acute viral rhinitis, acute sinusitis (viral or bacterial), allergic rhinitis, vasomotor rhinitis, nasal foreign body, congenital syphilis
Sore mouth and/ or throat	Aphthous stomatitis, herpetic gingivostomatitis, thrush, viral pharyngitis, Epstein-Barr virus (EBV)/mononucleosis, coxsackie virus, Streptococcal pharyngitis (definitive diagnosis requires culture), peritonsillar/retropharyngeal abscess, allergic rhinitis, postnasal drip, epiglottitis
Vomiting	Mechanical obstruction (non-bilious: pyloric stenosis, gastric web) (bilious: duodenal stenosis, malrotation, volvulus, intussusception), esophagitis, gastritis, duodenitis, gastroesophageal reflux, infection (viral or bacterial gastroenteritis, pyelonephritis/UTI, otitis media, pneumonia), central nervous system disorder (tumor, meningitis, increased intracranial pressure), metabolic disease (congenital adrenal hyperplasia [CAH], inborn error of metabolism, diabetic ketoacidosis), pregnancy

B. Weight, height, and head circumference should all be obtained at each visit during the first three years of life; utilize standard growth curves to assess growth pattern (Appendices I and II).

C. Take initial note of the child's overall appearance, with attention to any signs of distress; observation can be just as important as conversation and examination.

D. Give the child time to become familiar with the examiner.

E. Try to examine the child in a position that is most comfortable for him or her (e.g., parent's lap).

X. DIFFERENTIAL DIAGNOSIS (Table 29-7)

XI. LABORATORY STUDIES AND DIAGNOSTIC EVALUATIONS (Table 29-8)

XII. ACRONYMS AND ABBREVIATIONS (Table 29-9)

XIII. DEFINITIONS (Table 29-10)

XIV. SAMPLE H&P WRITE-UP

CC: "My baby has a fever and is fussy."

Table 29-3. COMMON PEDIATRIC DISEASES AND THEIR SYMPTOMS.

DISEASE	SYMPTOMS
Acute sinusitis (viral or bacterial)	Mucopurulent nasal discharge, night and day cough, malodorous breath (halitosis), rarely fever, sinus tenderness is uncommon
Acute viral rhinitis	Clear or mucoid rhinorrhea, congestion, cough, fever
Allergic rhinitis	Nasal itching, clear rhinorrhea, sneezing, itchy, watery eyes
Otitis externa	Ear pain, itching, swelling of external canal and tragus
Otitis media	Ear pain, other nonspecific symptoms such as rhinorrhea, cough, congestion, vomiting, fever, diarrhea
Pharyngitis	Sore throat, abdominal pain, headache, fine papular rash, lymphadenopathy, fever
Conjunctivitis	Itchy, watery eyes, conjunctival injection, discharge, normal vision
Viral gastroenteritis	Diarrhea without blood or mucous, vomiting, dehydration
Pneumonia	Cough, fever, chest pain, abdominal pain
Urinary tract infection	Dysuria in toilet trained, frequency, urgency, fever, vomiting, diarrhea

Table 29-4. GENERAL PEDIATRIC PHYSICAL EXAMINATION.

SYSTEM	PHYSICAL FINDINGS/CHARACTERISTICS
General	Note general appearance, including general development, ill or well, level of nourishment, level of comfort or discomfort, and response to examination and interaction with caregiver (cooperative, irritable with examination yet consolable, happy in parent's arms, smiling)
Skin	Check for color (cyanosis, jaundice, pallor), bruising, evidence of trauma, rashes, pigmented lesions, dermal and subcutaneous lesions, turgor, edema
Head	Size (circumference), symmetry, fontanelles, sutures, shape

Continued

Table 29-4. GENERAL PEDIATRIC PHYSICAL EXAMINATION—*cont'd*

System	Physical Findings/Characteristics
Ears	External (pinna and canal), position, examine tympanic membranes for color (ground-glass hue, yellow, erythematous), assess mobility, position (retracted, neutral, bulging), air bubbles, perforation, if PE tubes present, check for dislodgement, drainage, check hearing acuity
Eyes	Conjunctival erythema, discharge, excessive tearing, pupillary size, symmetry and reaction to light, photophobia, eye movements, visual acuity, nystagmus, ptosis, retina: red reflex, fundus, vessels, hemorrhage, cataracts
Nose	Symmetry, discharge, bleeding, flaring
Mouth	Color and consistency of lips, presence and hygiene of teeth, oral mucosal erythema, plaques, or lesions, hydration of mucosa (moist or dry)
Throat	Mucosal erythema and exudate, tonsillar symmetry, enlargement and exudate, postnasal drip, position of uvula
Neck	Position, range of motion, lymph nodes, thyroid, Brudzinski's sign, tonic neck reflex, palpate sternocleidomastoids, masses
Thorax	Symmetry, inspection of chest wall (e.g., intercostal retractions with breathing, masses, skin changes)
Breast	Observation, tenderness, discharge, redness, masses, Tanner stage (Sexual Maturity Rating)
Lungs	Breathing pattern, rate, effort, and quality, auscultation of breath sounds over anterior and posterior thorax (e.g., clear, wheezes, rales, rhonchi, grunting, rate) percussion for dullness, fremitus, splinting
Heart	Auscultation of rate, rhythm, presence of normal or abnormal S1 and S2, murmurs (systolic or diastolic, harsh or blowing, grade), friction rub, gallop, peripheral pulses, palpation (thrill, apex impulse, tenderness)
Abdomen	Inspection for size and symmetry (scaphoid, distended, peristaltic wave), auscultation for bowel sounds in four quadrants, distention or masses, hepatosplenomegaly, tenderness, rigidity, rebound, or guarding

Table 29-4—cont'd

System	Physical Findings/Characteristics
Genitalia	**Male**: Note presence of circumcision, foreskin, urethral opening (hypospadius), discharge, examine scrotum for testes including presence, size and contour, check for hydrocele and hernia, cremasteric reflex, trauma
	Female: Check for vaginal secretions, size of vaginal opening, labial adhesions, clitoral hypertrophy, trauma, Tanner stage should be noted
Anus	Erythema, fissures, bleeding, fistulas, prolapse, imperforate, tone, diaper rash
Musculoskeletal	Extremities: Symmetry, edema, muscle tone, contractures, atrophy, masses, clubbing, nail beds, capillary refill
	Joint: Erythema, heat, swelling, or limitation of movement Hip dislocation: Ortoloni and Barlow maneuver
	Spine and back: Assess overall posture, presence of curvature, sacral dimple/defect/cyst/hair tuft, scapulae
Neurologic	General: Level of consciousness, verbal comprehension appropriate for age, speech and communicative skills, cranial nerves, cerebellar function, motor function, reflexes

ID/Data Source: Nine-month-old female accompanied by her mother and father. The mother is the primary caretaker, and both parents are reliable historians.

HPI: M.N. is a nine-month-old white female who 2 days prior to admission (PTA) was noted to be more irritable, sleeping more, and have a decreased appetite. She felt a little warm, but no temperature was taken. One day PTA, child had four episodes of nonbilious, nonbloody emesis and further reduction in appetite. M.N. has continued to breast-feed regularly but has been uninterested in taking any solids. Early this morning, M.N.'s mother noted she was "hot" with a temperature of 103° (axillary), and she had three more episodes of emesis overnight. She received acetaminophen after the fever was discovered. Mother promptly brought the child to the clinic this a.m. M.N. has not had cough, runny nose, diarrhea, or known ill contacts. She only had one wet diaper yesterday, and her diaper was dry this a.m. Her weight was 8.6 kg at her nine-month-old well visit last week.

Table 29-5. MEAN RESPIRATORY RATES +/− 1 STANDARD DEVIATION.

AGE (YR)	BOYS	GIRLS	AGE (YR)	BOYS	GIRLS
0-1	31 +/−8	30 +/−6	9-10	19 +/−2	19 +/−2
1-2	26 +/−4	27 +/−4	10-11	19 +/−2	10 +/−2
2-3	25 +/−4	25 +/−3	11-12	19 +/−3	19 +/−3
3-4	24 +/−3	24 +/−3	12-13	19 +/−3	19 +/−2
4-5	23 +/−2	22 +/−2	13-14	19 +/−2	18 +/−2
5-6	22 +/−2	21 +/−2	14-15	18 +/−2	18 +/−3
6-7	21 +/−3	21 +/−3	15-16	17 +/−3	18 +/−3
7-8	20 +/−3	20 +/−2	16-17	17 +/−2	17 +/−3
8-9	20 +/−2	20 +/−2	17-18	16 +/−3	17 +/−3

Reproduced with permission from the publisher from Siberry GK, Iannone R. The Harriet Lane Handbook: A Manual for Pediatric House Officers, ed 15. St. Louis: Mosby, 2000.

Table 29-6. AGE-SPECIFIC HEART RATES (BEATS/MINUTE).

AGE	2%	MEAN	98%
<1 day	93	123	154
1-2 days	91	123	159
3-6 days	91	129	166
1-3 wk	107	148	182
1-2 mo	121	149	179
3-5 mo	106	141	186
6-11 mo	109	134	169
1-2 yr	89	119	151
3-4 yr	73	108	137
5-7 yr	65	100	133
8-11 yr	62	91	130
12-15 yr	60	85	119

Reproduced with permission from the publisher from Siberry GK, Iannone R. The Harriet Lane Handbook: A Manual for Pediatric House Officers, ed 15. St. Louis: Mosby, 2000.

Text continued on p. 629.

Table 29-7. COMMON PHYSICAL EXAMINATION FINDINGS AND ASSOCIATED DIAGNOSES.

SYSTEM	PHYSICAL EXAMINATION FINDING	POSSIBLE DIAGNOSES
Vital signs		
Pulse	Tachycardia	Fever, anxiety, sepsis, dehydration, pain
Blood pressure	Hypertension	Inappropriate BP cuff size, anxiety, obesity, essential, renal causes
Respiratory rate	Tachypnea	Fever, pain, anxiety, pneumonia, asthma, acidosis
Weight	Weight loss	Nutritional deprivation, inflammatory bowel disease (IBD), depression, diabetes mellitus, increased physical activity, chronic infections, eating disorder (e.g. anorexia nervosa)
Height	Abnormal linear growth velocity	Endocrinopathies (e.g., growth hormone deficiency, hypothyroid), genetic syndromes (e.g., Turner's), severe nutritional deprivation, IBD
HEENT		
Head	Macrocephaly	Familial, inaccurate measurement, hydrocephalus, fragile X
	Microcephaly	Congenital infections, familial, chromosomal abnormalities (e.g., Trisomy 18), syndromes (e.g., Prader-Willi), inaccurate measurement
	Bulging anterior fontanel	Hydrocephalus, meningitis, tumor
	Sunken anterior fontanel	Dehydration
	Abnormal shape	Benign positional plagiocephaly, craniosynostosis
Eyes	Absent red reflex (leukocoria)	Cataract, retinoblastoma, retinal detachment
	Abnormal corneal light reflex (Hirschberg test)	Congenital or acquired strabismus, syndrome (e.g., Apert's syndrome)
	Persistent watery eye from birth	Nasolacrimal duct obstruction

Continued

Table 29-7. COMMON PHYSICAL EXAMINATION FINDINGS AND ASSOCIATED DIAGNOSES—*cont'd*

System	Physical Examination Finding	Possible Diagnoses
Ears	Red tympanic membrane	Crying child, fever, flushing reaction from stimulation of canal, acute otitis media (AOM), otitis media with effusion (OME)
	Edematous auditory canal	Otitis externa, otitis media with secondary otitis externa secondary to rupture or draining PETs
Nose	Bleeding	Trauma (e.g., picking), allergy, von Willebrand disease, angiofibroma
	Nasal passage obstruction	Unilateral: Foreign body, polyp, choanal atresia Bilateral: Sinusitis, allergic rhinitis, polyps
Mouth	White plagues on buccal mucosa/tongue	Thrush, formula or breast milk
	Exudative, erythematous tonsils	Group A Streptococcus pharyngitis, mononucleosis, adenovirus
	Delayed dentition	Endocrinopathies (hypothyroidism), Down syndrome, achondroplasia
Face	Ptosis	Congenital ptosis, botulism, hydrocephalus, Horner syndrome
Neck		
Anterior Neck	Neck mass	Thyroglossal duct cyst, brachial cleft anomaly, enlarged thyroid, goiter
	Cervical adenopathy/adenitis	Infection (viral, bacterial, atypical mycobacterium, cat scratch disease), Kawasaki's, malignancy
	Torticollis	Congenital muscular, trauma, cervical adenitis, retropharyngeal abscess
Lungs	Wheezing	Asthma, bronchiolitis, foreign body, gastroesophageal reflux, cystic fibrosis, pneumonitis (e.g., *M. pneumoniae*)
	Rales	Pneumonia, bronchiolitis, foreign body, transient tachypnea of the newborn, congestive heart failure

	Stridor	Laryngo-tracheobronchitis (croup), foreign body, epiglottis, retropharyngeal or peritonsillar abscess
Chest	Intercostal muscular retractions	(See causes of wheezing, rales, stridor listed previously)
	Gynecomastia	Physiologic pubertal, transplacental passage of estrogen (neonatal), idiopathic, Klinefelter syndrome
Cardiovascular	Heart murmur	Flow murmur (Still's murmur), ventricular septal defect, peripheral pulmonic stenosis, other congenital heart defects
Abdomen	Splenomegaly	Viral infection (e.g., EBV), hemolytic disorder (e.g., sickle-cell anemia), tumors (e.g., leukemia)
	Hepatosplenomegaly	Congestive heart failure, sepsis, tumor (e.g., neuroblastoma), B-thalassemia, metabolic disorders (e.g., galactosemia), hepatitis, infection (e.g., malaria, amebiasis)
	Abdominal mass	Hydronephrosis, Wilm's tumor, neuroblastoma, fecal material, intussusception
Genitourinary		
Male	No palpable testicle in scrotal sac	Retractile, undescended, or intraabdominal testis, cryptorchism
Female	Vaginal bleeding	Menstruation, uterine/vaginal/cervical/ovarian pathology, dysfunctional/anovulatory uterine bleeding, endocrine (hormonal pathology), coagulopathy, medications, trauma, female genital self-multilation, Munchausen's syndrome
Skin	Jaundice	Physiologic neonatal, breast milk, hepatitis, drug-related
	Erythematous annular lesion with scales	Tinea corporis, nummular eczema, contact dermatitis

Continued

Table 29-7. COMMON PHYSICAL EXAMINATION FINDINGS AND ASSOCIATED DIAGNOSES—*cont'd*

SYSTEM	PHYSICAL EXAMINATION FINDING	POSSIBLE DIAGNOSES
	Fine, "sandpaper" macular-papular rash	Scarlet fever, viral exanthem
	Petechiae	Sepsis, DIC, ITP, trauma
	Ecchymoses	Injury, abuse, DIC, von Willebrand's disease
	Hypo/hyperpigmented patches	Neurocutaneous disorders (e.g., neurofibromatosis, tuberous sclerosis)
Lymphatics	Generalized, non-tender lymphadenopathy	Viral infections (e.g., EBV, CMV), leukemia, lymphoma
Extremities	Tender mass on tibial tuberosity	Osgood-Schlatter disease, osteosarcoma
	Limited abduction of hip	Congenital dysplasia of the hip
	In toeing	Metatarsus adductus, internal tibial torsion, femoral anteversion
	Toe walking	Normal variant, cerebral palsy, autism, Duchenne's muscular dystrophy
Neurologic	Ataxic gait	Acute cerebellar ataxia (e.g., post-varicella, Coxsackie virus), neoplasms (e.g., posterior fossa tumor, neuroblastoma), hereditary disorder (e.g., Friedreich's ataxia), ataxic cerebral palsy
	Generalized hypotonia	Inborn error of metabolism (e.g., hypothyroidism), benign congenital hypotonia, neuromuscular disorder (e.g., Werdnig-Hoffman disease), syndromes (e.g., Down syndrome), hypoxic-ischemic encephalopathy
	Asymmetric Moro reflex	Clavicle fracture, Erb's palsy

Table 29-8. SELECTED LABORATORY STUDIES AND DIAGNOSTIC EVALUATIONS.

STUDY/EVALUATION	PURPOSE/COMMENTS
Complete blood count	Evaluate red blood cells, white blood cells with differential, and platelet count
Urine analysis	Evaluate for specific gravity, hematuria, proteinuria, or evidence of bacteria, glucose, white or red blood cells
Purified protein derivative (PPD, Mantoux skin test)	Recommended if high index of suspicion for tuberculosis exposure or disease
Lead level	Recommended if risk factors exist for exposure to lead
Newborn state screening (tested at birth and generally repeated at 2-week visit)	Screen for genetically inherited metabolic disorders (e.g., sickle cell disease, congenital hypothyroid, galactosemia, maple syrup urine disease, cystic fibrosis), state mandated with variations in testing State to State
Newborn hearing screen	Screening for universal detection of hearing loss in infants less than 3 months of age (EOAE = evoked otoacoustic emissions or ABR = auditory brainstem response)

M.N. was seen this a.m. in the clinic, where her peripheral WBC was 20,000 and her catheterized urinalysis was nitrite and leukocyte esterase positive with numerous WBCs and bacteria on microscopy. Serum chemistries were normal other than bicarbonate of 16. After initial antibiotic and fluid management, she was referred for admission for further management of probable complicated urinary tract infection (urine culture pending) and moderate dehydration.

PAST MEDICAL AND SURGICAL HISTORY

Prenatal/Birth/Neonatal History: Pregnancy was without complications or medical concerns, followed by a spontaneous vaginal delivery at 38+ weeks. Prenatal ultrasounds were normal by the parents' report, including the kidneys. The nursery course was notable only for mild physiologic jaundice never requiring phototherapy. The child otherwise had a normal nursery course. Metabolic disease screens normal.

Growth/Development: She has met all developmental milestones with head circumference, length, and weight tracking at the 50th percentile since birth. She is just beginning to pull to a stand, feeds self Cheerios, plays "peek-a-boo," and "babbles."

Surgical History: None.

Table 29-9. PEDIATRIC ABBREVIATION AND ACRONYMS.

Acronym or Abbreviation	Term	Acronym or Abbreviation	Term
A&B	Apnea and bradycardia	**DI**	Diabetes insipidus
ABG	Arterial blood gas	**DTaP**	Diphtheria/tetanus/acellular Pertussis vaccine
AF	Anterior fontanelle	**ECMO**	Extracorporeal membrane oxygenation
AGA	Appropriate for gestational age	**EGA**	Estimated gestational age
ALL	Acute lymphoblastic leukemia	**FROM**	Full range of motion
ANC	Absolute neutrophil count	**GBS**	Group B streptococcus
AML	Acute myelogenous leukemia	**G tube**	Gastrostomy tube
BA	Bone age	**HAL**	Hyperalimentation
BAER	Brain stem audioevoked response	**HC**	Head circumference
BPD	Bronchopulmonary dysplasia	**HFOV**	High-frequency oscillatory ventilation
CDH	Congenital dislocation of the hip; Congenital diaphragmatic hernia	**HMD**	Hyaline membrane disease
CF	Cystic fibrosis	**HSP**	Henoch-Schönlein purpura
CHD	Congenital heart disease	**IDDM**	Insulin-dependent diabetes mellitus
CP	Cerebral palsy	**ITP**	Idiopathic thrombocytopenic purpura
DDST	Denver Developmental Screening Test	**IUGR**	Intrauterine growth retardation

Table 29-9—cont'd

Acronym or Abbreviation	Term	Acronym or Abbreviation	Term
IVH	Intraventricular hemorrhage	**SGA**	Small for gestational age
IVP	Intravenous pyelogram	**SIDS**	Sudden infant death syndrome
LGA	Large for gestational age	**SIADH**	Syndrome of inappropriate antidiuretic hormone secretion
LP	Lumbar puncture	**SVT**	Supraventricular tachycardia
NAD	No acute distress	**TEF**	Tracheoesophageal fistula
NEC	Necrotizing enterocolitis	**TOF**	Tetralogy of Fallot
NGT	Nasogastric tube	**TOGV**	Transposition of the great vessels
OFC	Occipitofrontal circumference	**TPN**	Total parenteral nutrition
OM	Otitis media	**UAC**	Umbilical artery catheter
PDA	Patent ductus arteriosus	**UPJ**	Ureteropelvic junction
PEG	Percutaneous endoscopic gastrostomy	**UTD**	Up-to-date
PPHN	Persistent pulmonary hypertension of the newborn	**UVC**	Umbilical venous catheter
PTA	Prior to admission	**VCUG**	Vesicocystourethrogram
RDS	Respiratory distress syndrome	**VSD**	Ventricular septal defect
RSV	Respiratory syncytial virus	**VUR**	Vesicoureteral reflux

Table 29-10. DEFINITIONS OF PEDIATRIC TERMS.

TERM	DEFINITION
APGAR Score	Numerical expression of condition of newborn infant (at 1 minute and 5 minutes following birth) based on heart rate, skin color, respiratory effort, muscle tone, and reflex irritability. A = Activity (muscle tone), P = Pulse (heart rate), G = Grimace (reflex irritability), A = Appearance (skin color), R = Respiration
Chalazion	Eyelid mass resulting from inflammation of meibomian glands
Dyslexia	Difficulty learning to read, write, and spell words despite ability to see and recognize letters; more frequently found in males
Enuresis	Involuntary discharge of urine, after age control should have been obtained; usually referring to night
Epiphysiolysis	Separation of epiphysis from bone
Fontanelles	Membrane-covered spaces remaining in incompletely ossified bone
Intussusception	Prolapse of part of intestine into lumen of adjoining part
Night terrors	Sudden awakening from deep sleep, inconsolable and amnestic later to the event (both distinguished from nightmares)
Phenylketonuria	Accumulation of phenylalanine resulting in mental retardation if not treated
Osteochondritis dessicans	Osteochondritis (inflammation of bone and cartilage) resulting in splitting of pieces of cartilage into joint
Pica	Compulsive eating of non-nutritive substances
Rhinorrhea	Discharge of nasal mucous
Scoliosis	Abnormal curvature of the spine
Tetralogy of Fallot	Combination of cardiac defects, consisting of pulmonary stenosis, interventricular septal defect, dextroposition of the great vessels so it overrides the ventricular septum, and right ventricular hypertrophy

Emergency/Trauma History: She has never been hospitalized, injured, or had an emergency room visit. She has had a couple of clinic visits for "colds" and one ear infection treated with amoxicillin approximately 2 months ago.

Travel/Exposure History: No travel since birth and is not in day care. They have one pet dog.

Medications, Allergies, and Adverse Reactions: No known allergies or adverse reactions to foods or medications. She takes a multivitamin with iron daily. Her mother's only medication is prenatal vitamins.

Pediatric Health Maintenance: M.N. has made the 2-week, 2-, 4-, and 12-month well-baby visits, and her immunizations are up-to-date per the medical record. Parents have safety locks on all cabinets with medications or poisons, with no concerns for a possible ingestion.

Nutrition/Diet: Other than breastfeeding four times per day, she eats rice cereal, jarred baby food vegetables and fruits, and is just starting some baby food with pureed meats.

Sleep Patterns: Typically sleeps through night other than last couple days since she has been ill.

Family History: Her family history is negative for chronic diseases on both sides. Mother denies having UTIs as a child. No family history of mental retardation, metabolic disease, or seizure disorders. No tobacco exposure. M.N. is an only child.

Social History: Lives with parents, 26-year-old father and 24-year-old mother. Describes stable and supportive family dynamics. Both parents have high school and some college education.

REVIEW OF SYSTEMS

General: See HPI.

Skin: No rashes, bumps, or bruising.

Eyes: Decreased tearing noted this morning by mother. No eye discharge or redness.

Ears: No tugging at the ears or discharge.

Nose: Denies rhinorrhea or epistaxis.

Mouth/throat: Denies hoarseness. Is afraid throat may be "sore" because of decreased appetite.

Dental: Her two bottom teeth came in about one month ago.

Neck: She has been moving her neck/head freely without apparent stiffness.

Cardiovascular: Denies cool extremities or cyanosis.

Respiratory: Denies cough, hemoptysis, phlegm, wheezing, or stridor.

GI: See HPI for emesis. However, denies diarrhea, constipation, change in bowel habits, melena, hematochezia, change in stool caliber, or jaundice. Last bowel movement was this a.m.

GU: See HPI for decreased frequency. Diapered infant, however, without apparent dysuria, hematuria, or malodorous or discolored urine. No vaginal discharge.

Musculoskeletal: Denies joint swelling, limited range of motion, erythema.

Neurologic: See HPI for irritability and increased sleepiness. However, oriented to parents, easily consoled, and vigorously resists examination.

PHYSICAL EXAMINATION

Vitals: BP: 92/60 Pulse: 130 Respirations: 32 Temp: 102.5°F (rectal) Height: 70 cm (50%) Weight: 7.9 kg (25-50%) (700 grams down from last week), Head circumference: 44 cm (50%).

General: Well-developed, well-nourished infant who is fussy with examination, vigorously opposes attempted separation from parent and examination. Easily consoled by parent after examination.

Skin: No lesions, rashes, petechiae. Normal to slightly reduced skin turgor.

Lymphatic: No palpable preauricular/postauricular/anterior cervical/posterior cervical/supraclavicular/inguinal nodes.

Head: Normocephalic, anterior fontanelle is soft and flat.

Eyes: PERRLA, EOMI, no conjunctival erythema or discharge.

Ears: TMs normal position, grey, normal mobility, translucent without effusions.

Nose: Septum midline, with nonfriable, nonhemorrhagic mucosa and no exudates.

Mouth/pharynx: Dry buccal and sublingual mucosa, no tonsil erythema or exudates, two lower incisors.

Neck: Full active and passive range of motion. Negative Brudzinski's sign.

Thorax/lungs: No retractions, lungs clear to auscultation with no rhonchi, wheezing, or rales.

Cardiovascular: Regular rate and rhythm, S1 and S2 normal with no murmur or gallop, femoral pulses are 2+/=, capillary refill = 2 seconds.

Abdomen: Active bowel sounds, no hepatosplenomegaly, difficult examination but not apparently tender when distracted.

GU: Normal female genitalia, no discharge or erythema, Tanner stage 1.

Rectal: Not performed.

Back: No costovertebral angle tenderness (CVAT).

Extremities: Full active range of motion of all extremities. No cyanosis, clubbing, or edema.

Neurologic: Mental: See general portion of PE. **Strength:** Not cooperative but apparently normal strength in extremities. **Reflexes:** DTRs 2+ bilateral at Achilles, patellar, biceps, without clonus, upgoing toes.

30

PREVENTIVE MEDICINE

Katerina M. Neuhauser, MD, PhD, MPH, Thomas S. Neuhauser, MD, and Eric H. Hanson, MD, MPH

I. GENERAL

A. Clinical Preventive Services

Clinical Preventive Services (CPS) focuses on health maintenance through screening examinations, immunizations, chemoprophylaxis, health education, and early intervention. All medical specialists should utilize CPS to target preventable diseases in their patient population. Doing so will help limit the physical and social dysfunction in symptomatic patients, minimize the occurrence of disease in the population, and thus help contain the rising cost of health care.

B. Levels of Prevention

1. Primary prevention.
   - **a.** This level of prevention focuses on reducing risk factors in otherwise healthy individuals.
   - **b.** Most primary prevention activities occur outside of the patient encounter.
     - **(1)** Health promotion and health education (e.g., classes, counseling, health fairs) attempt to improve the health of patients by stressing positive lifestyle changes (e.g., diet modification, exercise, stress management, smoking cessation).
     - **(2)** Health policies, health standards for food, water, and air, and health regulations (e.g., proper sewage and waste disposal) protect the health of the general population and the environment, and reduce the occurrence of disease in the populace (e.g., food and waterborne illnesses, reactive airway disease [RAD]).
       - **(a)** Fluoridation of water supplies helps prevent the development of dental caries in the general population.
       - **(b)** Iodized salt ensures that the populace has an adequate intake of iodine to prevent goiter.
       - **(c)** Ear protection devices reduce injuries in loud work environments.
       - **(d)** Helmets and hard hats protect bikers and construction workers.
       - **(e)** Seatbelts protect car occupants.
     - **(3)** Some primary prevention activities do occur in conjunction with the patient encounter (e.g.,

immunizations and chemoprophylaxis increases resistance to infectious diseases), and health education targets risky behavior (e.g., tobacco and alcohol usage, inadequate sleep, unhealthy diets, lack of exercise).

2. Secondary prevention.
   a. Secondary prevention generally occurs in conjunction with patient encounters.
   b. It focuses on identifying underlying medical problems in asymptomatic individuals; this early intervention may delay symptomatic manifestations in patients or limit the severity of their disease. It includes screening and education.
      (1) Screening for many congenital as well as benign and malignant disease processes as outlined by the U.S. Preventive Services Task Force (USPSTF).
      (2) Health education, targeting modifiable risk factors (e.g., diabetes, hypertension [HTN], cigarette smoking, hyperlipidemia, sedentary lifestyle) as opposed to nonmodifiable factors (e.g., gender, family history of myocardial infarction [MI]).
3. Tertiary prevention.
   a. This generally occurs in conjunction with patient encounters.
   b. Tertiary prevention focuses on ways to optimize the health of symptomatic patients.
      (1) Health education.
      (2) Medical and surgical intervention (disability limitation) or rehabilitation, which may help prevent disease progression.

II. HISTORY OF PRESENT ILLNESS

Does the patient have any current complaints? For each symptom, inquire about and note frequency, intensity, duration, and alleviating or aggravating factors. While interviewing the patient, identify the need for primary, secondary, or tertiary prevention services. Every patient encounter is an opportunity to apply preventive medicine.

III. PAST MEDICAL AND SURGICAL HISTORY

A. Past Medical History

1. Identify any chronic medical conditions or immunosuppressive disorders (e.g., diabetes, heart disease, cancer, human immunodeficiency virus [HIV]).
   a. Duration of medical conditions.
   b. Severity, intensity, and frequency of any accompanying symptoms.
   c. Medical complications related to inadequately treated or advanced diseases (e.g., retinopathy, colitis, paralysis).

2. Related hospitalizations, including when and where they occurred, lengths of stays, therapies, and sequelae.
3. Transfusions (what products, how much, sequelae).
4. Injuries.

B. Past Surgical History

1. Identify all surgeries for acute (e.g., appendicitis, organ repair following traumatic injury) and chronic (e.g., ulcerative colitis, diabetic complications) medical conditions.
   a. Type of surgery(ies) and when and where they occurred.
   b. Symptoms experienced before surgery (e.g., frequency and intensity of symptoms).
   c. Complications during surgery (e.g., transfusions, medical misadventures) or during recovery (e.g., infections, persistence of symptoms, neuropathy, paralysis).
2. Determine whether there were any related hospitalizations.

C. Childhood History

1. Identify all childhood-related diseases, injuries, hospitalizations, and immunizations.
2. Explore any congenital disease processes or anomalies (e.g., Potter's syndrome, sickle cell disease).

D. Occupational History

1. Identify present and past occupations.
2. Identify occupational injuries and illnesses present.
3. Assess for exposure to any harmful chemicals/unsafe working conditions (e.g., use of industrial dyes, construction work without access to safety harness).
4. Assess proper use of any personnel protective equipment.

E. Travel History

1. Explore travel within the continental United States or overseas. Provide summary of where, when, how long, and how frequently the individual has traveled.
2. Assess risk for exposure to unusual pathogens (e.g., cholera, amoebic dysentery, schistosomiasis) based on location and diet.
3. Determine whether any chemoprophylaxis or immunization(s) was required before traveling. If so, was the patient compliant?

F. Animal and Insect Exposure History

1. Identify recent exposure to infectious (mosquitoes, ticks, mites) or venomous insects (spiders, scorpions).
2. Identify recent exposure to potentially infectious or venomous animals (dogs, cats, raccoons, bats, birds, snakes, lizards).

IV. MEDICATIONS, ALLERGIES, AND ADVERSE REACTIONS

A. Determine the medications used for acute or chronic medical conditions, chemoprophylaxis, or health-related reasons. List all prescription medications, including chemoprophylactic agents, over-the-counter (OTC) medication, herbal preparations, and supplements.

B. Determine whether there are any allergic reactions to medication and annotate adverse reactions (e.g., rashes, anaphylaxis, nausea, vomiting, pruritis).

V. FAMILY HISTORY

A. **Medical History:** Obtain the present and past medical history of all immediate family members (e.g., parents, grandparents, siblings, and children).

B. **Three-Generation Genogram:** Develop a genogram summarizing the medical history of three generations of relatives (see Figure in Chapter 18, p. 339). Genograms are most helpful in outlining patterns of disease (e.g., early disease onset, male, inherited conditions).

VI. PSYCHOSOCIAL HISTORY

A. **Personal and Social History**

1. Determine the patient's race/ethnicity, which may predispose to certain medical conditions (e.g., African-Americans are at greater risk for some hemoglobin disorders such as sickle cell disease and thalassemia).
2. Assess impact of current illness on the activities of daily living (e.g., difficulty walking or driving).
3. Assess the effectiveness of support from family and friends (e.g., ability to find help when required).

B. **Behavioral History**

1. Diet: Is the patient obtaining the required dietary nutrients (e.g., eating well-balanced meals and not adhering to a fad diet)?
2. Exercise/recreation: Is the patient exercising? If so, identify the type of exercise, frequency, and duration.
3. Sleep patterns: Assess the patient's quality and length of sleep (e.g., enough rest to meet needs versus chronic exhaustion).
4. Social habits: Does the individual use tobacco (inquire about type, frequency, duration, pack-years) or alcohol (inquire about type, frequency of use, eye-opener, driving while intoxicated, blackouts)?

VII. PHYSICAL EXAMINATION

The general physical examination identifies the evidence, and the extent, of symptomatic disease. The physical examination findings, in concert with the history, help determine the need for CPS. Table 30-1 summarizes some of the medical findings and possible diagnoses that may suggest the need for CPS.

VIII. CLINICAL PREVENTIVE SERVICES

A. **Children and Adolescents (<18 years of age)**

1. For the latest screening recommendations, refer to the USPSTF, Department of Health and Human Services (DHHS), the American Academy of Pediatrics (AAP), or the Advisory Committee on Immunization Practices (ACIP), a section of the Centers for Disease Control and Prevention (CDC).
2. The CPS required for children and adolescents are based on patient age and associated medical conditions (Table 30-2).

Table 30-1. FINDINGS OF PHYSICAL EXAMINATION AND POSSIBLE DIAGNOSES.

System	Physical Examination Finding	Possible Diagnoses
Vital signs	Tachycardia	Cardiovascular, endocrine disorder, infectious disease
	Hypotension	Infectious disease/sepsis, endocrine disorder
	Tachypnea	Pulmonary disease (thromboembolic), infectious disease, pain/ anxiety
	Weight loss	Occult malignancy, hyperthyroidism, illicit drug use
	Fever	Infectious disease, endocrine disorder
HEENT	Retinal hemorrhages	Diabetes, HTN
	Icteric sclera	Underlying liver disease (e.g., alcohol)
	Hearing loss	Noise induced loss, otosclerosis, trauma
	Holes in nasal septum	Illicit drug use
	Bleeding gums	Poor dental hygiene, hematologic disorder
Neck	Thyroid enlargement or nodule	Goiter, thyroid disease
Lungs	Rhonchi, wheezes, focal inspiratory crackles	Occupational asthma, infectious disease (e.g., pneumonia)
Cardiovascular	Arrhythmia, chest pain	Thromboembolic disease, endocrine disorder (e.g., pheochromocytoma), infectious disease (e.g., endocarditis), atherosclerotic disease (e.g., myocardial infarction [MI])
Abdomen	Hepatosplenomegaly	Hematologic neoplasm, infectious disease, cancer (e.g., metastasis), gastrointestinal disease (e.g., cirrhosis)

Continued

Table 30-1. FINDINGS OF PHYSICAL EXAMINATION AND POSSIBLE DIAGNOSES—*cont'd*

System	Physical Examination Finding	Possible Diagnoses
Genitourinary	Costovertebral angle (CVA) tenderness	Kidney disease
	Vaginal bleeding	Gynecologic disease, spontaneous abortion
Skin	Eczematous dermatitis	Contact dermatitis (irritant versus allergic)
	Nodular lesions	Ultraviolet (UV)-induced skin cancers
	Urticaria	Allergic reactions
Extremities	Migratory arthralgia	Lyme disease
	Joint pain or swelling	Arthritis, arthropathy, infection (e.g., septic arthritis)
	Foot ulcers	Diabetes, infectious disease, neuropathy
Neurologic	Peripheral neuropathies	Underlying metabolic disorders, diabetes
	Erythema migrans (expanding red maculopapular lesion)	Lyme disease
Psychiatric	Abnormal mental status examination	Stress, overt psychiatric disease

3. Figure 30-1 outlines the immunization schedule, preventive counseling topics, and additional screening recommendations for children and adolescents by age group.

B. **Adults (>18 years)**

1. Table 30-3 lists some of the CPS required for adults based on age, gender, and existing medical condition(s).
2. Figure 30-2 outlines additional screening recommendations and preventive counseling topics for adults.

IX. VACCINATIONS

A. General

1. Diseases that are preventable by vaccination have essentially been eliminated in many highly industrialized nations; they do, however, still occur in lesser-developed nations.
2. Providers should review the immunization history of any patient who plans to travel to underdeveloped countries and query local public health officials or consult reference material (e.g., *Health Information for International Travel*) to determine whether any vaccinations or chemoprophylaxis are required.

Table 30-2. SCREENING BY RISK FACTOR CATEGORY BY AGE FOR INDIVIDUALS BETWEEN 0-18 YEARS OF AGE.

Risk Factor	Prevention Target Condition	Prevention Service and/or Referral
Newborn infants	Ophthalmia neonatorum (gonorrhea)	Ocular antibiotic prophylaxis
	Congenital hypothyroidism	Thyroid function tests (TFTs)
	Hemoglobinopathy	Hemoglobin electrophoresis, high pressure liquid chromatography (HPLC) or other comparable test
Newborn infants >1 day old	Phenylketonuria (PKU)	Blood phenylalanine level
Infants and toddlers	Iron-deficiency anemia	Complete blood count (CBC), serum ferritin, nutritional counseling, breast-feeding counseling
Children ages 3-4 years	Amblyopia and strabismus	Visual acuity screening, ocular alignment
Infants, children, and adolescents	Infectious diseases	Immunizations
Children and adolescents	Hypertension (HTN)	Blood pressure screening, nutritional counseling, exercise counseling
	Obesity, malnutrition	Obesity screening Nutritional screening Exercise counseling
	Unintentional injury	Counsel regarding lap belts, car seats, bicycle helmets, poison control phone number, syrup of ipecac, safe storage of drugs, firearms, toxic substances, matches
	Dental hygiene	Counsel regarding regular dental checks
	Tobacco-related complications	Tobacco counseling
Adolescents	Kyphoscoliosis	Visual inspection

Source: U.S. Department of Health and Human Services. Office of Public Health and Science and Office of Disease Prevention and Health Promotion. Put Prevention into Practice: Clinician's Handbook of Preventive Practice, ed 2, Washington, DC, 1998.

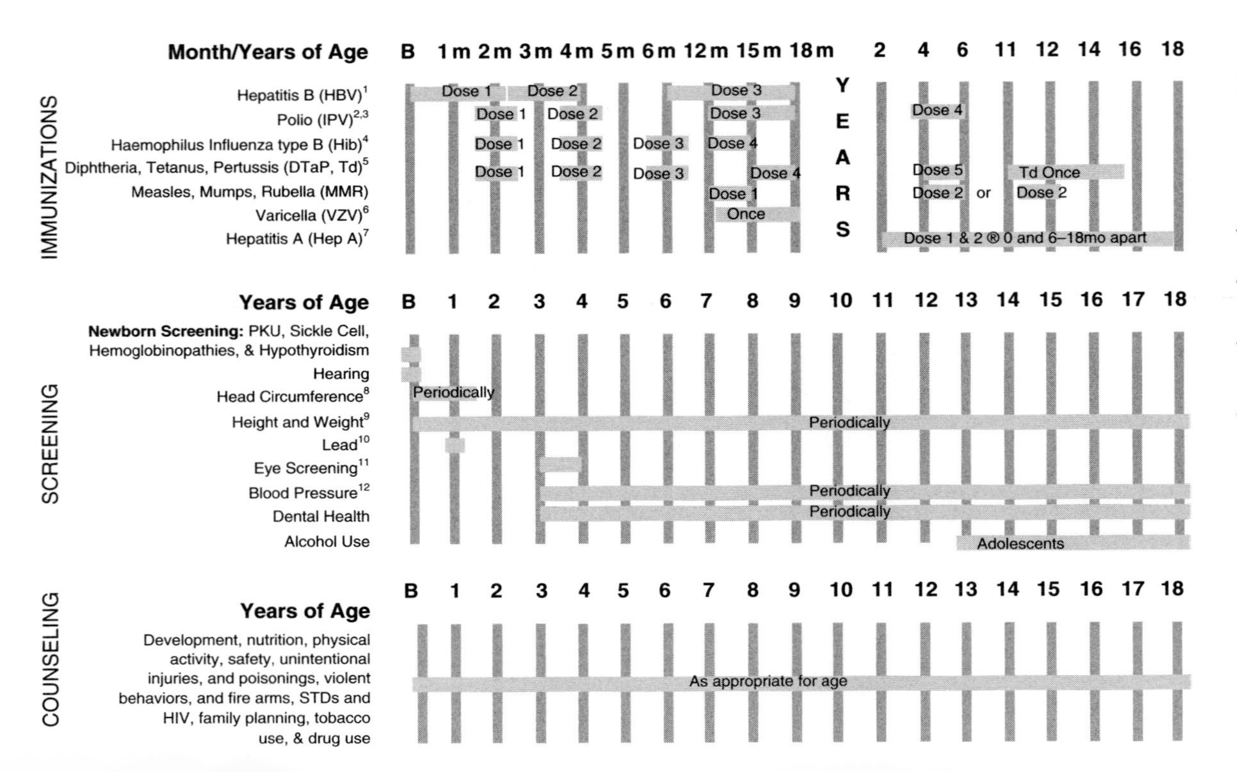
IMMUNIZATIONS
Month/Years of Age
B 1m 2m 3m 4m 5m 6m 12m 15m 18m 2 4 6 11 12 14 16 18
YEARS
Hepatitis B (HBV)1
Dose 1
Dose 2
Dose 3
Polio (IPV)2,3
Dose 1
Dose 2
Dose 3
Dose 4
Haemophilus Influenza type B (Hib)4
Dose 1
Dose 2
Dose 3
Dose 4
Diphtheria, Tetanus, Pertussis (DTaP, Td)5
Dose 1
Dose 2
Dose 3
Dose 4
Dose 5
Td Once
Measles, Mumps, Rubella (MMR)
Dose 1
Dose 2
or
Dose 2
Varicella (VZV)6
Once
Hepatitis A (Hep A)7
Dose 1 & 2 ® 0 and 6–18mo apart
SCREENING
Years of Age
B 1 2 3 4 5 6 7 8 9 10 11 12 13 14 15 16 17 18
Newborn Screening: PKU, Sickle Cell, Hemoglobinopathies, & Hypothyroidism
Hearing
Head Circumference8
Periodically
Height and Weight9
Periodically
Lead10
Eye Screening11
Blood Pressure12
Periodically
Dental Health
Periodically
Alcohol Use
Adolescents
COUNSELING
Years of Age
B 1 2 3 4 5 6 7 8 9 10 11 12 13 14 15 16 17 18
Development, nutrition, physical activity, safety, unintentional injuries, and poisonings, violent behaviors, and fire arms, STDs and HIV, family planning, tobacco use, & drug use
As appropriate for age

Figure 30-1 (opposing page). Clinical Preventive Services for Normal-Risk Children and Adolescents.

Recommended by most U.S. authorities.

[1]Hepatitis B vaccination scheduling can be flexible, and those not vaccinated in infancy may begin their series during any childhood visit. Those not immunized with the 3 doses should initiate or complete the series during the 11-12 year old visit.

[2]Schedules for polio vaccination vary depending on the vaccine combination chosen.

[3]CDC Publishes Updated Poliomyelitis Prevention Recommendations for the U.S. MMWR. 2000; 49:1-22.

[4]Number and periodicity of vaccinations may vary according to vaccine type.

[5]DTaP (diphtheria and pertussis toxoids and acellular pertussis) is the preferred vaccine for all doses. Whole cell DTP is an acceptable alternative.

[6]Children with a prior history of chicken pox do not need to be immunized. Children age 19 months to 12 years without a prior history of chickenpox should be vaccinated.

[7]Recommended in selected states or regions. Prevention of Hepatitis A Through Active or Passive Immunization: Recommendations of the Advisory Committee on Immunization Practices (ACIP). MMWR. 1999; 48(RR-12):1-37.

[8]Differences exist in recommendations for periodicity.

[9]Differences exist in age of onset and periodicity.

[10]In communities at established "low risk" for lead poisoning, targeted screening may be appropriate.

[11]Testing for strabismus is recommended by most authorities before or at 3 to 4 years of age. Routine visual acuity testing remains controversial.

[12]Differences exist in age of onset and periodicity.

Source: U.S. Department of Health and Human Services. Office of Public Health and Science of Office of Disease Prevention and Health Promotion. Put Prevention into Practice: Clinician's Handbook of Preventive Practice, ed. 2, Washington, D.C., 1998.

---

3. Vaccines.
   a. Vaccines are composed of toxoids or inactivated, live, or attenuated microorganisms. They confer *active immunity* to the individual. There is a rapid immune response to same/similar antigens at re-exposure. Table 30-4 provides a summary of some vaccines and their vaccine categories.
   b. Live vaccines (e.g., oral polio vaccine [OPV], measles, mumps, and rubella [MMR], yellow fever [YF]) should not be given to immunocompromised individuals or to women who are pregnant or lactating.

Category	Item	Ages (18–75 scale)	Recommendation
SCREENING	Blood Pressure, Height, Weight, Dental	18–75	Periodically
	Alcohol Use	18–75	Periodically
	Pap Smear[1]	18–75	Every 1 to 3 years: less frequently in same groups
	Cholesterol[2]	35–65	Men: Every 5 years
		40–65	Women: Every 5 years
	Mammography	50–70	Every 1 to 2 years
	Sigmoidoscopy and/or	50–75	Every 5 to 10 years
	Fecal Occult Blood	50–75	Yearly
	Vision, Hearing	65–75	Periodically
IMMUNIZATION	Tetanus-Diphtheria (Td)	18–75	Every 10 years
	Varicella (VZV)	18–75	Susceptibles only -- two doses
	Measles, Mumps, Rubella (MMR)[3]	18–50	Women of child-bearing age -- one dose
	Pneumococcal	65–75	One dose
	Influenza	65–75	Yearly
COUNSELING	**Women only:**		
	Calcium Intake	18–75	Periodically
	Folic Acid[4]	18–50	Women of childbearing age
	Hormone Replacement Therapy	40–75	Peri and post-meropausal women
	Mammography Screening	40–75	Periodically
	Men Only:		
	Prostate Cancer Screening	50–75	Periodically
	Both:		
	Tobacco cessation, drug and alcohol use, STDs and HIV, family planning, domestic violence, unintentional injuries, seat belt use, nutrition, physical activity, fall prevention, and polypharmacy (elderly)	18–75	Periodically

Figure 30-2 (opposing page). Clinical Preventive Services for Normal-Risk Adults.

Recommended by most US authorities.

[1]There is no upper age limit for pap smears, but regular testing in women over age 65 may be discontinued in those who have had regular screening with consistently normal results. Pap smears are not necessary in women who have undergone a hysterectomy in which the cervix was removed for reasons other than cervical cancer or its precursors.

[2]Some authorities initiate screening at age 19. Screening at less frequent intervals may be reasonable in low risk; individuals, including those with previously normal levels.

[3]MMR need only be given to women of childbearing age who lack documented evidence of immunization and are capable of becoming pregnant.

[4]Folic acid 0.4 mg per day is recommended for women of childbearing age who are capable of becoming pregnant.

Source: U.S. Department of Health and Human Services. Office of Public Health and Science and Office of Disease Prevention and Health Promotion. Put Prevention into Practice: Clinician's Handbook of Preventive Practice, ed. 2, Washington, D.C., 1998.

Table 30-3. SCREENING BY RISK FACTOR CATEGORY BY AGE AND GENDER FOR ADULTS.

Risk Factor	Prevention Target Condition	Preventive Services and/or Referral
All adults	Obesity	Obesity screening
	Hypertension (HTN)	Blood pressure screening
	Coronary heart disease (CHD)	Cholesterol screening
		Nutritional screening
		Exercise counseling
		Smoking cessation counseling
		Aspirin therapy (if indicated)
	Diabetes mellitus (DM)	Plasma glucose
	Malnutrition	Nutritional counseling

Continued

Table 30-3. SCREENING BY RISK FACTOR CATEGORY BY AGE AND GENDER FOR ADULTS—*cont'd*

Risk Factor	Prevention Target Condition	Preventive Services and/or Referral
	Dental disease	Dental check-ups
	Alcohol-related problems	Assess for problem drinking
	Injuries: intentional and unintentional, and related to drugs/alcohol	Counsel about various preventive measures
	Measles, mumps (persons born after 1956 only)	Serology for immune status (if no vaccination record), measles and mumps vaccines (if nonimmune)
Women of childbearing age	Neural tube defects	Folate
	Congenital rubella syndrome	Screen for rubella immunity (if no record of prior vaccination), rubella vaccine (if nonimmune)
Men 35-65 years Women 45-65 years	Elevated cholesterol	Cholesterol screening, nutritional counseling, exercise counseling, aspirin therapy (if indicated)
Women = 40 years of age	Breast cancer	Mammography, clinical breast examination
Men ages = 40 years of age	Prostate cancer	Digital rectal examination (DRE)* Prostate-specific antigen (PSA)*
Persons ages = 50 years	Colorectal cancer	Fecal occult blood test, sigmoidoscopy
All peri- and postmenopausal	Osteoporosis	Hormone replacement, nutritional counseling, exercise counseling

Table 30-3—cont'd

Risk Factor	Prevention Target Condition	Preventive Services and/or Referral
	CHD	Obesity screening, blood pressure screening, cholesterol screening, nutritional screening Exercise counseling, smoking cessation counseling, aspirin therapy (if indicated)
Persons = 60 years	Thyroid dysfunction	Thyroid function tests (TFTs)
Persons = 65 years	Influenza	Influenza vaccine
	Pneumococcal disease	Pneumococcal vaccine
	Tetanus	Check for last tetanus booster
	Visual problems including glaucoma	Referral for glaucoma screening
	Hearing impairment	Question regarding hearing
Persons >70 years with one or more of the following risk factors: psychoactive, cardiac or antihypertensive medication; impaired cognition, balance or strength	Falls	Counsel regarding home safety Assess vision Counsel regarding polypharmacy Assess for cognitive/ functional impairment

*Whether these procedures diminish the morbidity and mortality associated with prostate cancer is controversial.

Source: U.S. Department of Health and Human Services. Clinician's Handbook of Preventive Services: Put Prevention into Practice. Washington, DC: DHHS, Office of Public Health and Science, Office of Disease Prevention and Health Promotion, 1998.

Table 30-4. VACCINE CATEGORIES AND ASSOCIATED VACCINES AND/OR VACCINE COMPONENTS.

VACCINE CATEGORY	VACCINE AND/OR VACCINE COMPONENT
Inactivated bacterial vaccine	Pertussis typhoid (older version), anthrax, cholera, plague
Inactivated viral vaccine	Influenza inactivated poliomyelitis (IPV), hepatitis B (HBV), human diploid cell vaccine (HDCV) for rabies, Japanese encephalitis (JE)
Live attenuated bacterial vaccine	Bacillus Calmette-Guerin (BCG) for tuberculosis, typhoid: Ty21A (newer version)
Live attenuated viral vaccine	Oral poliomyelitis (OPV)
Live viral vaccine	Measles, mumps, rubella (MMR), varicella, yellow fever (YF)
Toxoid	Diphtheria, tetanus, meningococcal, haemophilus influenzae type b conjugate (Hib), pneumococcal

4. Some substances given to patients confer *passive immunity.* They provide limited protection (e.g., maternal antibodies protect infants from infection during their first few months of life; Hepatitis B immune globulin [HBIG] administered to individuals exposed to Hepatitis B temporarily protects them from developing active hepatitis).

B. Childhood Vaccinations

1. The AAP periodically publishes updates to their *Report of the Committee on Infectious Diseases,* which outlines immunization recommendations for infants and children. The ACIP periodically updates recommendations regarding immunization schedules, indications, and contraindications.
   a. There are varying schedules for some childhood vaccinations, including Hepatitis B virus (HBV); diphtheria, tetanus, pertussis (DTP); tetanus diphtheria (Td); inactivated poliomyelitis (IPV); *Haemophilus influenza* (Hib); and measles, mumps, rubella (MMR).
   b. The AAP does *not* consider the following conditions as contraindications to immunizing children:
      (1) Previous mild reactions.
      (2) Presence of nonspecific allergies.
      (3) Mild illness/diarrhea with low-grade fever in an otherwise healthy child.
      (4) Breast-feeding or pregnant household member(s).

2. Children and adolescents with chronic medical conditions (e.g., cancer, renal or hepatic disease, asplenia, or immunosuppressive disorders) should receive annual influenza vaccinations.

C. **Adult Vaccinations**

1. All adults should have received their childhood immunizations unless otherwise contraindicated.
2. Immunity conferred by some vaccinations (e.g., Td, MMR, HBV) wanes over time; consequently, at-risk individuals (e.g., health and child care workers, promiscuous individuals, intravenous [IV] drug users) require serum titers to ensure continued immunity. Those who are not immune will need booster shots in order to protect them from infection.
3. Elderly individuals (>65 years of age) or individuals with chronic medical conditions (e.g., chronic pulmonary or cardiac disease, cancer, renal, or hepatic disease, asplenia, or immunosuppressive disorders) should receive annual influenza vaccinations and at least one dose of the pneumococcal polysaccharide vaccine.

X. CHEMOPROPHYLACTIC AGENTS

Chemoprophylactic agents protect at-risk individuals from various infectious diseases (e.g., malaria, tuberculosis, sexually transmitted diseases [STDs], and meningococcal disease). Table 30-5 lists some chemoprophylactic agents and their indications.

XI. REPORTING OF NOTIFIABLE CONDITIONS

A. **Notifiable Conditions (Table 30-6):** Clinicians are required to report certain infectious diseases to their state public health

Table 30-5. PARTIAL LIST OF SOME CHEMOPROPHYLACTIC AGENTS AND THEIR INDICATIONS.

Chemoprophylactic Agents	Indication
Chloroquine phosphate or primaquine	For those traveling to underdeveloped countries with endemic malaria
Isoniazid (INH)	If there are no contraindications, it should be offered to those with positive intradermal purified protein derivative (PPD) tests or to those exposed to individuals with active tuberculosis
Rifampin	For those exposed to virulent meningococcal disease (e.g., meningitis or meningococcal sepsis)
Doxycycline and rocephin	For those who have been in sexual contact with a potentially infectious individual with syphilis and/or gonorrhea

PREV

Table 30-6. INFECTIOUS DISEASES DESIGNATED AS NOTIFIABLE AT THE U.S. NATIONAL LEVEL, 2002.

Acquired immunodeficiency syndrome (AIDS)	Mumps
Anthrax	Pertussis
Botulism	Plague
Brucellosis	Poliomyelitis, paralytic
Chancroid	Psittacosis
Chlamydia trachomatis, genital infections	Q Fever
Cholera	Rabies
Coccidiomycosis	Rocky Mountain spotted fever
Cryptosporidiosis	Rubella
Diphtheria	Rubella, congenital syndrome
Ehrlichiosis	Salmonellosis
Encephalitis, arboviral	Shigellosis
Enterohemorrhagic *Escherichia coli*	Streptococcal disease (invasive Group A)
Giardiasis	Streptococcal toxic-shock syndrome
Gonorrhea	*Streptococcus pneumoniae*, drug-resistant invasive disease
Haemophilus influenzae, invasive disease	*Streptococcus pneumoniae*, invasive, children <5 years
Hansen disease (leprosy)	Syphilis
Hantavirus pulmonary syndrome	Syphilis, congenital
Hemolytic uremic syndrome (HUS), post-diarrheal	Tetanus
Hepatitis, viral acute	Toxic-shock syndrome (TSS)
HIV infection	Trichinosis
Legionellosis	Tuberculosis (TB)
Listeriosis	Tularemia
Lyme Disease	Typhoid fever
Malaria	Varicella (deaths only)
Measles	Yellow fever
Meningococcal disease	

Source: Centers for Disease Control and Prevention. Division of Public Health Surveillance and Information. Epidemiology Program Office. Atlanta, 2002.

department; requirements differ slightly for each State. Providers should contact their respective state health department to obtain a current list of reportable events and procedures. The Council of State and Territorial Epidemiologists (CSTE) generates and periodically updates the list of nationally reportable infectious diseases. Access to the most current list can be obtained at the following website: *www.cdc.gov/epo/dphsi/PHS/infdis.htm*.

B. **Uses of Reported Information:** Public officials use reported information to determine the effectiveness of preventive measures, identify infection trends, find geographic clustering of cases, conduct contact tracing and community outreach efforts (identifying and educating exposed individuals and offering chemoprophylaxis to limit the spread of infection), and generate national summary statistics.

XII. **ACRONYMS AND ABBREVIATIONS (Table 30-7)**

Table 30-7. PREVENTIVE MEDICINE ACRONYMS AND ABBREVIATIONS.

Acronym or Abbreviation	Definition	Explanation
AHRQ	Agency for Healthcare Research and Quality	DDHS agency providing information on health care outcomes, quality, cost, use, and access
AZT	Azidothimidine	Drug used to fight HIV disease
AUDIT	Alcohol Use Disorders Identification Test	Alcohol screening questionnaire focusing on alcohol dependence and consequences of drinking
BSE	Breast self-examination	Breast examination by patient
CAGE	Cut down, annoyed, guilty, eye opener	Four-question survey to detect alcohol dependence
CBE	Clinical breast examination	Breast examination by provider
CBO	Community-based organization	Local organizations focused on population health

Continued

PREV

Table 30-7. PREVENTIVE MEDICINE ACRONYMS AND ABBREVIATIONS—*cont'd*

Acronym or Abbreviation	Definition	Explanation
CDC	Centers for Disease Control and Prevention	DHHS agency promoting health and quality of life by preventing and controlling disease, injury, and disability through partnerships, applied research, advocating sound public health policies, leadership, and training
CPS	Clinical Preventive Services	Screening examinations and counseling for medical conditions, immunizations, and chemoprophylaxis
DHHS	Department of Health and Human Services	U.S. government entity
DOT	Directly observed therapy	Part of some prevention initiatives, where the individual is observed taking medicines
DRE	Digital rectal examination	Rectal examination by provider; screening for prostate and colorectal cancer
FDA	Food and Drug Administration	DHHS agency that ensures the safety of foods and cosmetics, pharmaceuticals, biological products, and medical devices
HAART	Highly active antiretroviral treatment	Multidrug treatment for HIV infection
HBIG	Hepatitis B immune globulin	Chemoprophylaxis to protect persons exposed to hepatitis B virus via perinatal, percutaneous, sexual, or mucosal routes
HE/RR	Health education/risk reduction	Essential components to prevention initiatives

Table 30-7—cont'd

Acronym or Abbreviation	Definition	Explanation
HIV	Human immunodeficiency virus	Virus that causes AIDS
FOBT	Fecal occult blood test	Screening for colorectal cancer
HRIG	Human rabies immune globulin	Injection given in the gluteal muscle; along with wound cleansing and rabies vaccination series, it comprises part of postexposure rabies prophylaxis
HRSA	Health Resources and Services Administration	DHHS agency providing health resources for medically underserved populations
IDU	Injection drug use	Risk factor for AIDS, hepatitis, syphilis, etc.
HIS	Indian Health Service	DHHS agency providing services to American Indians and Alaskan Natives
INH	Isoniazid chemoprophylaxis	Postexposure prophylaxis for individuals exposed to *Mycobacterium tuberculosis*
MAST	Michigan Alcoholism Screening Test	Survey of alcohol dependence
MSM	Men who have sex with men	Risk factor for AIDS
NIH	National Institutes of Health	DHHS agency responsible for biomedical and behavioral research on diseases, human development, and aging
OI	Opportunistic infection	Infections that occur in patients with impaired host defenses, such as HIV-infected persons, transplant recipients, and elderly people

Continued

Table 30-7. PREVENTIVE MEDICINE ACRONYMS AND ABBREVIATIONS—*cont'd*

Acronym or Abbreviation	Definition	Explanation
PPD	Purified protein derivative	Intradermal injection used to detect infection with *M. tuberculosis* in asymptomatic individuals
PSA	Prostate-specific antigen	Screening test for prostate cancer
SAMHSA	Substance Abuse and Mental Health Services Administration	DHHS agency working to improve the quality and availability of substance abuse prevention, addiction treatment, and mental health services
SCHIPS	States Child Health Insurance Program	HCFA program providing health care coverage to children whose parents are not eligible for Medicaid
VCT	Voluntary counseling and testing	Part of various prevention initiatives

31

PSYCHIATRY

Brian Skop, MD, and Eric H. Hanson, MD, MPH

I. CHIEF COMPLAINT

A. Chief Complaint: Describe problem using patient's own words and include any complaints about the patient reported by other persons.

B. Identifying Data

1. Name, age, marital status.
2. Education level, occupational background, socioeconomic status, housing, religion.
3. Sources of information.
4. Referral sources.

II. HISTORY OF PRESENT ILLNESS

A. Reasons for Current Presentation

1. What symptoms are you currently experiencing? Be guided in your subsequent questions regarding symptoms by a review of Diagnostic and Statistical Manual of Mental Disorders (DSM-IV) signs and symptoms within the differential diagnoses being considered.
2. When did your symptoms begin (onset), and for what length of time have they occurred (duration)?
3. What external stressors do you think are contributing to your current condition?
4. What effects has your illness had on your family, work, and social interactions?
5. Have you received previous treatments for your condition, including hospitalizations, medications (type, dose, and duration of therapy), and psychotherapy? What was your response to these treatments, and who were the providing physicians or therapists?
6. Collateral history: Obtain with the consent of the patient from other individuals such as clinicians, relatives, friends, coworkers, or the police.

B. Psychiatric History

1. Have you been hospitalized for psychiatric or substance-related disorders? When? What type of treatment did you receive? Response to interventions?
2. What prescription medications have you taken in the past, including type, dose, duration of therapy, and provider?
3. What type of therapy have you received, and who were the providers?

4. Have you ever thought of committing suicide? Have you attempted suicide?
5. Have you experienced episodes of violence? Please describe.

III. PAST MEDICAL AND SURGICAL HISTORY

A. Past Medical History

1. What medical conditions do you currently have? What treatments have you received? With what response, including side effects?
2. Have you had a serious illness, such as seizures or central nervous system infections?
3. Female patient history: When was your last menstrual period? What, if any, premenstrual symptoms do you have? Have you ever been pregnant? Are you pregnant?
4. Are you sexually active? Do you use a contraceptive method? Which type?

B. Past Surgical History

1. Did your symptoms begin after a surgical procedure (e.g., bypass surgery and depression)?
2. Have you had an intracranial operation? Brain regions affected by intracranial operations, if known

C. Emergency and Trauma History

1. Have you ever had a head injury?
   - **a.** Did you lose consciousness?
   - **b.** Were you hospitalized?
   - **c.** Did your behavior change in any way following the injury?
2. Have you had other trauma or injuries? Emergency room visits and treatments?

D. Childhood History

1. Obtain birth and delivery history.
   - **a.** Intrauterine exposures to medications, toxins, or chemicals.
   - **b.** Complications with birth or delivery.
2. Development.
   - **a.** Where were you born?
   - **b.** What type of upbringing did you have?
   - **c.** Were you delayed in walking or talking or in any other developmental milestones?
   - **d.** How many siblings do you have (if any)? Were you a first-, middle, or last-born child?
   - **e.** Were your parents divorced or separated? Who raised you?
   - **f.** What type of relationships did you have with your primary relatives and caretakers?
   - **g.** Were you ever physically, sexually, or emotionally abused?
3. Did you have any serious childhood illnesses?

E. Occupational History

1. What is your current occupation?
2. How long have you been employed?

3. How satisfied are you with your job? Do you have any problems with your job?
4. Relationships with co-workers and boss.
5. What occupations/jobs have you held in the past? Why did you leave your previous positions?
6. Have you been exposed to any heavy metals, volatile chemicals, or infectious agents at work?

F. Travel History

1. Have you traveled to regions, or been in situations, where you might have been exposed to infectious agents that can affect the brain (e.g., New England and Lyme disease, Mexico and cysticercosis)?
2. Have you been exposed to any legal or illegal drugs during travel (e.g., arsenic-tainted drugs)?

G. Animal and Insect Exposure History: Have you been exposed to any animals or insects that might carry infectious diseases that infect the brain (e.g., mosquitoes and Venezuelan equine encephalitis, tsetse flies and sleeping sickness)?

IV. MEDICATIONS, ALLERGIES, AND ADVERSE REACTIONS

A. Medications

1. What prescription medications are you taking?
2. Are you taking any over-the-counter (OTC) medications, herbal preparations, or supplements?

B. Allergic or Adverse Reactions to Medications

V. HEALTH MAINTENANCE

A. Prevention

1. Have you ever sought or attended counseling?
   a. Concerning alcohol and other drugs: Have you ever found the need or been counseled to limit consumption? Have you received or been referred to treatment for abuse? Counsel to avoid driving while under the influence (DUI).
   b. Have you ever attended or been enrolled/sent to a tobacco cessation program?
2. Remain alert for depressive symptoms and suicide risk factors.

B. Diet

1. Have you lost or gained weight recently?
2. What is your typical diet? Is there any suggestion of vitamin deficiency (e.g., excessive alcohol intake leading to Vitamin B_{12} deficiency and memory deficits)?
3. Does the patient focus excessively on body weight or a specific region of the body?
4. Does the patient eat unusual substances (pica)? Are there signs of excessive restriction of eating, binging, or purging?

C. Exercise

1. How often do you exercise? For what length of time?
2. At what intensity do you exercise?

D. **Sleep Patterns**

1. How many hours do you sleep each night? Is your sleep restorative?
2. Do you have difficulty falling asleep? Do you wake up frequently throughout the night? Do you frequently awaken early?
3. Do you have night terrors?
4. Nightmares?
5. Do you snore or have apnea?
6. Do you sleepwalk?
7. Do you have episodes of suddenly falling asleep at unusual times (sleep attacks)?
8. Have you experienced temporary muscle weakness? Cataplexy: Transient attacks of muscle weakness while awake, often during times of excitement?
9. Do you have hallucinations while wakening (hypnopompic) or when falling asleep (hypnagogic)?
10. Do you have kicking (paroxysmal) leg movements?
11. Nocturnal seizure activity?
12. Do you make unusual movements while sleeping?

E. **Social Habits**

1. Do you use alcohol, tobacco, caffeine, or illicit drugs?
2. How much? For how long?
3. Has your use interfered with your work, relationships, or social activities?
4. Have you had any substance-related legal problems?
5. Have you acquired a tolerance to any substances (i.e., a decreased response to repeated doses of a drug or the need for increasing doses to achieve a response)?
6. Have you had withdrawal symptoms? How severe were they? What type (e.g., seizures, delirium tremens, hallucinations)?
7. Do you have any cravings?
8. Describe prior attempts to reduce use.
9. Have you had medical complications caused by previous substance use?

VI. **FAMILY HISTORY**

A. **First-Degree Relatives' Psychiatric History**

1. Have any relatives had psychiatric disorders?
2. What treatments did they receive?
3. What was the response to these treatments?
4. Were there any attempted or completed suicides?
5. Did any relatives abuse alcohol or other substances?

B. **First-Degree Relatives' Medical History**: Obtain family medical history, focusing on movement disorders, epilepsy, strokes, and hormonal diseases.

C. **Three-Generation Genogram**: Create a genogram focusing on any inherited, familial disorders and psychiatric disorders.

VII. PSYCHOSOCIAL HISTORY

A. Personal and Social History

1. Social history.
   a. What is your living situation? Do you live alone or with other people? Who? How many people and in what type of residence?
   b. What is your financial situation?
   c. What community activities do you participate in? Do you belong to any groups? What leisure activities do you engage in?
   d. Do you belong to any religion? Are you an active member? Do you regularly participate?
   e. What legal problems, if any, have you had?
2. Educational history.
   a. Highest level of achievement. High school diploma? College? Other?
   b. What type of grades did you receive in school?
   c. Did you have any academic or behavioral problems (e.g., truancy, suspension)?

B. Current Illness Effects on the Patient (explored in HPI)

C. Interpersonal and Sexual History

1. Are you heterosexual, homosexual, or bisexual?
2. Are you, or have you been, married or in a committed relationship? Length of time relationships lasted? If separated or divorced, why? Any children? How stable is your current family?

D. Family and Friends Support System: Assess degree to which patient's family and friends are supportive and the quality of these relationships.

E. Occupational Aspects of Illness: Assess whether this patient will be able to continue in previous occupation.

VIII. REVIEW OF SYSTEMS (Tables 31-1 and 31-2)

Review of physical symptoms that might indicate nonfunctional causes of the psychic complaints. Emphasis should be placed on chronic or episodic complaints and neurologic, endocrinologic, or psychosomatic elements. Should also include a review of symptoms from major psychiatric syndromes. (See the DSM-IV, published by the American Psychiatric Association, for full diagnostic criteria for psychiatric conditions.)

IX. PHYSICAL EXAMINATION

The general physical examination of a psychiatric patient should place special emphasis on the neurologic and mental status examination (Table 31-3). Individuals coping with physical illnesses are at increased risk for psychiatric comorbidity in general: Diabetes mellitus and coronary artery disease, for example, are associated with increased rates of major depression. Certain illnesses (e.g.,

Text continued on p. 671.

Table 31-1. GENERAL SYMPTOMS BY SYSTEM.

System	Symptoms
General and neurovegetative	Changes in appetite, weight loss or gain, changes in cold or heat tolerance, changes in sleep, changes in energy level, frequent infections, periods of lightheadedness, abnormal sweating
HEENT	Changes in hair coarseness or hair loss, change in skin tone, stigmas of alcohol dependence, facial hair in women, abnormal facies suggesting genetic or developmental disorder such as low-set ears and hypertelorism
Neck	Enlargement of the thyroid, tightness in the throat
Respiratory	Difficulty breathing or feeling short of breath
Cardiovascular	Chest discomfort, shortness of breath, palpitations
Gastrointestinal	Abdominal discomfort, nausea, vomiting, constipation, diarrhea, gastric bleeding, enlarged liver, cirrhosis
Genitourinary	Erectile and sexual functioning and sexual history, genital pain, risk factors for and symptoms of STDs, testicular and penis size
Obstetrics/ Gynecologic	Pelvic pain, clitoromegaly, breast enlargement in men, sexual functioning and sexual history, pain during intercourse, risk factors for and symptoms of STDs, premenstrual discomfort or changes in emotional state around menstrual cycle, pregnancy status and history, including emotional state during and after the pregnancy or any elective or spontaneous abortions
Hematopoietic	Symptoms of anemias
Lymphatic	Adenopathy
Musculoskeletal	Muscular atrophy or hypertrophy, long or short limb length, hyperflexibility
Neurologic	Paresthesia, dysesthesia, tremors, vertigo, dizziness, syncope, seizures, epilepsy, memory loss

Table 31-1—cont'd

System	Symptoms
Psychiatric	
Disorders usually first diagnosed in childhood	Mental retardation, learning disorders (reading, mathematics, written expression), developmental coordination disorder, communications disorders (expressive language, mixed receptive-expressive language disorder, phonologic disorder, stuttering), pervasive developmental disorders (autistic disorder, Rett's disorder, childhood disintegrative disorder), attention-deficit hyperactivity disorder, conduct disorder, oppositional defiant disorder, pica, rumination disorder, feeding disorder of infancy or early childhood, tic disorders (Tourette's syndrome, chronic motor or vocal tic disorder, transient tic disorder), encopresis, enuresis, separation anxiety disorder, selective mutism, reactive attachment disorder of infancy or early childhood, stereotypic movement disorder
Attention-deficit and behavior disorders	Problems maintaining attention and following through with tasks
Delirium, dementia, amnestic and cognitive disorders	Dementias (Alzheimer's, vascular, HIV/AIDS, head trauma, Parkinson's, Huntington's chorea, Pick's disease, Creutzfeldt-Jakob disease), delirium, amnestic disorders, cognitive disorders
Substance-related disorders	Abuse, dependence, substance-induced disorders (delirium, dementia, psychosis, mood, anxiety, sleep, sex)
Psychotic disorders	Schizophrenia, schizophreniform disorder, schizoaffective disorder, delusional disorder, and brief psychotic disorder, shared psychotic disorder
Mood disorders	Major depressive disorder, dysthymic disorder, bipolar I disorder, bipolar II disorder, cyclothymia
Anxiety disorders	Panic disorder with or without agoraphobia, agoraphobia, specific phobias, social phobia, obsessive-compulsive disorder, posttraumatic stress disorder, acute stress disorder, generalized anxiety disorder

Continued

Table 31-1. GENERAL SYMPTOMS BY SYSTEM—*cont'd*

System	Symptoms
Somatoform disorders	Somatization disorder, undifferentiated somatoform disorder, conversion disorder, pain disorder, hypochondriasis, body dysmorphic disorder
Factitious disorders	Feigning physical or psychological signs and symptoms to assume the sick role. Factitious disorder by proxy involves inducing the symptoms in another individual to vicariously assume the sick role
Dissociative disorders	Dissociative amnesia, dissociative fugue, dissociative identity disorder, depersonalization disorder
Sexual disorders	Dysfunction (hypoactive desire, aversion, female sexual arousal disorder, male erectile dysfunction, orgasmic disorders, premature ejaculation, dyspareunia, vaginismus), paraphilias (exhibitionism, fetishism, frotteurism, pedophilia, sexual masochism, sexual sadism, transvestic fetishism, voyeurism), gender identity disorder
Eating disorders	Anorexia nervosa, bulimia nervosa
Sleep disorders	Dyssomnias (insomnia, hypersomnia, narcolepsy, sleep apnea, circadian rhythm disorder), parasomnias (nightmares, sleep terrors, sleep walking)
Impulse disorders	Intermittent explosive disorder, kleptomania, gambling, trichotillomania, pyromania
Adjustment disorders	Emotional or behavioral response to a stress that is either excessive or causes significant psychosocial dysfunction
Personality disorders	Paranoid, schizoid, schizotypal, antisocial, borderline, histrionic, narcissistic, avoidant, dependent, obsessive-compulsive
v-codes	Conditions that bring an individual to see a psychiatrist that are not considered mental disorders, although they may accompany a mental disorder: psychological factors affecting a medical condition, medication-induced movement disorders, relationship problems, problems related to abuse, noncompliance with treatment, malingering, antisocial behavior, borderline intellectual functioning, age-related cognitive decline, bereavement, academic problem, occupational problem, identity problem, spiritual problem, acculturation problem, phase-of-life problem

Table 31-2. COMMON PSYCHIATRIC SYNDROMES AND THEIR SYMPTOMS.

DISORDER	SYMPTOMS
Attention-deficit/ hyperactivity disorder	Often displays six symptoms of inattention (careless mistakes, getting off task, does not listen well, does not follow through on instructions, avoiding difficult task, frequently loses things needed to accomplish tasks, easily distracted, forgetful) and/or often displays six symptoms of hyperactivity (fidgety, gets out of seat, runs and climbs excessively, inappropriate situations, loud during play and leisure activities, "on the go," talks excessively, blurts out answers before questions are completed, difficulty awaiting turn, interrupts). Symptoms present before age 7, seen in multiple settings, and cause significant impairment.
Conduct disorder	Pattern of behavior with at least three of the following present over the last year and at least one during the last month: Aggression to people and animals, destruction of property, deceitfulness or theft, serious violations of rules. If the individual is older than 18, criteria are not met for antisocial personality disorder.
Oppositional defiant disorder	Pattern of behavior lasting at least 6 months with a minimum four of the following symptoms being frequently present: Loses temper, argues with adults, refuses to comply with rules, deliberately annoys people, blames others, easily annoyed, angry, vindictive. If the individual is older than 18, criteria are not met for antisocial personality disorder. Does not meet criteria for conduct disorder and does not occur only in the context of a mood or psychotic disorder.
Delirium	Acute onset of disturbed consciousness and attention with associated cognitive problems resulting from a general medical condition, substance intoxication, or withdrawal.
Dementia	Gradual or subacute onset of cognitive deficits, including at least memory impairment and one of the following: Aphasia, apraxia, agnosia, or executive dysfunction. The most common etiology is Alzheimer's disease. Other causes include vascular, HIV, head trauma, Parkinson's, Huntington's disease, Pick's disease, Creutzfeldt-Jakob disease, substance-induced.

Continued

Table 31-2. COMMON PSYCHIATRIC SYNDROMES AND THEIR SYMPTOMS—*cont'd*

Disorder	Symptoms
Substance dependence	Over a 12-month period, three or more of the following: Tolerance, withdrawal, recurrent episodes where substance is taken in greater amounts or over longer periods than intended, unsuccessful attempts to cut down on substance use, excessive amounts of time using, obtaining, or recovering from substance use, negative impact on functioning because of substance use, persistent use despite knowing that psychological or physical problems arise from the substance use.
Substance abuse	Over 12-month period, one or more of the following causing significant dysfunction: Recurrent episodes where substance use causes a failure to fulfill major obligations, recurrent use in potentially hazardous situations, recurrent legal problems related to substance use, continued use despite the use causing or exacerbating interpersonal problems. Does not meet criteria for substance dependence.
Schizophrenia	A 6-month period with some of the following symptoms, including a 1-month period with at least two of the following: Delusions, hallucinations, disorganized speech, disorganized behavior, negative symptoms.
Major depressive episode	A 2-week period during which five of the following are present nearly every day, including either depressed mood or loss of interest: Depressed mood (in children and adolescents this can be an irritable mood), loss of interest or pleasure in most activities, appetite disturbance (reduced or increased), insomnia or hypersomnia, psychomotor retardation or agitation, loss of energy, worthlessness or excessive guilt, inability to concentrate or make decisions, recurrent suicidal thoughts.
Manic episode	One-week period of elated, irritable, or expansive mood with at least three (four if mood is irritable) of the following present: Grandiosity, reduced need for sleep, hyperverbal, flight of ideas or racing thoughts, distractible, increased goal-directed activity or kinetics, excessive involvement in pleasurable activities that have potentially serious consequences.

Table 31-2—cont'd

Disorder	Symptoms
Hypomanic episode	Four-day period of manic symptoms without severe social or occupational dysfunction and without the need for hospitalization.
Mixed episode	One-week period where symptoms of both manic and major depressive episodes are present.
Major depressive disorder	One or more major depressive episodes with no history of manic, hypomanic, or mixed episodes.
Dysthymic disorder	Two-year period (one year in children and adolescents) of depressed mood (may be irritable mood in children and adolescents) more days than not with two of the following: Appetite disturbance, sleep disturbance, low energy, low self-esteem, poor concentration or indecisiveness, or feelings of hopelessness.
Bipolar I disorder	Affective illness where there has been at least one manic or mixed episode either currently or in the past. Often one will see major depressive episodes and hypomanic episodes over the course of the illness.
Bipolar II disorder	Affective illness characterized by major depressive episodes and hypomanic episodes. There cannot be a history of full manic episodes.
Substance-induced mood disorder	Affective symptoms (depression, mania, hypomania) felt to be caused by substance or medication use. The diagnosis is listed with the name of the causative agent. For instance, cocaine-induced mood disorder with manic features.
Mood disorder caused by a general medical condition	Affective symptoms (depression, mania, hypomania) felt to be caused by a general medical condition. The diagnosis is listed with the name of the illness. For instance, mood disorder caused by stroke with depressive features.
Panic attack	Intense fear or discomfort accompanied by at least four of the following: Palpitations, sweating, trembling, difficulty breathing, feeling like one is choking, chest discomfort, abdominal distress, feeling lightheaded, dissociative symptoms, fear of going crazy, fear of dying, paresthesias, chills or flushing.

Continued

Table 31-2. COMMON PSYCHIATRIC SYNDROMES AND THEIR SYMPTOMS—*cont'd*

Disorder	Symptoms
Panic disorder with or without agoraphobia	Recurrent panic attacks that come "out of the blue" with subsequent intense fear of further attacks or worries about the implications of the attack. Agoraphobia (fear and avoidance of situations where escape might be difficult) is so frequently seen in those afflicted with panic disorder that its presence or absence is noted as part of the diagnosis.
Obsessive-compulsive disorder (OCD)	Recurrent obsessions (recurrent thoughts, impulses, or images that are intrusive and cause severe anxiety, e.g., urges to hit strangers and thoughts of infection) or compulsions (repetitive behaviors or mental acts to reduce anxiety usually caused by an obsession, e.g., hand washing, checking locks, and counting). These activities take up more than 1 hour a day of time or cause significant social or occupational impairment.
Posttraumatic stress disorder (PTSD)	At least one-month response to a traumatic event (defined as experiencing or witnessing an event that threatens or results in death, serious injury, or the violation of the physical integrity of self or others, where the event is experienced with intense fear) that includes: (1) Re-experiencing the event through intrusive memories of it, nightmares, flashbacks, intense psychological or physical distress when exposed to things that remind the victim of the incident; (2) avoidance of things or thoughts associated with the event or dissociative symptoms such as inability to remember aspects of the event, feeling detached, and feeling emotionally numb; (3) symptoms of increased arousal such as sleep disturbance, poor anger modulation, hypervigilance, and increased startle response.
Generalized anxiety disorder	Worry and anxiety over 50% of days associated with at least three of the following: Restlessness, easy fatigability, poor concentration, irritability, muscle tension, sleep disturbance.

Table 31-2—cont'd

Disorder	Symptoms
Anorexia nervosa	Refusal to maintain body weight so that weight is less than 85% of that expected for a given age and height; intense fear of weight gain despite low weight; disturbed perception of one's body habitus; and amenorrhea in postmenarcheal females.
Bulimia nervosa	Over at least a 3-month period, recurrent episodes (at least twice a week) of binge eating and behaviors (self-induced vomiting, excessive exercise, diuretic or laxative abuse) to prevent weight gain. Overly focused on body shape and weight.
Antisocial personality disorder	Pattern of behavior present since at least 15 years old where there is disregard for the rights of others, including at least three of the following: Repeated acts that are illegal, lying for personal profit or pleasure, impulsivity, repeated assaults, reckless disregard for the safety of others, repeated episodes of failing to sustain work or honor financial obligations, lack of remorse.
Borderline personality disorder	Pattern of unstable relationships, affect, self-image, and affect since at least early adulthood. Five or more of the following: Frantic efforts to avoid abandonment, pattern of unstable relationships, potentially damaging impulsivity, recurrent suicidal behavior or self-mutilation, affective instability, chronic feelings of emptiness, poor anger modulation, transient dissociation or stress-related paranoid ideation.
Histrionic personality disorder	Pattern of excessive emotionality and attention-seeking since at least early adulthood. Five or more of the following: Discomfort in situation where the individual is not the center of attention, seductive interactions, rapidly shifting and shallow emotions, frequent use of physical appearance to draw attention, speech is excessively impressionistic and lacking detail, dramatic, suggestible, misinterprets relationships to be more intimate than they actually are.

Continued

Table 31-2. COMMON PSYCHIATRIC SYNDROMES AND THEIR SYMPTOMS—*cont'd*

Disorder	Symptoms
Narcissistic personality disorder	Pattern of grandiosity, need for admiration, and lack of empathy since early adulthood. Five or more of the following: Grandiose sense of self-importance, fantasies of unlimited success, requires excessive admiration, sense of entitlement, interpersonally exploitative, lacks empathy, envious of others, and arrogant.
Obsessive-compulsive personality disorder	Pattern of preoccupation with orderliness, perfectionism, interpersonal control, lack of flexibility, openness, and efficiency since early adulthood. Four or more of the following: Preoccupied with details or rules to the degree that the point of the activity is lost, perfectionism that interferes with task completion, excessive devotion to work at the expense of friendships and leisure activities, inflexible about matters of morality and ethics, unable to discard worn-out objects even if they have no sentimental value, reluctant to delegate tasks, miserly spending with money viewed as something to be hoarded for future catastrophes, rigidity and stubbornness.
Dependent personality disorder	Pervasive pattern since early adulthood of needing to be taken care of that leads to submissiveness and fears of separation. Five or more of the following: Difficulty making decisions without excessive advice and reassurance, needs others to assume responsibility for most major areas of one's life, difficulty disagreeing because of fear of loss of the relationship, difficulty initiating projects because of lack of confidence, volunteers to do unpleasant tasks to obtain support from others, fears ability to care for self if alone, urgently seeks relationships when another relationship ends, preoccupied with fears of being left to care for oneself.

Table 31-3. FINDINGS OF PHYSICAL EXAMINATION AND POSSIBLE DIAGNOSES.

SYSTEM	PHYSICAL EXAMINATION FINDINGS	POSSIBLE DIAGNOSES
Vital signs and general	Cachexia	Eating disorders, major depression, inability to care for activities of daily living because of physical or mental illness, neglect or abuse
	Obesity	Eating disorder, Prader-Willi syndrome, major depression
	Autonomic instability	Neuroleptic malignant syndrome, malignant catatonia, substance intoxication or withdrawal, eating disorders
Skin/Hair/Nails	Abnormal patterns of hair loss	Trichotillomania
	Jaundice, telangiectasis	Alcohol dependence, end-stage liver disease related to drug abuse or sexually transmitted diseases
	Nail bed pitting	Eating disorders
	Lanugo	Eating disorders
	Needle tracks	IV drug abuse
	Tattoos and body piercing	Important to find out the meaning of tattoos and piercings. These can reflect antisocial and borderline personality traits
	Scars	Scars can indicate prior suicide attempts or self-mutilating behaviors that can accompany several different psychiatric disorders
	Hirsutism	Steroid dependence

Continued

Table 31-3. FINDINGS OF PHYSICAL EXAMINATION AND POSSIBLE DIAGNOSES—*cont'd*

System	Physical Examination Findings	Possible Diagnoses
HEENT	Abnormal facies	Fragile X, intrauterine alcohol exposure, Down syndrome, and other numerous genetic abnormalities
	Parotid enlargement	Eating disorders
	Dental enamel erosion	Eating disorders
	Perforated nasal septum	Cocaine dependence
	Miosis or mydriasis	Substance intoxication or withdrawal
	Omega sign (persistently furrowed brows)	Major depressive disorder
Cardiovascular	Midsystolic click	Mitral valve prolapse (MVP), which may be associated with panic disorder
Abdomen	Enlarged liver or small liver	Alcohol dependence
	Ascites	Alcohol dependence
Genitourinary	Enlarged testes	Fragile X syndrome
	Small testes	Alcohol dependence, steroid dependence
	Clitoromegaly	Steroid dependence
Extremities	Edema	Malnutrition resulting from alcohol dependence, eating disorders, inability to care for activities of daily living
Neurologic	Focal complaints with incongruent examination	Conversion disorder and other somatoform disorders
	Posturing	Catatonia, substance intoxication
	Rigidity	Neuroleptic malignant syndrome, substance intoxication, catatonia

Table 31-3—cont'd

System	Physical Examination Findings	Possible Diagnoses
	Cog wheeling, simian posture and shuffling gait, dystonia	Antipsychotic side effects
	Tardive movements	Antipsychotic side effects
	Tremor	Medication side effect, substance withdrawal

Table 31-4. MENTAL STATUS EXAMINATION OUTLINE.

A. Attitude toward examiner
B. Reliability of information
C. General appearance and behavior
D. Emotion
   1. Mood
   2. Affect
E. Speech/Language
F. Thought processes
G. Thought content
H. Cognition
I. Intelligence
J. Insight
K. Judgment

neurologic, autoimmune, and endocrinologic illnesses) can present with psychiatric symptoms or have psychiatric symptoms as part of their syndromes; other psychiatric illnesses are very much defined by physical complaints (e.g., somatoform disorders, panic attacks).

X. MENTAL STATUS EXAMINATION (Table 31-4 and Box 31-1)

A. Attitude Toward Examiner: Attitudes during the interview and examination (e.g., apathetic, passive, submissive, cooperative, flirtatious, obsequious, frank, guarded, withdrawn, evasive, irritable, angry, defensive, outspoken criticisms, hostile, suspicious, dramatic, manipulative, or indifferent).

B. Reliability of Information

1. Examiner's overall judgment of accuracy and completeness of source(s) of information.
2. Elements of presentation that may impair the transfer or content of information (e.g., disturbances in speech, extensive

PSYCH

Box 31-1. MINI-MENTAL STATE EXAMINATION.

Maximum score	
	Orientation
5	What is the (year) (season) (date) (day) (month)?
5	Where are we: (state) (county) (town) (hospital) (floor)?
	Registration
3	Name three objects. Ask the patient to repeat all three. Give one point for each correct answer. Repeat the objects until the patient learns all three. Record the number of trials.
	Attention and Calculation
5	Serial 7s. Subtract by 7s from 100 down to 65 (e.g., 100-93-86-79-72-65). Give one point for each correct answer. Alternatively may spell "world" backward.
	Recall
3	Ask for the three objects repeated above. Give one point for each object recalled.
	Language
9	Name a pencil and watch. (2 points) Repeat the following: "No ifs, ands, or buts." (1 point) Follow a three-stage command: "Take a paper in your right hand, fold it in half, and put it on the floor. (3 points) Read and obey the following: Close your eyes. (1 point) Write a sentence. (1 point) Copy a design or two intersecting pentagons. (1 point)
_____	**Total score**

Source: Folstein MF, Folstein SE, McHugh PR. Mini-mental state: A practical method for grading the cognitive state of patients for the clinician. J Psych Res 12:189-198, 1975.

use of defense mechanisms, preoccupation, failure to cooperate, psychosis, altered level of consciousness, and cognitive disorders).

C. General Appearance and Behavior

1. Physical appearance.
   - **a.** Apparent physical health.
   - **b.** Younger or older than stated age.
   - **c.** Physical deformities or limitations.
   - **d.** Personal hygiene.
   - **e.** Peculiarities in clothing, makeup, jewelry, hair, and accessories.
2. Eye contact: Avoids direct eye contact, has reduced eye contact, has intense eye contact, has "wide eyes," moves eyes toward distractions like hallucinations.
3. Posture: Body held rigid (stiff) or bizarre posture.
4. Motor activity: Purposeful or disorganized, stereotyped (repetitive, non-goal directed movements), graceful, tics, rituals, mannerisms, automatisms, dyskinesias, echopraxia (mirroring motor activity of those in the environment), attending to internal stimuli (responding to hallucinations or delusions), motor signs of anxiety or emotional state, psychomotor retardation (generalized slowing of activity and reactions), psychomotor excitement (generalized increased activity), waxy flexibility, or catalepsy (body stays in position into which it is positioned).

D. Emotion

1. Mood.
   - **a.** Pervasive and sustained emotional state (e.g., euphoric, elated, grandiose, happy, sad, depressed, anxious, worried, angry, irritable, frightened, worried, indifferent, apathetic, suspicious, or furious). Can use quote from patient.
   - **b.** Appropriateness of relationship between mood and content of thought.
2. Affect: Current expression of patient's emotional state through facial expression or motor activity.
   - **a.** Range: Degree to which facial expressions vary (e.g., full range, reactive, flat, blunted, intense).
   - **b.** Appropriateness of affect to mood and thought content (e.g., inappropriate, labile).

E. Speech and Language

1. Rate/pacing: Slow, moderate, or rapid.
2. Reaction time: Prompt, delayed, or hesitant.
3. Degree of spontaneity: Mute, minimal response to questions, reduced, increased, or pressured (uninterruptible).
4. Continuity: Sudden silences or changes of topic, prompt, hesitant.
5. Fluctuations: Monotonic, highly emotional.

6. Fluency: Observation of voice quality, articulation, and aphasia during the history.
   a. Dysarthria: Difficulty in articulating the individual sounds or the units (phenomes) of speech; f's, r's, g's, vowels, consonants, labials ("Pa", CN VII), gutturals ("Ka", CN X), and the linguals ("La", CN XII). Have patient say "Pa, Ka, La" or "Buttermilk."
   b. Dysphonia: Difficulty in producing the voice sound.
   c. Dysprosody: Difficulty with the stress of the syllables, inflections, pitch of voice, and the rhythm of the words. Difficulty conveying the emotional context of words.
   d. Dysphasia: Difficulty in expressing words as symbols of communication.
7. Coherency: Relevance to examiner's questions.
8. Volume: Soft to whisper, moderate, or loud to shouting.
9. Unusual patterns: Rhyming, echolalia (repeating words said in their presence), punning, difficulty in word finding, word salad, strange syntax, or neologisms (invention of new words).

F. **Thought Processes**

1. Description of the degree to which thoughts are connected together, the efficiency of thoughts, and the degree to which the thoughts are logical, deductive, and reality based. Normal thought processes are linear (connected), logical (reality-based and related in an understandable fashion), and goal directed (achieve an endpoint without a lot of detractors).
2. Examples of characteristic terms.
   a. Loosening of associations or derailed thoughts: There is no maintenance of subject. Thoughts shift continually between unrelated topics. At times speech can approach frank gibberish.
   b. Flight of ideas: Thoughts shift rapidly from one idea to the next. The new thought is weakly connected to the prior thought but not with a logical endpoint.
   c. Clang associations: Thoughts are connected by the sound of words or phrases rather than the meaning. Tends to have a musical or poetic quality but no meaning.
   d. Blocking: Thoughts are interrupted at illogical times. Usually there is a pause, and the thoughts seem to have been withdrawn from the patient's mind.
   e. Tangential: Thoughts are loosely connected but never reach an anticipated endpoint.
   f. Circumstantial: Thoughts wander toward the logical endpoint on a very indirect path. Content is overinclusive and full of unneeded detail.
   g. Perseveration: Repetition of one thought, or thoughts repetitively wander to the same idea.

h. Illogical: Thoughts have no logical connection and speech is disorganized.

i. Racing: Thoughts are being produced faster than they can be expressed.

j. Poverty of content: Speech lacks detail or substantive content.

k. Concrete: Thoughts are generally simple and do not reflect ability to abstract or understand complex ideas.

G. Thought Content

1. Thought content details should be described in this section or reference made to the HPI, if discussed there.
2. At a minimum, should comment on suicidal and violent ideations, plans, and intent at the time of the examination, as well as psychotic content. Also include thoughts expressed by the patient that help the reader of the examination get an understanding of the patient's illness and issues. For example: The patient was very pessimistic. He frequently spoke about how inadequate he was as a father.

a. Suicidal ideations.

(1) Do you have a plan?

(2) Do you have access to instruments necessary to carry out the plan?

(3) How intent on completing suicide are you?

(4) What preparations for suicide have you made (e.g., life insurance, giving items away)?

(5) Is there a suicide note?

(6) What changes or statements do you hope to make through suicide?

(7) Deterrents: What is stopping you from committing suicide (e.g., effects on family, religion, plans for the future)?

b. Homicidal or violent ideations.

(1) Do you have a plan?

(2) Do you have access to instruments necessary to carry out the plan?

(3) Is there a specific target?

(4) How intent on completing the violent act are you?

(5) What preparations for the act have you made (e.g., obtained a weapon, set up a meeting)?

(6) What changes do you hope to make through the violent act?

(7) To what extent does the patient understand the repercussions of completing the act (e.g., jail, getting shot by police)?

(8) Deterrents: What keeps you from carrying out this act (e.g., effects on family, legal problems)?

c. Hallucinations: False perceptions in the absence of real sensory stimulation.
   (1) Hallucinations can be auditory, visual, tactile, olfactory, or gustatory.
   (2) Describe the nature, quality, duration, exacerbators and relievers, and the effects on the patient's behavior.
   (3) For auditory hallucinations, describe the voice or voices if discernable, whether they are telling the patient to do something, and the degree to which the content of the hallucinations matches the mood of the patient (mood congruence). Examples of hallucination subtypes:
      (a) Command: Auditory hallucinations where the patient is directed to take some action.
      (b) Hypnopompic: Hallucinations occur during wakening.
      (c) Hypnagogic: Hallucinations occur when falling asleep.
      (d) Formication: The sensation of insects crawling on the skin often seen in drug withdrawal states.
      (e) Lilliputian: Things appear smaller than they really are.

d. Illusions: Misinterpretations of real sensory stimulations.

e. Delusions: Fixed false beliefs that cannot be explained by a person's background or culture. Delusions are often referred to as bizarre or nonbizarre depending on the degree to which they are possible in reality. Examples of delusion subtypes:
   (1) Paranoid: Themes of persecution (e.g., a belief by a patient that government agencies are pumping mind-controlling gases through his vents).
   (2) Grandiose: Delusion that one has special skills or qualities (e.g., a patient believes she has been selected to be God's lover).
   (3) Somatic: Delusion that body is diseased despite evidence to the contrary (e.g., a patient believes that he has serpents growing in his abdomen).
   (4) Jealousy: Delusion that mate is having an affair.
   (5) Erotomanic: Delusion by the patient that someone is in love with him.
   (6) Reference: Delusion by the patient that remarks or actions by others are directed toward him (e.g., patient believes a radio announcer is sending special messages to him alone that the world is coming to an end).
   (7) Control: Delusion by the patient that an outside force is controlling him.
   (8) Withdrawal: Delusion by the patient that an outside force is withdrawing his thoughts.

(9) Insertion: Delusion by the patient that thoughts are being inserted into his head.
(10) Guilt: Delusion by the patient that he has committed an unforgivable act.
(11) Folie à deux (shared delusion): Delusional belief that evolves in the context of a close relationship with one who has the delusion.

f. Obsessions: Repetitive ideas, impulses, or images that cause distress and anxiety. Patients with obsessions often develop compulsions (repetitive actions or mental exercises that relieve anxiety).

g. Ruminations: Thoughts on which the patient is overly focused, including helplessness, hopelessness, guilt, unworthiness, doubting and indecision, hypersexuality, and hyperreligiosity.

h. Somatizations: Focus on bodily complaints and pains usually in excess of the pathology present. Hypochondriacal ruminations are persistent fears of having a serious disease despite evidence to the contrary.

i. Dissociations: Depersonalization (feeling as though one has changed in some fashion), derealization (feeling as though the world has somehow changed), flashback phenomena, déjà vu, and jamais vu.

j. Phobic complaints: Specific fears of certain situations, people, or things. Subtypes:
(1) Agoraphobia: Fear of being in inescapable situations or in situations where one might not be able to obtain help.
(2) Social phobia: Fear of situations where one is likely to be scrutinized. Can be specific to performance-related situations or more generalized to fear of most social interactions.
(3) Specific phobia: Fear of certain situations (e.g., heights, flying, being in thunderstorms) or items (e.g., dogs, needles, wood).

H. Cognition

1. The most commonly used test of cognition is the Folstein Mini-Mental Status Examination (MMSE) (See Box 31-1).
2. The MMSE is less sensitive to frontal lobe functioning. Tests more specific to the frontal lobe include the following:
   a. Alternating sequence reproduction: Draw +0++0+++0 on a piece of paper and ask the patient to reproduce and continue the sequence.
   b. Verbal trails test: Ask the patient to repeat and continue the following sequence: 1, A, 2, B, 3, C.
   c. Go-no-go tasks: Ask the patient to raise his index finger in the air when the examiner touches his nose and ask the

patient to touch his nose when the examiner raises his finger in the air. The examiner then alternates raising his finger and touching his nose.

d. Luria hand movements: Demonstrate for the patient a pattern of making a fist, holding the hand on the side, and holding the hand palm down repeatedly, and then ask the patient to repeat this pattern.

e. Snout, suck, palmomental, and grasp reflexes.

I. Intelligence

1. Estimate the patient's intelligence based on educational level achieved, vocabulary, and ability to think abstractly (i.e., understand concepts, similarities, and proverbs).
2. Common proverbs: Test responses to common proverbs, such as "Don't cry over spilled milk." "A rolling stone gathers no moss." "People who live in glass houses should not throw stones."

J. Insight: Estimation of the patient's ability to recognize and understand own emotional, mental, or psychiatric problems or symptoms; awareness of situation, of own contributions to the illness, and the need for assistance.

K. Judgment: Ability to evaluate courses of action or interpret information based on life experiences.

1. It is often tested using simple questions such as "What would you do if you found a stamped envelope in the street?" and "What would you do if you smelled smoke in a movie theater?"
2. However, the examiner should also make an assessment based on the clinical interview, such as patient's awareness of social norms, ability to plan ahead, and ability to make reasonable decisions.

XI. PSYCHOLOGICAL TESTING AND FURTHER STUDIES

A. Commonly Used Psychological Tests (Table 31-5)

1. Psychological tests are often ordered for several reasons:
   a. Further clarify the differential diagnosis.
   b. Monitor the illness and effectiveness of treatment.
   c. Help develop a treatment plan.
   d. Assess functional strengths and weaknesses.
2. When ordering psychological testing, the physician should let the psychologist know what the goals of the testing are.
3. The psychologist selects the tests that are appropriate to these issues (e.g., to assess the effects of a head injury, the psychologist might choose to administer the Halstead-Reitan neuropsychological battery but not the Minnesota Multiphasic Personality Inventory).

B. Laboratory and Radiologic Data

1. Review prior laboratory tests for abnormalities that might indicate a general medical condition contributing to the clinical presentation or substance abuse. For instance, a low blood sugar can cause delirium.

Table 31-5. COMMON PSYCHOLOGICAL TESTS.

TEST	USES
Wechsler Intelligence Scales	There are three tests for different age groups. They provide verbal, performance, and full-scale intelligence quotient (IQ) scores
Halstead-Reitan	Neuropsychological battery
Luria-Nebraska	Neuropsychological battery
Wisconsin Card Sorting Test	Tests executive functioning (abstraction, set shifting)
Minnesota Multiphasic Personality Inventory-2 (MMPI-2)	Tests symptom patterns and personality on 13 scales. Self-reported but contains validity scales
Millon Clinical Multiaxial Inventory-II	Tests symptom patterns and personality on 25 scales. Self-reported but contains validity scales
Beck Depression Inventory (BDI)	Brief assessment of the intensity of depression symptoms. Self-reported. Often used to monitor treatment effectiveness
Hamilton Rating Scale for Depression (Ham-D)	Clinician-administered test of the intensity of depression symptoms. Often used to monitor treatment effectiveness
Beck Anxiety Inventory	Brief assessment of the intensity of anxiety symptoms. Self-reported. Often used to monitor treatment effectiveness
Hamilton Rating Scale for Anxiety (Ham-A)	Clinician-administered test of the intensity of anxiety symptoms. Often used to monitor treatment effectiveness
Yale-Brown Obsessive Compulsive Scale and Checklist (Y-BOCS)	Clinician-administered test of the intensity of obsessive compulsive disorder symptoms. Often used to monitor treatment effectiveness
Thematic Apperception Test	Projective test where the examinee is asked to tell a story about pictures presented to him or her by the examiner. Based on the responses, inferences about the psychodynamic functioning, such as reality testing and defense mechanisms, are made

Continued

Table 31-5. COMMON PSYCHOLOGICAL TESTS—cont'd

TEST	USES
Rorschach Inkblot Test	Projective test where the examinee is asked to comment on standard inkblots presented to him or her by the examiner. Based on the responses, inferences about the psychodynamic functioning, such as reality testing and defense mechanisms, are made

2. There is no standard battery of laboratory tests for psychiatric conditions. Laboratory and radiology testing is tailored to the individual presentation and differential diagnosis. For instance, if an individual with known schizophrenia and noncompliance presents with psychosis, the laboratory work-up could be minimal unless there is a suspicion of a complicating medical or substance use issue; however, if an elderly person presents with psychosis for the first time, a much more extensive work-up (e.g., blood counts, electrolytes, renal functions, liver functions, B_{12}, rapid plasma reagin [RPR], thyroid functions, electrocardiogram, and head imaging) would be indicated.

XII. FORMULATION

Assessment of the case is typically presented in the bio/psycho/social format. It is usually written in paragraph form and should comment on the patient's strengths and weaknesses.

A. **Biologic:** Biological components that contribute to the presentation (e.g., hereditary, substance use, medical conditions, and treatments).
B. **Psychological:** Developmental issues (e.g., abuse, observations of parental relationships) and defensive mechanisms (e.g., projection, denial, splitting).
C. **Social:** Environmental issues contributing to the presentation (e.g., job loss, financial problems, marital discord).

XIII. DIAGNOSTIC IMPRESSION

The DSM-IV provides a standard format for listing diagnoses:

A. **Axis I:** Most psychiatric disorders are listed on Axis I (e.g., major depressive disorder, recurrent, severe without psychotic features).
B. **Axis II:** Personality disorders (e.g., borderline personality disorder) and mental retardation are listed on Axis II.
C. **Axis III:** Lists physical conditions or treatments that may contribute to the psychiatric presentation (e.g., steroid therapy leading to mania).

D. Axis IV: Brief list of psychosocial and environmental stressors (e.g., occupational problems, marital discord, and financial problems).

E. Axis IV: Global Assessment of Functioning (GAF). This is a number from 0 to 100 that reflects the clinician's global estimate of how the patient is functioning currently and the highest level of functioning obtained over the last year. The DSM-IV has descriptions of what different scores on the GAF means: 0 = inadequate information; 1 = very severe symptoms; <50 = serious symptoms (e.g., suicidal thoughts or serious impairment in psychosocial functioning); 100 = superior functioning.

XIV. PROGNOSIS

Opinion about probable course, extent, and outcome of illness (e.g., "This is the patient's 10th hospitalization for an acute exacerbation of schizophrenia related to poor medication compliance and amphetamine dependence; his insight into his illness is poor. While over the short term in the control of an inpatient setting, he is likely to improve. His long-term prognosis is guarded.").

XV. TREATMENT PLAN

A. Gather collateral information (information from other sources to help clarify the diagnosis [e.g. family, co-workers, teachers]).

B. Indicate further work-up to be accomplished: Laboratory and radiology examinations, psychological testing, further observation.

C. Therapeutic interventions:

1. Inpatient, partial hospitalization, or outpatient.
2. Medication therapy.
3. Psychotherapy: individual, group, family, and/or milieu.
4. Interventions to improve patient's environment (e.g., Alcoholics Anonymous, boarding home, case management, Social Security Disability, vocational and education rehabilitation).

XVI. ACRONYMS AND ABBREVIATIONS (Table 31-6)

XVII. PSYCHIATRIC TERMS AND DEFINITIONS (Table 31-7)

XVIII. SAMPLE H&P WRITE-UP

CC: "I'm losing it."

Identifying Data: J.C. is a 25-year-old single white male. He lives alone and works at a local computer company in their product design department. He is seen with his girlfriend, who brought him to the emergency department. The emergency department physician is consulting Psychiatry at this time because J.C. has expressed suicidal thoughts.

HPI: J.C. reports that over the last 6 months he has had increasingly frequent bouts of anxiety. He reports that he feels shaky, his heart beats rapidly, he feels like he is having problems breathing, and he feels like he is going to pass out and like he needs to lie down. He has found it increasingly difficult to get out of his home and especially to go to work. As a result he has used all of his sick leave and has been told that he may be let go from his job if his absences continue. He relates that he likes his job and that he is very depressed about

Table 31-6. PSYCHIATRIC ACRONYMS AND ABBREVIATIONS.

Acronym or Abbreviation	Definition
SIG E CAPS	This is a screening commonly used to remember the symptoms of depression: **S**leep, **I**nterest in activities, excessive **G**uilt, **E**nergy, **C**oncentration, **A**ppetite, **P**sychomotor activity, **S**uicidal thoughts.
CAGE	This is a common screening for alcohol abuse: Efforts to **C**ut back, **A**nnoyance at others' comments about one's drinking, **G**uilt about the drinking, **E**ye-openers (drinking in the morning to cure a hangover).
SI	Suicidal ideation
HI	Homicidal ideation
LLGD	Abbreviation used in the Thought Process section of the Mental Status Examination: **L**inear, **L**ogical, and **G**oal **D**irected
DSM	Diagnostic and Statistical Manual of Mental Disorders
MDD	Major depressive disorder
BPD	Bipolar disorder
OCD	Obsessive-compulsive disorder
PTSD	Posttraumatic stress disorder
ADHD	Attention-deficit/hyperactivity disorder
MR	Mentally retarded
BIF	Borderline intellectual functioning
ODD	Oppositional defiant disorder
GAD	Generalized anxiety disorder

the situation. He reports that the first episode occurred after an argument with his father about his father's unwillingness to help his sister with college expenses. After this initial attack, the attacks seemed to come out of the blue. For the last month, he finds himself feeling overwhelmed by everything. He has withdrawn from most social activities. He is not sleeping. He feels lethargic. He is not eating and has lost 9 pounds. He acknowledges having thoughts that it would be better if he were dead. He has thought about shooting himself and has a gun at home. He does not desire to do this but feels he is likely to try if he loses his job. He reports that he is still hopeful that he can work through these problems and that he has promised his family and girlfriend that he will not hurt himself.

Table 31-7. PSYCHIATRIC TERMS.

TERM	DEFINITION
Agoraphobia	Fear and avoidance of situations where escape might be difficult
Cataplexy	Transient attacks of muscle weakness while awake, often during times of excitement
Catalepsy	State of unresponsiveness and waxy flexibility of the limbs
Echolalia	Repeating words said in their presence
Echopraxia	Mirroring motor activity of those in the environment
Frotteurism	Production of sexual excitement by rubbing against someone
Huntington's chorea	Inherited adult-onset progressive disease of the central nervous system, characterized by dementia and bizarre involuntary movements
Neologisms	Invention of new words
Pick's disease	A form of dementia characterized by a slowly progressive deterioration of social skills and changes in personality leading to impairment of intellect, memory, and language
Rett's disorder	A progressive syndrome of autism, dementia, ataxia, and purposeless hand movements; associated with hyperammonemia, principally in girls
Somatoform disorder	A group of disorders in which physical symptoms suggesting physical disorders for which there are no demonstrable organic findings or known physiologic mechanisms, and for which there is positive evidence, or a strong presumption that the symptoms are linked to psychological factors (e.g., hysteria, conversion disorder, hypochondriasis, and pain disorder)
Stereotyped movements	Repetitive, non-goal-directed movements
Tourette's syndrome	A neurologic disease of unknown cause that presents with multiple tics (uncontrolled behavior), associated with snorting, sniffing, and involuntary vocalizations. Explosive utterance of obscenities is common
Word salad	Production of words that have no goal direction or interrelatedness

His girlfriend relates that J.C. has become significantly worse over the last month. She reports that he has made several comments that he would be better off dead. Tonight she found him looking at his gun, and she convinced him to come to the emergency department. She reports that their relationship is good, although it has been strained by his mood and unwillingness to leave the home.

Psychiatric History: J.C. reports that he was in family counseling briefly during the period before his parents divorced. He was 10 years old at the time. He saw the counselor alone briefly after the divorce, but he is uncertain of the reason for this. He denies prior suicide attempts. He denies a history of violence.

PMHx: He reports that he has allergic rhinitis. He had a brief loss of consciousness following a motor vehicle accident when he was 16 years old. He reports he was taken to the hospital but released the same day. He does not believe this affected him. He denies any history of seizures or seizurelike activities. He denies HIV risk factors.

PSHx: He reports that he had sinus surgery seven years ago.

Childhood History: J.C. does not endorse developmental delays; though he stated he would need to ask his mother to be certain. He was born and raised in Chicago. He has two younger sisters. His father was a salesman and an alcoholic. J.C. reports that his father and mother often got into physical altercations when his father was drunk. He believes this ultimately led to their divorce when he was 10 years old. He reports his father would also often put him down and called him stupid. After the divorce, he would only infrequently see his father. He reports that he was and continues to be angry with his father. He denies physical or sexual abuse. He reports his mother was a homemaker. After the divorce, he and his sisters lived with her. They were very poor. He reports that he felt close to his mother: "She was always there for me."

Occupational History: J.C. denies occupational exposures.

Travel History: J.C. reports that he has not traveled recently because of his fear of leaving the home.

Animals and Insect Exposure History: He reports that he has a dog that is healthy. He is unaware of any insect bites.

Medications: Allegra 60 mg bid.

Allergies: He developed hives on penicillin as a child.

Health Maintenance: As previously noted, J.C. reports that he has not been eating well and his sleep has been off. He reports it takes him a long time to fall asleep and then he wakes up around 4 a.m. and cannot get back to sleep. He has been taking a multivitamin. He used to run 3 times a week but has not exercised for the last five months. He reports that he has been drinking a six-pack to a twelve-pack of beer every evening for the last 3 months. He denies alcohol-related arrests or a history of withdrawal symptoms. He states that he realizes he is drinking too much but felt it was the only way to cope with the anxiety. On occasion he drinks until he blacks out. Before the onset of the anxiety, he would only drink two to three beers on weekends. He has been drinking since he was in high school. He reports his mother and girlfriend have expressed concern about the drinking because he becomes more depressed and argumentative when he is intoxicated, and he has been unable to cut back. He acknowledges that hangovers are interfering with his job performance. He denies tobacco use. He does admit to smoking marijuana a few times a week since the anxiety started. Before this he reports he would use it at parties. He has been smoking since he was in high school. He reports that his girlfriend has been trying to get him to quit because she does not like his personality when he smokes. He denies other drug use except experimenting once with "shrooms."

Family History: J.C. reports that his father and paternal grandfather were alcoholics. He states he feels his mother suffered with depression but that she never sought treatment for this condition. He has a maternal aunt who was "crazy" and often in the psychiatric hospital. J.C. reports that his father has hypertension and heart disease.

Psychosocial History: J.C. lives alone in an apartment. He denies financial problems or legal problems. He reports that he is Christian but that he does not attend church. He lists his girlfriend, his mother, and a long-time friend as his main sources of support. He reports that he has other friends, but he does not consider them close friends. He reports that most of his friendships have been stable. He only speaks with his father twice a year. His main leisure activities before the anxiety were running and playing soccer. He has not done either of these activities for a few months. He reports that his soccer teammates no longer call him up because he is never willing to play.

He has a bachelor's degree in computer science from the University of Illinois. He reports that he was an average student, getting A's and B's. He reports that after his parents divorced, he was suspended once for fighting and cursing at the teachers. J.C. has been dating his girlfriend for 2 years. They are sexually active and monogamous. He is heterosexual. He denies a history of promiscuity. He reports he and his girlfriend had been talking about getting married until the last 6 months. He is not sure that he can be a good husband. He reports two other serious girlfriends. Both relationships lasted about 1 year and ended when he went from high school to college and when he graduated from college. He denies a history of abuse in his relationships.

J.C. has worked at his present position for 4 years. He reports he had some conflict with a supervisor 2 years ago over different ideas about a project. He thought about leaving at that time. Since then he has had no problems until the present situation. He reports he gets along with his co-workers and boss. He reports that he worked as a waiter in college and a bagboy in high school. He denies ever being fired from a job, and he left these jobs because of the school transitions.

Review of Systems: J.C. endorses the physical symptoms noted in the HPI during panic attacks. He also endorses that his sex drive has been poor and at times he has had problems maintaining an erection since the onset of the anxiety. He has also had more headaches. He reports these are a constant pain extending from the neck to the forehead. They tend to come at the end of the day and are helped by ibuprofen. He reports that he has had problems speaking in front of others most of his life. He gets anxious, tongue-tied, has palpitations, sweating, and a dry mouth. He reports that he tends to be a perfectionist and is orderly to the point that he loses track of the big picture. He believes that this trait is what led to the conflict with his boss a few years ago.

PHYSICAL EXAMINATION

Vital Signs: Temperature: 98.6°F, Respiratory rate: 16 breaths per minute, pulse: regular rhythm of 72, blood pressure: 125/65, height: 72 inches, and weight: 175 lbs.

Head and Neck (general): Normocephalic/atraumatic (NC/AT). Neck FROM, no lymphadenopathy. Trachea midline. Thyroid smooth without nodules or bruits. No carotid bruits. No JVD or HJR.

Eyes: Lids normal, conjunctivae are clear, and sclerae are non-icteric, PERRL (ADC), EOMI, full visual fields by confrontation. Fundoscopic examination reveals sharp disk margins, cup-to-disk (C/D) ratio less than 0.5, normal macula and venous pulsations.

Ears: No discharge noted, canals patent A.U. TMs normal landmarks, light reflex and mobility. Acuity grossly intact (to whispered voice). Weber midline, Rinne AC > BC.

Nose: No discharge noted. Nasal mucosa moist and pink. Septum midline and turbinates without polyps, swelling or inflammation. No frontal, ethmoidal, or maxillary tenderness.

Mouth: Lips, buccal mucosa, and gingiva moist and pink, without erythema, ulcerations, or petechiae. Tongue symmetrical without fissures or ulcerations.

Throat: Oropharynx (O/P) and tonsils without erythema or exudate.

Teeth: Normal dentition.

Chest (general): Symmetrical with equal expansion. No pain, tenderness, or masses upon palpation. No gynecomastia. Breasts and axilla without pain, tenderness, or masses upon palpation. No nipple retraction or inversion, erythema, or discharge. No axillary lymph nodes palpable.

Lungs: Lungs clear to auscultation and percussion (CTAP), breath sounds equal bilaterally. Normal chest symmetry/AP diameter without use of accessory muscles. No wheezes, rales (crackles), or rhonchi. No dullness to percussion.

Cardiovascular: Normal S1 and S2. Normal S2 splitting with inspiration. S3 and S4 absent. Regular rate without murmurs, rubs, heaves or thrills. Peripheral pulses symmetric and 2+ throughout.

Abdomen: S, NT, ND, NABS without hepatosplenomegaly (HSM). Liver edge was palpable and mildly tender. It was 15 cm at the right MCL by percussion. No masses palpable. No aortic pulsations. No peritoneal signs. No dilated veins, bruits, shifting dullness, or fluid wave. No suprapubic tenderness.

Back: Straight and symmetrical. No abnormal spinal curvatures. No costovertebral angle tenderness (CVAT).

Extremities: UE and LE symmetrical, FROM without joint tenderness, swelling, or deformity. No C/C/E (clubbing/cyanosis/edema). Pulses 2+ bilaterally.

Skin (Integument): Warm and dry. Normal turgor. No lesions, rashes, or petechiae.

Lymphatics: No cervical, axillary, or inguinal adenopathy.

Neurologic: Cranial Nerves II-XII intact by direct confrontation. Motor 5/5 strength throughout with good tone. Sensory intact throughout to pain, light touch, two-point discrimination, vibratory, and proprioception. Cerebellar function intact by finger to nose (F → N), heel to shin (H → S), and rapid alternating movements (RAMs). Gait is symmetrical and balanced (broad-based). Station: no drift, Romberg negative. Reflexes 2+ symmetrical. Babinski negative (down going). No asterixis.

Mental Status Examination: J.C. is a well-groomed, thin, white male. He is wearing jeans and a T-shirt. He maintains good eye contact. He is cooperative during the examination and relates well to the examiner. His kinetics are reduced. His mood is depressed and anxious. His affect is full range and consistent with his mood. He is frequently tearful. His speech is of low volume and the spontaneity is reduced. It is flat and monotone. It is fluent and coherent. J.C.'s thought processes are linear, logical, and goal directed. He tends to ruminate about being fired. He denies violent ideations, hallucinations, or delusions. He reports thoughts of suicide by shooting himself. He denies intent at this time, but reports the thoughts seem to be more frequent. He lists his mother and girlfriend as the main deterrents to following through with these thoughts.

J.C. scored 29 out of 30 on the Folstein Mini-Mental Status Examination. He missed one point for remembering only 2 of 3 items at five minutes. He was able to successfully do Luria hand movements and Go-No-Go tasks. His intelligence was estimated in the above average range based on his vocabulary and his ability to abstract. He was asked proverbs and gave the following responses: 1. *Don't cry over spilled milk* meant. "You can't change something once it is done." 2. *People who live in glass houses should not throw stones* meant "Don't say things to others before you see if they apply to you." His insight was judged to be good based on his understanding of the situation. His judgment was felt to be fair in that he was self-medicating with drugs and alcohol and had let his illness progress to a severe level but not sought help.

Psychological Testing: None had been accomplished.

Laboratory Testing: Electrolytes were within normal range. His liver functions were mildly elevated. He had a normal blood count. Thyroid function tests and a urine toxicology screen were pending. No radiological studies had been accomplished.

Formulation: J.C. is a 25-year-old male with depression associated with multiple neurovegetative symptoms and suicidal thoughts. He is having frequent panic attacks and agoraphobia. He has a family history of depression, substance abuse, and an unclear serious psychiatric disorder. He appears to be using alcohol and marijuana to alleviate some of his mood and anxiety symptoms. At this juncture he does not appear to have any medical conditions that would contribute to his presentation, and his overall good health and prior history of regular exercise are strengths.

From a psychological standpoint, he appears to have an anxious temperament. He is obsessive and likes structure. This style may in part be related to his upbringing, during which he appears to have felt the need to provide some stability for his family, which was stressed by his father's alcoholism. The conflict with his father that started this period of panic and depression was an effort by him to get his father to fulfill what J.C. felt was a family obligation. The panic attacks clearly are an affront to his usual defense mechanisms and are thus quite disruptive for him, as is the threat of job loss. Strengths include his ability to maintain stable relationships and employment. His reality testing is intact.

Social stressors include threatened job loss, ongoing conflict with his father, and social isolation caused by his agoraphobia. Strengths include a supportive girlfriend and mother, lack of financial problems, and stable housing.

Diagnostic Impression:

Axis I	Panic Disorder with Agoraphobia
	Major Depressive Disorder, Single Episode Severe
	Alcohol Dependence
	Cannabis Abuse
Axis II	Obsessive Compulsive Traits, rule out Obsessive Compulsive Personality Disorder
Axis III	Elevated Liver Function Tests and Hepatomegaly
Axis IV	Occupational Problems
Axis V	GAF present 35/highest the past year 65

32

PULMONOLOGY

Patricio G. Bruno, DO, Eric H. Hanson, MD, MPH, Thomas S. Neuhauser, MD, and Amro Y. Al-Astal, MD

I. CHIEF COMPLAINT

A. **Chief Complaint:** Usually focused on difficulty breathing or a complaint involving passage of air. Use the patient's own words.

B. **Identifying Data:** Name, age, gender, race/ethnicity, and location of evaluation.

II. HISTORY OF PRESENT ILLNESS

Determine if the chief complaint is attributable to a pulmonary problem or another system disorder manifesting with pulmonary symptoms.

A. **Seven Common Complaints Leading to a Pulmonology Evaluation**

1. Cough.
   a. When did the coughing start (onset)? How long has the cough persisted (duration: acute <3 weeks, subacute = 3 to 8 weeks, chronic >8 weeks)? Have there been significant changes in the severity of the cough over time (longitudinal pattern)?
   b. Is the cough better or worse in the morning or in the evening?
   c. Are you coughing at night (nocturnal cough)?
   d. Is there sputum or phlegm production with the cough? What does the sputum look like and how much are you coughing up? Is there any hemoptysis (i.e., expectoration of blood or of blood-stained sputum)?
   e. Is the cough associated with heartburn (gastroesophageal reflux disease [GERD]) or drainage in the throat (postnasal drip or sinusitis)?
   f. Do you smoke or use tobacco products (packs per day and duration of use)? Does anyone around you smoke?
   g. Is there a relationship of symptoms to work hours (possible workplace exposures)?
   h. Are you taking any medications (angiotensin-converting enzyme [ACE] inhibitors or beta-blockers)?
2. Shortness of breath (SOB).
   a. When did the SOB start (onset)? How long has the SOB persisted (duration)? Have there been significant changes in the SOB severity over time (longitudinal pattern)?
   b. Any relation to certain times of the day?

   c. Any relation of SOB to activities, and if so, which activities?
   d. Any relation to position (erect, supine, lateral)? Does resting or a recumbent position make the SOB better or worse (orthopnea or paroxysmal nocturnal dyspnea [PND])?
   e. Any dizziness or fatigue associated with the SOB?
3. Pain.
   a. Where is your pain located? On one or both sides of your chest (unilateral or bilateral)?
   b. How intense is the pain? Have the patient rank it from 0 to 10, with 10 being the most intense pain ever experienced. Give an example with 10 being equal to a traumatic amputation of an extremity.
   c. Any associated dyspnea (i.e., subjective difficult or distressed breathing) or SOB?
   d. Is the pain localized or diffuse, sharp or dull (qualify the pain)?
   e. Increased with inspiration (pleuritic pain)?
   f. Is there a history of trauma to the thoracic or abdominal regions?
4. Wheezing.
   a. Is the wheezing present on inspiration, expiration, or both?
   b. Do you know of factors that can trigger the wheezing (e.g., triggers can be cold, exercise, allergies/hay fever, foods, chemicals)? Any exacerbating factors that make an episode worse?
   c. Is the wheezing associated with an activity or location?
   d. Is the wheezing associated with ingestion of food shortly before onset?
   e. Is the wheezing associated with season of the year or temperature?
   f. What makes the wheezing better (alleviating factors)?
5. Snoring.
   a. Is the snoring of recent onset or is it long-term in duration?
   b. Do spouse or friends comment on how loud you snore and how frequently (quality and quantity)?
   c. Have there been any recent changes in the snoring pattern? Any worsening of the snoring since it started or was first noticed?
   d. Are you fatigued during the day? Do you have episodes of daytime sleepiness? Have you ever fallen asleep while driving or had a motor vehicle accident (MVA) because you were tired?
   e. Have you recently gained weight or lost weight?
6. Sputum production.
   a. When did the sputum production start (onset)? How long has the sputum production persisted (duration)? Have there

been significant changes in the sputum production over time (longitudinal pattern)?

b. Are there any associated fevers (>100.4°F)?
c. Is the sputum production greatest in the morning (timing)?
d. What is the color and have there been changes in color? Is the sputum bloody or blood streaked (quality)?
e. What is the amount produced in an hour or day? Has there been any change in that amount (quantity)?
f. Do you smoke or use tobacco products (packs per day and duration of use)? Does anyone around you smoke?
g. Is there a relationship of symptoms to work hours (possible workplace exposures)?

7. Hemoptysis.
   a. When did you start coughing up blood (onset)? How long has the hemoptysis persisted (duration)? Have there been significant changes in the amount of blood coughed up over time (longitudinal pattern)?
   b. How much blood have you coughed up (quantify the amount)?
   c. What is the color of the blood (bright red or black)? Did the blood clot or was it coagulated (look like coffee grounds)?
   d. Are there any associated fevers (>100.4°F) or chills?
   e. Have you lost any weight (wasting)?
   f. Do you experience chest pains, pleurisy, or other associated symptoms with the hemoptysis?
   g. Have you had any recent surgery (bronchoscopy)?
   h. Any recent inactivity or immobilization? Do you have any leg pains or swelling (deep venous thrombosis [DVT] and pulmonary embolism [PE])?
   i. Do you smoke or use tobacco products (packs per day and duration of use)? Does anyone around you smoke?
   j. Have you ever lived in a nursing home, prison, or on a farm? Have you traveled to other countries in the past?
   k. Do you have a history of tuberculosis (TB) exposure? Have you received isoniazid prophylaxis for TB skin test conversion?
   l. Are you taking any medications that thin the blood (nonsteroidal anti-inflammatory drugs [NSAIDS], coumadin)?
   m. Is there a family history of bleeding or clotting disorders?

B. Common Pulmonary Disorders Leading to a Pulmonology Evaluation

1. Asthma (reactive airway disease [RAD]): Paradoxical narrowing of the bronchi (mucus-plugged airways, inflammation, submucosal gland hyperplasia, smooth muscle hypertrophy) making breathing difficult.
   a. When did you first have symptoms of asthma (age of onset) or when were you diagnosed (onset)?

b. How long have you had asthma (duration)?
c. Have there been significant changes in the asthma symptoms over time (longitudinal pattern or progression)?
d. What symptoms do you commonly experience (episodes of wheezing, cough, fever, purulent sputum, dyspnea or SOB)? Have you had pneumonia or chronic obstructive pulmonary disease (COPD)? Do you experience recurrent episodes?
e. How many episodes of asthma exacerbation and hospitalizations per year?
f. Do you smoke or use tobacco products (packs per day and duration of use)? Does anyone around you smoke?
g. What factors are known to trigger an asthma attack? Examples of triggers are allergens (pollen, food, animal dander, medications), infectious, changes in temperature and humidity, emotional stress, foreign body aspiration, and exercise.
h. Is there a family history of asthma, hay fever/allergies, or atopic dermatitis?
i. Have you ever been intubated or had your breathing assisted by machine (ventilation)?
j. Have you used steroid treatments, home oxygen, or nebulizers in the past?
k. What medications are you taking currently? How often do you need rescue inhalers? Have you missed any recent doses?
l. Do you regularly check your peak flow? What is your normal peak flow?

2. Chronic obstructive pulmonary/lung disease: Two types (chronic bronchitis and emphysema) with progressive chronic airflow obstruction; irreversibility distinguishes from asthma. Patients often have both chronic bronchitis and emphysema symptoms.

a. Chronic bronchitis: Minimally reversible constriction of the bronchi with hypoventilation and chronic productive cough (3 months or more for 2 consecutive years).

(1) How long have you had the cough with sputum production? Is the sputum produced in large amounts (copious)? What is the color of the expectorant (yellow, green, or dirty gray [mucopurulent])?
(2) Do you smoke or use tobacco products (packs per day and duration of use)? Does anyone around you smoke?
(3) Do you have SOB with or without exertion (dyspnea)? Do you experience a feeling of "air hunger"? Do your extremities or lips turn blue or dusky? Patients with chronic bronchitis often are obese and have rapid,

shallow breathing, with perioral and extremity cyanosis ("blue bloater").

(4) How often do you have exacerbations? Have you been hospitalized or intubated?

(5) What medications are you taking (list dosages, frequency of use, and recent changes in treatment regimens)? Have you missed any doses of your medications? Are you using home oxygen?

b. Emphysema: Destruction of the alveolar septa with expansion of the air spaces and a decrease in lung compliance.

(1) How long have you had the cough (usually nonproductive cough)?

(2) Do you smoke or use tobacco products (packs per day and duration of use)? Does anyone around you smoke?

(3) Do you have SOB with or without exertion (dyspnea)? Patients with emphysema are frequently thin framed with a barrel chest deformity, have rapid, shallow breathing (pursed-lip breathing), and have a pink, flushed color ("pink puffer").

(4) How often do you have exacerbations? Have you been hospitalized or intubated?

(5) What medications are you taking (list dosages, frequency of use, and recent changes in treatment regimens)? Have you missed any doses of your medications? Are you using home oxygen?

(6) Do you have a family history of emphysema ($alpha_1$-antitrypsin deficiency) or alcohol abuse?

3. Interstitial Lung Disease (ILD): Distal lung parenchyma disease with alveolar wall inflammation and derangement; infiltration of lung tissue by fibrous tissue, infection, or inhaled agent.

a. Do you have SOB with or without exertion (dyspnea)? Patients frequently have a dry cough, rapid, shallow breathing, SOB, and dyspnea on exertion.

b. Do you have a cough? Is it productive of sputum?

c. Do you smoke or use tobacco products (packs per day and duration of use)? Does anyone around you smoke?

d. Do you have a history of autoimmune diseases (e.g., rheumatoid arthritis, systemic lupus erythematosus [SLE], Goodpasture's syndrome, myositis, systemic fibrosis, or inflammatory bowel disease [IBD]), collagen vascular disease, eosinophilic pneumonia, amyloidosis, or sarcoidosis?

e. Do you have a history of radiation exposure, dust exposure (inorganic dust: beryllium, silica, asbestos), fume or gas exposure, or other significant hobby or occupational exposures to chemicals or materials?

f. Have you had any recent surgeries (graft versus host reaction [GVHD] in transplant patients)?
g. Do you take medications (Nitrofurantoin; methotrexate)?
h. Is there a family history of similar lung conditions?

4. Pulmonary embolism (PE): Lodgment of a blood clot in the lumen of a pulmonary artery, causing a severe dysfunction in respiratory function (dyspnea) and pleuritic chest pain.
   a. When did the SOB start (onset)? How long has the SOB persisted (duration)? Have there been significant changes in the SOB severity over time?
   b. Does the chest pain change with respiration?
   c. Have you had a cough? Have you coughed up blood (hemoptysis)?
   d. Do you have any fevers or chills?
   e. Have you had any extended periods of inactivity or immobilization? Do you have any leg pains or swelling? Have you had a deep venous thrombosis (DVT) in the past?
   f. Any history of heart problems (heart failure, atrial fibrillation)?
   g. Are you pregnant?
   h. Any history of cancer (pancreatic, lung, genitourinary, stomach, breast, bone)?
   i. Any history of clotting disorders (hypercoagulability)? Any family history of clotting disorders?
   j. What medications are you taking (estrogens in oral contraceptives)?
5. Pneumonia (recurrent or complicated): Infection of the lungs with consolidation.
   a. Have bouts with pneumonia been a recurrent problem? When were the episodes and how were they treated?
   b. Have you been hospitalized for pneumonia? Were you ever intubated?
   c. What symptoms did you experience and in what settings were the pneumonias acquired (community versus hospital-acquired)?
      (1) Community-acquired pneumonia is characterized by sudden chills, high fevers, pleuritic, localizing chest pain, SOB, and a productive cough.
      (2) Atypical pneumonia ("walking pneumonia") is characterized by slow, progressive weakness with exertional dyspnea, nagging, nonproductive cough, low-grade fever (although not necessary), and extrapulmonary symptoms (e.g., nausea, vomiting, diarrhea, headache).
   d. Have you ever used intravenous (IV) drugs (risk factor for AIDS)?
   e. Do you have diabetes, heart failure, COPD, asthma, alcoholism, or immunosuppression? Have you used steroids? Have you ever been exposed to TB?
   f. Have you received a pneumococcal vaccination and been vaccinated yearly for influenza?

III. PAST MEDICAL AND SURGICAL HISTORY

A. Past Medical History

1. Have you been diagnosed with a chronic medical condition (list diagnoses with date of onset, current status, responses to interventions, complications or sequelae)?
2. Were you ever hospitalized? For what reason? When?
3. Any history of ventilation assistance (intubations) and steroid treatment?

B. Past Surgical History: Although all past surgeries should be evaluated, surgeries that affect cardiopulmonary function (e.g., coronary artery bypass graft [CABG], pleurodesis for pneumothorax, lung biopsy, and thoracotomy) require in-depth evaluation.

C. Emergency and Trauma History

1. History of hospitalization for pulmonary problems such as asthma, COPD, ILD, pneumothorax, PE, and pneumonias.
2. Any history of injuries, accidents, or fractures (list dates and sequelae/complications)?

D. Childhood History

1. What childhood illnesses did you have? Did you ever have bronchiolitis, epiglottitis, asthma, or recurrent pneumonias?
2. Were you born prematurely? Were there any complications from the early birth?
3. Did you, or do you, have any inherited or congenital disease processes (cystic fibrosis [CF], alpha$_1$-antitrypsin deficiency, atopic dermatitis, ciliary dyskinesia, familial idiopathic fibrosis, yellow nail syndrome, Ehler-Danlos syndrome, Gaucher's disease (types 1, 2, 3), hereditary hemorrhagic telangiectasia, Marfan's syndrome, immunodeficiency syndromes, neurofibromatosis type I (e.g., von Recklinghausen's disease, tuberous sclerosis [TS])?

E. Occupational History: The standard occupational history delineates all past employment, usually starting with the present and working backward systematically. The occupational history should include environmental exposures outside of the workplace (e.g., hobbies, neighborhood, or in the home).

1. Have you ever been exposed to asbestos, beryllium, silica, radon, coal, mercury, pesticides, or other toxins? Exposure to these substances can cause pneumonoconioses and hypersensitivity pneumonitis. Pneumonoconioses are the dust diseases of the lung (Table 32-1).
2. History of respiratory symptoms from work-related exposure (Table 32-2).

F. Travel History

1. Where have you traveled? It is important to identify past travels to TB-endemic areas such as Africa, Asia, and Latin America.
2. Have you ever had a positive TB skin test (purified protein derivative [PPD])? If the TB skin test was positive, were you treated with isoniazid?

Table 32-1. SOURCES AND PRESENTATIONS OF PNEUMONOCONIOSES.

Dust Particle	Common Exposure Sites	Associated Disease	Clinical Presentation
Coal	Coal mining	Coal worker's pneumoconiosis	Productive cough, dyspnea with impaired pulmonary function. May or may not have radiographic changes. CXR shows nodularity with possible cavitations. Melanoptysis (black sputum) may occur with cavitations
Asbestos	Miners, textile workers, renovation and construction workers (formerly used in most buildings as a flame retardant)	Asbestosis	Cough, dyspnea, bibasilar fine crackles CXR: Irregular opacities at lung bases Carcinogen leading to throat and lung cancer
Silica	Mining, sandblasting, foundry work, pottery making, quarrying	Silicosis	Air-flow obstruction and lung restriction (increased risk of mycobacterial infection), fever, weight loss CXR: Small nodules in upper lobes may have compensatory hyperinflation of lower lobes
Beryllium	Aerospace industry, nuclear industry	Berylliosis	Granulomatous disease with chronic cough of slow onset; genetic marker (HLA-Dpbeta1) associated with increased risk of disease

Table 32-2. COMMON OCCUPATIONAL-RELATED DISEASES.

Exposure	Diseases or Disorders
Asbestosis	Pulmonary fibrosis, mesothelioma
Asthma	Baker asthma, grain farmer asthma, cosmetic and plastic industry asthma, etc
Berylliosis	Granulomatous lung disease, sarcoid-like illness
Cadmium exposure	Emphysema
Hard metal disease	Giant cell pneumonia
High-altitude pulmonary edema	Noncardiogenic pulmonary edema
Irritant inhalant injury	Diffuse alveolar damage (DAD) (acute respiratory distress syndrome[ARDS])
Paraquat injury (pesticide)	Pulmonary edema (acute), pulmonary fibrosis (chronic)
Silicosis (acute)	Pulmonary alveolar proteinosis
Silicosis (chronic)	Pulmonary fibrosis, progressive massive fibrosis, TB
Spanish toxic oil syndrome	Plexigenic pulmonary arteriopathy, (pulmonary hypertension)
Uranium mining, coke oven work	Lung carcinogenesis

3. Have you had a bacillus Calmette-Guérin (BCG) vaccination (if born outside the United States)?

G. Animal and Insect Exposure History

1. Zoonoses.
2. Are you sensitive or allergic to pollens, spores, or other irritants that may trigger pulmonary reactions or disease processes?
3. Do you have birds (hypersensitivity pneumonitis), cats, dogs, or other exotic animals as pets?

IV. MEDICATIONS, ALLERGIES, AND ADVERSE REACTIONS

A. Medications

1. Are you currently taking any prescription medications?
   - **a.** Cardiac and pulmonary?
     - **(1)** ACE inhibitors and aspirin? Both can cause cough and exacerbation of pulmonary symptoms.
     - **(2)** Beta-blocker in patients with bronchospasm?
   - **b.** Use of inhalers, both prescription and over-the-counter (OTC) medications?

Table 32-3. PRESENTATIONS OF INFECTIOUS AGENTS TRANSMITTED BY ANIMAL VECTORS/RESERVOIR HOSTS.

Disease	Infective Agent	Clinical Presentation	Vector/Reservoir Host
Psittacosis	Chlamydia psittaci	Pneumonia	Aerosols from birds
Tularemia	Francisella tularensis	Pneumonia with hilar nodes, cutaneous ulcers, pleural effusions	Rabbits in winter and ticks in summer
Mycoplasma arginini	Mycoplasma arginini	Pneumonia, sepsis	Sheep, goats
Foot and mouth disease	Aphthovirus	Oral vesicles, cold symptoms	Cloven-hooded animals
Plague	Yersinia pestis	Inguinal lymphadenopathy, bubonic plague, hilar adenopathy	Fleas from prairie dogs, squirrels, rats
Hantavirus	Hantavirus	Symptoms of upper respiratory infection (URI) or pneumonia, ARDS	Deer mice excrement

c. Recent or frequent use of antibiotics? Reason and how they were obtained?

d. Oral contraceptives (estrogen)?

2. Do you take OTC cough and cold medications? Frequency and duration?
3. Herbal preparations?
4. Supplements such as appetite suppressants?

B. **Allergies to Medications and Side Effects**

1. History of shortness of breath or tightening sensation in the throat after medication use?
2. Inquire about medication allergies such as penicillin and cephalosporins.
3. Do you have any food allergies, especially shellfish?
4. Are you allergic to aspirin, other NSAIDs (e.g., aspirin triad: asthma, nasal polyps, and sinusitis, which indicates allergic diathesis)?

C. **Adverse Reactions to Medications**

1. Have you had rashes or hives after medication use?
2. Vague gastrointestinal symptoms in the absence of the above are usually a side effect of medication and not a true allergic reaction.

V. HEALTH MAINTENANCE

A. Prevention

1. Have you received a pneumococcal vaccine?
   a. Streptococcal pneumoniae is the most common bacterial cause of community-acquired pneumonia, acute exacerbation of chronic bronchitis and otitis media; it carries a high mortality rate in certain populations.
   b. Vaccine is effective in reducing the infection rate by 70% to 85%.
   c. Target groups for pneumococcal immunization: Older age, especially >65 years, COPD, chronic cardiovascular disease, alcoholism, diabetes mellitus (DM), cirrhosis, nephrotic syndrome, renal failure, immune deficiency (including immunosuppressive therapy, corticosteroids, organ transplantation, human immunodeficiency virus (HIV), and Hodgkin lymphoma.
2. Do you receive seasonal influenza vaccinations?
   a. Influenza virus not only causes high economical burden due to work absence but also has a high mortality rate among certain populations (e.g., pandemic Influenza A season in 1918 caused 20 million deaths).
   b. Vaccine is effective in reducing the infection rate by 70% to 90%.
   c. Target groups for influenza immunization:
      (1) High-risk groups:
         (a) Adults and children with chronic pulmonary or cardiovascular disease, including asthma.

(b) Residents of chronic care facilities and nursing homes.

(c) Adults and children with chronic metabolic disease (renal insufficiency, anemia, DM, immunosuppression).

(2) Children and teenagers receiving long-term aspirin therapy.

(3) Health care providers with high-risk patient contact.

(4) Household contacts of high-risk persons.

(5) Adults who provide essential community services (police, firefighters).

(6) Any person who wants to reduce risk of influenza infection.

3. Have you ever tried to stop smoking? More than 80% of lung cancers are attributed to tobacco exposure, with a 20-fold increase in the relative risk for lung cancer for current smokers versus nonsmokers.

B. Diet

1. Assessing risk factors for aspiration is important in young children and elderly.
2. Toddlers should not be given small candy and nuts (especially peanuts).

C. Exercise/Recreation

1. What type of exercise do you engage in? At what level of endurance? Exercise-induced asthma may limit athletic activities in children and teens, thereby limiting both physical and psychosocial development.
2. Do you experience fatigue or wheezing during or after exercising? Symptoms of exercise-induced asthma include cough, early fatigue, and wheezing.

D. Sleep Patterns: What is your normal sleep pattern? Any recent changes? Episodes of apnea, loud snoring, and extreme daytime somnolence can be pathologic signs of obstructive sleep apnea (OSA).

E. Social Habits

1. Do you smoke?
   a. Number of packs smoked per day (20 cigarettes/pack) times how many years the person has been smoking (pack-years).
   b. Additional types of smoking (cigars, pipe, cannabis or marijuana) and other types of tobacco use (snuff or chew).
   c. Passive (secondary) smoke: Use in family, friends.
   d. Past history of smoking. If the patient denies smoking, ask them if they ever smoked, and if so, how much, for how long, and when did they quit.
2. Do you drink alcohol? What type, how much, and for how long?
   a. Alcoholism increases the risk of pneumonia.

b. Social drinking means something very different to different people. A good rule of thumb is to exaggerate when asking how much; for example, ask them if they drink 3 or 4 six-packs of beer per night "socially."
c. Have patient answer the CAGE questionnaire (Table 32-4).

Table 32-4. CAGE QUESTIONNAIRE.

C	Have you ever felt you ought to **C**ut down on your drinking?
A	Have people **A**nnoyed you by criticizing your drinking?
G	Have you ever felt bad or **G**uilty about your drinking?
E	Have you ever had a drink in the morning (**E**ye opener) to steady your nerves or to get rid of a hangover?

3. Have you used drugs?
   a. Inquire about past and current drug use.
      (1) Intravenous drug use carries with it the risk of HIV and hepatitis contagion.
      (2) Cocaine use can lead to pleuritis, which can mimic pneumonia as well as upper respiratory symptoms of coryza. Often, chronic use leads to nasal septal erosion.
      (3) If positive IV drug use, ask about ingredients; sometimes IV drugs are mixed with talc, which can cause ILD-like disease.
   b. Oral contraceptives and appetite suppressant use.

VI. FAMILY HISTORY

A. First-Degree Relatives' Medical History

1. Have any first-degree relatives had lung cancer? If so, what treatment did they receive with what outcome?
2. Have any relatives had malignancies of other organs?
3. Asthma, COPD, or recurrent pneumonias?
4. Did they have cardiac disease?
5. Diabetes?
6. Autoimmune diseases?
7. Sleep apnea?

B. Three-Generation Genogram is indicated. Some pulmonary disease processes may be inherited or be seen as part of a syndrome.

VII. PSYCHOSOCIAL HISTORY

A. Personal and Social History

1. Where were you born (country and city)? Religious affiliation? Race/ethnicity background?
2. Are you married or have a significant other? Do you have any children?
3. What level of education have you attained (e.g., years of schooling, college and advanced degrees)?

4. Where do you currently reside (including physical layout of the home and living conditions)? Important for smoking history of the patient and of relatives and close friends (second-hand exposure).

B. **Current Illness Effects on the Patient**
   1. How has the illness affected your life? Assess adaptation and acceptance of life changes.
   2. Assess for depression: May increase mortality and decrease patient compliance.
   3. Has your illness affected your employment? How?
   4. Do you have any special needs (e.g., handicapped parking sticker, portable oxygen, home health care needs)?

C. **Interpersonal and Sexual History**
   1. Identify risk factors for sexually transmitted diseases (STDs), HIV, and TB.
      a. Patients with risk factors for STD (multiple partners, unprotected sex) should be offered STD screening.
      b. Patients who have risk factors for TB exposure (health care workers, homeless, patients with exposure history) should be offered annual PPD testing.
   2. Patients with history of marijuana and cocaine use should be identified (bronchial irritants).

D. **Family Support**
   1. The patient's support system should be identified and encouraged.
   2. For children, it is important to properly instruct child care providers in the proper use of inhalers and signs of treatment failure that warrant immediate medical care.
   3. In older patients, disease-specific symptoms (SOB, incessant cough) should be discussed with patients' families.

VIII. **REVIEW OF SYSTEMS (Tables 32-5, 32-6, and 32-7)**

Table 32-5. PULMONARY REVIEW OF SYMPTOMS BY SYSTEM.

SYSTEM	SYMPTOMS
General	Fatigue, appetite, sleep and sleep apnea, snoring, weight
HEENT	Sore throat, dysphagia, history of rhinitis, sinusitis, postnasal drip, URI
Neck	Pain, swelling, mass, history of surgery (e.g., tracheostomy, thyroidectomy)
Cardiovascular	Chest pain, angina, congestive heart failure (CHF), valvular disease, HTN, syncope, arrhythmias/palpitations, positional or exercise-related shortness of breath, hypertension, exercise tolerance

Table 32-5—cont'd

System	Symptoms
Chest/Pulmonary	Acute bronchitis/pneumonia, shortness of breath, asthma (severity, inhalers used, ED treatment history), smoking and COPD, cough, airway/pulmonary surgery, recent URI, recurrent URIs
Gastrointestinal	Ulcers, GERD (can present as cough or chest pain), gastrointestinal (GI) bleeding, "heartburn" as undiagnosed cardiac disease, abdominal pain, problem swallowing (possible obstruction or mass), cough when swallowing, choking while eating (tracheoesophageal fistula, especially in infants)
Hepatic	Right upper quadrant fullness/pain, jugulovenous distension (JVD), abdominal distention (ascites), which can indicate right-sided heart failure
Obstetrics/ Gynecologic	SOB in pregnancy (can be physiologic from increased ventilation or increased intra-abdominal pressure later in pregnancy) or a sign of HTN, as with preeclampsia (second and third trimesters), pleuritic cough, tachycardia (pulmonary embolism)
Genitourinary	Adequate urine output, hematuria
Hematologic/ Oncologic	Unusual bleeding, epistaxis, hemoptysis, fatigue, shortness of breath, pallor, chest pain, history of blood transfusion
Musculoskeletal	Kyphoscoliosis, spinal stenosis (can inhibit normal thoracic cage motion and labor breathing), rib fractures, signs of wasting (which could clue you into cancer or AIDS), bone pain (cancer), arthralgia or arthritis (in connective tissue disorder)
Skin	Clubbing, petechiae, rashes (viral exanthems)
Endocrine	Thyroid masses, recent weight gain or loss (paraneoplastic syndromes seen with lung cancers), bone pain
Neurologic	Excessive tiredness, falling asleep during the day (sleep apnea vs. narcolepsy), hyperventilation (anxiety, central nervous system [CNS] disorder), progressive debilitation (multiple sclerosis [MS], amyotrophic lateral sclerosis [ALS], myasthenia gravis [MG], which eventually leads to respiratory failure)

Continued

Table 32-5. PULMONARY REVIEW OF SYMPTOMS BY SYSTEM—*cont'd*

System	Symptoms
Psychiatric	Anxiety leading to hyperventilation, depression, somatoform disorders
Infectious disease	Fevers, temporal pattern of fevers, associated symptoms of cough, diaphoresis, hemoptysis, pleuritic chest pain, characteristics of onset (gradual vs. sudden)
Immunizations	Full complement of pediatric vaccinations, including varicella, hepatitis A virus (HAV) and hepatitis B virus (HBV) series, pneumococcal and influenza vaccines (especially in elderly and those with comorbidities such as COPD)

Table 32-6. NONSPECIFIC SYMPTOMS AND THEIR PULMONARY DISEASES.

Symptom	Diseases
Cough, dry	TB, atypical pneumonia, malignancy, pulmonary fibrosis
Hemoptysis	Bronchitis, malignancy, TB, granulomatous disease, bronchiectasis, vasculitis, mitral stenosis, pneumonia (staphylococcus)
Pain	Pneumonia, pleuritis, PE, trauma, cardiac causes (e.g., myocardial infarction, aortic dissection), gastrointestinal causes (e.g., esophagitis, acid reflux)
Shortness of breath	COPD, asthma, PE, pulmonary hypertension, ILD, CHF
Snoring	OSA, large tonsils, redundant soft palate, large adenoid tissue, septum deformity
Sputum	Pneumonia, chronic bronchitis, asthma, lung abscess, malignancy
Tachypnea	Diabetes (e.g., ketotic state), asthma, chronic bronchitis, emphysema, pulmonary hypertension, ILD, pulmonary embolus
Wheezing	Asthma, extrabronchial mass effect, bronchiolitis in the young, reactive airway disease

Table 32-7. COMMON PULMONARY DISEASES AND THEIR SYMPTOMS.

DISEASE	SYMPTOMS
Asthma	Wheezing, cough, purulent sputum, fevers, chills, SOB, intercostal retractions, hypoxia
Chronic bronchitis	Chronic (>3 months for 2 consecutive years), productive cough of purulent sputum and dyspnea. "Blue bloater" with rapid, shallow breathing (pursed-lip breathing), obesity, perioral and extremity cyanosis
Emphysema	Nonproductive cough, mild to modest dyspnea and dyspnea on exertion. "Pink puffer" with rapid, shallow breathing, thin frame (can have a barrel chest deformity but usually with weight loss), and skin color is pink and flushed
Tuberculosis (TB)	Hemoptysis, night sweats, weight loss, low grade fever
Community-acquired pneumonia	Sudden chill, high fevers, pleuritic, localizing chest pain, shortness of breath, productive cough
Atypical pneumonia (walking pneumonia)	Slowly, progressive weakness with shortness of breath on exertion, nagging, nonproductive cough, low-grade fever (although not necessary), many extrapulmonary symptoms (e.g., nausea, vomiting, diarrhea, headache)
Interstitial lung disease (ILD)	Dry cough, rapid, shallow breathing, shortness of breath, exertional hypoxia

IX. PHYSICAL EXAMINATION

The physical examination should be complete. Clusters of physical findings for common pulmonary conditions are to be used as a guide to form a differential diagnosis (Table 32-8). Isolated findings do not usually give a diagnosis; a differential is developed from a synthesis of a good history, physical, and medical knowledge.

A. **Classic Physical Findings in Some Common Pulmonary Disorders (Table 32-9).**

B. **Lung Examination:** Each examination should include the following:
   1. **Inspection/Observation:** General comfort (distressed, diaphoretic), breathing pattern: rate, rhythm, depth of breathing (regular, labored, pursed lips), position (upright, tripod position), retractions and use of accessory muscles (scalenes or

Text continued on p. 712.

Table 32-8. FINDINGS OF PULMONARY-FOCUSED PHYSICAL EXAMINATION.

System	Physical Examination Finding	Possible Diagnoses
General/vital signs	Tripod position	Position of respiratory distress; the patient will lean forward resting hands on knees
Pulse	Bradycardia	Benign, sick sinus syndrome, heart block, beta-blocker use
	Tachycardia	Essential arrhythmia, fever, hypoxia, PE, atrial fibrillation, supraventricular tachycardia, atrial flutter, atrial flutter with 2 : 1 block
Blood pressure	Hypotension	Vascular collapse (carbon dioxide intoxication), benign, drug toxicity, hypovolemia, adrenal insufficiency, shock (e.g., cardiac, hypovolumic, septic, anaphylactic)
	Hypertension	Essential, renal artery stenosis, pheochromocytoma (risk factor for heart failure, which can lead to right heart failure with pulmonary hypertension and pulmonary symptoms)
	Pulmonary hypertension	Congential heart disease (CHD) (left-to-right shunt), chronic PE, fibrosis, hypoxia, idiopathic
Respiratory rate	Bradypnea	Central dysfunction such as a brain tumor, stroke in the respiratory centers (opioid overdose)
	Tachypnea	Obstructive process (COPD), restrictive disease, anxiety, pulmonary embolus, hypoxia secondary to pneumonia, shock, empyema, pneumothorax, metabolic acidosis, aspirin toxicity (most causes of respiratory compromise will lead to tachypnea, a normal compensatory response; it should not be ignored or immediately attributed to an anxious state)
Temperature	Fever	Infection, inflammation, malignancy, drug fever

HEENT		
Eyes	Papilledema	Hypoxia, hypercapnia
Mouth	Perioral cyanosis	Hypoxia, perfusion deficiencies, methemoglobinemia
	Pursed lips	Generally a sign of increased respiratory effort; funneling air by increasing the transit time
	Infected teeth/gums	Aspiration pneumonitis, lung abscess
Neck	Jugular venous distention (JVD)	JVD suggests right heart failure with venous backup, which may indicate pulmonary pathology
	Thyromegaly	Thyroid dysfunction; hyperthyroidism can present with tachypnea and tachycardia
Lungs	Breath sounds, decreased	Impaired air movement (bronchial obstruction, emphysema), insulation/impaired sound transmission (pleural effusion/thickening, pneumothorax, obesity)
	Breath sounds, increased	Atelectasis, consolidation, fibrosis, infarct, pneumonia, tumor
	Flat percussion	Massive atelectasis, lobar pneumonia, pleural effusion, pneumonectomy
	Dull percussion	Atelectasis, consolidation, enlarged heart, fibrosis, neoplasm, pleural effusion, pleural thickening, pulmonary edema
	Hyper-resonant percussion	Acute asthma, emphysema, pneumothorax
	Normal percussion	Bronchitis, healthy lung
	Rales (crackles)	"Crackles" suggesting fluid in the alveoli; discrete finding with atelectasis, bronchitis, emphysema, pneumonia, pulmonary edema, ILD ("velcro" rales with idiopathic pulmonary fibrosis [IPF])

Continued

Table 32-8. FINDINGS OF PULMONARY-FOCUSED PHYSICAL EXAMINATION—*cont'd*

System	Physical Examination Finding	Possible Diagnoses
	Rhonchi	Loud low-pitched bubbling with expiration (may be inspiration) with bronchitis, emphysema, pneumonia, pulmonary edema
	Rub	Grating vibration with pericarditis, peripheral pneumonia, pleurisy, PE, TB
	Stridor	Inspiratory wheeze associated with upper airway obstruction in croup, vocal cord edema, tracheal stenosis, epiglottitis, foreign body, tumor
	Tympany	Large pulmonary cavity, massive (tension) pneumothorax
	Wheezes	"Wheezing," suggests an obstructive process such as asthma or exacerbated COPD. Remember: "all that wheezes is not asthma." Differential should include aspiration, pneumonia, bronchitis, extrabronchial masses that may show an obstructive picture
Chest wall	Barrel chest	A chest permanently resembling the shape of a barrel; increased AP diameter roughly equaling the lateral diameter; usually with some degree of kyphosis; seen in cases of emphysema
	Dowager's hump	Thoracic kyphoscoliosis (combination of kyphosis and scoliosis, lateral curving of the spine)
	Pectus carinatum	Congenital narrow thorax with increased anteroposterior diameter as the sternum protrudes from the chest wall

	Pectus excavatum	Congenital retraction of the chest wall toward the spine and deformed lower costal cartilages involving the inferior sternum and xiphoid process
	Thoracic levoscoliosis	Lateral curvature of the thoracic spine to the left
	Thoracic dextroscoliosis	Lateral curvature of the thoracic spine to the right
Cardiovascular	Loud P2	Pulmonary hypertension
	Murmurs	May be benign, or could signal a more serious condition. Attempt to localize, characterize time in relation to the heart cycle, radiation, change with respiration, and develop a differential accordingly
	Splitting S2	Normal variant caused by later closing of pulmonic valve. Usually during inspiration because of prolonged right heart ejection of blood from right ventricle (remember fixed splitting in atrial septal defect [ASD])
Abdomen	Hepatomegaly	Hepatitis, right heart failure (together with JVD suggests such a picture), malignancy (common site of metastasis)
	Significant abdominal distention/girth	Many etiologies from obesity to malignancy (ascites). Increased intraabdominal pressure can labor breathing via interference with diaphragmatic movement. Obesity is also a risk factor for sleep apnea
Skin/nails	Clubbing	A trademark finding for pulmonary disease (unknown mechanism of action) but often clues you in to longstanding pulmonary pathology, such as cystic fibrosis, non-small-cell lung cancer, chronic hypoxia (pulmonary arteriovenous fistula, congenital heart disease with right-to-left shunt). Can be benign normal variant in some people
	Stains on fingers/teeth	Cigarette smoking
	Flushing	Hypoxia/carbon dioxide intoxication

Continued

Table 32-8. FINDINGS OF PULMONARY-FOCUSED PHYSICAL EXAMINATION—*cont'd*

System	Physical Examination Finding	Possible Diagnoses
Spine	Kyphosis	A posterior curvature of the thoracic spine usually the result of a disease (lung disease, Paget's disease) or a congenital problem
	Scoliosis	A congenital lateral curvature of the spine
Extremities	Extremity cyanosis	Hypoxic states manifested by cold, bluish gray extremities; an ominous sign. Check capillary refill time (normal 2-4 seconds) to differentiate between a hypoxic versus hypoperfusion state. Causes include hypoventilation, pulmonary hypotension, pulmonary edema, ILD
	Extremity edema	Distinguish anasarca, nondependent edema (generally nonpitting: Seen with hypoproteinemic states such as with end-stage malignancy/wasting) vs. pitting dependent edema secondary to fluid overload (seen in congestive heart failure exacerbation). In bed-ridden patient, dependent edema is seen in the sacral areas and the back (dependent parts) versus the lower extremities (ambulatory patients)
	Homan's sign	Pain in the calf with dorsiflexion of the foot with a deep venous thrombosis (DVT)
Neurologic	Coma	Hypoxia (multiple disease processes), carbon dioxide retention

Table 32-9. PHYSICAL FINDINGS IN PULMONARY DISORDERS.

DISORDER	INSPECTION	PALPATION	PERCUSSION	AUSCULTATION
Atelectasis (lobar obstruction)	Decreased chest expansion (same side), increased respiratory rate (RR), tracheal deviation (same side)	Decreased fremitus	Dullness or flatness	Decreased or absent breath sounds, rales (subcrepitant), whispered pectoriloquy
Bronchial asthma (acute attack)	Hyperinflation; use of accessory muscles	Impaired expansion; decreased fremitus	Hyperresonance; low diaphragm	Prolonged expiration; inspiratory and expiratory wheezes
Consolidation (pneumonia)	Possible lag or splinting on affected side, increased RR, fever	Increased fremitus	Dullness	Bronchial breath sounds; bronchophony; pectoriloquy; crackles
Pleural effusion (large)	Lag on affected side (same side), increased RR, tracheal deviation (opposite side)	Decreased fremitus; trachea and heart shifted away from affected side	Dullness or flatness (may be only way to distinguish from pneumothorax)	Decreased or absent breath sounds, egophony (above effusion)
Pneumothorax (complete)	Lag on affected side, increased RR, cyanosis, tracheal deviation (opposite if tension)	Absent fremitus	Hyperresonant or tympany	Decreased or absent breath sounds

sternocleidomastoids), color around lips and nail beds (cyanotic, dusky), ability to speak (complete sentences or few words per breath), audible noises (wheezing or gurgling), and appearance: increased anteroposterior (AP) chest diameter or obvious chest deformities (lag or splinting on affected side, hyperinflation [barrel chest], kyphosis, scoliosis).

2. **Palpation:** Evaluate for normal chest expansion or excursion (asymmetry with air or fluid in the lungs); tactile fremitus with hands on patient (see below), assess tracheal position; investigating areas of tenderness or deformity (rib fracture give-way, subcutaneous emphysema).
3. **Percussion:** Normal resonance, dullness (fluid- or tissue-filled cavity), hyper-resonant (emphysema, pneumothorax), diaphragmatic excursion.
4. **Auscultation:** Assess for vesicular, bronchial, and bronchovesicular sounds; areas of absent breath sounds, inspiratory and expiratory wheezes or other adventitious breath sounds (crackles/rales, rubs, stridor), bronchophony, egophony, and pectoriloquy.
   - **a.** Clear to auscultation and percussion (CTAP), breath sounds equal bilaterally.
   - **b.** Equal diaphragmatic excursion posterior midscapular line.
   - **c.** Voice transmission tests.
     - **(1)** Tactile fremitus.
       - **(a)** Ask the patient to say "99" in a normal voice and palpate an area of the lung.
       - **(b)** Increased transmission in one area can indicate an area of consolidation or increased fluid in the lung.
       - **(c)** Decreased fremitus indicates air or fluid outside the lung obstructing the transmission.
     - **(2)** Whispered pectoriloquy.
       - **(a)** Ask the patient to whisper "99" and listen with the stethoscope.
       - **(b)** Faint sounds are normal.
       - **(c)** Increased transmission in one area can indicate an area of consolidation.
     - **(3)** Egophony.
       - **(a)** Ask the patient to say "ee" several times.
       - **(b)** Listen with the stethoscope and you should hear a muffled "ee" sound.
       - **(c)** If you hear an "ay" sound, this is referred to as egophony, indicating consolidation.
   - **d.** Note adventitious (extra) lung sounds and diagram their locations.
     - **(1)** Wheezes: High pitched and "musical" in quality.
     - **(2)** Rales or crackles: Fine/coarse crackles.

(3) Stridor: Inspiratory noise usually associated with upper airway obstruction.
(4) Rhonchi: "Snoring" or "gurgling" quality.
(5) Pleural rubs.

X. DIFFERENTIAL DIAGNOSIS (Tables 32-10 and 32-11)

Table 32-10. DIFFERENTIAL DIAGNOSIS ACCORDING TO THE PULMONARY DISORDER.

DISORDER	DIFFERENTIAL DIAGNOSIS
Asthma	Bronchitis, COPD, pneumonia, CHF, anaphylaxis, upper airway obstruction, endobronchial tumors, carcinoid
Chronic obstructive pulmonary disease (COPD)	Chronic bronchitis, asthma, pneumonia, CHF, $alpha_1$-antitrypsin deficiency, cystic fibrosis
Metabolic acidosis (anion-gap)	Lactic acidosis (infections, muscle breakdown), ketoacidosis (diabetes), uremic acidosis (renal failure), salicylate toxicity, paraldehyde ingestion, methanol ingestion, ethylene glycol ingestion
Metabolic acidosis (non-anion gap)	Renal causes: Renal tubular acidosis (RTA) type II (proximal tubular), dilutional acidosis, carbonic anhydrase inhibitors, primary hyperparathyroidism, distal RTAI, distal RTA IV, diuretics GI causes: Small bowel surgery, diarrhea Other: Parenteral hyperalimentation
Pneumonia	Asthma, COPD, bronchitis, CHF, malignancy, pulmonary embolism, viral infection
Pulmonary embolism	CHF, MI, pneumonia, pulmonary edema, asthma, COPD, hyperventilation, aspiration of a foreign body
Respiratory acidosis	Central respiratory failure, general anesthesia, sedative overdose, obstructive lung disease, restrictive lung disease, pneumonia (severe), neuromuscular diseases (Guillain-Barré, myasthenia gravis)
Respiratory alkalosis	Hyperventilation (hyperventilation syndrome, anxiety disorder), neurologic disorders (trauma, infections, CNS malignancies, cerebrovascular accidents [CVAs]); it is often a compensatory response to a metabolic acidosis

Table 32-11. DIFFERENTIAL DIAGNOSIS ACCORDING TO FUNCTIONAL PULMONARY FINDING.

Functional Pulmonary Finding	Characteristic Test Findings	Differential Diagnosis
Obstructive ventilation	Reduced FEV1/VC %	Chronic bronchitis, asthma, bronchiectasis, mucous gland hyperplasia, emphysema
Restrictive ventilation	Reduced TLC, VC. Increased/ Normal FEV1/VC %	Obesity, kyphoscoliosis, Guillain-Barré syndrome and other neuromuscular diseases, pleural thickening, malignancy, pleural effusions, cardiomegaly, lobectomy or partial lobectomy
Ventilation abnormalities	VQ mismatch with decreased ventilation	Pneumonia, atelectasis, pleural effusions, ARDS, ILD
Perfusion abnormalities	VQ mismatch with decreased perfusion	PE, cancer, amniotic fluid emboli, fat emboli
Arterial hypoxia	Low PO_2, Low O_2 saturation	Low FIO_2 (high attitude) Hypoventilation Diffusion abnormality V-Q mismatch Right-to-left shunt Low mixed venous O_2 tension (shock)

XI. LABORATORY STUDIES AND DIAGNOSTIC EVALUATIONS

A. Pulse Oximetry

1. Optimal method at determining arterial saturation of blood, highly precise with little random variability.
2. Values below 90% will not reflect partial pressure changes of oxygen in arterial blood accurately.

B. Arterial Blood Gas (ABG)

1. Useful for assessment of acid-base balance.
2. Routine monitoring of blood gases without a change in the clinical condition is not warranted.

C. Electrolytes and Acid-Base Balance: Acid-base (intake/output of hydrogen ions) regulated by plasma (bicarbonate, proteins, inorganic phosphorous), red blood cells (RBCs: bicarbonate, proteins, inorganic phosphates, hemoglobin) renal hydrogen excretion (weak acids), and renal reabsorption of bicarbonate.

D. **Serologies:** Assessment for specific organisms.

E. **Sputum Examination**
   1. Culture: Assessment for identification of pathogens (bacterial, fungal, viral).
   2. Exfoliative cytology (assess for carcinoma, organisms, eosinophils, hemosiderin).

F. **Thoracentesis:** Diagnostic or therapeutic procedure to remove fluid from the chest cavity using a hollow-bore needle.

G. **Diagnostic Imaging (Radiologic) Studies**
   1. Chest x-ray (CXR) is the most ordered radiologic study and is very helpful in the initial assessment of the pulmonary disease process (e.g., infiltrate, effusion, edema), as well as looking at other structures (e.g., heart, bone).
   2. Computed tomography (CT) scan is very useful for delineating disease processes that are not or are only partially suspected by the CXR (e.g., nodules, masses, infiltrates, mediastinal lymph nodes).
   3. High-resolution computed tomography (HRCT) is very useful for delineating disease processes that involve the interstitium (e.g., pulmonary fibrosis).
   4. Magnetic resonance imaging (MRI) is very useful for delineating disease processes that involve the posterior mediastinum (neuroma, neurofibroma), the apex of the lung (Pancoast tumor), or the major blood vessels and the heart.
   5. Ventilation-perfusion scan (V/Q scan) is helpful in evaluating patients suspected to have pulmonary embolism.
   6. Pulmonary angiogram: Gold standard test for the diagnosis of PE.
   7. Arteriogram is used sometimes for evaluation of hemoptysis.

H. **Bronchoscopy**
   1. Direct visualization of pulmonary tree.
   2. Biopsy/cytologic (aspiration, brush) assessment of any lesions.
   3. Cultures, as appropriate.

I. **Assessment of Pulmonary Function**
   1. Spirometry is a very useful, simple test to evaluate and follow up patients with pulmonary diseases, especially those with obstructive lung disease (e.g., COPD, asthma).

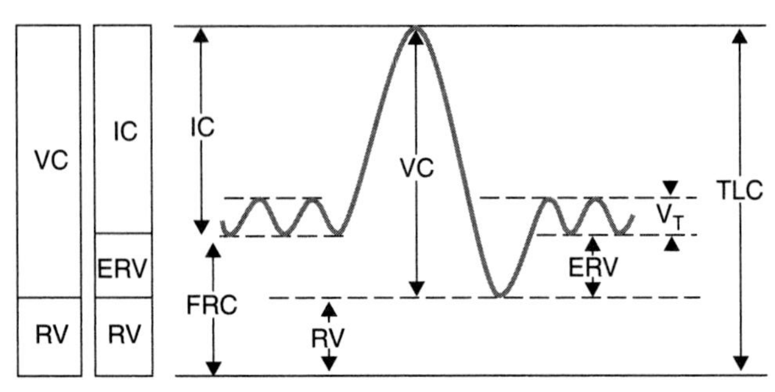

Lung volumes, shown by block diagrams *(left)* and by a spirographic tracing *(right)*. TLC = total lung capacity; VC = vital capacity; RV = residual volume; IC = inspiratory capacity; ERV = expiratory reserve volume; FRC = functional residual capacity; V_T = tidal volume.

2. Pulmonary function test (PFT): Used for evaluation and follow up of patients with obstructive (such as COPD, asthma) or restrictive lung disease (e.g., pulmonary fibrosis).
3. Cardiopulmonary exercise testing: Used to evaluate the limiting factor for patient's symptoms (e.g., SOB), cardiac versus pulmonary, and is very important in disability issues.

XII. ACRONYMS AND ABBREVIATIONS (Table 32-12)

XIII. DEFINITIONS (Table 32-13)

XIV. SAMPLE H&P WRITE-UP

CC: "I'm coughing up blood."

HPI: A.R. is a 61-year-old white male with a long history of smoking (60 pack-years) and coronary artery disease (CAD). He was initially evaluated in the ED 2 weeks ago with complaints of cough and yellow, greenish sputum of 3 days' duration. Work-up at that time showed acute bronchitis, and he was given antibiotics, with partial response. A few days ago he started to notice blood streaks in his sputum. He denied any previous episodes of hemoptysis, shortness of breath, chest pain, and night sweats, and any change in weight or appetite. He also denied use of IV or OTC drugs.

PMHx: CAD, acute myocardial infarction (MI) 4 years ago.

PSHx: Coronary artery bypass graft (CABG) 4 years ago.

Emergency and Trauma History: Besides his recent visit due to bronchitis, he was seen at the time he suffered his acute MI (4 years ago).

Childhood History: Chicken pox at age 4. He denies any other childhood illnesses.

MEDICATIONS: Aspirin, beta-blocker, ACE inhibitor, and prn nitrate. He denies use of herbal supplements/vitamins and any allergies/adverse reactions to medications.

Text continued on p. 722.

Table 32-12. PULMONARY-FOCUSED ACRONYMS AND ABBREVIATIONS.

Acronym or Abbreviation	Term	Acronym or Abbreviation	Term
ABG	Arterial blood gas	**CNS**	Central nervous system
ACE	Angiotensin-converting enzyme	**CO**	Cardiac output
ADH	Antidiuretic hormone	**COPD**	Chronic obstructive pulmonary disease
ALS	Amyotrophic lateral sclerosis	**COX-2**	Cyclo-oxygenase subtype 2 receptor (analgesia)
Ambu	Brand name of bag-valve-mask device	**CPAP**	Continuous positive airway pressure
ANS	Autonomic nervous system	**CPB**	Cardiopulmonary bypass
AR	Aortic regurgitation	**CPR**	Cardiopulmonary resuscitation
ARDS	Adult respiratory distress syndrome	**CRF**	Chronic renal failure
AS	Aortic stenosis	**CSF**	Cerebrospinal fluid
ASA	Aspirin (acetyl salicylic acid)	**CVP**	Central venous pressure
ASD	Atrial septum defect	**CXR**	Chest x-ray
AV	Aortic valve	**DIC**	Disseminated intravascular coagulation
Beta	Receptor subtype, autonomic nervous system	**ECG**	Electrocardiogram
BE	Base excess	**EF**	Ejection fraction
BP	Blood pressure	**EJ**	External jugular vein
CABG	Coronary artery bypass graft	**EMLA**	Eutectic mixture of local anesthetics (topical agent)
CAD	Coronary artery disease	**Epi**	Epinephrine
CBF	Cerebral blood flow (or coronary blood flow)	**$ETCO_2$**	End-tidal carbon dioxide
CHF	Congestive heart failure	**ETT**	Endotracheal tube

Continued

Table 32-12. PULMONARY-FOCUSED ACRONYMS AND ABBREVIATIONS—*cont'd*

Acronym or Abbreviation	Term	Acronym or Abbreviation	Term
Fa/Fi	Fraction of alveolar to fraction inspired gas ratio	**NO**	Nitric oxide
FEV	Forced expiratory volume	**N_2O**	Nitrous oxide (anesthetic)
FIO_2	Fraction of inspired oxygen	**NPO**	Nil per os (nothing by mouth)
FRC	Functional residual capacity	**NSAID**	Nonsteroidal anti-inflammatory drug
FROM	Full range of motion	**NTP**	Sodium nitroprusside
FVC	Forced vital capacity	**O_2**	Oxygen
HCT	Hematocrit	**OR**	Operating room
Hespan	Brand name for hetastarch plasma expander	**OCP**	Oral contraceptive pill
HR	Heart rate	**PAC**	Premature atrial contractions
HTN	Hypertension	**PACU**	Postanesthesia care unit (or recovery room)
IABP	Intra-aortic balloon pump	**PCA**	Patient-controlled analgesia
IBD	Inflammatory bowel disease	**PCO_2**	Partial pressure of carbon dioxide
ICU	Intensive care unit	**PCWP**	Pulmonary capillary wedge pressure
IDDM	Insulin-dependent diabetes mellitus	**PDPH**	Postdural puncture headache
IJ	Internal jugular (vein)	**PEEP**	Positive end-expiratory pressure
ILD	Interstitial lung disease	**pH**	Power of hydrogen
IM	Intramuscular	**PRBC**	Packed red blood cells
IMV	Intermittent mandatory ventilation	**PT**	Prothrombin time

IPF	Idiopathic pulmonary fibrosis	**PTT**	Partial thromboplastin time
IV	Intravenous	**PVC**	Premature ventricular contractions
K	Potassium	**PVR**	Pulmonary vascular resistance
LA	Left atrium	**RA**	Right atrium
LE	Lower extremity	**RR**	Respiratory rate
L3-4	Third and fourth lumbar vertebrae	**RSD**	Reflex sympathetic dystrophy
Lead II	Second lead of ECG, monitored for rhythm	**RV**	Right ventricle
LMA	Laryngeal mask airway	**SLE**	Systemic lupus erythematosus
LV	Left ventricle	**SpO_2**	Oxygen saturation
LVEDP	Left ventricular end-diastolic pressure	**S2**	Second heart sound
MG	Myasthenia gravis	**ST**	Sinus tachycardia
MI	Myocardial infarction	**SVR**	Systemic vascular resistance
mmHg	Millimeters of mercury (pressure)	**SVT**	Supraventricular tachycardia
Modified V5 lead	ECG lead used to monitor for ischemia	**T**	Temperature
MR	Mitral regurgitation	**T-piece**	Breathing circuit used sometimes for weaning
MRI	Magnetic resonance imaging	**TLC**	Total lung capacity
Mu receptor	Morphine receptor in brain and spinal cord	**TR**	Tricuspid regurgitation
MV	Mechanical ventilation	**UE**	Upper extremity
MVP	Mitral valve prolapse	**VF**	Ventricular fibrillation
NIDDM	Non-insulin-dependent diabetes mellitus	**V/Q**	Ventilation/perfusion
NMDA	N-methyl-D-aspartate (receptor)	**VT**	Ventricular tachycardia
NMJ	Neuromuscular junction	**WPW**	Wolff-Parkinson White syndrome
Norepi	Norepinephrine (Levophed)		

Table 32-13. PULMONOLOGY-SPECIFIC TERMS AND DEFINITIONS.

Term	Definition
A-a gradient	Arterial-alveolar gradient
Alveolar ventilation	Volume of fresh gas entering alveoli each minute
Anatomic dead space	Airway conduction system; no gas exchange takes place (e.g., bronchi)
Apnea	Period of cessation of breathing
Bradypnea	Slow respiratory rate (less than 8 breaths per minute)
Biot's breathing	Ataxic breathing, unpredictable irregularity
Bronchial (normal breath sound)	Normal sound over the manubrium
Bronchophony	A modification of the voice sounds, by which they are intensified and heightened in pitch; observed in auscultation of the chest in certain cases of intrathoracic disease
Bronchovesicular (normal breath sound)	Normal breath sounds over the carina area and between the upper scapulae
Cheyne-Stokes breathing	Periods of no breathing with alternating crescendo-decrescendo periodic breathing
Compliance	Refers to elasticity of lungs and chest wall
Cyanosis	Bluish discoloration of skin usually caused by low blood perfusion and/or hypoxic state
Dyspnea	Sensation of respiratory distress
Egophony	The sound of a patient's voice so modified as to resemble the bleating of a goat, heard on applying the ear to the chest in certain diseases within its cavity, as in pleurisy with effusion
Forced expiratory volume	Maximal air exhaled during forced expiration, over 1 second
Fremitus	Palpable vibrations while patient talks
Functional residual capacity	Normal resting lung volume
Hypercapnia	Excess of carbon dioxide in the blood
Hyperpnea	Deep breathing
Inspiratory capacity	Maximal volume that can be expired from the resting level
Orthopnea	When a person can only breath easily when sitting straight (propped up with pillows at night) or standing erect

Table 32-13—cont'd

Term	Definition
Paroxysmal nocturnal dyspnea (PND)	Acute dyspnea suddenly at night, usually waking the patient after an hour or two of sleep; caused by pulmonary congestion with or without edema that results from left-sided heart failure following immobilization of fluid from dependent areas after lying down
Paradoxical movement	Movement of diaphragm up on inspiration, rather than down as expected; caused by paralysis of this muscle
Pectoriloquy	The distinct articulation of the sounds of a patient's voice, heard on applying the ear to the chest in auscultation; usually indicates some morbid change in the lungs or pleural cavity
Perfusion	Passage of a fluid through the vessels of a specific organ
Physiologic dead space	Calculation based on assumption, reduction of PCO_2 in expired air is caused by underperfused alveoli
Physiologic shunt	Calculation made with assumption, all hypoxemia caused by blood passing through unventilated alveoli
Pulmonary blood flow	Equal to the total cardiac output
Rhonchi	Deep wheezing
Rales	Crackling sounds (crackles)
Residual volume	Air remaining in lung after maximal exhalation
Respiratory acidosis	Impaired gas exchange, resulting in decreased blood pH
Respiratory alkalosis	Decreased PCO_2 usually related to increased ventilation, resulting in increased blood pH
Restrictive lung disease	Lung disease associated with loss of elasticity of lung
Shunted blood	Blood that has bypassed ventilated areas
Stridor	Inspiratory noise
Tachypnea	Rapid breathing (greater than 14 breaths per minute)
Total lung capacity	Total volume of gas in lung after full inspiration

Continued

Table 32-13. PULMONOLOGY-SPECIFIC TERMS AND DEFINITIONS—*cont'd*

TERM	DEFINITION
Ventilation	Exchange of air between the lungs and the ambient air. Pulmonary ventilation (measured in liters per minute) refers to the total exchange. Alveolar ventilation refers to the effective ventilation of the alveoli, in which gas exchange with the blood takes place
Ventilation/ Perfusion ratio	Ratio of alveolar ventilation to simultaneous alveolar capillary blood flow in any part of the lung (liters of gas per liter of blood)
Vesicular (normal breath sound)	Normal breath sounds over most of the lungs
Vital capacity	Maximal air forcibly exhaled after deep inspiration

HEALTH MAINTENANCE

Prevention: The patient has had a colonoscopy at age 55 and received his influenza vaccination 6 months ago.

Diet: Patient admits to an irregular diet, comprised primarily of fast food and canned goods. He denied any recent change in weight or appetite.

Exercise: The patient does not exercise.

Sleep Patterns: The patient wakes up one time to void. He denied snoring, a.m. headache, or daytime sleepiness.

Social Habits: The patient gives a history of smoking 1 1/2 packs a day for 40 years (60 pack-years), but quit 4 years ago (since his MI). He denies drinking or use of IV or other recreational drugs.

FAMILY HISTORY

First-Degree Relatives' Medical History: The patient's father was healthy "until he died of old age." The patient's mother is alive (81 years) with adult-onset diabetes and hypertension (HTN). He has no siblings.

PSYCHOSOCIAL HISTORY

Personal and Social History: The patient is Caucasian. He is married, has 2 children (28, 21), owns a house, and was a school principal until his retirement 4 years ago.

TRAVEL AND EXPOSURE HISTORY

He spent most of his life in southern Ohio; as a child had close contact to his grandfather, who died of TB.

REVIEW OF SYSTEMS

General: Fatigue. No weight change, fever, chills, or sweats.

HEENT/Neck: No hoarseness, history of radiation, cancers, or epistaxis.

Gastrointestinal: No change in bowel habits, nausea, vomiting, or change in stool color.

Cardiovascular: No tachycardia, palpitations, orthopnea, paroxysmal nocturnal dyspnea, chest pain, claudication, or pedal edema.

Respiratory: As above.

Genitourinary: No dysuria, urinary urgency, urinary tract infections, or malignancies.

Hematologic/lymphatic: No easy bruising or bleeding tendencies or anemia.

Endocrine: No polyuria, polydipsia, polyphagia, thyroid disease, or hair loss. Positive for recent problems with impotence.

Skin: No rash or pigmentary changes.

Neuropsychiatric: Intermittent headaches. No history of seizures, somnolence, paraesthesias, numbness/tingling in extremities, or ataxia.

Musculoskeletal: Occasional back discomfort. No weakness. No bone pain.

Extremities: No edema or swelling.

PHYSICAL EXAMINATION

Vital Signs: T 99.0°F P 74 BP 136/92 RR 16 Weight 182 lbs. No orthostatic changes.

General: Slightly anxious white male, not in acute distress.

HEENT: No jaundice. No nystagmus. Pupils equal and reactive to light. No oral lesions, cheilitis, or glossitis.

Neck: No thyroid enlargement. Jugular venous pulse (JVP) not elevated.

Lungs: Scattered rhonchi mainly at the rt. apex, no wheezes, rales. No dullness to percussion. No egophony. Not using the accessory muscles.

Chest: Scar of mediastinotomy, well healed, increased AP diameter.

Cardiovascular: Normal S1 and S2. Regular rate and rhythm. No murmur, no jugular venous distension (JVD).

Abdomen: No abnormal colorations or palpable masses. Spleen and liver not palpable. No bruits. No costovertebral angle tenderness (CVAT).

Digital rectal exam (DRE): Negative for occult blood. No masses. Sphincter tone normal.

Skin: No petechiae, rashes, or telangiectasias. No clubbing.

Extremities: No edema, peripheral pulses palpable all over.

Neurologic: Oriented to person, place, and time. Cranial nerve examination normal. No focal sensory or motor deficits noted, negative cerebellar signs.

33

GENERAL SURGERY

William P. Butler, MD, MTM&H, FACS

I. CHIEF COMPLAINT

A. Who, What, When, Where, and How Template for CC and Chronology

1. Who: Obtain patient demographics (i.e., name, age, gender, race/ethnicity).
2. What: Find out the problem (e.g., belly pain, inguinal bulge, breast mass, car accident).
3. When: Know the problem's chronology.
   - **a.** When did the problem begin?
   - **b.** Has the problem changed since it began?
   - **c.** How long has the problem really been a problem?
4. Where: Know the problem's location both physically and geographically (e.g., belly pain at the picnic, inguinal bulge at work, breast mass in the shower, car accident on the interstate).
5. How: Know the circumstances surrounding the problem (e.g., belly pain at the picnic after eating potato salad, inguinal bulge at work after lifting a heavy barrel, breast lump in the shower during self-examination, car accident on the interstate involving a high-speed head-on collision).

B. Identifying Data: Obtain name, age, gender, race/ethnicity; admission date, time and site.

II. HISTORY OF PRESENT ILLNESS

A. Who, What, When, Where, and How Template for the HPI

1. Who: Is the patient the only individual affected?
2. What: Detailed characterization of the problem.
   - **a.** What is the nature of your pain? Is it constant, intermittent, or migratory?
   - **b.** What type of pain do you have? Is it sharp, boring, or achy?
   - **c.** Has there been a change in the quality of your pain? Can anything make it better or worse? Have you had similar pain in the past?
   - **d.** Is the pain accompanied by nausea, vomiting, diarrhea, or other symptoms?
3. When: Chronology and progression of problem.
   - **a.** When did the pain begin (onset)?
   - **b.** Has it worsened or lessened over time?
   - **c.** Has it changed in character over time?

4. Where: Specifics of the problem's location.
    a. What is the specific location of the pain?
    b. Do you have accompanying pain elsewhere?
5. How: Specific circumstances of the problem.
    a. What was happening when the problem began?
    b. What has happened since?
    c. What made you seek medical care when you did have the pain?

III. PAST MEDICAL AND SURGICAL HISTORY

A. **Past Medical History:** This information can be obtained quickly and efficiently if approached systemically.
1. General: Are you in general good health? If not, explain.
2. HEENT: Have you had any head, ears, eyes, nose, or throat problems?
3. Neck: Have you had neck problems or endocrine problems?
4. CV: Have you had any heart, blood vessel, or blood problems?
5. Chest/Breast: Lung problems, breast problems?
6. Back: Back problems, endocrine problems?
7. Abdomen: Gastrointestinal problems?
8. Rectum: Rectal problems?
9. Genitourinary/Pelvic: Genitourinary problems, gynecologic problems?
10. Extremities: Musculoskeletal problems?
11. Skin: Dermatologic problems, lymph node problems?
12. Neurologic: Neurologic problems, psychiatric problems?
13. Miscellaneous: Anything else that crops up in the discussions.

B. **Past Surgical History**
1. What, if any, surgical procedures have you undergone? What were the diagnoses, procedures, responses to interventions, operative and postoperative complications or sequelae, dates, hospitals, anesthesia types (local, spinal, general), and anesthetic complications?
2. Have you undergone any obstetric surgical procedures? What were the methods of delivery (vaginal or Caesarean), complications of labor and delivery, anesthesia types (local, spinal, general), and anesthetic complications?

C. **Emergency and Trauma History**
1. Have you been hospitalized? What were the dates, diagnoses, degrees of severity, durations, doctors, hospitals, treatments, medications, complications, and sequelae.
2. Have you had any transfusions? What were the dates, total number, and known complications (e.g., HIV, hepatitis)?
3. Have you had any trauma or injuries? Have you had any serious sprains or fractures? Document limitations of range of motion, deformities, disabilities, and weaknesses. If a motor vehicle accident (MVA), what type of vehicle was involved, what was your position in the vehicle, what was the speed of

the vehicle, what was the deceleration force, were restraints or other protective measures (e.g., air bags) used?

D. **Childhood History**

1. What childhood illnesses and injuries did you have? Patients are usually aware of most unusual childhood diseases, but they may not remember the specific name (e.g., rheumatic fever, rubella).
2. Assess for emergency treatments and trauma in childhood (e.g., hospitalizations and injuries).

E. **Occupational History**

1. What is your occupation? Is it sedentary or does it involve exercise or labor?
2. Did your problem arise on the job (e.g., hernia caused by lifting or abdominal tear caused by twisting with load)?
3. Did your problem get worse while on the job (e.g., wrist pain at the computer in carpal tunnel syndrome; Crohn's disease flare-up in high-stress scenario)?

F. **Travel History:** Have you traveled within the United States? Have you traveled to foreign countries? The answers may suggest the presence of certain infectious disease etiologies (e.g., malaria and Africa, traveler's diarrhea and Mexico).

IV. MEDICATIONS, ALLERGIES, AND ADVERSE REACTIONS

A. **Medications**

1. What prescription medications are you taking? What are the indications, last doses, durations of use, and possible drug interactions? When did you begin taking the medications? Have you made any changes in taking them? Annotate date started and regimen changes.
2. Are you taking any over-the-counter (OTC) medications, including analgesics, laxatives, sleeping medications, vitamins or nutritional supplements (sometimes these substances are tainted with arsenic and lead), herbal preparations, and diet pills?
3. Are you using any alternative medicine therapies?

B. **Allergies and Adverse Reactions**

1. Do you have any allergies to medication?
   a. What was your allergic reaction (e.g., respiratory or neurologic manifestations)?
   b. How was the allergic reaction treated?
2. Differentiate between allergic manifestations and adverse reactions. Obtain information about any medication and nonmedication allergies and adverse reaction, along with the specifics (e.g., "allergic to penicillin and I get total body swelling").

V. HEALTH MAINTENANCE

A. **Prevention**

1. Patients older than 50 years of age: Screening for colorectal cancer is recommended with annual fecal occult blood testing

(FOBT) or flexible sigmoidoscopy (periodicity is unspecified) or both.

2. Patient's with hereditary syndromes associated with high risk of colon cancer (e.g., familial polyposis) require frequent monitoring and intensive education.

B. **Current Illness Effects on the Patient:** How has your illness affected your day-to-day activities (e.g., job, recreation, nutrition)?

C. **Diet:** What is your normal diet pattern? What has your diet been since the illness began?

D. **Exercise:** Is your job sedentary or does it involve labor? What type of recreational activities do you engage in? Sedentary? Sports? Aerobic or anaerobic?

E. **Sleep Patterns:** What is your normal sleep pattern? What has your sleep pattern been since the illness began?

F. **Social Habits:** Do you use tobacco, alcohol, or recreational drugs? Never refrain from the opportunity to encourage smoking cessation and alcohol moderation.

VI. FAMILY HISTORY

A. **First-Degree Relatives' Medical History:** Always inquire about heart disease, kidney disease, hypertension, diabetes, and cancer. Any one of these maladies can have a significant impact when approaching surgical disease.

B. **Three-Generation Genogram:** Expand family history to create a third-degree family genogram if increased susceptibility (genetic predisposition) is known to occur with the disease or syndrome.

VII. PSYCHOSOCIAL HISTORY

A. **Personal and Social History**

1. What is the patient's race? Race may suggest increased risk (susceptibility) to certain disorders: African-American and sickle cell disease; American Indian (especially Pima) and gallbladder disease.
2. What is the patient's ethnicity? Ethnicity may suggest certain problems: North European Jewish and metabolic disorders; first-generation Chinese Americans and heavy use of herbal remedies.

B. **Interpersonal and Sexual History:** Inquire about any interference with sexual life patient may be having. This might suggest certain problems (e.g., hernias in male and low-grade pelvic inflammatory disease in females).

C. **Family Support**

1. Is family present?
2. Does family confirm the problem?
3. Is family supportive of and nurturing toward the patient?
4. Does the family exacerbate or contribute to the problem?

D. **Occupational Aspects of the Illness:** Assess how the illness has affected the patient's physical or job functioning (i.e., adaptation).

VIII. REVIEW OF SYSTEMS (Tables 33-1 to 33-3)

Table 33-1. GENERAL SURGERY SYMPTOMS BY SYSTEM.

System	Symptoms
General	Current overall health
HEENT	Headaches, head lumps, seizures; ringing in the ears, hearing loss, vertigo; blurred vision, double vision, swollen eyes, black eyes; congestion, colds, discharge; sinus pain (frontal, maxillary), nasal discharge, epistaxis; hoarseness, sore throat; difficulty swallowing, painful swallowing; regurgitation, acid taste, halitosis; excessive salivation
Neck	Lumps, soreness; thyroid swelling, thyroid pain, recent weight changes, slowing/speeding of life; neck vibrations; neck fistulas' draining
CV	Palpitations, rapid heart, irregular beating, chest pain; any arm/leg vibrations; any excess bleeding/bruising
Chest	Shortness of breath, wheezing, cough, asthma, pneumonia
Breasts	Breast lumps, discharges, skin changes, menstrual variations, underarm lymph nodes
Back	Pain or aches, lumps, costovertebral angle pain
Abdomen	Pain, nausea, vomiting, diarrhea, distention; hematemesis; heartburn; appetite changes; bowel movement/flatulence changes; excess constipation/looseness; inguinal lumps, inguinal pain
Rectum	Bleeding, pain, discharge; painful defecation; black stool, blood in stool, mucous floating in stool or foul-smelling stools; protrusions, lumps; change in stool color
GU/Pelvic	Suprapubic/pelvic pain; pain with voiding; urine with debris, air, blood; frequency; genital ulcers; vaginal discharge, pain; menstrual history; pregnancy (very important)
Extremities	Muscle pain, joint pain; any swelling; any arm/leg pain at rest or with exertion; lymph nodes in axilla and groin; nonhealing ulcers; change in skin color; numbness and/or tingling
Skin	Rashes, itching, blisters, bruising; color (pale, yellow, sallow); lumps under the arms/in the groin
Neurologic	Mental status changes; changes in motor/sensory status; coordination changes
Miscellaneous	Exposures to chemicals, foods; any other people similarly ill; any similar difficulty in the past

Table 33-2. NONSPECIFIC SYMPTOMS AND THEIR GENERAL SURGERY DISEASES.

SYMPTOMS	DISEASES
Dysphagia	Tonsillitis, foreign body, diverticula, reflux, achalasia, thyroid, cancer
Nausea, vomiting	Obstruction, peptic ulcer disease, gastritis, gallbladder disease, cancer
Constipation	Obstruction, dehydration, irritable bowel, diverticulitis, cancer
Diarrhea	Irritable bowel, inflammatory bowel, diverticulitis, GI bleeding
Fever	Appendicitis, cholecystitis, perforated ulcer, diverticulitis, abscess
Skin color changes	Pale (anemia), yellow (hepatitis, biliary obstruction, cirrhosis, cancer)
Abdominal pain (general)	Obstruction, peptic ulcer disease, pancreatitis, intussusception, small bowel pathology (volvulus, tumor), bowel infarction, achalasia, reflux, hiatal hernia, hyperparathyroidism, aortic aneurysm, hernia, cancer
Right upper quadrant (RUQ)	Cholecystitis, common duct disease, hepatitis, cirrhosis, Fitz-Hugh-Curtis syndrome, pancreatitis, peptic ulcer disease, gastritis, cancer
Left upper quadrant (LUQ)	Peptic ulcer disease, leaking gastric ulcer, splenic infarct, hemopoietic splenic disease, splenic rupture, pancreatitis, colonic volvulus, cancer
Right lower quadrant (RLQ)	Appendicitis, Meckel's diverticulitis, inflammatory bowel, ovarian disease/torsion, ectopic pregnancy, renal/ureteral stone, hernia, cancer
Left lower quadrant (LLQ)	Diverticulitis, inflammatory bowel, ovarian/torsion disease, hernia, leaking gastric ulcer, renal/ureteral stone, cancer

This review concentrates on present time. Is there any other ongoing system problem that might complicate the presenting problem? It is important to record both pertinent positives and pertinent negatives.

IX. PHYSICAL EXAMINATION (Table 33-4)

When performing the neurologic examination in a general surgery context, the goal is not to delineate specific lesions and their loca-

Text continued on p. 741.

Table 33-3. COMMON GENERAL SURGERY DISEASES AND THEIR SYMPTOMS.

Disease	Symptoms
Appendicitis	RLQ pain (classically shifting from periumbilical), nausea, vomiting, anorexia, inconstant symptoms (fever, diarrhea, constipation, distention)
Cholecystitis	RUQ pain, nausea, vomiting, anorexia, fatty food intolerance, fever, bloating, flatulence, loose stools, inconstant symptoms (jaundice, distention)
Diverticulitis	LLQ pain, diarrhea and/or constipation, fever, inconstant symptoms (tenesmus, blood per rectum, debris/air in urine [indicates fistula])
Breast cancer	Nonpainful lump, nonmobile lump, nipple bleeding (more common with benign intraductal papilloma), skin/nipple retraction, peau d'orange

Table 33-4. FINDINGS OF SURGICAL PHYSICAL EXAMINATION AND POSSIBLE DIAGNOSES.

System	Physical Examination Finding	Possible Diagnoses
General	Patient lies extremely still	Peritonitis (perforated ulcer)
	Patient constantly moving	Colic (cholecystitis, kidney stone)
	Diaphoresis	Condition with severe pain
Vitals		
Pulse	Bradycardia	Decompensation, shock
	Tachycardia	Volume depletion, inflammatory process, infectious process
Blood pressure	Low and/or orthostatic	Dehydration, volume depletion
	High	Endocrine pathology

Table 33-4—cont'd

System	Physical Examination Finding	Possible Diagnoses
	Narrowed pulse pressure	Cardiac tamponade
Respiratory rate	Low	Decompensation, shock
	High	Pneumothorax, hemothorax
Weight	Recent weight loss	Cancer, endocrine pathology
	Recent weight gain	Endocrine pathology
HEENT		
Head	Mastoid bruising	Basilar skull fracture
Eyes	Double vision, blurred vision	Ocular muscle entrapment
	Orbital discontinuity	Orbital fracture
	Nystagmus, vertigo	Tympanic membrane (TM) rupture
	Fundi (papilledema)	Increased intracranial pressure
Ears	Retracted TM	Barotrauma
	Blood behind TM	Barotrauma, basilar skull fracture
Nose	Nasal discharge, redness, deformity	Cocaine abuse, cancer
	Septal ulceration	Cocaine abuse, cancer
Mouth	Throat asymmetry	Peritonsillar abscess
	Color: White	Leukoplakia, candidiasis
	Black spots	Peutz-Jaegers disease, Addison's disease
	Magenta (red tongue)	Vitamin B deficiency
	Discharge, swelling	Abscess
	Ulceration	Aphthous, uremia, cancer
	Hypersalivation	Epiglottitis, severe pertonsillar abscess, esophageal foreign body

Continued

Table 33-4. FINDINGS OF SURGICAL PHYSICAL EXAMINATION AND POSSIBLE DIAGNOSES—*cont'd*

System	Physical Examination Finding	Possible Diagnoses
Face	Raccoon eye sign	Basilar skull fracture
	Unilateral eye swellings	Periorbital cellulitis
	Cheek swelling/mass	Parotiditis, parotid gland tumor
Neck	Cervical, submental, posterior auricular nodes	Lymphoma, Hodgkin lymphoma, metastatic cancer
	Troisier's sign (Virchow's node)	Metastatic gastric cancer
	Upper lateral mass (transilluminates)	Cystic hygroma
	Carotid palpation: Mass	Carotid body tumor
	Auscultation with thrills and bruits	Atherosclerotic carotid disease
	Jugular venous distention	Cardiac tamponade, pneumothorax
	Tracheal deviation	Pneumothorax, hemothorax
	Fistulous opening: Lateral to midline	Branchial cleft fistula (cyst)
	Fistulous opening: Anterior midline	Thyroglossal duct fistula (cyst)
Thyroid	Thyroid palpation (two methods): From behind with bilateral index and middle fingers or in front with bilateral thumbs allows simultaneous inspection with palpation)	
	Painless, enlarged	Grave's disease
	Painful, enlarged or shrunken	Hashimoto's thyroiditis
	Thyroid nodule	Adenoma, cyst, cancer

Table 33-4—cont'd

System	Physical Examination Finding	Possible Diagnoses
Chest	Rales, rhonchi, and wheezes	Atelectasis, pneumonia, tracheal-bronchial foreign body
	Shortness of breath	Pneumothorax, partial airway block
	Hyperresonance	Pneumothorax, large lung bleb
	Diminished breath sounds	Pneumothorax, hemothorax, chylothorax, pneumonia
	Hyporesonance	Hemothorax, chylothorax, pneumonia
Breasts	*BREAST PALPATION* Use two hands taking the index, middle, and ring fingers of one hand to gently palpate from the outer breast to the nipple in a circular pattern, while the other hand stabilizes the breast	
	Asymmetry	Mammary hypertrophy, cancer, normal variant
	Tender, mobile mass	Cyst
	Nontender, mobile mass	Fibroadenoma
	Nontender, nonmobile mass	Cancer
	Erythematous skin	Inflammatory breast cancer
	Peau d'orange skin	Cancer in skin lymphatics
	Skin retraction/dimpling	Cancer
	Nipple retraction	Cancer

Continued

Table 33-4. FINDINGS OF SURGICAL PHYSICAL EXAMINATION AND POSSIBLE DIAGNOSES—_cont'd_

System	Physical Examination Finding	Possible Diagnoses
Areola	Gently milk each quadrant to express any discharge, noting color, location, smell, texture, blood (hemoccult for blood)	White: milk (endocrine disease) Straw: cyst (menstrual variant) Red: blood (intraductal papilloma, cancer)
	Axillary and supraclavicular nodes	Metastatic cancer
	Aspirated breast mass	No fluid: fibroadenoma, cancer Straw fluid: cystic
Cardiovascular	Murmurs, gallops	Valvular heart disease
	Rubs	Pericardial heart disease
	Muffled heart sounds	Cardiac tamponade
	Cardiac thrills	Ventricular aneurysm
	Peripheral pulse bruits	Atherosclerotic vascular disease, peripheral aneurisms
	Palpate radial, brachial, femoral, popliteal, dorsalis pedis, and posterior tibial pulses	Obstructive vascular disease
Abdomen	Inspect for symmetry, distention, masses, bruising	
	Auscultate bowel sounds	Normal: rumbling Obstructive: tinkling, borborygmi Peritonitis: silence
	Solid organs percussion Liver (>2-3 fingerbreadths below costal margin)	 Hepatitis, cirrhosis, abscess, echinococcal cyst, cancer
	Spleen (below costal margin)	Hematopoietic disease, rupture, portal hypertension, cancer

Table 33-4—cont'd

SYSTEM	PHYSICAL EXAMINATION FINDING	POSSIBLE DIAGNOSES
	Fluid wave Puddle sign	Ascites, bile, chyle Ascites, bile, chyle
	Distention	Fluid, obstruction, paralytic ileus, megacolon, mass
	Palpate beginning away from any pain (*ask patient to point out any localized pain*), noting symmetry, distention, masses, tenderness	
	Guarding: Voluntary muscle tightness to protect from palpatory pain	Muscle tear, localized inflammation (appendicitis, cholecystitis), cancer
	Rebound (Blumberg's sign): Pain with light percussion or pain on quick release of gentle palpation denoting peritoneal irritation	Localized inflammation (ovarian torsion, diverticulitis), penetrating peptic ulcer, cancer
	Rigidity: Painful belly with muscles that are involuntarily boardlike and rigid denoting severe, generalized peritoneal inflammation	Generalized inflammation (ruptured abscess, perforated peptic ulcer, perforated cancer, ruptured aortic aneurysm)
Nonspecific abdominal location	Gastrointestinal (esophagus, stomach, small bowel, colon), pancreas, abdominal wall, aorta, pancreas	Obstruction, peptic ulcer disease, pancreatitis, intussusception, small bowel pathology (volvulus, tumor), bowel infarction, achalasia, reflux, hiatal hernia, hyperparathyroidism, aortic aneurysm, umbilical/inguinal umbilical/inguinal hernia, cancer

Continued

Table 33-4. FINDINGS OF SURGICAL PHYSICAL EXAMINATION AND POSSIBLE DIAGNOSES—*cont'd*

System	Physical Examination Finding	Possible Diagnoses
	Carnett's sign	Abdominal wall (muscle tear, hematoma)
	Caput medusae	Portal hypertension
	Sister Mary Joseph sign	Metastatic gastric cancer
	Puddle sign	Ascites, chyle, blood
Right upper quadrant (RUQ)	Liver, gallbladder, duodenum, stomach, pancreas, transverse colon, and hepatic flexure of the colon	Cholecystitis, common duct disease, hepatitis, cirrhosis, liver abscess, Fitz-Hugh-Curtis syndrome, pancreatitis, pancreatic pseudocyst, peptic ulcer disease (gastric or duodenal), penetrating duodenal ulcer, gastritis, bile acid reflux, hepatic flexure syndrome, irritable bowel, inflammatory bowel, umbilical hernia, cancer
	Courvoisier's sign	Pancreatic cancer
	Murphy's sign	Acute cholecystitis
	Cullen's sign	Ectopic pregnancy, hemorrhagic pancreatitis
Left upper quadrant (LUQ)	Spleen, stomach, pancreas, transverse colon, and splenic flexure of the colon	Peptic ulcer disease, leaking gastric ulcer, splenic infarct, hemopoietic splenic disease, splenic rupture, pancreatitis, pancreatic pseudocyst, colonic volvulus, splenic flexure syndrome, irritable bowel, inflammatory bowel, umbilical hernia, cancer

Table 33-4—cont'd

SYSTEM	PHYSICAL EXAMINATION FINDING	POSSIBLE DIAGNOSES
	Kenawy's sign	Bilharzial portal hypertension
Right lower quadrant (RLQ)	Cecum, appendix, ileum, right ovary, uterus, right kidney with ureter, and bladder	Leaking duodenal ulcer, appendicitis, Meckel's diverticulitis, irritable bowel, inflammatory bowel, ovarian disease/torsion, ectopic pregnancy, renal /ureteral stone, umbilical/inguinal hernia, cancer
	McBurney's sign	Appendicitis
	Obturator sign	Retroperitoneal appendicitis
	Psoas sign	Retroperitoneal appendicitis
	Rovsing's sign (referred rebound)	Appendicitis
Left lower quadrant (LLQ)	Descending colon, sigmoid colon, bladder, uterus, left ovary	Leaking gastric ulcer, diverticulitis, irritable bowel, inflammatory bowel, ovarian disease/torsion, umbilical/inguinal hernia, renal/ureteral stone, cancer
Rectum	External masses	Hemorrhoids, hypertrophied anal papilla, abscess, cancer
	Internal masses	Hemorrhoids, hypertrophied anal papilla, abscess, cancer
	Blumer's shelf	Metastatic gastric cancer
	Pain	Anal fissure, abscess, hemorrhoids

Continued

Table 33-4. FINDINGS OF SURGICAL PHYSICAL EXAMINATION AND POSSIBLE DIAGNOSES—cont'd

System	Physical Examination Finding	Possible Diagnoses
	Drainage	
	Without openings	Rectal prolapse, inflammatory bowel
	With openings	Fistula-in-ano (Goddsall's Line)
	Poor sphincter tone	Neurologic disorder, trauma
	Bleeding (red or hemoccult)	Polyps, Meckel's diverticulum, inflammatory bowel, diverticulosis, cancer
	Melena	Upper GI bleeding (gastritis, peptic ulcer disease, Mallory-Weiss tear), varices, hemobilia, cancer
Back/spine	Vertebral discomfort	Compressed vertebra, infection
	Paravertebral discomfort	Paravertebral muscle spasm
	Costovertebral angle tenderness (CVAT)	Renal stone, pyelonephritis, kidney disease, lumbar hernia, cancer
	Grey Turner's sign	Ruptured aortic aneurysm, hemorrhagic pancreatitis
Genitourinary		
Male	Urethral discharge	Sexually transmitted disease, perforative diverticulitis
	Urethral bleeding	Urethral papilloma, urethral trauma
	Hematuria	Renal/ureteral stone, renal/ureteral trauma, bladder trauma, cystitis, perforative diverticulitis, cancer

Table 33-4—cont'd

System	Physical Examination Finding	Possible Diagnoses
	Penile ulcer	Sexually transmitted disease, cancer
	Inguinal mass (above inguinal crease)	Direct/indirect/ pantaloon hernia, lymphadenopathy
	Inguinal mass (below inguinal crease)	Femoral hernia
	Scrotal mass	Hydrocele (transilluminates), varicocele, cancer
	Testicular pain	Epididymitis, appendices testis torsion, testicular torsion, cancer
Female	Urethral discharge	Sexually transmitted disease, perforative diverticulitis
	Urethral bleeding	Urethral papilloma, urethral trauma
	Labial ulcer	Sexually transmitted disease, cancer
	Labial mass	Bartholin abscess, Bartholin cyst, cancer
	Inguinal mass (above inguinal crease)	Direct/indirect/ pantaloon hernia, lymphadenopathy
	Inguinal mass (below inguinal crease)	Femoral hernia
	Chandelier sign	Pelvic inflammatory disease
	Adnexal mass (with or without pain)	Ovarian cyst, tuboovarian abscess, ectopic pregnancy, cancer
	Krukenberg tumor	Metastatic gastric cancer
Skin	Sweat (diaphoresis)	Pain is present
	Pallor	Anemia, volume depletion
	Erythema	Inflammation with local infection

Continued

Table 33-4. FINDINGS OF SURGICAL PHYSICAL EXAMINATION AND POSSIBLE DIAGNOSES—*cont'd*

System	Physical Examination Finding	Possible Diagnoses
	Rashes (color, macular, papular)	Medication allergy
	Blistering	Burns, Stevens-Johnson syndrome
	Bruising	Coagulation disorder, trauma
	Heat	Fever is present
	Petechiae	Vascular fragility, general sepsis, meningococcemia
	Neck, axillary, supraclavicular, epitrochlear, groin nodes	Lymphoma, Hodgkin's disease, metastatic cancer
Extremities	Symmetry and function	
	Masses	Dermatofibroma, sebaceous cyst, lipoma, synovial cyst, sarcoma, aneurysm
	Pain (with or without swelling)	Abscess, tendon/ligament rupture, compartment syndrome
	Deformity	Bone cyst, fracture, periosteal hematoma, tendon/ligament rupture
Neurologic	Mental status	Alert and oriented?
	Cranial nerves	I-XII normal?
	Motor	Upper and lower extremity equal bilaterally?
	Sensory	Upper and lower extremity equal bilaterally?
	Coordination	Upper or lower extremity coordination, ataxia?
	Reflexes	Upper and lower extremity equal bilaterally?

tions. The goal is to discover abnormalities. Thus a thorough and repeatable examination can be performed in about 4 to 5 minutes. It is important to remember to never examine the "hurting" area initially. Always begin as far as possible from the point of interest.

X. DIFFERENTIAL DIAGNOSIS (Table 33-5)

In general surgery, diagnosis and pathology are often directly related to anatomy, particularly in patients with abdominal pain. It must be the first consideration when developing any differential diagnosis.

XI. LABORATORY STUDIES AND DIAGNOSTIC EVALUATIONS

Laboratory and radiologic examinations must be tailored to the complaint and the physical findings. All blood, urine, radiologic, and sonographic examinations are performed to clarify and confirm the tentative diagnosis. As a result, excess testing is avoided.

A. **Common Blood Tests:** Complete blood count (CBC), electrolytes, blood urea nitrogen (BUN), creatinine, blood sugar, urinalysis, amylase, lipase, and liver function tests.

B. **Common Diagnostic Imaging Exams:** Chest x-ray (posterior to anterior and lateral), abdominal series (flatplate with upright or left lateral decubitus), and computed tomography (CT) scan (evaluation of masses). Sonographic examinations are usually ordered to evaluate the gallbladder, pancreas, right lower quadrant (RLQ), and adnexa.

XII. ACRONYMS AND ABBREVIATIONS (Table 33-6)

XIII. DEFINITIONS (Table 33-7)

XIV. SAMPLE H&P WRITE-UP

CC: W.F., a 25-year-old white female, complains of 12 hours of "belly pain that I first noticed yesterday afternoon during our company picnic . . . after I ate two large burgers."

HPI: She notes that the pain began as a mild ache around her belly button. It has gradually worsened almost to the point of doubling her over. Although it was relatively mild and intermittent early on, it is now sharp and unremitting. In addition, most of the pain is now in her right lower belly. She feels better when lying still. She notes no other pains; however, she describes a mild, intermittent nausea, and she is very concerned that the pain is not going away. Of note, she relates that no one else at the picnic has gotten ill.

MHx: Unremarkable.

SHx: No prior surgeries for patient or family.

Medications: None.

Allergies: NKA (no known allergies, medicines or otherwise).

HEALTH MAINTENANCE

Cigarettes: Nonsmoker.

ETOH: Nondrinker.

Family History: Mother with eczema.

ROS: Excellent general health; had a cold about a week ago, now recovered; no respiratory illnesses; no past problem with bleeding or bruising, but did notice a small bruise around the belly button; no

Text continued on p. 747.

Table 33-5. DIFFERENTIAL DIAGNOSIS OF COMMON GENERAL SURGERY DISORDERS.

Finding	Differential Diagnosis
Right upper quadrant pain (RUQ)	Cholecystitis, common duct disease, hepatitis, cirrhosis, Fitz-Hugh-Curtis syndrome, pancreatitis, peptic ulcer disease, gastritis, cancer
Left upper quadrant pain (LUQ)	Peptic ulcer disease, leaking gastric ulcer, splenic infarct, hemopoietic splenic disease, splenic rupture, pancreatitis, colonic volvulus, cancer
Right lower quadrant pain (RLQ)	Appendicitis, Meckel's diverticulitis, inflammatory bowel disease, ovarian disease/torsion, ectopic pregnancy, renal/ureteral stone, hernia, cancer
Left lower quadrant pain (LLQ)	Diverticulitis, inflammatory bowel disease, ovarian disease/torsion, hernia, leaking gastric ulcer, renal/ureteral stone, cancer
Non-surgical abdominal pain	Pneumonia, acute porphyria, systemic lupus erythematosus, congestive heart failure (liver capsule distention), hepatitis, mononucleosis, sickle cell disease, lead poisoning, black widow spider bite
Breast lump	Cystic disease, fibroadenoma, hemangioma, leiomyoma, neurofibroma, granular cell tumor, galactocele, sarcoidosis, fat necrosis, abscess, foreign body reaction, cancer
Inguinal mass	Inguinal hernia (direct, indirect, pantaloon), femoral hernia, lymphadenopathy, femoral artery aneurysm, sebaceous cyst abscess, sexually transmitted disease
Thyroid mass	Follicular adenoma, follicular cyst, adenomatous goiter, localized hyperplasia, thyroiditis, cancer (papillary, follicular, medullary, anaplastic), lymphoma, metastatic cancer
Jaundice	Biliary atresia, cholelithiasis, choledocholithiasis, pancreatitis, pancreatic cancer, bile duct/ampulla of Vater cancer, lymphoma, sarcoidosis, hepatitis, hemolysis, sepsis, Gilbert's disease, drugs

Table 33-6. GENERAL SURGERY ACRONYMS AND ABBREVIATIONS.

Acronym or Abbreviation	Term	Acronym or Abbreviation	Term
AFP	Alpha fetoprotein	**CMF**	Cytoxan, methotrexate, 5-fluorouracil
AGE	Air gas embolism; arterial gas embolism	**CMV**	Cytomegalovirus
AKA	Above the knee amputation	**COPD**	Chronic obstructive pulmonary disease
APR	Abdominoperineal resection	**CPAP**	Continuous positive airway pressure
ARDS	Adult respiratory distress syndrome	**DCI**	Decompression illness (decompression sickness [DCS] and air or arterial gas embolism [AGE])
ARF	Acute renal failure	**DCS**	Decompression sickness
ASA	Aspirin; American Society of Anesthesiologists	**DIC**	Disseminated intravascular coagulation
ASD	Atrial septal defect	**DIP**	Distal interphalangeal joint
ATN	Acute tubular necrosis	**DPG 2,3**	DPG 2,3 diphosphoglyceric acid
BEE	Basal energy expenditure	**DPL**	Diagnostic peritoneal lavage
BER	Basal electrical rhythm	**DTs**	Delerium tremens
BKA	Below-the-knee amputation	**DVT**	Deep venous thrombosis
BMI	Body mass index	**ECF**	Extracellular fluid
Ca	Cancer	**ECMO**	Extracorporeal membrane oxygenation
CABG	Coronary artery bypass graft	**ED**	Emergency department
CAPD	Chronic ambulatory peritoneal dialysis	**EOM**	Extraocular muscles
CEA	Carcinoembryonic antigen	**ER**	Emergency room; estrogen receptor

Continued

Table 33-6. GENERAL SURGERY ACRONYMS AND ABBREVIATIONS—cont'd

Acronym or Abbreviation	Term	Acronym or Abbreviation	Term
Fem pop	Femoral popliteal bypass graft	**OSHA**	Occupational Safety and Health Administration
FFP	Fresh frozen plasma	**PDA**	Patent ductus arteriosus
GB	Gallbladder	**PE**	Pulmonary embolus
GCS	Glasgow Coma Scale	**PEEP**	Positive end-expiratory pressure
GERD	Gastroesophageal reflux disease	**PERRLA**	Pupils round and reactive to light and accommodation
GFR	Glomerular filtration rate	**PFT**	Pulmonary function tests
HAV	Hepatitis A virus	**PgR**	Progesterone receptor
HBV	Hepatitis B virus	**PIP**	Proximal interphalangeal joint
HCC	Hepatocellular carcinoma	**PPN**	Peripheral parenteral nutrition
HCV	Hepatitis C virus	**PSA**	Prostatic-specific antigen
HDV	Hepatitis D virus	**PT**	Prothrombin time
HEV	Hepatitis E virus	**PTCA**	Percutaneous transluminal coronary angioplasty
HIV	Human immunodeficiency virus	**PTFE**	Polytetrafluoroethylene
HR	Heart rate (pulse)	**PTH**	Parathormone
IABP	Intraaortic balloon pump	**PTT**	Partial thromboplastin time

ICF	Intracellular fluid	**RDI**	Respiratory distress index
ICP	Intracranial pressure	**RIH**	Right inguinal hernia
IE ratio	Inspiratory-to-expiratory ratio	**RR**	Respiratory rate
INH	Isoniazid	**RRR**	Regular rate and rhythm
IL	Interluekin	**SVT**	Supraventricular tachycardia
ITP	Immune thrombocytopenic purpura	**TBSA**	Total body surface area
Lap	Exploratory laparotomy	**TEF**	Tracheoesophageal fistula
Lap chole	Laparoscopic cholecystectomy	**TFT**	Thyroid function tests
LES	Lower esophageal sphincter	**TIA**	Transient ischemic attack
LFT	Liver function tests	**TNM**	Tumor Node Metastasis Staging System
LIH	Left inguinal hernia	**TPN**	Total parenteral nutrition
MAC	Minimal alveolar concentration	**TTP**	Thrombotic thrombocytopenic purpura
MCP	Metacarpophalangeal joint	**US**	Ultrasound
MEN	Multiple endocrine neoplasia	**VBG**	Vertical-banded gastroplasty
MHC	Major histocompatibility complex	**VIP**	Vasoactive intestinal peptide
MODS	Multiple organ dysfunction syndrome	**VQ scan**	Ventilation perfusion scan
NIOSH	National Institute for Occupational Safety and Health	**VSD**	Ventricular septal defect
NSE	Neuron-specific enolase	**ZE**	Zollinger Ellison Syndrome

Table 33-7. GENERAL SURGERY TERMS.

TERM	DEFINITION
Battle's sign	Mastoid bruising suggesting basilar skull fracture
Blumberg's sign	Pain with light percussion or pain on quick release of gentle palpation denoting peritoneal irritation (rebound tenderness)
Blumer's shelf	Anterior rectal mass classically associated with metastatic gastric cancer (or any GI cancer)
Carnett's sign	Tender abdomen to palpation as the patient lifts his or her head, denoting abdominal source of pain
Chandelier sign	Exquisite anterior-placed pain with motion of cervix with pelvic inflammatory disease
Courvoisier's sign	Nontender palpable gallbladder with jaundice commonly associated with pancreatic cancer
Cullen's sign	Periumbilical bruising associated with ectopic pregnancy and hemorrhagic pancreatitis
Fitz-Hugh-Curtis syndrome	RUQ pain associated with liver-diaphragm adhesions formed during pelvic inflammatory disease (chlamydial and/or gonococcal infections)
Fluid wave	Tapping one side of the abdomen and feeling the impulse on the other side of the abdomen; denotes ascites
Goodsall's line	Anterior-placed tracts lead directly to rectum while posterior-placed tracts curve in a horseshoe fashion to open in the midline rectum
Grey Turner's sign	Flank bruising associated with ruptured aortic aneurysm and hemorrhagic pancreatitis
Hepatic flexure syndrome	RUQ pain associated with a temporarily trapped pocket of gas at the hepatic flexure; relief with abdominal massage is common
Kenawy's sign	Splenomegaly found with bilharzial (schistosomiasis) cirrhosis
Krukenberg tumor	Ovarian mass classically associated with metastatic gastric cancer (or any GI cancer)

Table 33-7—cont'd

TERM	DEFINITION
McBurney's sign	Point tenderness at McBurney's point (two-thirds from umbilicus to anterior-superior iliac spine): appendicitis
Murphy's sign	Inspiratory arrest with RUQ deep palpation: acute cholecystitis
Obturator sign	Pain with rotation of flexed thigh: inflammation around the internal obturator muscle (retroperitoneal appendicitis)
Pantaloon hernia	Combination of direct and indirect hernia
Psoas sign	Pain with thigh extension: inflammation around the psoas muscle (retroperitoneal appendicitis)
Puddle sign	Patient on hand and knees; flick side of abdomen with finger while listening with stethoscope; by moving diaphragm over dependent abdomen can delineate fluid collections (used to detect small amounts of ascites)
Raccoon eye sign	Bilateral black eyes suggesting basilar skull fracture
Rovsing's sign (also known as "referred rebound")	Palpatory pressure in the LLQ elicits pain in the RLQ; often associated with appendicitis
Sister Mary Joseph sign	Umbilical mass classically associated with metastatic gastric cancer (or any GI cancer)
Splenic flexure syndrome	LUQ pain associated with a temporarily trapped pocket of gas at the splenic flexure; relief with abdominal massage is common
Troisier's sign (also known as Virchow's node)	Enlarged left supraclavicular lymph nodes classically associated with metastatic gastric cancer (or any GI cancer)

costovertebral angle pain; mild nausea without vomiting, constipation, or diarrhea; no urinary pain or frequency; no vaginal discharges; married using condoms for birth control and is presently in midcycle; appropriate concern for this never-before-experienced problem.

PHYSICAL EXAMINATION

Vital Signs: Unremarkable.

General: Pleasant but uncomfortable lady.

HEENT: Head, ears, eyes unremarkable; nose without discharge; no throat redness, swelling, or exudates.

Neck: Soft, supple without masses; no nodes palpated; carotid pulses normal.

CV: Regular rate and rhythm without murmurs, gallops, tachycardia.

Chest/Breast: Clear to auscultation and percussion without rales, rhonchi, or wheezes; breasts unremarkable.

Back: No vertebral or costovertebral angle tenderness (CVAT).

Abdomen: Normal bowel sounds; generally soft and nontender except in the right lower quadrant, where there is localized tenderness to deep palpation and rebound to percussion; guarding is present; no distention, masses, or organomegaly noted.

Rectum: No masses; no cervical motion pain, but there is pain to the right anteriorly; no blood.

GU/Pelvic: Gentle bimanual examination revealed pain in the right adnexa; no masses or discharges noted.

Extremities: Unremarkable.

Skin: Unremarkable.

Neurologic: Normal.

LABS

Blood: White blood cell count is 13,800 with 87% polymorphonuclear cells.

Urine: Urinalysis is normal; pregnancy test is positive.

Sonogram: Right adnexal mass with fluid in the cul-de-sac.

DX: Right-sided ectopic pregnancy: The patient is 25-year-old female who is sexually active using condoms for birth control, suggesting possible ectopic pregnancy. She is presently midcycle, suggesting ruptured follicular cyst. Yesterday, the pain began periumbilical, but today is localized in the right lower quadrant with guarding and rebound, suggesting appendicitis. A periumbilical bruise suggests ectopic pregnancy. The rectal/pelvic examination is consistent with both an ectopic pregnancy and appendicitis. She additionally notes a recent viral illness, suggesting mesenteric adenitis (this is a diagnosis of exclusion; it is considered once the more serious considerations are eliminated). **White blood cell count** is consistent with both ectopic pregnancy and appendicitis. **Pregnancy test** is positive, consistent with ectopic pregnancy and appendicitis. **Sonogram** revealed a right adnexal mass with fluid in the cul-de-sac, suggesting a bleeding ectopic pregnancy.

PLAN: Take patient to the operating room as soon as possible; the most likely diagnosis of ruptured ectopic pregnancy requires an operation.

XV. ADMISSION TEMPLATE

When a patient is admitted to the surgical service, but does not immediately go to the operating room, orders must be written. These orders are an extension of your history and physical examination. As such, they must reflect what you think is going on, what you think is needed, and what you want to happen. This template is a checklist to ensure that you do not omit anything:

D Diagnosis
C Condition (e.g., critical, stable)
V Vital signs frequency; special examination frequency (e.g., nursing neurologic check)
A Activity (e.g., bed rest, bathroom privileges, no limitation)
N Nutrition (e.g., clear liquids, regular diet, no food)
D Drugs (e.g., intravenous fluids, pain medicines, antibiotics)
L Laboratory exams (e.g., blood, urine)
I Intake and output (e.g., measure amounts)
S Stool (e.g., hemoccult)
M Miscellaneous (e.g., parameters requiring physician notification)

34

UROLOGY

R. Clay McDonough III, MD, and Jay T. Bishoff, MD

I. CHIEF COMPLAINT

A. Chief Complaint: Use the patient's own words. Chronology is often very important with urology patients and is usually recorded within the chief complaint.

B. Identifying Data: Obtain patient's name, age, gender, race/ethnicity, and location of evaluation/admission.

II. HISTORY OF PRESENT ILLNESS

For each of the following symptoms, ask about the following characteristics: Onset, duration, frequency, distributions, radiation, alleviating factors, exacerbating factors, and treatments.

A. Urinary Symptoms

1. Irritative symptoms are often associated with infection, inflammation, or cancer.
   - **a.** Are you awakening at night to urinate (nocturia)? If so, how many times during the night? Significant nocturia is more than two times per night.
   - **b.** How often do you urinate during the day (frequency)? Significant frequency is voiding at least every 2 hours.
   - **c.** Do you need to urinate immediately to avoid incontinence (urgency)?
   - **d.** Do you have pain or a burning sensation when urinating (dysuria)?
2. Obstructive symptoms are associated with obstruction of the lower urinary tract.
   - **a.** Do you have difficulty initiating stream of urine (hesitancy)?
   - **b.** Is there a decrease in force or caliber of urine stream?
   - **c.** Is voiding incomplete?
   - **d.** Any terminal dribbling?
   - **e.** Is your stream interrupted?
3. Hematuria: Patients with hematuria need examination of their urine, cystoendoscopy, and intravenous urography (explained later in this chapter). All such patients should be referred to a urologist for these studies.
   - **a.** Have you seen blood in your urine (gross hematuria)?
   - **b.** Has blood in your urine been noted in urinalysis only (microscopic hematuria)?
   - **c.** Does the blood appear at the beginning of the stream, at the end of the stream, or throughout the entire urine stream (timing)?

4. Incontinence.
   a. Do you experience incontinence when coughing, sneezing, or on Valsalva maneuver? Stress incontinence is associated with increases in intra-abdominal pressure.
   b. Do you have a strong urge to void before incontinence episode (urge incontinence)?
   c. Do you have involuntary loss of urine when your bladder is full? Overflow incontinence is associated with obstructive symptoms.

B. **Genitourinary Sources of Pain**

1. Kidney: Typically in the flank, usually colicky, associated with nausea and vomiting.
2. Ureteral: Colicky, can radiate from flank to scrotum/vagina.
3. Bladder: Suprapubic, often associated with irritative symptoms.
4. Prostate: Vague perineal/rectal pain, abdominal or pelvic pain.
5. Testicle: Local pain, may radiate to abdomen.

C. **Urethral Discharge:** Often associated with sexually transmitted disease (e.g., gonorrhea, Chlamydia, syphilis).

D. **Sexual Function**

1. Can you obtain and maintain erection sufficient for penetration (erectile function)?
2. Do you have any children (fertility)?
3. Do you reach orgasm before penetration or immediately after penetration? Premature ejaculation is often misinterpreted as erectile dysfunction by patients?
4. Is your sexual desire (libido) or sexual appetite normal? Important to know if present with erectile dysfunction.

III. PAST MEDICAL AND SURGICAL HISTORY

A. **Past Medical History**

1. Have you had any sexually transmitted diseases (STDs)?
2. Do you have diabetes?
3. Have you been diagnosed with hypertension (HTN)?
4. Have you had any neurologic or renal disease?
5. Have you had kidney stones (renal calculi)? If so, what were the diagnostic evaluations or analyses of the collected stones?

B. **Past Surgical History**

1. Have you undergone any previous urologic surgeries? When and with what results (sequelae)?
2. Have you had any previous abdominal surgeries?

C. **Emergency and Trauma History**

1. Have you received blood transfusions? Did you have a reaction to the transfusion? Were there any complications?
2. Have you visited an emergency room for urologic complaints? What type of complaints were they? When and which hospitals?
3. Have you had a traumatic injury?

D. Childhood Development and Illnesses

1. Was your genital development normal? Ambiguous? Undescended testis?
2. Testicular femininization syndrome?
3. Did you have vesicoureteral reflux (VUR)? Was it treated medically or surgically?

E. Occupational History

1. Are you exposed to any industrial dyes (e.g., aniline dyes) at work? Workers who are exposed to aniline dyes or who work in the rubber industry have a higher incidence of transitional cell carcinoma of the bladder.
2. Have you been exposed to thorotrast? Thorotrast was used as a radiologic agent until the 1950s.

F. Travel History: Do you travel within the United States? To foreign countries? Schistosomiasis is endemic in some counties, and may predispose to bladder cancer.

IV. MEDICATIONS, ALLERGIES, AND ADVERSE REACTIONS

A. Medications

1. Are you taking any of the following prescription medications: Antihypertensives, cold medicines, hormones, hormone blocker(s), anticoagulants, anticholinergics, 5-alpha reductase inhibitors, medicines for erectile dysfunction?
2. Are you taking over-the-counter (OTC) medications? Abuse of some analgesics may cause kidney disease.
3. Any herbal preparations? Saw palmetto is a common herbal treatment for benign prostatic hypertrophy (BPH).
4. Any supplements? Studies are currently underway to determine whether Vitamin E and selenium can prevent the development of prostate cancer.

B. Allergies to Medications and the Side Effects

1. Is the patient on medications that may affect therapy? Some drugs may interfere with surgery (e.g., anticoagulants).
2. Is the patient on a drug that may cause cancer?
3. Have you had an allergic reaction to prior medicines (classic example of penicillin and cross-reactivity with penicillin derivatives/cephalosporins)?
4. Have you experienced intolerable side effects to any medications (e.g., unable to achieve erection with some antihypertensives or constipation and dry mouth with anticholinergics)?

V. HEALTH MAINTENANCE

A. Prevention

1. Have you received immunizations? This is primarily important in the pediatric population. Contracting mumps can lead to orchitis and potential infertility.
2. How often have you had a digital rectal examination (DRE)?
   a. Do you have annual DREs (men aged 40 to 50 years)?

b. Do you have annual DREs and prostate-specific antigen (PSA) screening test? PSA is a serum screening test for prostate cancer (men older than age 50; men older than age 40 if they have a positive first-degree family history or if of African-American descent because both of these increase the risk of prostate cancer)?

3. Have you had a PSA screening test? This test is thought to be responsible for prostate cancer presenting at an earlier stage now; data on survival benefit, however, is still pending.

B. **Diet:** What is your regular diet? How much fat does it contain? The higher fat content in the American diet is a possible contributor to the higher risk of prostate cancer when compared to Eastern Asian countries.

C. **Exercise/Recreation:** What type of exercise and recreational activities do you regularly engage in? Exercise tolerance is important in the cardiac evaluation of patients with cardiac risks who are to undergo surgery.

D. **Sleep Patterns:** Have your sleeping habits changed? Note changes because they can be related to nocturia.

E. **Social Habits**

1. Do you use tobacco? What form, how much, and for how long? Smoking is linked to increased risk of urothelial carcinoma and renal carcinoma, as well as peripheral vascular disease (PVD) and impotence.
2. Do you drink alcohol? What type, how much, and for how long? Alcohol abuse can result in autonomic and peripheral neuropathy, which may interfere with urinary function or cause impotence.
3. Do you use any illicit drugs? Marijuana is a common cause of testicular atrophy and impotence. Cocaine abuse can cause priapism or prolonged erection.

VI. FAMILY HISTORY

A. **First-Degree Relatives' Medical History**

1. Have any of your first-degree male relatives had prostate cancer? Eight to ten percent of men with prostate cancer have a familial form that develops earlier than the more common form.
2. Have any first-degree relatives had renal cell cancer? The familial tendency to develop renal cell carcinoma has been linked to a genetic anomaly on chromosome number 3; it also may be seen in association with certain syndromes.
3. Have any relatives had infertility problems? While working up infertility, it is important to determine if either partner has previously reproduced.

B. **Three-Generation Genogram:** Are there any familial genetic diseases? Many familial genetic diseases (e.g., von Hippel Lindau) and certain autosomal-dominant polycystic diseases can have renal manifestations.

VII. PSYCHOSOCIAL HISTORY

A. Personal and Social History

1. What is your country of birth? The risk of prostate cancer varies in different countries. Squamous cell carcinoma of the bladder has a much higher risk in Egypt because of exposure to schistosomiasis.
2. What is your race/ethnicity? African-American males have a higher risk of prostate cancer and tend to have a more aggressive course of the disease.

B. Current Illness Effects on the Patient

1. Do you understand your illness and all of the treatment options available (e.g., surgery versus radiation therapy or medical treatment, transplant versus dialysis)?
2. Do you have any employment concerns?
3. Will you be able to afford the recommended medications?

C. Interpersonal and Sexual History

1. Are you sexually active?
2. Do you have more than one partner? What precautions, if any, do you take against contracting an STD?
3. Have you ever had any STD? If so, it may be necessary to notify public health departments and partners.

D. Family Support

1. Does your family understand your illness?
2. Ascertain whether supplemental home care will be necessary (e.g., home health care worker to care for wounds, change bandages, and implement outpatient Foley catheter use and changes).
3. Will genetic counseling be necessary (e.g., von Hippel Lindau, tuberous sclerosis)?

E. Occupational Aspects of Illness

1. Are you able to continue working at your current job? A patient who needs frequent dialysis, for example, might not be able to hold a full-time job)?
2. Do you have any transportation concerns?

VIII. REVIEW OF SYSTEMS (Tables 34-1 to 34-3)

IX. PHYSICAL EXAMINATION (Table 34-4)

A. Penis

1. Presence of foreskin and retractability. Inability to retract foreskin entirely (i.e., phimosis), inability to put the foreskin over the glans penis (i.e., paraphimosis).
2. Location of urethral meatus.
   a. Hypospadias: Meatus on the ventral surface of the penis.
   b. Epispadias: Meatus located on the dorsal surface of the penis.

Table 34-1. GENERAL UROLOGY SYMPTOMS BY SYSTEM.

System	Symptoms
General	Fatigue, change in weight, fever/chills
Cardiovascular	Palpitations, tachycardia, chest pain, dyspnea on exertion (DOE), orthopnea, paroxysmal nocturnal dyspnea (PND)
Chest	Breast development, enlargement, pain or tenderness, nipple discharge
Gastrointestinal	Diarrhea, constipation, emesis, nausea
Obstetrics/ Gynecologic	Age of onset of menstruation, regularity, duration, and quantity of menstrual flow, prior pregnancy, change in libido, infertility, secondary sexual characteristics
Lymphatic	Lower extremity edema
Hematologic	History of deep venous thrombosis (DVT), pulmonary embolism (PE), anemia, hematologic malignancy
Neurologic	History of stroke, TIA, neurologic injury and pattern of deficits
Miscellaneous	History of reaction to anesthetics

3. Palpation for plaques/strictures.
   a. Peyronie's disease manifests as a fibrous plaque on the tunica albuginea of the corpora cavernosa, causing penile curvature with erection.
   b. Urethral stricture can sometimes be associated with fibrosis of the corpora spongiosum.
4. Discharge is often associated with urethritis.
5. Skin changes.
   a. Condyloma is thought to be caused by human papilloma virus.
   b. Balanitis xerotica obliterans (BYO) is a white patch located on the glans penis with atrophic epidermis and underlying hypocellular region on microscopic examination.
   c. Carcinoma-in-situ is seen as red on the penis.
   d. Invasive carcinoma appears as a papillary or ulcerative lesion present on the penis.

B. Testicles

1. Size.
   a. Normal range.
   b. Atrophy can occur after mumps orchitis, surgery, or torsion.
   c. Enlargement can occur with testicular mass or inflammation.

Table 34-2. NONSPECIFIC SYMPTOMS AND THEIR UROLOGIC DISEASES.

Symptoms	Diseases
Flank pain	Common symptom of urolithiasis; may be present with renal cell carcinoma
Hematuria	Can be secondary to infection, urolithiasis, or malignancy anywhere along the urinary tract
Incontinence of urine	Can be caused by both anatomic or neurologic abnormalities
Irritative urinary symptoms (nocturia, frequency, dysuria, hesitancy)	Often associated with infection, inflammation, or cancer
Obstructive urinary symptoms (hesitancy, decreased force/caliber of stream, incomplete voiding, terminal dribbling, interrupted stream)	Associated with obstruction of the lower urinary tract: prostate, urethra
Pneumaturia	Secondary to enterovesical fistula; may be caused by carcinoma, diverticulitis, and inflammatory bowel disease
Suprapubic pain	Bladder infection, interstitial cystitis, urinary retention
Premature ejaculation	Typically psychogenic in origin; important to differentiate from impotence
Testicular pain	Testicular torsion, torsion of testicular appendages, trauma, epididymitis
Urethral discharge	Often associated with sexually transmitted disease, can be related to urethral carcinoma

   d. Absence can be caused by failure of the testicle to descend into the scrotum (cryptorchidism).

2. Masses.
   a. Solid masses are regarded as malignant tumors until proved otherwise.
   b. Hydrocele is a fluid collection next to the testicle proper, which will transilluminate.

Table 34-3. COMMON UROLOGIC DISEASES AND THEIR SYMPTOMS.

Disease	Symptoms
Benign prostatic hypertrophy	Frequency, hesitancy, dysuria, nocturia, retention
Bladder cancer (most commonly transitional cell carcinoma)	Hematuria, lower extremity edema with lymphatic metastases, frequency, urgency
Cystitis	Dysuria, frequency, nocturia, hematuria
Epididymitis	Testicular pain, swelling, scrotal erythema, dysuria, urethral discharge
Erectile dysfunction	Inability to achieve or maintain an erection
Hydrocele	Scrotal mass, pain, difficulty with ambulation
Incontinence	Loss of urine secondary to increases in abdominal pressure, inability to suppress urgency, or constant leakage of urine
Prostate cancer	Often asymptomatic until metastatic. Metastatic disease can present with bone pain or lower extremity neurologic changes
Renal cell carcinoma	Flank pain, hematuria, abdominal mass
Spermatocele	Pain, scrotal mass
Testicular cancer	Testicular mass (often painless)
Testicular torsion	Acute testicular pain, swelling, scrotal erythema
Urolithiasis	Flank pain, scrotal pain, hematuria, dysuria
Varicocele	Pain, scrotal mass (often described as a "bag of worms"), infertility

3. Tenderness.
- **a.** Epididymitis/orchitis is caused by bacterial or viral (e.g., mumps) infection.
- **b.** Torsion is a twisting of the testicle on the spermatic cord that impairs blood flow. This is a true urologic emergency requiring surgical intervention within 4 hours.
- **c.** Trauma may be associated with a hematocele.

4. Spermatic cord.
- **a.** Spermatocele is a painless cystic mass above and posterior to testis.

Table 34-4. FINDINGS OF UROLOGIC PHYSICAL EXAMINATION AND POSSIBLE DIAGNOSES.

System	Physical Examination Finding	Possible Diagnoses
Vital signs		
Pulse	Tachycardia	Trauma, infection, pulmonary embolus
Blood pressure	Hypertension	Aldosteronoma, pheochromocytoma, Cushing's disease/syndrome, idiopathic
	Hypotension	Volume loss with trauma, sepsis, myocardial infarction, antihypertensive medications
Respiratory rate	Tachypnea	Pulmonary embolus, pneumonia
Weight	Cachexia	Malignancy
	Obesity	Cushing's disease/syndrome
Height	Tall eunichoid stature	Klinefelter's syndrome
	Short stature female	Turner's syndrome
Neck	Adenopathy	Solid tumor malignancy, infection, lymphoma
Abdomen	Masses	Malignancy
	Lower abdominal pain	Urinary retention, cystitis (e.g., infectious)
	Scars	Previous surgery
Flank	Pain	Carcinoma (e.g., kidney), pyelonephritis, urolithiasis
Genitourinary		
Male	Testicular mass	Torsion, tumor
	Discharge	Urethritis (e.g., STD, Reiter's syndrome)
	Testicular pain	Testicular/appendage torsion, epididymitis, trauma
	Scrotal mass	Hydrocoele, varicocoele, spermatocele

Table 34-4—cont'd

System	Physical Examination Finding	Possible Diagnoses
	Testicular absence	Cryptorchidism, prior surgical removal
	Testicular atrophy	Aging, previous torsion, previous surgery, previous mumps orchitis
	Penile plaque	Peyronie's disease
	Phimosis	Penile carcinoma, balanitis, idiopathic
Female	Anterior vaginal mass	Cystocele
	Posterior vaginal mass	Rectocele, enterocele
Rectal	Prostate nodule	BPH, prostate cancer
	Prostatic enlargement	BPH, prostate cancer
Skin	Genital vesicular lesions	Herpes simplex virus (HSV)
	Genital papillary masses	Condyloma, Kaposi's sarcoma, squamous cell carcinoma
	Genital ulcerations	Squamous cell carcinoma, candidiasis, chancroid, syphilis
Lymphatics	Inguinal lymphadenopathy	Metastatic tumor, GU infection, penile cancer
Extremities	Edema	DVT, renal cell carcinoma invading the inferior vena cava, cardiovascular disease, poor nutritional status, renal failure
	Decreased peripheral pulses	Hypotension, peripheral vascular disease
Neurologic	Incontinence	Idiopathic, multiple sclerosis, spinal cord injury
	Abnormal visual fields (with erectile dysfunction)	Prolactinoma

b. Varicocele is the dilatation of the pampiniform plexis above the testis, often described as a "bag of worms." Most common on the left side and can affect fertility and cause pain.

C. **Prostate: Digital Rectal Exam (DRE)**

1. Size: Often enlarged in older men and associated with benign prostatic hyperplasia or hypertrophy (BPH).
2. Symmetry: Asymmetry can be associated with BPH or prostate cancer.
3. Nodules: Often associated with prostate cancer.
4. Consistency: Prostate should be uniform; indurated areas are suspicious for prostate cancer.
5. Invasion into other structures: Prostate cancer concern.
6. Seminal vesicles are normally difficult to palpate, but sometimes can be palpated with invasion from prostate cancer.
7. Abnormalities of the prostate on DRE should be referred to a urologist for biopsy.

X. DIFFERENTIAL DIAGNOSIS (Table 34-5)

XI. LABORATORY STUDIES AND DIAGNOSTIC EVALUATIONS

A. Blood and Serum Labs

1. Prostate-specific antigen (PSA).
   a. Glycoprotein secreted by prostate cells normally functions in liquefaction of semen.
   b. Serum values may be elevated (>4 ng/mL) with BPH or prostate cancer.
   c. Should be checked yearly in males older than age 50 and males older than age 40 with a family history of prostate cancer.

Table 34-5. UROLOGIC DIFFERENTIAL DIAGNOSIS BY SYSTEM.

SYSTEM	POSSIBLE DIAGNOSES
Bladder	Cystitis, malignancy, urolithiasis
Kidney	Renal tumor, renal cystic disease, urolithiasis, pyelonephritis
Penis	Phimosis, paraphimosis, Peyronie's disease, priapism, hypospadias, carcinoma
Prostate	Carcinoma, benign prostatic hyperplasia (BPH), acute/chronic prostatitis
Scrotum/Testicles	Malignancy, torsion, hydrocele, varicocele
Ureter	Malignancy, urolithiasis
Urethra	Urethritis, malignancy, incontinence

d. Elevated PSA should be referred to a urologist for prostate biopsy.
2. Serum studies.
a. Blood urea nitrogen (BUN) and serum creatinine are helpful in assessing renal function.
b. Serum electrolytes may be abnormal with multiple medical diseases, including kidney disorders, adrenal disorders, and endocrine disorders.
3. Complete blood count (CBC).
a. Anemia may be present with renal failure.
b. Erythrocytosis can be associated with renal cell cancer.
4. Hormone studies.
a. Testosterone may be decreased in infertile and impotent patients; should be checked in the impotent patient with decreased libido.
b. Leutinizing hormone (LH) and follicle-stimulating hormone (FSH) abnormalities indicate a pituitary abnormality in the sex steroid axis.

B. Urine studies

1. Urine dipstick examination.
a. Color: An abnormal color may be caused by medications, diet, hematuria, or myoglobinuria.
b. Specific gravity: Normal range = 1.003-1.030; this is an assessment of the concentration of urine.
c. pH: Average range = 5.5-6.5. High pH is seen with urea-splitting bacterial infection; low pH is associated with uric acid stone formation, metabolic acidosis, or renal tubular acidosis.
d. Protein: Primarily albumin. Elevation indicates renal disease such as glomerulonephropathy.
e. Glucose: Positive glucose tests indicate spillage of glucose into the urine that overwhelms tubular reabsorption; this is seen with poorly controlled diabetes.
f. Hemoglobin: Positive hemoglobin indicates hematuria or myoglobinuria; microscopic examination for red blood cells is necessary for differentiation.
g. Nitrites: Positive for coagulase-splitting bacteria; suggestive for >100,000 organisms per mL.
h. Leukoesterase is produced by granulocytic leukocytes and indicates pyuria.
i. Ketones are produced in the serum during breakdown of body fat with insufficient carbohydrate stores. Dipstick tests identify only acetoacetic acid and not acetone or beta-hydroxybutryic acid.
j. Bilirubin: Conjugated bilirubin appears in the urine when the liver is unable to convert it to urobilinogen with intrinsic liver disease or bile duct obstruction. Elevated

urobilinogen can be seen with hemolysis or hepatocellular disease.

2. Urine microscopic examination.
   a. Bacteria indicates infection or colonization of the urinary tract.
   b. Leukocytes, white blood cells (WBCs), in the urine show the presence of inflammation, which may be caused by infection or urolithiasis.
   c. Red blood cells (RBCs): More than 3 RBCs per high-power field in the urine is abnormal. In the absence of trauma or infection, the patient should be referred to a urologist for evaluation to rule out malignancy.
   d. Epithelial cells (epis): High numbers of epis indicate contamination of the specimen from the vagina in females or the distal urethra in males. Abnormal epis may indicate a malignant process.
   e. Casts, formed in the distal tubules, can be made of white cells, red cells, epithelial cells, or protein.
   f. Crystals may help in the diagnosis of urolithiasis by differentiating types of urinary tract stones.
   g. Other organisms: Yeast or trichomonads indicate infection with these organisms.
3. Urine culture.
   a. Urinary tract infections generally grow >100,000 bacteria per mL but may be symptomatic and clinically significant with fewer organism.
   b. Culture can identify particular organisms and antibiotic sensitivities.
   c. Multiple organisms can indicate contamination of the urine specimen.
4. Urine electrolytes.
   a. Abnormalities can indicate renal or endocrine medical disease.
   b. Abnormalities of some electrolytes (such as calcium) can predispose the patient to stone formation.

C. Radiographic Studies

1. Kidneys-urethra-bladder (KUB).
   a. Identifies calcifications in the urinary tract that could have multiple causes, including urolithiasis, nephrocalcinosis, cancer, or cystic disease of the kidney.
   b. May show renal outlines.
   c. Loss of psoas shadow indicates overlying inflammation.
   d. Bowel gas pattern can be assessed.
   e. Allows identification of bony abnormalities, including spinal dysraphism.
2. Intravenous pyelogram (IVP): A series of films that are taken before and after administration of intravenous contrast.

a. Provides better definition of renal outlines: Position, size, and shape of kidneys can be assessed.
b. Defines the collecting system as the contrast is excreted to show obstruction, structural abnormalities, and filling defects.
c. Provides an assessment of how well the bladder empties (after patient voids contrast).

3. Retrograde urethrogram: A contrast instilled through the urethra toward the bladder).
   a. Useful in trauma to evaluate urethral disruption.
   b. Can also define location and size of urethral strictures.
4. Voiding cystourethrogram: Plain films taken as patient voids after instillation of contrast into the patients' bladder.
   a. Can demonstrate degree of reflux into the ureters.
   b. May show bladder abnormalities such as diverticula or ureterocoeles.
5. Ultrasound (US).
   a. Used to assess most portions of the urinary tract.
   b. Can demonstrate renal cysts or hydronephrosis.
   c. Transrectal ultrasound can evaluate the prostate and help guide biopsies.
   d. Testicular ultrasound can help define masses and cysts, as well as provide assessment of testicular blood flow. This is a mandatory study in the evaluation of testicular torsion.
6. Computed tomography (CT).
   a. Improves tissue contrast resolution over plain radiographs.
   b. Nonenhanced CT can be used to demonstrate ureteral calculi and associated obstruction.
   c. Can define renal masses, hematomas, and renal cysts.
   d. Can identify lymphadenopathy in the evaluation of urologic malignancies.
7. Nuclear medicine studies.
   a. Renal scan provides estimation of renal function.
   b. Renal scan may also demonstrate obstruction of collecting system.
   c. Bone scans can show evidence of metastatic disease.
   d. Testicular scans can demonstrate decreased testicular blood flow with testicular torsion or increased flow with inflammation.

XII. EPONYMS, ACRONYMS, AND ABBREVIATIONS (Table 34-6)

XIII. DEFINITIONS (Table 34-7)

XIV. SAMPLE H&P WRITE-UP

CC: "I've been urinating blood for the past week."

HPI: J.R. is a 45-year-old African-American male who has complained of gross hematuria over the past 7 days. He has never had similar symptoms previously. He denies any pain related to his bleeding. He denies any recent trauma. He is voiding without difficulty and

Table 34-6. UROLOGY EPONYMS, ACRONYMS, AND ABBREVIATIONS.

Acronym or Abbreviation	Term	Acronym or Abbreviation	Term
BPH	Benign prostatic hyperplasia, benign prostatic hypertrophy	**PSA**	Prostate-specific antigen
BXO	Balanitis xerotica obliterans	**PVS**	Pubovaginal sling
CAH	Congenital adrenal hyperplasia	**RCCa**	Renal cell carcinoma
CaP	Carcinoma of the prostate	**RPLND**	Retropubic lymph node dissection
CVAT	Costovertebral angle tenderness	**RPP**	Radical perineal prostatectomy
DI	Detrusor instability	**RRP**	Radical retropubic prostatectomy
DRE	Digital rectal examination	**SCCa**	Squamous cell carcinoma
ED	Erectile dysfunction	**SP tube**	Suprapubic tube
ESWL	Extracorporeal shock wave lithotripsy	**STD**	Sexually transmitted disease
GU	Genitourinary	**TCCa**	Transitional cell carcinoma
HIV	Human immunodeficiency virus	**TRUS**	Transrectal ultrasound
HSV	Herpes simplex virus	**TUIP**	Transurethral incision of the prostate
IC	Interstitial cystitis	**TURP**	Transurethral resection of the prostate
IVP	Intravenous pyelogram	**UA**	Urinalysis
LUTS	Lower urinary tract symptoms	**US**	Ultrasound
MPLND	Modified pelvic lymph node dissection	**UTI**	Urinary tract infection
NGB	Neurogenic bladder	**VCUG**	Voiding cystourethrogram
NS	Nerve sparing	**VHL**	Von Hippel Lindau syndrome
NSGCT	Nonseminomatous germ cell tumor	**VUR**	Vesicoureteral reflux
PCKD	Polycystic kidney disease	**VV**	Vasovasostomy

Table 34-7. UROLOGY TERMS.

Term	Definition
Balanitis xerotica obliterans	White patch located on the glans penis with atrophic epidermis and underlying hypocellular region on microscopic examination
Cystitis	Inflammation of the urinary bladder
Dysuria	Burning or painful urination
Epispadias	Urethral meatus located on the dorsal surface of the penis
Frequency	Voiding more times than normal during waking hours; significant frequency is voiding at least every 2 hours
Hesitancy	Difficulty initiating stream
Hydrocele	A fluid collection next to testicle proper, which will transilluminate
Hypospadias	Urethral meatus located on ventral surface of the penis
Orchitis	Inflammation of the testicle
Paraphimosis	Inability to put the foreskin over the glans penis
Peyronie's disease	Fibrous plaque on the tunica albuginea of the corpora cavernosa, causing penile curvature with erection
Phimosis	Inability to retract foreskin entirely
Pneumaturia	Air in the urine
Priapism	Prolonged painful erection; treatment needed to prevent later impotence
Spermatocele	Painless cystic mass above and posterior to testis
Urgency	Need to urinate immediately to avoid incontinence
Urolithiasis	Stone disease of the urinary tract
Varicocele	Dilatation of the pampiniform plexis above testis, often described as a "bag of worms"

not passing any clots. He has never had any kidney stones and denies any current fevers. He has no history of any hematologic disorders (including sickle cell disease/trait).

PMHx: Hypertension for 10 years. Beta-blocker treatment for 4 years.

PSHx: Vasectomy at age 30, uncomplicated.

Childhood History: Unremarkable.

Occupational History: Patient denies ever working in the dye or rubber industry. He currently works as a bank clerk.

Travel History: Patient denies any foreign travel. He has lived his entire life in the United States.

Medications: Patient is on a beta-blocker for his hypertension.

Health Maintenance: He receives an annual prostate cancer screening with a DRE and PSA secondary to his ethnic status and increased risk of prostate cancer. All DREs and PSAs reported by patients as normal.

Family History: The patient's father has Von Hippel Lindau syndrome and has been diagnosed previously with renal cell carcinoma.

Psychosocial History: He denies any history of STDs. He currently smokes 1 ppd of cigarettes and has been doing so for 20 years. He reports rare alcohol use and denies any drug use.

REVIEW OF SYSTEMS

General: Unplanned five-pound weight loss over the past 3 months. Denies fatigue.

HEENT/Neck: No visual changes.

Respiratory: No cough, dyspnea, or shortness of breath.

Cardiovascular: No tachycardia, palpitations, orthopnea, or paroxysmal nocturnal dyspnea. Denies chest pain.

Gastrointestinal: No nausea, vomiting. No constipation, diarrhea. No GI bleeding.

Genitourinary: As per HPI.

Hematologic/Lymphatic: No easy bruising. No history of any bleeding diathesis.

Endocrine: No history of diabetes.

Skin: No rash.

Neurologic: No history of seizures. No weakness.

Musculoskeletal: Denies any bone pain. No complaints of back pain.

Extremities: Complains of mild bilateral lower extremity swelling. No history of DVT.

PHYSICAL EXAMINATION

Vitals: T 99°F P 70 BP 145/60 RR 18 Weight 180 lbs.

HEENT: Normocephalic, atraumatic. Oropharynx clear. No adenopathy.

Neck: Thyroid within normal limits without masses.

Lungs: Clear to auscultation bilaterally without wheezes, rales, rhonchi.

Cardiovascular: Normal S1 and S2. Regular rate and rhythm.

Abdomen: Soft, nontender, nondistended with normal bowel sounds. No palpable masses. No inguinal hernia bilaterally. No costovertebral angle (CVA) tenderness.

Genitourinary: Normal circumcised phallus without lesion. Testes descended bilaterally, both of normal size, shape, consistency. No varicocele, hydrocele, spermatocele present. No testicular masses.

Rectal: Normal sphincter tone. Prostate minimally enlarged with normal consistency. No rectal masses. No prostatic fluctuance. Stool negative for hemoglobin.

Skin: Unremarkable.

Extremities: No clubbing, cyanosis present. 2+ pitting edema noted of both lower extremities up to the knees.

Neurologic: Normal gait. Alert, oriented ×3. Deep tendon reflexes are equal and symmetric. Normal strength in all four extremities.

III

FOCUSED HISTORY AND PHYSICAL EXAMINATION

35

ALCOHOL SCREENING

T.M. Worner, MD, and Eric H. Hanson, MD, MPH

I. CHIEF COMPLAINT

A. Chief Complaint

1. Use patient's own words for the chief complaint or reason for admission.
2. Onset of symptoms and duration, alleviating or exacerbating factors.

B. Identifying Data: Obtain name, age, date of birth, gender, place of birth, race/ethnicity of patient, educational level, marital status, number of dependents, other names used by the patient, source/reliability of information, and admission date/time/site.

II. HISTORY OF PRESENT ILLNESS

A. Opening Questions

1. Do you drink alcohol (beer, wine, distilled liquor)?
2. If yes, consider the CAGE questionnaire as a standard approach (Table 35-1).
3. If no, "Most people do drink alcohol, is there any reason why you don't drink?"

B. Drinking History

1. How old were you when you had your first drink? What did you drink and how much?
2. At what age did you first get drunk? What were you drinking and how much?
3. What is the longest period of sobriety you've had (when alcohol was available). Why were you abstaining?
4. At what age did you begin drinking regularly? What did you drink and how much?
5. Self-perception: Do you feel you are a "normal" drinker?
6. Others' perceptions: Do friends and relatives feel you are a "normal" drinker?

C. Frequency of Drinking

1. When was your last drink? What was it and how much did you drink?
2. What factors cause you to start and to stop drinking?
3. Have you ever cut down on your drinking? (Be aware that reduction or cessation of alcohol is often the result of injury, intercurrent illness, or alcohol-related diseases.)
4. Do you go on drinking "binges" (episodic drinking)?
5. Do you spend excessive amounts of time thinking about alcohol or planning drinking episodes?
6. Do you drink only at night or at a definite time daily?

Table 35-1. CAGE QUESTIONNAIRE.*

Questions	Scoring	Sensitivity	Specificity	Probability
Have you ever felt you ought to **Cut** down on your drinking?	**One Positive**	0.85	0.89	62% positive predictive value patient has alcohol disorder
Have people **Annoyed** you by criticizing your drinking?	**Two Positive**	0.75	0.96	82% positive predictive value patient has alcohol disorder
Have you ever felt bad or **Guilty** about your drinking?	**Three Positive**	0.51	0.997	99% positive predictive value patient has alcohol disorder
Have you ever had a drink first thing in the morning to steady your nerves or get rid of a hangover (**Eye opener**)?	**Four Positive**	0.20	1.00	100% positive predictive value patient has alcohol disorder

*Based on 31% prevalence of alcoholism in inpatient general medicine, orthopedics, and surgery patients. Adapted from Mayfield et al. The CAGE questionnaire: Validation of a new alcoholism screening instrument. Am J Psychiatry 131(10):1121-1123, 1974; and Bush et al. Screening for alcohol abuse using the CAGE questionnaire. Am J Medicine, 1987;82:231-235.

D. **Type of Alcohol**
1. What do you drink (e.g., beer, wine, alcohol ["hard liquor"])?
2. What is your drink of preference?
3. Do you drink nonbeverage alcohol (e.g., cologne, mouthwash)?

E. **Quantity**
1. How much do you drink (size of your glass or suggest an amount)?
2. How much do you need to drink to get drunk?
3. What is the most you drank in one sitting?
4. How much do you spend on alcohol per week/month (may help quantify)?
5. Does it take more alcohol now to make you drunk (i.e., tolerance)?

F. **Patterns**
1. Do you drink alone?
2. Do you sneak or hide drinks?

G. **Lifestyle and Psychological Effects: Relationships**
1. Has your drinking caused marital or relationship difficulties? Is drinking making your home life unhappy?
2. Does your spouse or significant other drink? What is your spouse's or family member's attitude toward drinking?
3. Has anyone suggested that you decrease your drinking (e.g., family members or a doctor)?
4. Do any of your friends or family members ever worry or complain about your drinking?
5. Is there a history of drinking problems in your family?
6. Does drinking make you careless of your family's welfare?

H. **Lifestyle and Psychological Effects: Legal**
1. Have you driven while intoxicated?
2. Have you had any auto accidents related to your drinking?
3. Has your drinking resulted in spouse or family physical abuse? Fights?
4. Have you had financial problems as a result of drinking?

I. **Lifestyle and Psychological Effects: Occupational**
1. Have you ever gotten into trouble at work because of your drinking?
2. Have you been disciplined at work?
3. Do you avoid supervisors at work?
4. Have you been late to work (or absent) as a result of drinking, especially on Mondays?
5. Has your ambition or income level decreased since you began drinking?

J. **Lifestyle and Psychological Effects: Medical**
1. Have you ever been treated by a physician as a result of drinking?
2. Have you ever been to a hospital as a result of drinking?
3. Have you used alcohol against medical advice?

4. Have you ever taken Antabuse, Lithium, Carbamezepine, Acamprosate, Naltrexone (ReVia®), Ondansetron (Zofran®), Sertraline (Zoloft®) or Buspirone?
5. While drinking, have you ever had loss of control, inappropriate outbursts, problems remembering events, or personality changes?
6. Have you ever experienced any of the following symptoms: Hand tremors, severe shakes, loss of appetite, upset stomach, nausea/vomiting, rapid/irregular heartbeat, weakness, irritability, restlessness, sweats, nightmares, seizures/fits/convulsions, seeing/hearing things that were not there? (All of these symptoms may result from alcohol withdrawal.)

K. Signs and Symptoms of Alcohol Abuse and/or Withdrawal

1. Early effects: Agitation, anxiety, restlessness, tremor, anorexia, diaphoresis, and insomnia. Usually 0 to 48 hours post-ethanol or following significant reduction in alcohol consumption; peak of symptoms 24 to 36 hours and risk of seizures usually 6 to 48 hours.
2. Late or major effects: Extreme overactivity (speech, psychomotor, autonomic), confusion, and disorientation. Usually 24 to 150 hours post-ethanol; peak of symptoms 72 to 96 hours and is potentially life threatening.
3. Describe quality/character, quantity/intensity, setting/precipitating factors, alleviating/aggravating factors, course/progression/variations.

L. Associated Signs of Alcohol Abuse and/or Alcohol Withdrawal

1. Defense mechanisms: Denial, repression, rationalization, minimizing, direction-inappropriate anger, memory distortions (e.g., denial, alcoholic blackout, out of touch with reality and severity of disease).
2. Describe quality/character, quantity/intensity, setting/precipitating factors, alleviating/aggravating factors, course/progression/variations.

M. Treatment

1. Outpatient or inpatient treatment.
2. Hospitalization and treatment of acute episodes.
3. Alcoholics Anonymous (AA) or Al-Anon program.
4. Alternative therapies (e.g., herbs, acupuncture).
5. Treatment for other drug abuse and withdrawal (prescription and "illicit").

III. PAST MEDICAL AND SURGICAL HISTORY

For each medical or surgical illness, obtain the following information.

A. Past Medical History (Adult Illnesses)

1. Diagnosis.
2. Date of onset and progression.
3. Responses to interventions.
4. Complications or sequelae.

5. Hospitalizations.
6. Physicians.
7. Medications.
8. Assess severity of concurrent illnesses.

B. Past Surgical History

1. Diagnosis.
2. Procedures.
3. Responses to interventions.
4. Operative and postoperative complications or sequelae.
5. Hospitals and clinics; ambulatory or inpatient.
6. Date of procedures.
7. Anesthesia (types, adverse reactions, and complications).

C. Emergency History

1. Have you ever been injured or broken any bones as a result of drinking?
2. Have you ever been hospitalized or admitted to any other institution as a result of drinking, other than for alcohol treatment (e.g., treatment for injuries resulting from an alcohol-related car accident, injuries sustained fighting while intoxicated)?

D. Childhood History

1. Where did you grow up? Describe childhood, family background, and religious background.
2. Did you have any unusual childhood illnesses? If so, how severe were they?

E. Occupational History

1. What is your occupation? What jobs have you held?
2. Are you exposed to chemicals, hazardous materials, or noise at your workplace?
3. Is patient unemployed or underemployed?

F. Travel History

IV. MEDICATIONS, ALLERGIES, AND ADVERSE REACTIONS

A. Medications: Metabolism of many drugs is affected by chronic and heavy alcohol consumption. Doses of these medications may need to be altered following cessation of alcohol in order to prevent adverse effects.

1. What prescription medications are you taking? Note indications, last doses, duration of use, and possible drug interactions. Annotate date started and regimen changes. A medications list at the bottom of the HPI or within the medical history section is helpful.
2. See Section II, J, 4.3. What over-the-counter (OTC) medications are you taking?
3. Herbal preparations or alternative medicine therapies?

B. Allergic Reactions and Adverse Reactions

1. Any problems with nonsteroid anti-inflammatory drugs (NSAIDS) (e.g., stomach upset, gastrointestinal bleeding, kidney problems)?

2. Any reactions to certain antibiotics (e.g., swelling, airway constriction, development of rash)?

V. HEALTH MAINTENANCE

A. Prevention

1. Have you ever attended an alcohol/drug awareness program (e.g., health education in high school, college courses)?
2. Have you received all appropriate vaccines/boosters?
3. When was your last blood pressure check? Cholesterol/blood sugar screening? What did they show?
4. When was your last physical examination? What did it show?
5. Have you ever been tested for human immunodeficiency virus (HIV)?

B. Diet

1. What is your typical diet?
2. What have you eaten in the last 24 hours?
3. Do you have any dietary restrictions?
4. Do you consume caffeine-containing beverages and foods?
5. Do you drink alcohol in the morning?
6. What is your daily caloric intake from alcohol?

C. Exercise/Recreation

1. Do you exercise? What types of exercise (e.g., aerobic)?
2. How often do you exercise?
3. For what period of time?
4. At what intensity (how measured)?

D. Sleep Patterns

1. How many hours of sleep do you get each night? Usual pattern?
2. Do you nap regularly? Patterns?
3. Do you have difficulty falling asleep or insomnia?
4. Do you take any products to help you fall asleep?
5. Do you use alcohol to induce sleep?
6. Do you awake during the night? Why (e.g., pain, micturition)?
7. Do you have nightmares?

E. Social Habits

1. Alcohol (see HPI).
2. Do you use tobacco? What type? How much? For how long?
3. See Section V, B, 4. Do you take diet pills?
4. Do you use illicit or recreational drugs? Which ones? Any adverse reactions from use?

VI. FAMILY HISTORY

A. Family Members' History

1. Does spouse or significant other drink alcohol or use drugs? Create a three-generation family tree, including especially those members who use alcohol. Please note that other medical con-

ditions, such as unspecified liver disease or bipolar disorder, may also indicate alcoholism.

2. Assess family enabling (i.e., family system revolves around the sick member, protecting and allowing the person to continue the destructive pattern).
3. Have any family members participated in alcohol-related studies?

VII. PSYCHOSOCIAL HISTORY

A. Personal and Social History

1. Where do you currently reside?
   - **a.** What is the physical layout of the home and living conditions (e.g., 3 bedroom, 1 bath, 8 occupants)?
   - **b.** Have alcohol and drugs been removed from the home?
   - **c.** What is patient's socioeconomic status?
2. What social involvement do you have on a regular basis? Describe a typical day.

B. Current Illness Effects on the Patient

1. Address the patient's perception of the severity of the illness (e.g., Do you perceive a problem? Have you considered the long-term effects of alcohol abuse? Have you considered making changes to avoid or ameliorate future problems?).
2. Address death and dying issues, as applicable (e.g., Have you thought about dying? If you are unable to care for yourself, have you made arrangements for somebody to care for you? Have you considered hospice care?).
3. Are advanced directives in place (e.g., Have you considered a power of attorney if you are unable to make decisions for yourself? Who would you consider? Do you have a will? How aggressive do you want or expect medical care to be if you are incapacitated and possibly may not recover? Do you want your life extended by machines? Do you want aggressive resuscitation in the event of cardiopulmonary arrest?)?

C. Interpersonal and Sexual History

1. Does this disorder interfere with any part of your personal or sexual life? Use discreet questioning only when applicable.
2. Evaluate adverse medication effects as a source of sexual dysfunction.
3. Evaluate alcohol and illicit drugs as a source of sexual dysfunction.

D. Family Support

1. What sources of support does the patient have?
2. Is the family informed about this illness?
3. Is the family involved in Al-Anon or Al-a-Teen?
4. Proximity of family and important phone numbers (helpful when information is needed or if information must be relayed to family).

E. Occupational Aspects of the Illness

1. What stressors or problems do you have with your job or other workers? Do you drink or use drugs with co-workers? At work or elsewhere?
2. Does the patient need occupational therapy or physical therapy?

VIII. REVIEW OF SYSTEMS (Tables 35-2, 35-3, 35-4)

Table 35-2. GENERAL ALCOHOL-RELATED DISEASE SYMPTOMS AND SIGNS BY SYSTEM.

System	Symptoms/Signs
General	Fatigue, change in weight, insomnia, trauma (review each system for alcohol-related incidents)
Systemic	Hypertension, hyperlipidemia, cancer, gout, diabetes mellitus (current or past history)
HEENT	Swelling (parotid gland), epistaxis, change in vision (double vision, floaters, night vision impairment), change in voice, dental hygiene, oral lesions (e.g., erythroplakia, leukoplakia)
Cardiovascular	Palpitations, tachycardia, chest pain, dyspnea on exertion (DOE), orthopnea, paroxysmal nocturnal dyspnea (PND)
Chest	Breast development, enlargement, pain or tenderness, nipple discharge, date and result of last mammogram, rib fractures (past or current)
Respiratory	Fever, shortness of breath, chest pain, recurrent pneumonia, tuberculosis, isoniazid (INH) treatment for positive PPD
Gastrointestinal	Diarrhea, steatorrhea, constipation, emesis, nausea, hematemesis, hematochezia, dysphagia, heartburn, jaundice, anorexia, appetite changes, abdominal pain, peptic ulcer disease, Mallory-Weiss tear, variceal disorder, pancreatitis, hepatitis (biopsy done?), cirrhosis (biopsy diagnosis), other liver disease (specify)
Genitourinary	Polyuria, libido (sexual appetite)/loss of libido, erectile/ejaculatory dysfunction in men, morning erections, infertility
Hematopoietic	Bleeding disorders, bruising tendencies, anemia (especially macrocytic)
Lymphatic	Lymphadenopathy (swelling or lumps in neck, armpits, groin)

Table 35-2—cont'd

System	Symptoms/Signs
Obstetrics/ Gynecologic	Age of onset of menstruation, regularity, duration, and quantity of menstrual flow, obstetric history (prior pregnancy, abortions, miscarriages, including complications), libido (sexual appetite)/change in libido, infertility, secondary sexual characteristics, date and results of last Pap smear
Musculoskeletal	Proximal muscle weakness (difficulty climbing stairs), muscle tenderness, joint pain, gout, fractures, deformities, osteoporosis (male)
Neuro-psychiatric	Peripheral neuropathy, paresthesias, tremor (familial), anxiety, depression, suicidal or homicidal ideations, delirium, hallucinations, psychiatric or mood disorder, seizures (rule out withdrawal)
Skin	Striae, easy bruising, change in distribution of hair growth (men), bleeding tendencies, rashes, color change (jaundice or pallor), Casal's necklace (advanced pellagra)
Extremities	Tremor, paresthesia, ulcers, swelling (edema)
Laboratory history (abnormal)	Macrocytosis, elevated liver function tests (LFTs), especially SGOT, unexplained isolated GGTP elevation, elevated uric acid, blood alcohol ever >300 mg/dL, blood alcohol >150 mg/dL in absence of the appearance of intoxication, odor of alcohol on breath at time of physical examination

Table 35-3. NON-SPECIFIC SYMPTOMS AND SIGNS AND ALCOHOL-RELATED DISEASES.

Symptom/Sign	Possible Diseases
Abdominal pain	Pancreatitis, gastritis, peptic ulcer disease, alcoholic acidosis, hepatitis (alcoholic or viral), portal hypertension (splenomegaly), Budd-Chiari syndrome (occlusion of the hepatic vein), Zieve's syndrome (hemolytic anemia and hyperlipidemia complicate alcohol related liver disease), peritonitis, carcinoma (metastatic or primary)

Continued

Table 35-3. NON-SPECIFIC SYMPTOMS AND SIGNS AND ALCOHOL-RELATED DISEASES—*cont'd*

Symptom/Sign	Possible Diseases
Amenorrhea or oligomenorrhea	Anorexia nervosa, liver disease, direct effect alcohol
Anemia	Nutritional deficiency (especially folate), iron deficiency secondary to gastrointestinal bleeding, hemolytic with stomatocytosis, direct bone marrow toxicity
Anorexia	Acidosis, malignancy, gastritis, hepatitis, cirrhosis, sepsis, tuberculosis, depression, early alcohol withdrawal syndrome, continued alcohol consumption, medication or illicit drug use
Constipation	Colonic neoplasm, medication effect (licit/illicit)
Dementia	Wernicke-Korsakoff syndrome, direct alcohol toxicity, subdural hematoma, depression
Depression	Common in first few days following alcohol withdrawal, common during excessive alcohol intake, hepatitis (viral)
Diarrhea	Pancreatitis, malabsorption syndrome, sepsis, intestinal effect of alcohol, medication effect (licit/illicit), nutritional deficiency (e.g., pellagra)
Fever	Sepsis, severe withdrawal syndrome, alcoholic hepatitis, hyperthermia syndrome
Gynecomastia	Liver disease, medications (e.g., marijuana, aldosterone)
Hair changes	Female escutcheon in male (liver disease)
Hallucinations	Severe alcoholic withdrawal syndrome (i.e., delirium tremens), chronic alcoholic hallucinosis, underlying psychiatric disorder (e.g., schizophrenia), illicit drug abuse
Headache	Subarachnoid hemorrhage, subdural hematoma, meningitis, abscess
Hypothermia	Cold exposure, sepsis
Insomnia	Alcohol withdrawal syndrome, sleep apnea syndrome
Libido changes	Direct effect alcohol, liver disease
Nervousness or tremor	Alcohol withdrawal syndrome, withdrawal syndrome other medications (illicit), familial essential tremor, hepatic encephalopathy (cirrhosis)

Table 35-3—cont'd

Symptom/Sign	Possible Diseases
Palpitations	"Holiday heart syndrome," cardiomyopathy, beriberi, alcohol withdrawal syndrome
Polyuria	Diabetes insipidus, hypokalemia
Seizures	Alcohol withdrawal syndrome, noncompliance with anticonvulsant regimen, illicit drug abuse, central nervous system (CNS) pathology (meningitis, subdural, trauma, CVA, subarachnoid hemorrhage [SAH], tumor), pellagra
Skin changes	Dupuytren's contracture, plethora, bruising, petechiae, ecchymoses (trauma, thrombocytopenia, splenomegaly, decompensated liver disease), Caput Medusa (cirrhosis), telangiectasia, palmer erythema, spider angioma (liver disease), rosacea, flushed facies, diaphoresis, jaundice (liver disease, hemolysis), cigarette burns on hands or chest, "tracks" (IV drug abuse), pellagra (Casal's necklace)
Weakness and fatigue	Hypokalemia, hypoglycemia, alcoholic myopathy, depression
Weight gain	Ascites (liver disease, pancreatic disease, peritonitis, metastatic carcinoma), peripheral edema (malnutrition, decompensated cardiac or pulmonary disease)
Weight loss	Anorexia nervosa, liver disease, carcinoma, inadequate caloric intake, sepsis, pancreatic insufficiency, severe lung disease, cardiac disease

IX. PHYSICAL EXAMINATION (Table 35-5)

X. LABORATORY STUDIES AND DIAGNOSTIC EVALUATIONS (Table 35-6)

XI. ACRONYMS AND ABBREVIATIONS (Table 35-7)

XII. DEFINITIONS (Table 35-8)

XIII. SAMPLE H&P WRITE-UP

CC: "My boss sent me."

HPI: J.R. is a divorced 40-year-old white American male. Treatment was mandated by his employer. He has no physical complaints. He currently consumes one quart of scotch daily. He began drinking at age 16. Initially, he consumed a six-pack of beer on Saturdays and

Table 35-4. COMMON ALCOHOL-RELATED DISEASES AND THEIR SYMPTOMS AND SIGNS.

DISEASES	SYMPTOMS AND SIGNS
Cirrhosis, decompensated	Abdominal pain, abdominal mass (splenomegaly), abdominal swelling, weight loss, weight gain (ascites), jaundice, anorexia, weakness, hematemesis, gynecomastia, skin lesions (telangiectasia, spider angioma), shortness of breath (vascular ectasias of lung)
Fetal alcohol syndrome	Small cranium (microcephaly), low nasal bridge, flat midface, short palpebral fissures, indistinct philtrum, thin upper lip, small jaw (micrognathia)
Hepatitis	Abdominal pain, fever, anorexia, fatigue, jaundice, weight loss, hematemesis
"Holiday heart syndrome"	Palpitations, tachycardia, light-headedness, chest pain, shortness of breath
Pancreatitis	Abdominal pain, steatorrhea, diarrhea, weight loss, abdominal distention
Peripheral neuropathy	Glove/stocking paresthesia, numbness of hands/feet, dystrophic nail changes, difficulty walking (can't feel the ground)
Withdrawal syndrome	Anxiety, tremor, agitation, restlessness, diaphoresis, anorexia, insomnia, hallucinosis, fever, tachycardia, palpitations, seizures

Sundays. He increased his consumption to one pint of alcohol daily at age 25. He has been drinking a quart of scotch daily since age 35. He denies withdrawal symptoms, including seizures. A "friend" took him to an AA meeting a year ago. He denies other treatment for alcoholism.

PMHx: At a recent employment examination, was told of hypertension and abnormal "liver tests." He denies any known exposure to Hepatitis A, B, or C or to TB or HIV.

PSHx: None.

Emergency and Trauma History: Fell, fracturing his ribs several years ago. He denies prior hospitalizations or blood transfusions.

Childhood History: Denies childhood illnesses.

Occupational History: Completed Masters in Business Administration (MBA). Currently employed as "middle-management" in pharmaceutical company, but job is "on the line." Previously employed as

Text continued on p. 795.

Table 35-5. FINDINGS AND POSSIBLE ALCOHOL-RELATED DIAGNOSES

System	Physical Examination Findings	Possible Diagnoses
Vital signs		
Pulse	Tachycardia	Alcohol withdrawal, cardiomyopathy, "holiday heart syndrome," anemia, beriberi, acute blood loss (trauma, gastrointestinal bleeding), dehydration
	Arrhythmia	Alcohol withdrawal, cardiomyopathy, "holiday heart syndrome"
Temperature	Fever	Severe alcohol withdrawal syndrome (delirium tremens), hepatitis, sepsis, hyperthermia syndrome
Blood Pressure	Orthostatic	Blood loss (trauma, gastrointestinal bleeding), dehydration, contraction alkalosis
	Hypertension	Alcohol withdrawal, rebound clonidine withdrawal (opiate detoxification)
Weight	Gradual weight loss	Carcinoma (colon, esophageal, hepatic, breast, pulmonary), liver disease (cirrhosis hepatitis), tuberculosis, pancreatic insufficiency, cardiomyopathy, inadequate caloric intake, concomitant illicit drug use

Continued

Table 35-5. FINDINGS AND POSSIBLE ALCOHOL-RELATED DIAGNOSES—*cont'd*

System	Physical Examination Findings	Possible Diagnoses
	Gradual weight gain	Decompensated liver disease (ascites), cardiac decompensation (edema)
General appearance		
Age	Appears older than stated age	Chronic alcohol consumption
Mental status		
Orientation	Disoriented	Alcohol withdrawal syndrome, decompensated liver disease, Wernicke-Korsakoff syndrome, alcoholic dementia, alcoholic acidosis, hyponatremia, alcohol intoxication, trauma (subdural, epidural), CNS lesions (SAH, CVA), concomitant drug use (licit or illicit)
HEENT		
Head	Burr holes	Status post (S/P) subdural evacuation
	Microcephaly, low nasal bridge, flat midface, short palpebral fissures, indistinct philtrum, thin upper lip, micrognathia	Fetal Alcohol Syndrome (FAS may be present in adults; ethnicity must be considered)
	Parotid gland swelling	Alcoholism

Table 35-5—cont'd

System	Physical Examination Findings	Possible Diagnoses
Eyes	Jaundice	Liver disease (alcoholic or viral hepatitis, cirrhosis), hemolytic anemia (Zieve's syndrome)
	Pallor	Chronic gastrointestinal blood loss, inadequate iron or folate intake, sideroblastic anemia
	Nystagmus	Alcohol withdrawal, Wernicke's syndrome, cerebellar degeneration
	Gaze palsies	Wernicke's syndrome
	Retinal or conjunctival hemorrhages	Trauma, coagulopathy (liver disease), nutritional deficiency (inadequate intake), hypertension
	Lipemia retinalis	Hyperlipidemia
	Raccoon sign: Periorbital ecchymosis	Basilar skull fracture
Ears	Battle's sign: Ecchymosis over mastoid process Hemotympanum	Basilar skull fracture
Nose	Septal perforation	Cocaine insufflation
	Rhinophyma	Alcoholism
Mouth	Torus palatini	Alcoholism
	Enamel loss posteriorly	Anorexia nervosa
	Tongue tremor	Alcohol withdrawal, familial tremor
	Erythroplakia	Rule out carcinoma
	Leukoplakia	Rule out carcinoma
	Bleeding/inflamed gums	Malnutrition/vitamin deficiency; coagulopathy

Continued

Table 35-5. FINDINGS AND POSSIBLE ALCOHOL-RELATED DIAGNOSES—*cont'd*

System	Physical Examination Findings	Possible Diagnoses
Neck		
Throat	Hoarseness	Rule out laryngeal carcinoma
	Absent gag reflex	Anorexia nervosa
Lung	Rales or wheezing	Decompensated cardiomyopathy, decompensated liver disease (cirrhosis or severe hepatitis)
Chest		
Thorax	Gynecomastia (male patients)	Alcoholic liver disease, illicit drug use (e.g., marijuana), drug side effect (e.g., aldosterone)
	Breast atrophy (females)	Alcoholism
	Rib deformity (old fractures)	Past alcohol intoxication
Breasts	Mass	Rule out carcinoma
Cardiovascular		
	Tachycardia	Alcohol withdrawal, "holiday heart syndrome," cardiomyopathy, dehydration, anemia, acute blood loss (trauma, gastrointestinal bleeding), beriberi
	Arrhythmia	Alcohol withdrawal, cardiomyopathy, "holiday heart syndrome"
	Cardiomegaly	Cardiomyopathy, beriberi
	S3, S4	Cardiomyopathy

Table 35-5—cont'd

System	Physical Examination Findings	Possible Diagnoses
Abdomen	Ascites	Decompensated liver disease (cirrhosis, severe alcoholic hepatitis), Budd-Chiari, bacterial peritonitis, tuberculous ascites, cardiomyopathy, pancreatic ascites
	Hepatomegaly	Alcoholic liver disease (steatosis, hepatitis, cirrhosis), viral liver disease, Zieve's syndrome, hepatocellular carcinoma
	Splenomegaly	Portal hypertension
	Caput Medusa	Cirrhosis
	Grey-Cullen sign	Severe necrotizing pancreatitis
	Turner's Sign	Severe necrotizing pancreatitis
	Murphy's sign	Cholecystitis
	Sister Mary Joseph's sign	Metastatic gastric carcinoma
GU		
Male	Small testis	Alcoholism
Rectum	Guaiac test positive	Gastritis, esophagitis, hemorrhoids, gastrointestinal carcinoma
Skin	Tracks	Intravenous drug abuse
	Cigarette burns on fingers	Alcoholism
	Petechiae	Thrombocytopenia, splenomegaly, malnutrition (vitamin deficiency)

Continued

Table 35-5. FINDINGS AND POSSIBLE ALCOHOL-RELATED DIAGNOSES—*cont'd*

System	Physical Examination Findings	Possible Diagnoses
	Ecchymoses	Liver disease with coagulopathy, thrombocytopenia, trauma while intoxicated
	Spider angioma	Liver disease
	Jaundice	Liver disease, hemolytic anemia (Zieve's syndrome)
	Casal's necklace	Advanced pellagra
Extremities	Palmer erythema	Liver disease
	Dupuytren's contracture	Alcoholism
	Muscle atrophy	Alcoholic myopathy
	Peripheral neuropathy	Alcoholic neuropathy, Vitamin B_{12} deficiency, folate deficiency
	Peripheral edema	Decompensated liver disease, beriberi, decompensated cardiomyopathy
Neurologic	Dementia	Wernicke-Korsakoff syndrome, alcohol withdrawal syndrome, subdural hematoma, nutritional deficiency, depression
	Hallucinations	Alcohol withdrawal syndrome, Wernicke-Korsakoff syndrome, chronic alcoholic hallucinosis, underlying psychiatric disorder (e.g., schizophrenia), concomitant illicit drug use
	Gaze paralysis	Wernicke's syndrome

Table 35-5—cont'd

System	Physical Examination Findings	Possible Diagnoses
	Nystagmus	Wernicke's syndrome, cerebellar degeneration
	Tremor	Alcohol withdrawal, familial essential tremor
	Proximal muscle weakness	Alcoholic myopathy, rhabdomyolysis
	Peripheral neuropathy	Alcoholic peripheral neuropathy, vitamin deficiency (thiamin, B_{12}.)
	Decreased deep tendon reflexes (DTRs)	Alcoholic peripheral neuropathy, vitamin deficiency (thiamin, B_{12})
	Cerebellar ataxia	Cerebellar degeneration

Table 35-6. ALCOHOL-RELATED LABORATORY STUDIES AND DIAGNOSTIC EVALUATIONS.

Tests	Indicative of Alcoholism
Alcohol (blood or breath)	Blood alcohol >300 mg/dL, blood alcohol >150 mg/dL in absence of the appearance of intoxication, odor of alcohol on breath at time of physical examination are markers of alcohol dependence
Complete blood count (CBC)	Macrocytosis in absence of B_{12} or folate deficiency is marker for alcoholism Thrombocytopenia (rule out hypersplenism or alcoholism)
Chemistry profile	Elevated LFTs, especially SGOT (AST), unexplained isolated GGTP elevation, elevated uric acid
Liver biopsy	Histopathological documentation of liver disease in presence of abnormal liver chemistries
Urine toxicology	Observe urine for toxicology to exclude concomitant drug abuse

Table 35-7. ALCOHOL-RELATED ACRONYMS.

Acronym	Definition
AA	Alcoholics Anonymous: Self-help group, based on 12 steps to recovery
Al-Anon	Self-help group for spouses or for adult "significant others" of alcoholics
CAGE	Four-item screening tool, used to diagnose alcoholism (*vide supra*)
DTs	Delirium tremens
FAS	Fetal alcohol syndrome

Table 35-8. ALCOHOL SCREENING TERMS.

Term	Definition
Alcoholism	Extreme pathologic dependence on alcohol that is marked by socially unacceptable behaviors. It is a chronic illness that starts slowly and may begin at any age. Almost all organ systems are affected. Mortality caused by accidents (e.g., DWI) is as common as death caused by liver disease. Sudden cessation or significant reduction in alcohol consumption, either voluntarily or because of intercurrent illness, may result in a withdrawal syndrome (*vide infra*). There is no single treatment of the alcoholic. A variety of medications are currently in clinical trials. Outpatient treatment, Alcoholics Anonymous, acupuncture, and "physician advice" are all currently included in the treatment armamentarium. Disulfiram (Antabuse) and electroshock are rarely used today.
Alcohol dependence	DSM-IV criteria with three or more of the following: tolerance, withdrawal, large amounts over a long period, unsuccessful efforts to cut down, time spent in obtaining the substance replaces social, occupational or recreational activities, and continued use despite adverse consequences.

Table 35-8—cont'd

TERM	DEFINITION
Alcohol abuse	DSM-IV criteria with one or more of the following: failure to fulfill major obligations, use when physically hazardous, recurrent legal problems, and recurrent social or interpersonal problems.
Alcohol intoxication	DSM-IV criteria: Clinically significant maladaptive behavioral or psychological changes (e.g., inappropriate sexual or aggressive behavior, mood lability, impaired judgment, impaired social or occupational functioning) that developed during, or shortly after, alcohol ingestion. One (or more) of the following signs, developing during, or shortly after, alcohol use: slurred speech, incoordination, unsteady gait, nystagmus, impairment in attention or memory, or stupor or coma.
Alcohol poisoning	Poisoning resulting from consumption of alcohol, as ethyl, isopropyl, or methyl. Ethyl alcohol (grain alcohol) is in whiskies, brandy, gin, and other drinks. In most cases, it is lethal only if very large amounts are consumed in a short time (e.g., hazing). Isopropyl alcohol, found in cosmetics, "rubbing alcohol," and solvents, is more poisonous, and drinking 8 ounces may cause respiratory distress or heart failure. Methyl alcohol (wood alcohol), found in paint removers, antifreeze, fuels, and copying fluids, is very poisonous. It may cause nausea, vomiting, mild CNS depression, respiratory difficulties, weakness, abdominal pain, blindness, and metabolic acidosis. Death may come after drinking only 2 ounces. Treatment includes gastric aspiration, giving sodium bicarbonate and glucose intravenously, and, if necessary, blood dialysis (hemodialysis). More recently, intravenous ethanol or 4-methylpyrazole has been used therapeutically.

Continued

Table 35-8. ALCOHOL SCREENING TERMS—*cont'd*

Term	Definition
Alcohol withdrawal	Symptoms and signs that result from sudden cessation or marked reduction in alcohol consumption. The early, mild withdrawal syndrome is characterized by weakness, tachycardia, anorexia, anxiety, diaphoresis, tremor, very brisk reflexes, seizures, and seeing and hearing things that are not there (hallucinations). The most severe withdrawal syndrome is known as delirium tremens (DTs) (*vide infra*). Caution must be used in medicating the patient because drug metabolism may vary, depending on the clinical state (i.e., drinking or abstinence).
Caput Medusa	From caput (head) Medusa (a mythological character whose scalp consisted of a mass of serpents): Term used to describe the pattern of varicose veins radiating from the umbilicus in persons with cirrhosis of the liver and portal hypertension.
Delirium tremens (DTs)	Serious and sometimes fatal psychotic reaction to the sudden withdrawal or marked reduction in alcohol intake. It may follow an alcoholic binge during which no food was eaten. It can also be triggered by a head injury, infection, or withdrawal of alcohol after extended drinking. Initial symptoms include loss of appetite and difficulty in sleeping. This is followed by excitement, mental confusion, hallucinations, fear, and anxiety. There may also be body tremors, fever, increased heart rate, diaphoresis, stomach pain, and chest pain. The episode generally lasts from 3 to 5 days and is a medical emergency. A deep sleep often follows. Sedatives and tranquilizers are useful for calming the patient.
Delusion	An immovable illusion; a false belief or wrong judgment.

Table 35-8—cont'd

TERM	DEFINITION
Dupuytren's contracture	Progressive, painless thickening and tightening of the fascial tissue surrounding the tendons and ligaments of the palm. It causes the fourth and fifth fingers to bend into the palm and resist extension. Tendons and nerves are not involved. Although the condition begins in one hand, both hands may be affected. Of unknown cause, it is most frequent in middle-aged males.
Fetal alcohol syndrome (FAS)	Clinical syndrome, usually diagnosed in infancy or childhood, characterized by microcephaly, low nasal bridge, flat midface, short palpebral fissures, indistinct philtrum, thin upper lip, micrognathia.
Gynecomastia	Abnormal swelling of one or both breasts in men. The condition is usually temporary and harmless. It may be caused by hormonal imbalance, tumors of the testis or pituitary, drugs containing estrogen or steroids, or failure of the liver to metabolize estrogens in the bloodstream.
Hallucinations	A subjective perception of what does not exist. During alcohol withdrawal, most commonly visual, but may be auditory. Typically animate and frightening to the patient. A chronic auditory form may occur.
Palmar erythema	A fixed, diffuse erythema, most predominant on the hypothenar eminence. The thenar prominence may be less intensely involved. In severe cases, the palmar tips of the digits may be reddened. The condition occurs most commonly in liver disease and pregnancy.
Spider angioma	A blood vessel disorder, marked by a central, raised fiery red dot the size of a pinhead, from which small blood vessels radiate. If the central body is pressed with a pencil tip, the radicles fade. They fill centrifugally as soon as the pressure is removed. Spider angiomas are often linked with high estrogen levels such as occur in pregnancy or when the liver is diseased and unable to detoxify estrogens.

Continued

Table 35-8. ALCOHOL SCREENING TERMS—*cont'd*

TERM	DEFINITION
Telangiectasia	Permanent widening of groups of superficial capillaries and small vessels (venules). Common causes include damage due to excess sunlight, excessive levels of female hormones, collagen vascular diseases, and other skin diseases, such as rosacea.
Wernicke's encephalopathy	Characterized by ophthalmoplegia (double vision, nystagmus, gaze palsies), ataxia (difficulty walking), and confusion, which may be mild or severe. It is caused by a deficiency of thiamine. Pathologic changes (edema, bleeding, and cellular degeneration) occur in several brain regions, including the hypothalamus, mammillary bodies, and tissues surrounding ventricles and aqueducts. Alcoholism, excessive vomiting (e.g., hyperemesis gravidarum), and malabsorption are predisposing factors.
Withdrawal symptoms	Unpleasant, sometimes life-threatening bodily changes that occur when some drugs are acutely withdrawn after long-term, regular use. The effects may occur after use of a narcotic, tranquilizer, stimulant, barbiturate, alcohol, or other substance on which the person has become physically or psychologically dependent.
Withdrawal signs	Physical or psychological manifestations resulting from the immediate cessation of both prescription and nonprescription drugs, including alcohol. See alcohol withdrawal (*supra vide*).
Zieve's syndrome	Symptom complex occurring in patients with excessive consumption of alcohol, characterized by hemolytic anemia, severe hyperlipoproteinemia, transient jaundice, and abdominal pain. More prevalent in middle-aged male patients.

"executive" in a biotechnology company. He is unable to explain his demotion.

Travel History: Vacations in Europe and Caribbean.

Animal and Insect Exposure History: Lives in area endemic for Lyme disease.

Medications: Uses acetaminophen for pain as needed. Denies allergies to medications.

HEALTH MAINTENANCE

Prevention: He received all childhood vaccines. He has not received Lyme vaccine. His last tetanus shot was more than 10 years ago. Has yearly "check-up."

Diet: Was advised to decrease salt intake and alcohol intake at last physical examination.

Exercise: Denies regular physical exercise.

Sleep patterns: For more than a year, awakens frequently with "bad dreams."

Social habits: Smokes 1 ppd for 30 years. Has never tried to stop. Denies illicit drug use. See HPI for alcohol consumption.

FAMILY HISTORY

First-Degree Relatives' Medical History: Father is alcoholic; sister died of unknown liver disease at age 45; brother hospitalized for pancreatitis last year. Mother is healthy. He is not in contact with his children or other siblings.

Three-Generation Genogram: He is not in contact with his children. He is not aware of genetic diseases or traits in his immediate family. History is not reliable because of lack of family contact.

PSYCHOSOCIAL HISTORY

Personal and Social History: Lives alone and is socially isolated.

REVIEW OF SYSTEMS

General: 10-pound weight loss over the past year; told of elevated blood pressure at last annual examination; results of blood lipids pending; no history of gout or cancer.

HEENT/Neck: No changes in vision; no epistaxis; denies change in voice; no routine dental care.

Respiratory: No history of pneumonia or tuberculosis; PPD was negative last year; does not fall asleep at work during the day. Admits to nonproductive AM cough for "years." Denies SOB.

Cardiovascular: Denies chest pain, dyspnea, orthopnea, paroxysmal nocturnal dyspnea, palpitations, or tachycardia.

Endocrine: Has mild breast swelling and pain; denies history of diabetes mellitus.

Gastrointestinal: Denies abdominal pain, hematemesis, hematochezia, steatorrhea, diarrhea, dysphagia, or heartburn. His appetite has been poor for several months. He does not eat regular meals. He denies a history of peptic ulcer disease or pancreatitis. He was told of abnormal "liver tests" at last annual "check-up."

Genitourinary: Denies impotence, loss of libido, or polyuria.

Hematologic/Lymphatic: Denies bleeding or easy bruising. Denies history of anemia or blood disorders. Denies swelling in neck, axilla, or groin.

Skin: Denies jaundice or pallor, petechiae, striae, rashes, or change is pattern of hair distribution. Denies diaphoresis.

Neuro-Psychiatric: Denies tremors or family history of tremors; denies history of seizures; denies hallucinations, depression, anxiety, suicidal, or homicidal ideations. Denies paresthesias of hands/feet or difficulty walking. Has never been treated for a psychiatric problem.

Musculoskeletal: Fractured ribs (*vide supra*): Denies muscle weakness or tenderness. Denies joint pain or history of gout. Has never been evaluated for osteoporosis.

Extremities: Denies swelling of legs. Denies ulcers of lower extremities. Denies tremors of hands.

PHYSICAL EXAMINATION

Vital Signs: T 98.8°F P 110 BP 180/100 RR 20 Weight 140 lbs. Height 6 ft.

Alcohol level pending.

General Appearance and Mental Status: Poorly nourished WM, A&O ×4, anxious, diaphoretic, appears older than stated age, poorly cooperative.

HEENT: No evidence FAS. No parotid enlargement; eyes: atraumatic, no jaundice, mild horizontal nystagmus, no gaze palsy, no lipemia retinalis; nose: no septal perforation; mouth: no torus palatini; odor of alcohol on breath; teeth: no posterior enamel loss; no oral lesions; no leukoplakia/erythroplakia; no bleeding/inflammation gums; dental hygiene fair; throat: no hoarseness; gag reflex intact.

Chest (general): Bony rib deformity consistent with previous fracture, palpable left posterior ribs 8-10, nontender to palpation.

Breasts: Minimally enlarged bilaterally, without masses. Mild tenderness to palpation.

Lungs: Increased AP diameter. Slightly distant breath sounds, with coarse rhonchi bilaterally to auscultation; no rales; no wheezing.

Cardiovascular: S_1 and S_2 distant. No S_3 or S_4. Tachycardia; No murmur.

Abdomen: Soft, nontender to palpation and percussion, without masses. Bowel sounds active. Liver palpable 3 cm below right costal margin (RCM), smooth edge, without nodules, masses, or bruit, span 16 cm. No splenomegaly. No ascites.

Genitalia: Penis without lesions. No testicular atrophy.

Rectum/Prostate: Stool brown, guaiac negative. Prostate—normal size, shape, and consistency.

Extremities: Mild resting tremor. No asterixis, Dupuytren's contracture, or palmer erythema. No muscle atrophy or tenderness, no peripheral edema.

Skin (Integument): No spider angioma, no jaundice, no caput medusa, no ecchymoses, no petechiae, no rash, no "tracks"; fingers "nicotine stained," with slight clubbing.

Lymphatics: No adenopathy.

Neurologic: Mental status: A&O ×4; no hallucinosis; poorly cooperative for tests of higher intellectual functioning (e.g., serial 7s); cranial nerves II-XII WNL. Sensory: Uncooperative for sensory examination. Motor: WNL, without muscular atrophy or tenderness; DTRs: 3+/4DTR bilaterally lower extremities, 4+/4 upper extremities. Cerebellar: no gait ataxia; Finger → nose WNL; no dysmetria. Babinski downgoing bilaterally; see also extremities and HEENT *supra vide*.

36

EPIDEMIOLOGY

Katerina M. Neuhauser, MD, PhD, MPH,
Thomas S. Neuhauser, MD, Roger Gibson, MD, and
Jill Feig, MD, MPH

I. OVERVIEW OF EPIDEMIOLOGY

Descriptive epidemiology characterizes the distribution of health-related events in a specific population by person, place, and time. It uses case reports, case series, or cross-sectional studies to generate hypotheses that can be tested later using more sophisticated study designs.

Analytical epidemiology identifies associations between specific factors that can influence the occurrence of health-related observations—the why and how of such events. It tests hypotheses through either observational (e.g., case-control, cohort studies) or experimental study designs.

II. NATURAL HISTORY OF DISEASE MODEL: DIAGRAM OF DISEASE MODEL

This model shows the interrelationships among four factors: agent, host, environment, and vector.

A. Host

1. Individual who is at risk for a specific disease or illness.
2. Susceptibility to disease or illness depends on the interaction of four variables: genotype, nutritional status, immune status, and social behavior. These variables affect host resistance.

B. Agent

1. Infectious organism or factor that can cause a specific disease or illness.
2. It includes allergens, vaccines, antibiotics, foods, and infectious organisms (bacteria, viruses, fungi, or parasites).

C. Environment

1. The home, work, or outdoor surroundings in which the host is found.
2. The environment influences the probability of an agent or vector causing infection or disease in a host (e.g., sanitation, effective sewage or waste disposal, water purification units).
3. The overall health (e.g., nutritional status) of a population depends partly on the political climate or the economic stability of that population.

D. Vector

1. Carrier or other means by which an infective agent that causes disease is transferred to a host.

2. Usually biologic entities such as insects (e.g., mosquitoes), arthropods (e.g., ticks), or animals (e.g., raccoons).
3. Possibly groups (e.g., vendors of heroin or cocaine) or objects (e.g., needles contaminated with agents associated disease).

III. DEFINITIONS

A. **Incidence (Incident Cases):** Frequency (number) of new occurrences of disease, injury, or death in a defined population over a specified period of time.

B. **Point Prevalence (Prevalence Cases):** Frequency of all individuals with a specified disease or condition at a particular point in time.

C. **Period Prevalence:** Frequency of all individuals with a specified disease or condition (incident and prevalence cases) over a specified time interval.

D. **Cohort:** A defined group of individuals followed over a period of time to determine the incidence of a risk event (e.g., disease, injury, or death).

E. **Risk:** Proportion of individuals who undergo a risk event during a specified time interval.

F. **Rate:** Frequency of a specific health event that occurs in a defined time period divided by the population at risk.

1. Unlike raw numbers, rates adjust for differences in the size of populations studied.
2. For populations that fluctuate over time (e.g., monthly or yearly), the average population or the midpoint population are used in the rate calculations.
3. Rates are multiplied by a constant multiplier (any multiple of 10) in order to make them easier to understand, discuss, and compare. Typical constant multiplier values are 1000, 10,000, and 100,000.

$$R = \frac{\text{Frequency of specific health event}}{\text{Population at risk (during specified time interval)}} \times \text{constant multipler}$$

G. **Incidence Rate (IR):** Number of incident cases in a population divided by population at risk during a defined study period.

$$IR = \frac{\text{Number of incident cases}}{\text{Population at risk (during specified time interval)}} \times \text{constant multipler}$$

H. **Cumulative Incidence (CI):** Sum of incidence rates over several time intervals.

$$CI = (IR_1 + IR_2 + IR_3 + IR_X) \times \text{constant multiplier}$$

I. **Prevalence Rate (PR):** Proportion (usually a percentage) of a population with a new or previously identified disease or condition at a particular point in time.

$$PR = \frac{\text{Number of incident and prevalent cases}}{\text{Total population at a particular point in time}} \times 100$$

J. **Crude Rates:** Rates in a study population that have not been adjusted for specific group characteristics (e.g., age, race, or sex).

K. **Standardized (Adjusted) Rates:** Rates that have been adjusted for specific group characteristics; adjusted rates allow comparison of populations with differing group characteristics.

IV. **MEASURES OF DISEASE FREQUENCY**

A. **Epidemic:** The frequency of a health event in a human population exceeds its expected frequency (e.g., foodborne illnesses, heart disease, cancer, violence, reproductive hazards, psychiatric conditions).

B. **Endemic:** The frequency of a health event in human populations within a given geographic area is at the expected level.

C. **Pandemic:** An epidemic that encompasses large numbers of people across multiple countries or continents.

D. **Epizootic:** The frequency of disease in the animal population within a given geographic location exceeds the expected frequency.

E. **Enzootic:** The frequency of disease in animals within a given geographic location is firmly established and at the expected level.

V. **DIAGNOSTIC TESTING (Table 36-1)**

A. **True-Positive (Cell A):** Test reflects the "true" positive disease status of the individual.

B. **True-Negative (Cell D):** Test reflects the "true" negative disease status of the individual.

Table 36-1. STANDARD 2 × 2 TABLE COMPARING THE TEST RESULTS AND THE TRUE DISEASE STATUS OF THE SUBJECTS TESTED

		TRUE DISEASE STATUS		
		Diseased	Nondiseased	Total
	Positive	a_{TP}	b_{FP}	$a + b$
TEST RESULT	Negative	c_{FN}	d_{TN}	$c + d$
	Total	$a + c$	$b + d$	$a + b + c + d$

Interpretation of the cells is as follows:

a = subjects with a true-positive test result
b = subjects with a false-positive test result
c = subjects with a false-negative test result
d = subjects with a true-negative test result

$a + b$ = all subjects with a positive test result
$c + d$ = all subjects with a negative test result
$a + c$ = all subjects with the disease
$b + d$ = all subjects without the disease

$a + b + c + d$ = all study subjects

C. **False-Positive (Cell B):** Test incorrectly identifies an individual without disease as having disease.

D. **False-Negative (Cell C):** Test incorrectly identifies an individual with disease as not having disease.

E. **Sensitivity:** Percentage of persons with a condition of interest that has a positive test result. The higher the sensitivity of the test, the more likely the test will detect individuals with the condition.

$$\text{Sensitivity} = \frac{\text{True-Positives (a)}}{\text{True-Positives + False-Positives (a + c)}} \times 100$$

F. **Specificity:** Proportion of persons without the condition of interest who have a negative test result. The higher the specificity of a test, the less likely individuals without the condition will be positive. Generally, as specificity increases, sensitivity decreases and vice versa.

$$\text{Sensitivity} = \frac{\text{True-Negatives (d)}}{\text{True-Negatives + False-Positives (d + b)}} \times 100$$

G. **Positive Predictive Value (PPV):** Percentage of persons with positive test results whom actually have the condition of interest; in other words, the probability that a condition is present if the test result is positive.

$$\text{PPV+} = \frac{\text{True-Positives (a)}}{\text{True-Positives + False-Positives (a + b)}} \times 100$$

H. **Negative Predictive Value (NPV):** Percentage of persons with negative test results who do not have the condition of interest; in other words, the probability that a condition is present if the test result is negative.

$$\text{NPV}- = \frac{\text{True-Negatives (d)}}{\text{True-Negatives + False-Negatives (d + c)}} \times 100$$

VI. CAUSALITY MODEL

A. General

1. Medical researchers identify associations between the condition of interest and risk factor(s) or protective factor(s).
   a. Risk factors are characteristics (e.g., age, race, smoking history) that place an individual at risk.
   b. Protective factors are characteristics that reduce the likelihood that an individual will have a particular disease or condition.
2. Presence of a statistically significant finding does not prove causation.

B. **Determining Causality:** Research results are evaluated scientifically to determine if there is evidence of causation for statistically significant results.

1. Investigation of statistical association. Mill's Canons is a set of criteria whereby the more that are met, the greater the likeli-

EPI

hood that the statistically significant association has a causal relationship.

a. Strength of association: Strong associations (high odds ratios or relative risks, or very significant p-values) suggest causality.

b. Biologically plausible: The association should be possible based on knowledge of biology.

c. Biologic gradient: As individuals are exposed to more risk factors, their risk of contracting the medical condition increases.

d. Consistency: Other investigators should have demonstrated similar associations with similar risk or protective factors. Highly consistent data will actually demonstrate associations across different time frames and populations.

2. Investigation of temporal relationships.

a. The individual must have been exposed to the risk factor(s) before the development of the medical condition being investigated.

b. Temporal relationships are not necessarily clear-cut. Different individuals exposed to the same risk factor may require different levels of exposure (e.g., time, dose) before they experience a health event.

c. Elimination of alternative explanations. All scientific explanations regarding significant or non-significant findings are tentative because it is not possible to account for all possibilities in any study design.

C. **Factors Affecting Causal Relationships:** Causal research has many pitfalls that can lead researchers to draw wrong conclusions.

1. Bias (differential error) results from a flaw in the study design whereby analyzed data are consistently deviated or distorted in one direction. This affects interpretation of associations (e.g., weakening true associations, changing the direction of true associations, or producing spurious associations).

a. Measurement bias occurs when baseline or follow-up data are collected imprecisely (e.g., subjects all wore shoes when height measurements were taken).

b. Recall bias occurs when data describing past events are collected in such a manner that the data are distorted.

(1) It may occur when individuals completing a survey cannot easily quantify their answers (e.g., how many total workdays did you lose last year, or list all of the foods you ate over the last week).

(2) It may also occur when subjects remember specific details of past events differently. For example, subjects who have had an adverse outcome (e.g., spontaneous abortion, disability) are more likely to recall risk-associated factors than those who have not.

c. Selection bias occurs when subjects are not randomly selected into study groups.
  (1) For example, if given a choice, diseased individuals may prefer to be in an experimental group receiving an experimental medication rather than in a control group receiving a control medication.
  (2) If subjects choose their study groups, these groups would not be comparable because study results may reflect the differing group characteristics and not the efficacy of the medication under investigation.

2. Random error (chance or non-differential error).
   a. Errors are randomly distributed among each study group; these errors usually do not affect the results of a study, unless the statistical power of the study was low.
   b. This could occur if the study population was too small to detect any statistical difference among the study groups.
3. Confounding.
   a. Occurs when study design chosen does not take into account all potential causal factors; causal factors not investigated become confounders that bias study results.
   b. For instance, although an individual's risk for myocardial infarction (MI) is positively associated with the individual's percentage of gray hair, it is not a causal factor—age is.
4. Synergism.
   a. Occurs when two causal variables interact in such a way that the combined effect is greater than the individual effect.
   b. For instance, lung cancer is associated with both smoking and asbestos exposure, but the risk of developing this malignancy is much greater if both causal risk factors are present at the same time.
5. Effect modification (interaction).
   a. Occurs when a third variable changes the strength of association between two causal variables.
   b. For example, low birth weight (defined as 2500 grams or less) is associated with teenage pregnancy and smoking.

VII. PUBLIC HEALTH SURVEILLANCE

A. A systematic method for establishing **baseline** (usual) rates or patterns of health events in a population and monitoring these rates over time.

B. **Prevention** initiatives in the community are often based on data obtained from passive (the majority) or active surveillance systems.
   1. Passive surveillance system.
      a. All reporting officials (e.g., physicians, laboratories, and hospitals) are required to report specific diseases to their state health department.
      b. Health agencies do not track down reporting officials to ensure that they provide the required data. Consequently,

the data may not reflect the true rates of health events in the population.

2. Active surveillance system.
   a. Health agencies exert "continuous pressure" on reporting officials to collect timely and accurate data.
   b. Data more accurately depicts general population trends.
   c. It is a more labor-intensive and costly system to maintain than a passive surveillance system.

VIII. INVESTIGATION OF A LOCAL EPIDEMIC (OUTBREAK)

A. Definitions

1. Attack rate (AR): Proportion of exposed individuals who acquire the disease divided by the total population at risk.

$$AR = \frac{\text{Number of new cases in exposed population}}{\text{Total number of persons exposed to a particular outbreak}} \times 100$$

2. Case fatality ratio (CFR): Proportion of clinically ill persons who die. Higher CFRs reflect more virulent infections.

B. Procedures for Investigation: Public Health officials investigate the etiology of an outbreak and establish methods to contain the spread of infection. The general approach is as follows:

1. Establish the existence of an epidemic.
   a. Confirm the presence of cases (those individuals with symptoms or disease) by talking with providers and laboratory personnel.
   b. Review data from surveillance systems to determine if the number of cases is more than what would be expected for that time of year at that particular location.
   c. Identify the presumptive diagnosis and possible etiologic agent based on the constellation of symptoms in affected individuals (e.g., high temperature, nausea, vomiting, diarrhea, abdominal pain).
2. Establish the case definition: Specific set of criteria that will be used to identify other cases.
   a. Specific set of criteria includes where the infection occurred, time frame within which the infection occurred, and likely symptoms that infected individuals may present with (e.g., any individual who ate at Bobby's Restaurant between January 28 and February 1 with symptoms of nausea or vomiting).
   b. Case definitions are initially broad to ensure that all of the cases are captured; they are refined as more data become available throughout the course of the investigation.
3. Characterize the nature of the epidemic by plotting an epidemic time curve.
   a. Plot the number of new cases (y-axis) by the time of onset of symptoms (x-axis).
   b. Common source exposure: The epidemic time curve spikes

if many individuals came into contact with a point source (responsible entity).

   c. Propagated outbreak: The epidemic curve would have a more prolonged and irregular pattern if the outbreak was the result of person-to-person spread.

4. If the causative organism is known, determine the probable time of exposure using the epidemic time curve. For example, assume that the causative organism had an incubation period of 1 to 9 days and the first case was seen on September 1, 2000 and the last case on September 10, 2000. The shortest incubation period (1 day) is applied to the first case. One day before the first case is August 31, 2000. The longest incubation period (9 days) is applied to the last case; 9 days before September 10, 2000 would be September 1, 2000. Consequently, the exposure would have occurred between August 31, 2000 and September 1, 2000.
5. Generate hypotheses to explain the pattern of spread (e.g., point source or propagating) and the mode of transmission (e.g., respiratory, fecal-oral, vector-borne, skin-to-skin) of suspected organisms.
6. Test hypotheses by obtaining additional information.
   a. Consider conducting a case-control study in which cases (those affected) are compared to controls (asymptomatic persons with similar characteristics to the cases: e.g., ate at the same restaurant during the time cases were exposed to the offending organism). This study will hopefully elicit specific differences between the two groups (e.g., cases were three times more likely to have eaten potato salad).
   b. Consider reviewing medical records of subjects.
   c. Consider collecting labs from subjects (e.g., blood, stool).
   d. Consider collecting environmental specimens (e.g., specific food items).
7. Initiate control measures that will hopefully contain the spread of infection. Types of interventions include the following:
   a. Treatment of infected individuals (e.g., tuberculosis [TB]).
   b. Prophylaxis of affected and/or unaffected individuals presumed to be at risk using medicines (e.g., antimalarial drugs) or immunizations (e.g., hepatitis A vaccination).
   c. Vector control measures (e.g., aerial spraying to kill mosquitoes).
   d. Sanitation measures (e.g., super-chlorination of water supply to kill pathogenic organisms).
8. Monitor the effectiveness of control measures in preventing recurrences.

37

ETHICAL CONSIDERATIONS

Gail A. van Norman, MD

I. INFORMED CONSENT

Laws and the principles of ethical medical practice require obtaining informed consent before performing medical treatment and procedures. **Competent patients** have both legal and moral rights to refuse medical therapy, even when it might be lifesaving. **Appropriate information** must be provided to patients about the treatment or procedure, including reasons for it, alternative treatments, risks of treatment (including the risks of nontreatment), and common or serious potential complications. **Voluntary consent** must be given by a competent patient. When the voluntariness of consent, or the ability to decide about medical therapy, is in doubt, examination of the patient focuses on elements of the history and physical examination that support or refute the patient's ability to consent to or refuse treatment.

A. **Chief Complaint:** Ensure that complaint coincides with the patient's condition and the procedure to be completed.

B. **Identifying Data**
   1. What is the patient's age? In most states, patients younger than age 18 require special circumstances, such as legal emancipation from their parents, to give consent for medical procedures.
   2. Is the patient pregnant? In many states, patients younger than age 18 can legally consent to medical care that is related to their pregnancy.
   3. Is consent for the treatment of mental illness, a sexually transmitted disease, or substance abuse? Is consent for contraceptive prescription or device? In many states, it is legal for patients younger than age 18 to consent to medical treatment without parental knowledge or approval.
   4. What is the patient's native language? Whenever possible, the patient's native language should be used to discuss treatment or procedures.
   5. If interpreters are used to communicate with the patient, what is their relation to the patient? It is advisable to use interpreters who are not members of the patient's immediate family.
   6. If other persons are present during discussion with patient, who are they and what is their relationship to the patient?

C. **Past Medical and Surgery History:** Table 37-1 contains symptoms and conditions about which a patient should be asked before obtaining informed consent from the patient.

Table 37-1. MEDICAL AND SURGICAL HISTORY CHARACTERISTICS THAT MIGHT AFFECT ABILITY TO PARTICIPATE IN INFORMED CONSENT.

SYSTEM OR CONDITION	CURRENT AND PAST MEDICAL DIAGNOSES
General	Sleep deprivation, trauma, hypothermia, "ICU psychosis"
Respiratory	Acute respiratory distress and failure (acute changes in pH, PAO_2, $PaCO_2$ may affect mental function; chronic changes generally do not)
Gastrointestinal	Acute or chronic liver disease, severe nausea and vomiting
Renal disease and electrolyte disorders	Acute or chronic renal failure, significant uremia, hypo- or hypercalcemia, hyponatremia, hyperosmolarity, hypomagnesemia
Neuropsychiatric	Hallucinations, extreme anxiety reaction, mental illness (especially alcoholic dementia or encephalopathy), organic brain syndromes, anatomy abnormalities of the brain (e.g., hydrocephalus, tumor, trauma), diagnosis of dementia, Alzheimer's, depression or other mood disorders, seizures (may be a symptom of substance withdrawal), mental retardation or other mental handicap, aphasia, dysarthria, (may make communication difficult) cerebrovascular disease, Parkinson's disease
Endocrine	Thyroid abnormalities, diabetes (diabetic ketoacidosis [DKA], hypoglycemia, hyperosmolar hyperglycemia)
Nutritional status	Vitamin deficiency (e.g., thiamin, niacin, B_{12})
Medications	Antidepressants, anxiolytics, analgesics, thyroid medication, weight-loss medications, insulin, steroids
Substance abuse	Present or past alcohol abuse, present or past significant marijuana use, current use of amphetamines, current use of narcotics, cocaine, steroids, barbiturates
Exposure to infectious agents	Syphilis, Jacob-Creutzfeldt, malaria, meningococcus, bacterial or viral encephalitis
Toxin exposure	Unusual foods, exposure to volatile petroleum derivatives, carbon monoxide, heavy metal exposure

D. Psychosocial History

1. Personal and social history.
   a. Religious background: Does the patient practice a religion with alternative beliefs about medical care (e.g., Jehovah's Witness or Christian Scientist)? Does the patient have strong religious beliefs about certain aspects of care (e.g., a practicing Catholic might strongly oppose the termination of a pregnancy)?
   b. Cultural background: Are there cultural issues that might significantly affect the informed consent process? Address cultural beliefs that may affect portions or all of the procedure.
2. Family support.
   a. What is the patient's marital status? Are there any children? Siblings?
   b. Is the patient socially isolated or is there a supportive family structure?

E. Focused Physical and Laboratory Examination: Direct the examination toward detection of conditions that might lead to impaired mental functioning or diminished capacity to make medical decisions. The presence of physical findings is not sufficient indication of impaired competence, and any such findings must be accompanied by evidence of diminished capacity (Table 37-2).

F. Indicators of Capacity to Consent

1. Discussion of the procedure with the patient: The following elements indicate that the patient has the capacity to consent to medical treatment, even when the patient does not have capacity to carry out other tasks, such as money management. Orientation to date and place are less important; many patients with mild dementia, for example, will still have the capacity to give informed consent.
   a. Can the patient describe the proposed procedure and the reasons for it?
   b. Does the patient appear to understand the potential risks of the treatment and of nontreatment?
   c. Does the patient understand alternative treatments, if any?
   d. Does the patient express a decision about the treatment?
   e. Does the decision appear at least in part related to information conveyed in the conversation (e.g., "I don't want my leg amputated even though I might die because I don't want to live without a leg," uses appropriate information, while "I don't want my leg amputated because the house is blue" does not)?
2. Patient's behavior.
   a. Does the patient appear to be confused or hallucinating?
   b. Does the patient appear very anxious? Anxiety can prevent a patient from assimilating information necessary for informed consent.

Table 37-2. INFORMED CONSENT—FOCUSED PHYSICAL EXAMINATION.	
SYSTEM OR CONDITION	PHYSICAL EXAMINATION FINDINGS TO LOOK FOR
Vital signs	Severe hypotension, tachycardia, hypothermia, fever
Cardiovascular	Respiratory distress, tachypnea, stridor, low SAO_2, wheezing, rales, diminished breath sounds (may indicate the presence of acute respiratory failure), ABG with findings of severe hypoxemia ($PAO_2 < 45$-50 mmHg) or acute respiratory acidosis
Gastrointestinal	Severe jaundice or ascites, elevated bilirubin
Renal disease	Severely elevated BUN, creatinine, decreased or increased serum calcium, decreased serum sodium, decreased serum magnesium
Endocrine	Tachycardia or bradycardia, depressed or brisk deep tendon reflexes, ketone odor to breath, elevated thyroid hormone levels, severe hyperglycemia (glucose above 400 mg/dL), presence of serum ketones, decreased serum pH
Neuropsychiatric	Focal motor or sensory findings suggestive of anatomic brain lesion or acute CVA, asterixis, tremor, dysarthria, aphasia, severely depressed or inappropriate affect (e.g., somnolence, agitation, incoherence)
Vitamin deficiency	Megaloblastic anemia, cardiac failure, ataxia, nystagmus, peripheral neuropathy, photosensitive dermatitis
Substance abuse	Pinpoint or dilated pupils, decreased respiratory rate, tachycardia or bradycardia, hypertension
Toxin exposure	"Cherry red" appearance to skin or mucous membranes (carbon monoxide exposure), Kaiser-Fleischer rings (e.g., copper, heavy metal intoxication)

c. Is the patient in significant pain? Pain can interfere with the patient's ability to discuss and comprehend the treatment.
d. Does the patient appear somnolent? Sedating medications and certain medical conditions can interfere with a patient's ability to discuss and comprehend treatment.

3. Patient's social contacts.
   a. Are family members concerned about the patient's ability to give consent?
   b. Does the patient's primary care provider have concerns about the patient's ability to give consent?

G. Indicators of Coercion

1. Pressure from others: Are family members or friends, including church members, reluctant to allow the patient to be interviewed outside of their presence? This may indicate that the patient would render a different decision if free from their influence. Does the patient in fact express a different decision when interviewed alone?
2. Severity of pain: Is the patient in significant pain? The patient may render a decision that he or she feels is most likely to gain rapid treatment for pain.
3. Drug-seeking behavior: Is the patient withdrawing from alcohol or other substance? The patient may render a decision that he or she feels is most likely to gain access to drugs for the treatment of withdrawal.

H. Discussion of Medical Procedures

1. Describe proposed procedure and reasonable alternatives.
2. Describe risks of the procedure.
   a. Common risks, even if consequences are minor.
   b. Uncommon risks that have severe consequences, such as significant injury or death.
   c. Risks of nontreatment.
   d. Risks that may be of special relevance to the individual patient.

II. ADVANCED DIRECTIVES AND SURROGATE DECISION MAKERS

In many cases, health care decisions must be made precisely at the time when patients are incapacitated by disease or medical therapy and cannot express their wishes. Ethicists and legal experts agree that when competence cannot be restored through medical therapy in a timely fashion, patients' wishes may still be expressed via advanced directives, which are legal specification of a patient's wishes with regard to health care decisions that have been executed by the patient before incapacitation or by surrogate decision makers appointed by the patient or by legal hierarchy. Questions about advanced directives should be asked when taking the social history of any hospitalized patient.

A. Patient History: Issues to discuss before hospital admission or when patient has a serious illness.

1. Does the patient have someone designated to make health care decisions for him or her? Do you have contact information for that person?
2. Are there any persons the patient specifically excludes from being involved in health care decisions?
3. If the patient has a living will or durable power of attorney, is a copy present in the chart?
4. In the absence of a legal document, whom does the patient suggest you contact for serious health care questions?
5. Does the patient have specific wishes regarding resuscitation in the event of cardiac arrest?

B. **Advanced Directive Documents**

1. A living will specifies the wishes of the patient regarding specific medical interventions, such as mechanical ventilation, CPR, intravenous hydration, and nutrition.
2. A Durable Power of Attorney or Durable Power of Health Attorney is the legal designation of a specific person or persons to make health care decisions. This document must be signed by witnesses and should be notarized if possible.

C. **Surrogate Decision Maker:** A person with legal power to make health care decisions for an incompetent patient in the absence of a living will.

1. Persons who qualify as surrogate decision-makers.
   a. Person designated by the patient (durable power of attorney or durable power of health attorney).
   b. Person designated by law (in the absence of a living will or durable power of attorney). Although the exact order of relatives varies among states, the following order is most common.
      (1) Spouse.
      (2) Children, if all are unanimous.
      (3) Parents, if both agree.
      (4) Siblings, if all are unanimous.
   c. Guardian-ad-litem is a person specially designated by court order. Guardian may be appointed when the patient's family cannot come to an agreement or when the best interests of the patient are in question.
2. Appropriate circumstances for use of a surrogate decision maker.
   a. Patient suffers from condition, injury, or illness that, in the opinion of medical experts, will permanently impair the capacity to make medical decisions.
   b. Patient suffers from injury or illness that results in temporary impairment of capacity to make medical decisions that, in the opinion of medical experts, must be made within a particular period before competence can be restored (e.g., emergency medical therapy).
   c. Patient is too young to make medical decisions.

3. Circumstance in which use of a surrogate decision maker is inappropriate.
   a. Patient is competent to make the medical decision, although suffering from mild dementia or other condition that impairs ability to make other types of decisions.
   b. Patient is temporarily incapacitated but can be restored to competence within a time frame that will allow appropriate medical intervention (e.g., with a patient who is overly sedated but has no emergent health condition about which a decision must be made immediately, the decision can be delayed until the patient is capable of deciding. Note: A lightly sedated patient may be competent).
   c. Patient is incapacitated but has clear advanced directives.
4. Qualifications of surrogate decision makers: To make medical decisions for others, surrogate decision makers must possess certain qualities.
   a. Ability to make reasoned judgments.
   b. Adequate knowledge and information about the issues involved.
   c. Emotional stability.
   d. Commitment to the patient's interests with no conflict of interest and under no controlling influence of those who might not act in the patient's best interests.

III. DO-NOT-RESUSCITATE (DNR) ORDERS

A. **Overview:** Physicians are ethically obligated to respect a wish to refuse life-sustaining treatment if it is expressed by a competent patient (see Informed Consent), indicated in an advanced directive, or made by the appropriate surrogate decision maker. Because DNR orders encompass a wide range of potential therapies, discussion with the patient should establish which procedures might be acceptable to the patient and which would not be acceptable. DNR wishes should again be discussed in the setting of special procedures or surgery and if the patient's status changes.

1. Circumstances under which a DNR order can be entered into a patient's chart.
   a. Competent patient or appropriate surrogate desires a DNR order.
   b. Health care team determines that resuscitation attempts would be futile (i.e., resuscitation would not succeed, even in the short term).
2. Deciding on and documenting a DNR order.
   a. Patient must be given appropriate information regarding the risks and benefits of resuscitation and of nonresuscitation.
   b. Discussion of which procedures may be considered by the patient or surrogates as a resuscitation situation.
      (1) Chest compressions.
      (2) Direct current (DC) countershock or pacing.

(3) Intubation and mechanical ventilation.
(4) Mask ventilation or mouth-to-mouth resuscitation.
(5) Administration of vasoactive drugs, such as epinephrine, dopamine, and lidocaine.
(6) Placement of invasive intravenous lines and monitors (central venous pressure [CVP], pulmonary artery [PA] catheters, and arterial lines).
(7) Placement of nasogastric (NG) tubes and feeding tubes.

B. DNR in the Setting of Special Procedures and Surgery

1. DNR order status before surgery: The American Society of Anesthesiologists, the American College of Surgeons, and the Association of Operating Room Nurses agree that automatic suspension of DNR orders during surgery is not consistent with ethical medical practice, and clarification and discussion of the DNR order status should occur before the patient undergoes surgery or special procedure.
   a. Many therapies considered "resuscitation" in other hospital settings, such as mechanical ventilation and administration of vasoactive drugs, are a routine or even required part of anesthetic and surgical care and do not necessarily violate a DNR order.
   b. Requiring patients to agree to CPR to obtain therapies that can only be given in the OR is coercive.
   c. Resuscitation carries a much more favorable risk-to-benefit ratio in the OR than elsewhere for the following reasons:
      (1) Arrest is witnessed.
      (2) Cause of arrest is known and usually reversible (e.g., drug-induced, hemorrhage).
      (3) Survival to pre-arrest state from OR causes is 92%, compared with 8% to 14% elsewhere in the hospital.
   d. Different patient expectations in the OR: Most patients expect to survive the operation, even if long-term survival is uncertain.
   e. Refusal of resuscitation does not and should not equate with refusal of all other medical and surgical care.
2. For patients undergoing surgery who have DNR orders.
   a. Alert the anesthesiologist of the presence of a DNR order and ask that the patient be seen preoperatively.
   b. Alert the surgical team of the presence of a DNR order.
   c. Inform the patient or their surrogate decision maker that the anesthesiologist will want to discuss the DNR order with them before surgery.

C. DNR Order Documentation: DNR orders should include the following information:

1. Rationale for the DNR order.
2. Risks and benefits of resuscitation and nonresuscitation that were discussed with the patient or appropriate surrogate.

3. Procedures that will be acceptable to the patient.
4. Procedures that will not be acceptable to the patient.
5. Signature of the patient or surrogate.
6. Instead of designating specific procedures, the patient may express general goals for therapy, allowing the health care team to determine the specific implementation procedures. The patient's general goals and wishes should be documented.

38

NUTRITIONAL STATUS EVALUATION

Donald F. Kirby, MD, FACP, FACN, FACG, CNSP, CPNS

NUTRITION STATUS EVALUATION COMPONENTS

I. Chief Complaint
II. History of Present Illness
  A. Medical and Weight History
  B. Dietary History
  C. Family History
  D. Medication History
III. Physical Examination
IV. Laboratory Studies and Diagnostic Evaluations
  A. Body Composition Measurements
    1. Anthropometric measurements
    2. Hydrostatic weighing
    3. Isotope measurements
    4. Infrared reactance
    5. Bioelectrical impedance
    6. Air-displacement plethysmography
  B. Biochemical Measurements
    1. Plasma proteins
      (a) Albumin
      (b) Transferrin
      (c) Prealbumin
    2. Urinary measurements
      (a) Creatinine-height index
      (b) 3-Methylhistidine
  C. Immunologic Tests
    1. Total lymphocyte count
    2. Skin tests for delayed hypersensitivity
V. Summary of Standard Nutrition Assessment
VI. Malnutrition
VII. Definitions

All patients who are interviewed and examined should have their nutritional status considered. As physicians counsel more patients on how to optimize their health and wellness, patients will hopefully turn to them for nutritional advice. Practitioners should be prepared to assess nutritional status and to seek help as necessary to improve the care of their patients.

I. HISTORY OF PRESENT ILLNESS

A. **Past Medical and Weight History:** By keeping nutritional problems in the differential diagnosis, a thorough H&P can help identify patients who are at high risk for adverse outcomes where nutrition may play a role.

1. Height and weight history: A measured height and weight are preferable to a patient's report.
2. Comparison of height and weight to standardized tables or Body Mass Index tables is advisable (Table 38-1).
3. Body mass index (BMI) = weight in kg/height in m^2). BMI is considered a good measurement of obesity because there is a high correlation between total body fat and obesity. It can have limitations in very short-statured people, and some athletes who have large muscle mass with little fat can be misclassified.
4. Weight-to-height comparison: A quick way to calculate a rough weight-to-height comparison is as follows: Men, 106 lbs. for the first 5 feet and 6 lbs. for each inch thereafter; women, 100 lbs. for first 5 feet and 5 lbs. for each inch thereafter.
5. Percentage of ideal body weight: Obtain history of patient's usual body weight (UBW) and compare it to their Ideal Body Weight (IBW) and their Present Body Weight (PBW). Calculate % IBW (% IBW = PBW/IBW × 100) and % UBW (% UBW = PBW/UBW × 100).
6. Fluid status: Note whether the patient's present weight is affected by fluid status. Is the patient dehydrated or fluid overloaded?
7. Is there evidence of recent weight loss? If yes, was it intentional? Consider cancer in all patients with unintentional weight loss, but further evaluation may elucidate another etiology.

B. **Diet History:** Physicians should interview patients about their normal dietary practices. Consultation with a registered dietitian can define the patient's present practices and help the patient implement what the physician feels might be the most efficacious dietary plan.

C. **Family History:** Obtain age, sex, health status (if deceased, cause of death), and chronic disease(s) of patient's family.

D. **Medication History**

1. What medications are the patient currently taking?
2. Are there any potential drug-drug or drug-nutrient interactions?
3. Is the patient taking over-the-counter (OTC) weight loss medications or herbal preparations?

II. PHYSICAL EXAMINATION

This examination may provide important information about a patient's underlying nutritional state. Areas to consider, and some of the findings that might be seen, are listed in Table 38-2.

Table 38-1. BODY MASS INDEX TABLE.

	NORMAL						OVERWEIGHT					OBESE										EXTREME OBESITY														
BMI	19	20	21	22	23	24	25	26	27	28	29	30	31	32	33	34	35	36	37	38	39	40	41	42	43	44	45	46	47	48	49	50	51	52	53	54
HEIGHT (INCHES)	BODY WEIGHT (POUNDS)																																			
58	91	96	100	105	110	115	119	124	129	134	138	143	148	153	158	162	167	172	177	181	186	191	196	201	205	210	215	220	224	229	234	239	244	248	253	258
59	94	99	104	109	114	119	124	128	133	138	143	148	153	158	163	168	173	178	183	188	193	198	203	208	212	217	222	227	232	237	242	247	252	257	262	267
60	97	102	107	112	118	123	128	133	138	143	148	153	158	163	168	174	179	184	189	194	199	204	209	215	220	225	230	235	240	245	250	255	261	266	271	276
61	100	106	111	116	122	127	132	137	143	148	153	158	164	169	174	180	185	190	195	201	206	211	217	222	227	232	238	243	248	254	259	264	269	275	280	285
62	104	109	115	120	126	131	136	142	147	153	158	164	169	175	180	186	191	196	202	207	213	218	224	229	235	240	246	251	256	262	267	273	278	284	289	295
63	107	113	118	124	130	135	141	146	152	158	163	169	175	180	186	191	197	203	208	214	220	225	231	237	242	248	254	259	265	270	278	282	287	293	299	304
64	110	116	122	128	134	140	145	151	157	163	169	174	180	186	192	197	204	209	215	221	227	232	238	244	250	256	262	267	273	279	285	291	296	302	308	314
65	114	120	126	132	138	144	150	156	162	168	174	180	186	192	198	204	210	216	222	228	234	240	246	252	258	264	270	276	282	288	294	300	306	312	318	324
66	118	124	130	136	142	148	155	161	167	173	179	186	192	198	204	210	216	223	229	235	241	247	253	260	266	272	278	284	291	297	303	309	315	322	328	334
67	121	127	134	140	146	153	159	166	172	178	185	191	198	204	211	217	223	230	236	242	249	255	261	268	274	280	287	293	299	306	312	319	325	331	338	344
68	125	131	138	144	151	158	164	171	177	184	190	197	203	210	216	223	230	236	243	249	256	262	269	276	282	289	295	302	308	315	322	328	335	341	348	354
69	128	135	142	149	155	162	169	176	182	189	196	203	209	216	223	230	236	243	250	257	263	270	277	284	291	297	304	311	318	324	331	338	345	351	358	365
70	132	139	146	153	160	167	174	181	188	195	202	209	216	222	229	236	243	250	257	264	271	278	285	292	299	306	313	320	327	334	342	348	355	362	369	376
71	136	143	150	157	165	172	179	186	193	200	208	215	222	229	236	243	250	257	265	272	279	286	293	301	308	315	322	329	338	343	351	358	365	372	379	386
72	140	147	154	162	169	177	194	191	199	206	213	221	228	235	242	250	258	265	272	279	287	294	302	309	316	324	331	338	346	353	361	368	375	383	390	397
73	144	151	159	166	174	182	189	197	204	212	219	227	235	242	250	257	265	272	280	288	295	302	310	318	325	333	340	348	355	363	371	378	386	393	401	408
74	148	155	163	171	179	186	194	202	210	218	225	233	241	249	256	264	272	280	287	295	303	311	319	326	334	342	350	358	365	373	381	389	396	404	412	420
75	152	160	168	176	184	192	200	208	216	224	232	240	248	256	264	272	279	287	295	303	311	319	327	335	343	351	359	367	375	383	391	399	407	415	423	431
76	156	164	172	180	189	197	205	213	221	230	238	246	254	263	271	279	287	295	304	312	320	328	336	344	353	361	369	377	385	394	402	410	418	426	435	443

Source: Adapted from *Clinical Guidelines on the Identification, Evaluation, and Treatment of Overweight and Obesity in Adults: The Evidence Report*.

Table 38-2. PHYSICAL EXAMINATION FINDINGS AND POSSIBLE NUTRIENT DEFICIENCIES.

System	Sign/Symptom	Potential Nutrient Deficiency
HEENT		
Hair	Easy pluckability	Protein, essential fatty acids
	Lackluster	Protein, zinc
	Loss	Zinc, essential fatty acids, biotin
	Pigmentation	Protein, copper
Eyes	Bitot's spot's, corneal irritation, dry eyes, night blindness	Varying degrees of Vitamin A deficiency
	Corneal vascularization	Riboflavin
Temporal region	Bitemporal wasting	Calorie and protein deficits
Mouth	Cheilosis	Pyridoxine, riboflavin, iron
	Inflammation	Pyridoxine, riboflavin, iron
	Tongue inflammation	Pyridoxine, zinc, niacin, folate, Vitamin B_{12}
	Magenta tongue	Riboflavin
	Fissured tongue	Niacin
	Nose-lip dryness	Niacin, pyridoxine, riboflavin
	Swollen, bleeding gums	Vitamin C
	Angular stomatitis	Riboflavin
Neck	Casal's necklace	Niacin
Heart	Congestive heart failure or cardiomegaly	Possible thiamin deficiency
	Heart degeneration	Possible selenium deficiency
Abdomen	Enlarged liver	"Classic" protein malnutrition = Kwashiorkor
Extremities	Subcutaneous fat loss	Calorie deficit
	Muscle wasting	Calorie and protein deficits
	Edema	Protein deficit or sodium excess
	Osteomalacia, bone pain, rickets	Vitamin D

Table 38-2—cont'd

SYSTEM	SIGN/SYMPTOM	POTENTIAL NUTRIENT DEFICIENCY
	Bone pain	Vitamin C
	Koilonychia (spoon nails)	Iron
	Muehrcke's lines*	Hypoalbuminemia
	Tetany	Calcium, magnesium
Skin	Dry and scaling	Vitamin A, essential fatty acids, zinc
	Petechiae/ecchymoses	Vitamin C and Vitamin K
	Follicular hyperkeratosis	Vitamin A, essential fatty acids
	Bilateral dermatitis	Niacin, zinc
Neurologic	Dementia/disorientation	Niacin, thiamin
	Confabulation	Thiamin
	Peripheral neuropathy	Thiamin, pyridoxine[†], Vitamin B_{12}

*Muehrcke's Lines = paired bands of pallor that appear in the nail bed.
[†]Both deficiency and excess may cause disease.

III. LABORATORY STUDIES AND DIAGNOSTIC EVALUATIONS

A. **Body Composition Measurements:** Low-technology, easy, and highly available methods, such as anthropometric measurements, provide information on body composition. Alternately, methods using more sophisticated technology that involves special equipment may be expensive and not always readily available. See what is available at your institution.

1. Anthropometric measurements, which can be done easily by the practitioner or ancillary staff, can provide rough estimates of the body's energy stores.
   a. Although many body areas may be measured and compared, the most commonly used area for nutrition assessment is the upper arm.
      (1) Midpoint: Use a tape measure to measure from the acromion process to the olecranon process. Find the midpoint.
      (2) Mid-arm circumference (MAC): From the midpoint, measure the circumference of the arm.
   b. Triceps skin fold (TSF): A special measuring calipers is used to grasp the skin and subcutaneous fat overlying the triceps muscle. This measurement can be compared to tables to obtain an estimate of fat stores.

c. Mid-arm muscle circumference (MAMC): This number reflects the protein stored in the body and is calculated using the following formula: MAMC = MAC (cm)—[0.314 × TSF (mm)].
   (1) Unfortunately, this technique cannot account for the genetic differences in bone size in different sexes or ethnic backgrounds.
   (2) Advantages of this technique are that it is easy to learn, inexpensive to perform, and has wide applicability.

2. Other techniques: It is worthwhile to be familiar with some other available anthropometric techniques, although they tend to focus more on the amount of body fat present.
   a. Hydrostatic weighing: Currently the "gold standard" for determining body density, from which body fat can accurately be determined.
   b. Isotope measurements: By using different tracers, fat-free mass and total body protein can be determined.
   c. Infrared reactance: This method irradiates a person's tissues with a spectrum of infrared radiation. Depending on the tissue's composition, certain absorptive and reflective properties can be compared to known data. Ultimately, this is another method for determining body fat.
   d. Bioelectrical impedance: By passing a small current between body surface electrodes, the body resistance or impedance can be estimated. In well patients, this is becoming an increasingly common method for determining fat mass. It is not as valid a measurement in critically ill patients.
   e. Air-displacement plethysmography: This method determines body volume by placing the patient into a chamber and measuring the reduction in chamber volume induced by the displacement of a fixed air volume.

B. Biochemical Measurements

1. Plasma proteins: Commonly used tests that are often quoted as "markers of nutrition," although they are not. Instead, they reflect different metabolic processes in the body and help determine a patient's nutritional risk.
   a. Albumin is a commonly measured plasma protein that has a half-life of approximately 21 days. It accounts for 70% of the colloid osmotic pressure of plasma and is a transport protein for vitamins, many administered medications, and many other molecules.
   b. Transferrin has a half-life of approximately 7 to 10 days. It may be more sensitive than albumin to changes in protein synthesis of the liver, but it can be affected by iron overload or deficiency, pernicious anemia, pregnancy, and chronic infection.

c. Prealbumin has a half-life of approximately 2 days. It may reflect efforts to refeed. It is a more expensive test that is not as readily available as the albumin test. This appears to be commonly used for patients who receive total parenteral nutrition (TPN).

2. Urinary measurements: These tests usually are limited by the need for an accurate 24-hour urinary collection and are not done routinely at this time.
   a. Creatinine-height index is a measure of lean body mass. When there is no rapid muscle breakdown, a fixed amount of creatinine is produced from creatine. Certain injuries and medications, renal insufficiency, and dietary meat intake may affect this measurement.
   b. 3-Methylhistidine is a myofibrillar protein that is released during protein catabolism and excreted unchanged in the urine. This measurement reflects total muscle mass. It is not commonly used.

C. **Immunologic Tests**

1. Total lymphocyte count (TLC).
   a. TLC is often readily available in most hospitalized patients.
   b. It has been correlated with cellular immune function.
   c. Low counts may be associated with protein depletion or deficits in immune system responsiveness.
   d. The TLC is calculated as follows:

$$\text{TLC} = \text{White Blood Count} \times \%\ \text{lymphocytes}$$

   e. Many nonnutritional conditions are known to alter this number, but usually counts of less than 800 cells/mm^3 indicate ill patients at heightened immune risk.

2. Delayed hypersensitivity (skin tests).
   a. These tests are performed as intradermal injections of recall antigens to see if the body responds. When a tuberculosis skin test (purified protein derivative [PPD]) is performed, it is often compared to several other antigens on the opposite arm, such as candida, trichophyton, and mumps.
   b. A positive response to any of these antigens suggests that part of the body's cellular immunity is actively functioning.
   c. Anergy is the lack of response to PPD and a series of recall antigens.
   d. When combined with the serum albumin, knowledge of the patient's ability to respond to skin tests can have predictive value for surgical risk. A normal serum albumin and response to skin tests predicts a low incidence of morbidity and mortality for elective surgery. However, a low serum albumin and anergy portends a 3 to 5 times higher risk of morbidity and mortality. (Incidentally, this is how albumin got its fame as a "nutrition marker.")

IV. SUMMARY OF STANDARD NUTRITION ASSESSMENT

After obtaining all of the information for a nutritional assessment, a patient can be categorized into one of three general categories: undernourished, normally nourished, and overnourished. It is important to note that obesity is the largest form of malnutrition in the United States.

V. MALNUTRITION (Tables 38-3 and 38-4)

Table 38-3. MALNUTRITION DEFINITIONS.

TERM	DEFINITION
Marasmus	Represents simple starvation. The body adapts to a chronic state of insufficient caloric intake. It may take months to years to develop. The patient looks like a "skeleton" with marked muscle wasting and little subcutaneous fat. These patients usually do not have edema. Their visceral proteins are usually maintained because they can cannibalize their muscles to support their protein needs.
Classic Kwashiorkor	Characteristically seen in developing nations or where there has been famine, but less often seen in industrialized nations. It is the body's response to insufficient protein intake but usually sufficient calories for energy. A predominant feature is painless, pitting edema of the feet and legs, but can involve the upper extremities and the face.
Immunorepressive malnutrition (hypoalbuminemic malnutrition)	Much more common in the U.S. and is characterized by a normal-appearing patient who has a low albumin and depressed delayed hypersensitivity reaction to skin tests. This patient has had the liver pathway for albumin turned off by cytokines, such as interleukins 1 and 6. This condition is typified by a high degree of metabolic stress that perpetuates the body's response.
Mixed malnutrition	Potentially an even more severe condition because it takes a marasmic host and adds metabolic stress that yields a patient who is at very high risk for morbidity or mortality.

Table 38-4. ASSESSMENT FEATURES IN MALNUTRITION.

	Marasmus	Kwashiorkor (Immunorepressive Malnutrition or Hypoalbuminemic Malnutrition)	Mixed Malnutrition
Nutritional intake	Decreased calorie intake	Decreased protein intake and stress	Decreased calorie and protein intakes plus stress
Time course to develop	Months to years	Weeks to months	Weeks
Physical exam	Cachetic fat depletion muscle wasting	May look well nourished	Cachetic, may have edema, giving more normal appearance
ANTHROPOMETRIC MEASUREMENTS			
TSF	Depressed	Relatively preserved	Variable
MAC	Depressed	Relatively preserved	Variable
Weight for height	Depressed	Relatively preserved	Variable
Skin test responses	Normal or depressed	Depressed	Depressed
VISCERAL PROTEINS			
Albumin	Relatively normal	Low	Low
Transferrin	Relatively normal	Low	Low
Total lymphocyte count	Relatively normal	Low	Low

Based in part on Silberman H. Parenteral and Enteral Nutrition, ed 2. Norwalk, CT: Appleton & Lange, 1989; p. 55. Reprinted with permission from Foxx-Orenstein A, Kirby DF. Malnutrition and refeeding. In Kirby DF, Dudrick SJ (eds), Practical Handbook of Nutrition in Clinical Practice. Boca Raton, FL: CRC Press, 1994; pp. 18–30.

VI. DEFINITIONS (Table 38-5)

Table 38-5. ADDITIONAL NUTRITION-FOCUSED DEFINITIONS.

Term	Definition
Overnourished	Overnourished can also be nutritional assessment diagnosis
Overweight	More than 20% above one's IBW or a BMI > 27
Obese	BMI > 30 and is associated with several medical problems, including hypertension, diabetes, restrictive lung disease, hyperlipidemia, coronary heart disease, increased risk of certain cancers, osteoarthritis, sleep apnea, depression, job prejudice and decreased longevity
Angular stomatitis	Fissuring at the angles of the mouth
Bitot's spots	Represent an advanced phase of Vitamin A deficiency where there is a heaping up of desquamated, keratinized epithelial cells; corneal vascularization: riboflavin deficiency
Casal's necklace	A bandlike eruption around the neck associated with niacin deficiency
Cheilosis	Vertical fissuring of the lips
Magenta tongue	Smooth, purplish-red tongue

39

TOBACCO SCREENING

Katerina M. Neuhauser, MD, PhD, MPH, Thomas S. Neuhauser MD, and Eric H. Hanson, MD, MPH

I. CHIEF COMPLAINT

A. **Chief Complaint:** Why is the patient here? Use the patient's own words (e.g., "My wife is pregnant and wants me to quit smoking.").

B. **Identifying Data:** Obtain name, age (date of birth), marital status, number of dependents, educational level, date and site of clinical visit or admission.

II. APRROACH TO SMOKING CESSATION

A. Proactive Provider Tobacco Cessation Involvement

1. Physicians should ask all patients: "Do you use tobacco?" "Do you want to quit?"
2. Those patients who indicate a desire to stop should have their concerns and barriers to stopping addressed (e.g., current/future health, family support network).
3. The health, social, and economic benefits of tobacco cessation should be stressed.
4. Patients should be encouraged to set a "quit date."
5. Self-help materials should be offered and drug therapy prescribed (if not contraindicated).
6. Clinicians should also review withdrawal symptoms with their patient (e.g., craving, difficulty concentrating, fatigue, headaches, shaking, nausea) and potential countermeasures.
7. Success can be improved with scheduled follow-up visits and referral to approved tobacco cessation programs or support groups.
8. Individuals who have not yet committed to tobacco cessation should be queried again at follow-up visits.

B. **Transtheoretical Model:** A five-stage model used in the process of tobacco cessation.

1. Precontemplation: Patient has no interest in tobacco cessation. Clinician should address tobacco cessation at next clinical appointment.
2. Contemplation: Patient has given serious thought to quitting but is not ready to make a serious attempt: "Yes, I am ready to quit, but the stress at work is too great." Clinician should address tobacco cessation again at the next clinical visit.
3. Preparation: Patient expresses serious intention to quit within the next month and may have tried to quit within the past 12 months. Clinician should facilitate tobacco cessation through

medication, referral to tobacco cessation programs, and counseling.

4. Action: Patient has taken steps to quit (e.g., joined a tobacco cessation program, paired with a quitting buddy, started using nicotine replacement products). Clinician should support the efforts to quit by discussing the patient's concerns or barriers to quitting and encouraging the patient to join a support group.
5. Maintenance of cessation: Former user is aware of the danger of relapse and has taken steps to remain tobacco free. Clinician should support the patient's efforts (e.g., support group, relaxation therapy, stress management classes).

III. HISTORY OF PRESENT ILLNESS

A. Use of Tobacco

1. Are you currently using tobacco?
2. Have you ever used tobacco?
3. What type (cigarettes, cloves, cigars, chew/smokeless tobacco)?
4. How much? Daily use and circumstances?
5. For how many years?
6. How old where you when you started?
7. How much do you spend on tobacco? Monthly and yearly costs?
8. Under what circumstances do you use tobacco?
9. Do you drink alcohol? What type? How much and how often?
10. Do you use other non-prescribed substances, including caffeine? What are they? How much and how often?
11. Have you attempted to stop using tobacco? (If no, move to Intervention section)
12. For how long (months or years) did you quit?
13. What method(s) did you use to quit?

B. Lifestyle and Psychologic Effects

1. What effect has tobacco use had on your general health?
2. Are you aware of any disability caused by tobacco use? Long-term effects?
3. What is your present occupation? Previous occupations?
4. What family, work, economic, or other life stressors are you currently experiencing?
5. Has your sleep pattern changed (disturbances by symptoms)?
6. Have your recreational activities changed?

C. Past Medical History

1. Have you had any illnesses that may be associated with your tobacco use?
2. Identify contraindications to drugs used to assist in tobacco cessation.

D. Family History: Have any family members had a malignancy, chronic obstructive pulmonary disease (COPD), addiction, or cardiovascular disease (CVD)?

E. Medications
1. What prescribed and over-the-counter (OTC) medications are you currently taking?
2. Have you had any allergies or adverse reactions to medications (e.g., nausea after taking medication, adhesive or tape allergy).

IV. REVIEW OF SYSTEMS (Table 39-1)

Table 39-1. TOBACCO-RELATED SYMPTOMS AND SYSTEMS AFFECTED.

SYSTEM	SYMPTOMS
General and neurovegetative	Malignancy (specify types), insomnia, syncope, weight loss, loss of appetite (anorexia), night sweats, fever, weakness/fatigue
HEENT	Allergies, recurrent ear infections/pain/discharge, dental problems, oral pain, sore throat, hoarseness, voice changes, nasal discharge, obstruction, or epistaxis
Skin	Baldness, skin color, pigmentation, bruising, bleeding, clubbing of digits
Respiratory	Cough (productive or nonproductive), hemoptysis, chest pain (with or without radiation), shortness of breath (SOB), dyspnea, wheezing, orthopnea, pleurisy, bronchitis, asthma, pneumonia
Cardiovascular	Chest pain (with or without radiation, quality, duration, activity that precipitates episodes), tachycardia, palpitations, exertional dyspnea, orthopnea, cyanosis, leg pain/claudication (quality, duration, activity that precipitates events), paroxysmal nocturnal dyspnea (PND), foot swelling
Gastrointestinal	Symptoms of reflux or abdominal pain, dysphagia, hematemesis
Genitourinary	Erectile dysfunction, hematuria, pelvic pain, flank pain, nocturia
Obstetrics and Gynecology	Low birth-weight infants
Infectious disease	Frequent infections/colds/pneumonia
Musculoskeletal	Chronic pain
Neuropsychiatric	History of addiction, insomnia, or mental illness
Hematopoietic	Lymphadenopathy, thrombosis

V. PHYSICAL EXAMINATION (Table 39-2)

Table 39-2. TOBACCO-RELATED PHYSICAL EXAMINATION.

System	Symptoms
Vital signs and General	Note blood pressure, pulse, respirations, cachexia
HEENT	Note discolorations, ulcerations, odor, masses
Cardiovascular	Auscultate for heart sounds/dysrhythmias/ murmurs, check position of heart, pulses, jugulovenous distension, cyanosis, edema, consider performing an ECG on all current/ex-smokers
Pulmonary	Note abnormal breath sounds (crackles/rales, wheezes, rhonchi, rubs), resonance/ hyperresonance, thoracic deformities, chest movement, tracheal deviation, mass(es), percussion
Other	Chest x-ray, as indicated by history and review of systems (ROS)

VI. DEFINITIONS (Table 39-3)

Table 39-3. TOBACCO-RELATED TERMS AND ACRONYMS.

Term or Acronym	Definition
COPD	Chronic obstructive pulmonary disease
Fagerstrom test	Survey administered to determine nicotine dependence
Nicotine withdrawal symptoms	Includes depression, frustration, anger, irritability, trouble sleeping, difficulty concentrating, restlessness, headache, tiredness, and increased appetite
NRT	Nicotine replacement therapy (e.g., patches, gum, nasal spray)
Pack year history	Number of packs per day multiplied by the number of years smoked

VII. TOBACCO INTERVENTIONS

A. Tobacco's Addictive Properties

1. Users develop both a physiologic and psychologic dependence to nicotine.
2. A constant supply of nicotine in the blood is required to prevent the onset of withdrawal symptoms that occur because of the physiologic dependence.
3. After two weeks of abstinence, patients no longer experience withdrawal symptoms, but they do continue to experience craving, which is an uncontrollable desire for cigarettes that results from an even more powerful psychologic dependence.
4. Regular use of tobacco becomes integrated into patients' daily routines, including part of their social network.
   a. Tobacco users develop triggers (events that result in the urge to use tobacco, e.g., drinking coffee, talking on the phone, driving a car).
   b. Tobacco helps users cope with stress (e.g., taking a cigarette break when anxious), alleviate boredom (e.g., smoking is something to do), or just relax (e.g., smoking while reading).
   c. The psychologic dependence must be targeted if an individual is going to be successful.
   d. Only 10% of smokers who "quit cold turkey" are smoke-free after one year.
5. Successful tobacco cessation programs often incorporate behavior modification techniques into their program.
   a. Identification of environmental cues associated with tobacco use.
   b. Modification of behavior to make cues ineffective (e.g., avoidance, relaxation techniques).
   c. Reinforcement of positive behavior patterns.
6. Programs that incorporate use of nicotine replacement products are generally more successful than those that don't because their use allows patients to focus on their behavior patterns. Regardless, most patients make several attempts at stopping before they succeed.

B. Counseling

1. Clinicians should face the patient (either sitting or standing) and maintain eye contact.
2. There should be no physical barriers (e.g., desk, wall).
3. Begin with a brief, unambiguous, and informative statement such as "As your health care provider, I advise you to quit smoking."
4. Briefly review the pertinent health, social, and economic benefits of quitting.
5. If the patient is not contemplating stopping, provide motivation again at the next visit. If the patient expresses a desire to stop, delve into patient's concerns or barriers, negotiate a "quit

date," review withdrawal symptoms, discuss use of medications, support finding a "quitting buddy" to increase chance of succeeding, and encourage entrance into a certified tobacco cessation program or support group.

6. Counseling can be accomplished in either group or individual sessions.

VIII. BACKGROUND ON TOBACCO

A. Costs of Tobacco Use

1. Use of tobacco products is the primary cause of preventable disease and death in the United States.
2. Tobacco use costs the health care system more than $50 billion each year.
3. Use results in more than 430,000 deaths per year (approximately 1 of every 5 deaths are tobacco-related).
4. Use promotes atherosclerosis and is thereby a leading risk factor for heart disease, which causes 100,000 deaths per year), cerebrovascular disease (CVD), which results in 23,000 deaths per year, and peripheral vascular disease (PVD).
5. Tobacco use has been associated with approximately 148,000 cancer-related deaths annually, particularly malignancies of the lung, trachea, bronchus, larynx, pharynx, oral cavity, and esophagus.
6. Risk for pancreatic, kidney, bladder, and cervical malignancies are increased.
7. Use is associated with respiratory illness, including COPD and pneumonia.

B. Benefits of Tobacco Sensation: Many studies have demonstrated improvement in health risks with tobacco cessation.

1. Following discontinuation, smoking-related elevations of the pulse rate and blood pressure (BP) return to normal, circulation improves, and carbon monoxide (CO) levels in the blood decline.
2. Cessation reduces COPD mortality rates, respiratory symptoms, and infections.
3. Risk of dying from cardiovascular heart disease or having a myocardial infarction (MI) is halved within a year of stopping.
4. After 5 years of abstinence, the risk of acquiring oral or pharyngeal cancer is 50% of that of current smokers.
5. After 10 years of remaining smoke-free, lung cancer risk is halved; after 15 years, the risk approaches that of nonsmokers.

C. Attempts at Quitting

1. More than 70% of the 50 million current tobacco users in the United States have made at least one attempt to quit; 50% of tobacco users try to quit each year. Attempts are generally more successful with the encouragement and support of providers.
2. Only 50% of current smokers have been urged to quit by their providers. Clinicians may feel reluctant to intervene because of

lack of confidence regarding counseling on tobacco cessation, lack of patient interest, lack of financial reimbursement, insufficient time, or inadequate staff support.

3. Most medical schools do not require clinical training in tobacco cessation. Only 21 % of currently practicing physicians feel adequately trained to help their patients quit using tobacco.

IX. DOCUMENTATION

For medical and legal purposes, be sure that all aspects of the patient encounter are well documented in the SOAP(P) format, highlighting pertinent examination findings and interventions.

Sample Note in SOAP(P) Format

Name: ID #:
Date of Visit: Allergies:
Vitals: T: P: R: BP:
Medications:

Subjective:

Reason for visit: Tobacco Screening.

1. Type of product.
2. Use and circumstances.
3. Monthly cost.
4. Years used and age at first use.
5. Past medical history and family history: Hypertension (HTN), cardiovascular disease, peripheral vascular disease (PVD), bronchitis, asthma, environmental allergies, recurrent ear infections, erectile dysfunction, dental problems, cancer, other problems.
6. Alcohol and other non-prescribed substances.
7. Prior cessation attempts.
8. Method of cessation and length of abstinence.

Objective:

Ear-Nose-Throat (ENT) exam:
Cardiovascular exam:
Pulmonary exam:
Other (as indicated by history):

Assessment: Tobacco Use Disorder.

Plan: Advised patient to stop tobacco use. Provided information on self-help and group therapy and discussed additional medication options. Patient (will/will not) set quit date. Follow-up by (telephone/appointment) in “x” weeks.

Prevention (P2): Discussed triad of addiction and ways to stop or decrease use of all three (cigarettes, alcohol, and caffeine).

Bibliography

SECTION I ESSENTIALS OF THE HISTORY AND PHYSICAL EXAMINATION

CHAPTER 1 HISTORY AND PHYSICAL EXAMINATION (H&P) ESSENTIALS

Burnside, McGlynn. Physical Diagnosis. ed 17. Baltimore: Williams and Wilkins, 1987.

Gomella LG. Clinician's Pocket Reference: The Scut Monkey's Handbook. Norwalk, Conn: Appleton and Lange, 1989.

Krupp MA, Tierney LM, Jawetz E, Roe RL, Camargo CA. Physicians Handbook. ed 21. Los Altos, Calif: Lange Medical Publications, 1985;26-29.

Macklis RM, Mendelson ME, Mudge GH. Manual of Introductory Clinical Medicine. A Student-to-Student Guide, ed 2. Boston: Little, Brown and Co (LBSM), 1989;5-20.

Novey DW. Rapid Access Guide to the Physical Examination. Chicago: Year Book Medical Publishers, 1988.

Rothwell W. "Sample PE Write Up, PE" H & P Cards. A Pocket Reference to the Adult History and Physical Examination. Rochester, Minn: Medical Imagineering, 1989.

Rothwell W. "Adult History" H & P Cards. A Pocket Reference to the Adult History and Physical Examination. Rochester, Minn: Medical Imagineering, 1989.

CHAPTER 2 RECORDING LABORATORY VALUES AND DIAGNOSTIC INFORMATION, AND CONVERSION TABLES

Krupp MA, Tierney LM, Jawetz E, Roe RL, Camargo CA. Physicians Handbook, ed 21. Los Altos, Calif: Lange Medical Publications, 1985;156.

Lentner C (ed). Geigy Scientific Tables, ed 8. West Caldwell, NJ: Ciba-Geigy Corporation, 1984;3:78-90, 210.

CHAPTER 3 ASSESSMENT AND PLAN FORMULATION

Braunwald E, Isselbacher JK, Petersdorf RG, Wilson JD, Martin JB, Fauci AS (eds). Harrison's Principles of Internal Medicine, ed 11. New York: McGraw-Hill Book Co, 1987;141-144, 149-153, 905-915.

Eisenberg MS, Cummins RO. Blue Book of Medical Diagnosis. Philadelphia: WB Saunders, 1986;37-45.

Krupp MA, Tierney LM, Jawetz E, Roe RL, Camargo CA. Physicians Handbook, ed 21. Los Altos, Calif: Lange Medical Publications, 1985;29-32.

Macklis RM, Mendelson ME, Mudge GH. Manual of Introductory Clinical Medicine. A Student-to-Student Guide. ed 2. Boston: Little, Brown and Co (LBSM), 1988;131-143.

Wolcott BW. Basic decisions in emergency department cases: a logical approach. JACEP. April 1978;7:149-151.

CHAPTER 4 CHARTWORK GUIDELINES

Gomella LG. Clinician's Pocket Reference, ed 6. Norwalk, Conn: Appleton and Lange, 1989;17-20.

CHAPTER 5 PRESENTATION OF MEDICAL CASES

Cotran RS et al. Robbins Pathologic Basis of Disease, ed 5. Philadelphia: WB Saunders, 1994;111-112.

Myers A. Medicine, ed 3. Baltimore: Williams and Wilkins, 1997;137.
Rosen P et al (eds). Emergency Medicine: Concepts and Clinical Practice, ed 3. St. Louis: Mosby-Year Book, 1992;1770-1800.

CHAPTER 6 DEATH CERTIFICATION

Selby D, Clark B, Cina S. Accuracy of death certification in two tertiary care military hospitals. Military Med 1999;164(12):897-899.
Froede RC (ed). Handbook of Forensic Pathology, ed 2. Northfield, Ill: College of American Pathologists, 2003.
Hanzlick R (ed). The Medical Cause of Death Manual. Northfield, Ill: College of American Pathologists, 1994.
Medical Certifier Instructions for selected items on the U.S. Standard Death Certificate. Retrieved from www.cdc.gov/nchs/about/major/dvs/vital_certs_rev/death1_and_instruc_2_5_acc.pdf.

SECTION II SPECIALTY HISTORY AND PHYSICAL EXAMINATION

CHAPTER 8 ANESTHESIA

Barash PG, Cullen BF, Stoelting RK (eds). Clinical Anesthesia, ed 2. Philadelphia: JB Lippincott, 1992.
Braunwald E et al (eds). Harrison's Principles of Internal Medicine, ed 15. New York: McGraw-Hill, 2001.
O'Hara DA. Heal the Pain, Comfort the Spirit. Philadelphia: University of Pennsylvania Press, 2002.
Stoelting RK, Miller RD. Basics of Anesthesia, ed 3. New York: Churchill Livingstone, 1994.

CHAPTER 9 CARDIOLOGY

Braunwald E (ed). Heart Disease: A Textbook of Cardiovascular Medicine, ed 5. Philadelphia: WB Saunders, 1997.
Constant J. Bedside Cardiology, ed 5. Baltimore: Lippincott Williams & Wilkins, 1999.
DeGowin RL. DeGowin's Diagnostic Examination, ed 6. New York: McGraw-Hill, 1994.
Georgetown University School of Medicine. The Essentials of the Cardiovascular Examination, A student's handout developed by the Division of Cardiology, 1992.
Harvey WP. Cardiac Pearls. Newton, NJ: Laennec Publishing, 1993.
Lembo NJ. Bedside diagnosis of systolic murmurs. N Engl J Med 1988;38(24):1572.
Seidel HM (ed). Mosby's Guide to Physical Examination, ed 4. St. Louis: Mosby, 1999.
Wyngaarden JB (ed). Cecil Textbook of Medicine, ed 19. Philadelphia: WB Saunders, 1992.

CHAPTER 10 DERMATOLOGY

Clinical Dermatology: A Color Guide to Diagnosis and Therapy.
Kusch SL. Clinical Dermatology: A Manual of Differential Diagnosis. Westwood Pharmaceuticals Inc.

CHAPTER 11 EMERGENCY MEDICINE (TRAUMA ASSESSMENT FOCUS)

American College of Surgeons Committee and Subcommittee on Trauma Members. Advanced Trauma Life Support Student Manual. Chicago: American College of Surgeons, 1989.

American College of Surgeons Committee on Trauma Brent Eastman and Subcommittee on Advanced Trauma Life Support of the American College of Surgeons Committee on Trauma 1988-1992, Advanced Trauma Life Support Reference Manual. Chicago: American College of Surgeons, 1994.

Saunders C, Ao MT (eds). Current Emergency Diagnosis and Treatment: The Multiply Injured Patient (Donald D. Trunkey), ed 4. Lange Medical Book.

Tintinalli (Ruiz E, author of section). Emergency Medicine, ed 3;906-909.

CHAPTER 12 ENDOCRINOLOGY

Baxter JD. Introduction to Endocrinology: Basic and Clinical Endocrinology, ed 6. New York: McGraw-Hill Medical Publishing, 1997;27-28.

Becker KL (ed). Principles and Practice of Endocrinology and Metabolism, ed 2. Philadelphia: Lippincott, 1995.

DeGowin RL. DeGowin & DeGowin. Bedside Diagnostic Examination, ed 5. New York: Macmillan, 1981;884-969.

Mahley RW, Weisraber KH, Farese RV Jr. Disorders of lipid metabolism. In Williams RH, Foster DW, Kronenberg HM, Lason PR, Wilson JD (eds), Williams Textbook of Endocrinology, ed 9. Philadelphia: W.B. Saunders, 1998;1125-1136.

McCulloch DK. Evaluation of the Diabetic Foot. Chevy Chase, Md: UpToDate Inc., 1999.

Wartofsky L. The thyroid gland. In Principles and Practice of Endocrinology and Metabolism, ed 2. Philadelphia: Lippincott, 1995;278-280.

CHAPTER 14 GYNECOLOGY

Berek JS, Adashi EY, Hillard PA. Novak's Gynecology, ed 12. Williams and Wilkins, 1996.

Mishell DR, Stenchever MA, Droegemueller W, Herbst A. Comprehensive Gynecology, ed 3. Mosby, 1997.

Scott JR, DiSaia PJ, Hammond CB, Spellacy WN. Danforth's Obsterics and Gynecology, ed 7. JB Lippincott, 1994.

CHAPTER 15 HEMATOLOGY

McKenna R. Acute leukemias. In C Kjeldsberg (ed), Practical Diagnosis of Hematologic Disorders, ed 2. Chicago: ASCP Press, 1995;355-440.

Meideros LJ, Carr J. Overview of the role of molecular methods in the diagnosis of malignant lymphomas. Arch Pathol Lab Med 1999;123:1189-1207.

Perkins S, Foucar K. Anemias. In C Kjeldsberg (ed), Practical Diagnosis of Hematologic Disorders, ed 2. Chicago: ASCP Press, 1995;3-224.

Peterson P. Myeloproliferative disorders. In C Kjeldsberg (ed), Practical Diagnosis of Hematologic Disorders, ed 2. Chicago: ASCP Press, 1995;441-490.

Rodgers G. Bleeding disorders. In C Kjeldsberg (ed), Practical Diagnosis of Hematologic Disorders, ed 2. Chicago: ASCP Press, 1995;625-722.

Rodgers G. Thrombotic disorders. In C Kjeldsberg (ed), Practical Diagnosis of Hematologic Disorders, ed 2. Chicago: ASCP Press, 1995;723-744.

Triplett DA. Coagulation abnormalities. In KD McClatchey (ed), Clinical Laboratory Medicine. Baltimore: Williams and Wilkins, 1997;1081-1099.

CHAPTER 16 INFECTIOUS DISEASE

Durack D, Street A. Fever of unknown origin-reexamined and redefined. In Remington J, Swartz M (eds), Current Clinical Topics of Infectious Diseases. St. Louis: Mosby Year Book, 1991;35.

IDSA Practice Guidelines Committee. Clin Infect Dis 1997;25:574-583.

Petersdorf RG, Beeson PB. Fever of unexplained origin. Report on 100 cases Medicine 1961;40.

Speck EL, Murray HW. Fever and fever of unknown etiology. In Reese RE, Betts RF (eds), A Practical Approach to Infectious Diseases, ed 3. Boston: Little, Brown and Company, 1991;1-15.

CHAPTER 18 INTERNAL MEDICINE AND FAMILY PRACTICE

Marino PL. The ICU Book, ed 2. Baltimore: Williams and Wilkins, 1998.
Parrillo JE, Dellinger RP (eds). Critical Care Medicine: Principles of Diagnosis and Management in the Adult, ed 2. Philadelphia: Mosby, 2001.
Shoemaker WC (ed). Textbook of Critical Care, ed 4. Philadelphia: Saunders, 2000.

CHAPTER 19 NEONATOLOGY

Behrman RE, Kliegman R, Jenson HB. Nelson Textbook of Pediatrics, ed 16. Philadelphia: WB Saunders, 2000.
Fanaroff AA, Martin RJ. Neonatal-Perinatal Medicine: Diseases of the Fetus and Infant, ed 7. St. Louis: Mosby-Year Book, 2001.
Avroy A, Gomella TL, Cunningham MD, Eyal FG, Zenk KE. Neonatology: Management, Procedures, On-Call Problems, Diseases, and Drugs, ed 4. New York: McGraw-Hill Professional Publishing, 1999.
Siberry GK, Iannone R, Childs C. The Harriet Lane Handbook: A Manual for Pediatric House Officers, ed 15. St. Louis: Mosby-Year Book, 2000.
Swartz MH. Textbook of Physical Diagnosis: History and Examination, ed 2. Philadelphia: WB Saunders, 1997.
Zitelli BJ, Davis HW. Atlas of Pediatric Physical Diagnosis, ed 3. St. Louis, Mosby-Year Book, 1997.

CHAPTER 20 NEPHROLOGY

Massory and Glassock's Textbook of Nephrology.
Manual of Nephrology, edited by Robert Schrier.
Primer on Kidney Diseases, NKF, edited Arthur Greenberg.
Nephrology House Officer Series, edited by C. Craig Tischer.
The Principles and Practice of Nephrology, edited by Harry R. Jacobson, et al.
Pathophysiology of Renal Disease, edited by Burton D. Rose.

CHAPTER 21 NEUROLOGY

Anderson JE. Grant's Atlas of Anatomy, ed 8. Baltimore, Md: Williams and Wilkins, 1983.
DeGroot J, Chusid JG. Correlative Neuroanatomy, ed 20. East Norwalk, Conn: Appleton and Lange, 1988;382-383, 408-413.
DeMeyer WE. Technique of the Neurologic Examination: A Programmed Text, ed 4. New York: McGraw-Hill, 1993.
DeMeyer W. Neuroanatomy. The National Medical Series for Independent Study. Media, Penn: John Wiley and Sons;1988:355-361.
Fuller G. Neurological Examination Made Easy, ed 2. New York: Churchill Livingstone, 1999.
Haerer A. DeJong's The Neurologic Examination, ed 5. Philadelphia: Lippincott Williams & Wilkins, 1992.
Hoppenfeld S. Orthopaedic Neurology. A Diagnostic Guide to Neurologic Levels. Philadelphia, Penn: JB Lippincott Co;1977:2.
Hoppenfeld S. Physical Examination of the Spine and Extremities. Norwalk, Conn: Appleton-Century-Crofts;1976:119.
Weiner HL. Neurology for the House Officer. Baltimore, Md: Williams and Wilkins, 1983.

CHAPTER 22 OBSTETRICS

American College of Obstetricians and Gynecologists. The Obstetrician-Gynecologist and Primary-Preventive Health Care. ACOG, 1993.
Cruikshank DP, Wigton TR, Hays PM. Maternal physiology in pregnancy. In Gabbe SG, Niebyl JR, Simpson JL (eds), Obstetrics: Normal and Problem Pregnancies, ed 3. New York: Churchill Livingstone, 1996.
Fuchs AR. Physiology and endocrinology of lactation. In Gabbe SG, Niebyl JR, Simpson JL (eds), Obstetrics: Normal and Problem Pregnancies, ed 3. New York: Churchill Livingstone, 1996.

Gordon MC, Landon MB. Dermatologic disorders. In Gabbe SG, Niebyl JR, Simpson JL (eds), Obstetrics: Normal and Problem Pregnancies, ed 3. New York: Churchill Livingstone, 1996.

Johnson TRB, Walker MA, Niebyl JR. Preconception and prenatal care. In Gabbe SG, Niebyl JR, Simpson JL (eds), Obstetrics: Normal and Problem Pregnancies, ed 3. New York: Churchill Livingstone, 1996.

Sever LE, Mortensen ME. Teratology and the epidemiology of birth defects: Occupational and environmental perspectives. In Gabbe SG, Niebyl JR, Simpson JL (eds), Obstetrics: Normal and Problem Pregnancies, ed 3. New York: Churchill Livingstone, 1996.

CHAPTER 23 OCCUPATIONAL MEDICINE

Centers for Disease Control and Prevention, Office of Communication, Facts about Occupational Injuries, Sept 12, 1997. www.cdc.gov/od/oc/media/fact/safety.htm.

Greaves WW (ed). Occupational and Environmental Medicine "Pearls" of the Specialty. Beverly: OEM Press;1996.

Kusnetz S, Hutchinson MK. A Guide to the Work-Relatedness of Disease (revised edition), U.S. Department of Health, Education, and Welfare, Public Health Service, Centers for Disease Control and Prevention, National Institute for Occupational Safety and Health, January 1979.

LaDou J. Occupational and Environmental Medicine, A Lange Medical Book, ed 2. Appleton and Lange, A Simon and Schuster Company, Stamford, Conn;1997.

McCunney RJ (ed). Practical Approach to Occupational and Environmental Medicine, ed 2. Boston: Little, Brown and Company;1994.

Rom WN (ed). Environmental and Occupational Medicine, ed 3. Philadelphia: Lippincott-Raven;1998.

Wallace RB, Doebbeling BN, Last JM. Maxcy-Rosenau-Last, Public Health and Preventive Medicine, ed 14. Appleton and Lange, Stamford, Conn;1998.

CHAPTER 24 ONCOLOGY

Carlson HE, Lowitz BB, Casciato DA. Endocrine neoplasms. In Casciato DA, Lowitz BB (eds), Manual of Clinical Oncology, ed 3. Boston: Little, Brown and Company;268-287.

Einhorn LH, Lowitz BB. Testicular cancer. In Casciato DA, Lowitz BB (eds), Manual of Clinical Oncology, ed 3. Boston: Little, Brown and Company;228-236.

Farias-Eisner RO, Walker DL, Berek JS. Gynecologic cancers. In Casciato DA, Lowitz BB (eds), Manual of Clinical Oncology, ed 3. Boston: Little, Brown and Company;200-227.

Figlin RA, deKernion JB. Urinary tract cancers. In Casciato DA, Lowitz BB (eds), Manual of Clinical Oncology, ed 3. Boston: Little, Brown and Company;237-257.

Haskell CM, Casciato DA. Breast cancer. In Casciato DA, Lowitz BB (eds), Manual of Clinical Oncology, ed 3. Boston: Little, Brown and Company;183-199.

Mack EE. Neurologic tumors. In Casciato DA, Lowitz BB (eds), Manual of Clinical Oncology, ed 3. Boston: Little, Brown and Company;258-267.

Parker RG, Rice DH, Casciato DA. Head and neck cancers. In Casciato DA, Lowitz BB (eds), Manual of Clinical Oncology, ed 3. Boston: Little, Brown and Company;1995:113-132.

Rosen PJ. Hodgkin's disease and malignant lymphoma. In Casciato DA, Lowitz BB (eds), Manual of Clinical Oncology, ed 3. Boston: Little, Brown and Company;347-385.

Tabbarah HJ, Lowitz BB, Livingston RB. Lung cancer. In Casciato DA, Lowitz BB (eds), Manual of Clinical Oncology, ed 3. Boston: Little, Brown and Company;133-144.

Tabbarah HJ. Gastrointestinal tract cancers. In Casciato DA, Lowitz BB (eds), Manual of Clinical Oncology, ed 3. Boston: Little, Brown and Company;145-182.

Wagner RF, Casciato DA. Skin cancers. In Casciato DA, Lowitz BB (eds), Manual of Clinical Oncology, ed 3. Boston: Little, Brown and Company;288-299.

CHAPTER 25 OPHTHALMOLOGY

Basic and Clinical Science Course 2001-2002, American Academy of Ophthalmology.

The Wills Eye Manuel, ed 3. Lippincott Williams and Wilkins.

CHAPTER 26 ORTHOPEDICS

Greene WB (ed). Essentials of Musculoskeletal Care, ed 2. Rosemont, Ill: American Academy of Orthopaedic Surgeons, 2000.
Iverson LD, Clawson DK. Manual of Acute Orthopaedic Therapeutics. Boston: Little, Brown and Co, 1987.
Hoppenfeld S, Hutton R. Physical Examination of the Spine and Extremities. New York: Appleton-Century-Crofts, 1976.
Hoppenfeld S. Orthopaedic Neurology. A Diagnostic Guide to Neurologic Levels. Philadelphia: JB Lippincott Co, 1977.
Magee DJ. Orthopedic Physical Assessment, ed 2. Philadelphia: WB Saunders, 1992.
Mercier LR. Practical Orthopedics, ed 2. Chicago: Yearbook Medical Publishers Inc, 1987.
Snider RK, editor. Essentials of Musculoskeletal Care, American Academy of Orthopaedic Surgeons, Rosemont, Ill: 1997.
Wadsworth CT. Manual Examination and Treatment of the Spine and Extremities. Baltimore, Md: Williams and Wilkins, 1988.
Wilson FC, Lin PP. General Orthopaedics. New York: McGraw Hill Co., 1997.

CHAPTER 28 PATHOLOGY (AUTOPSY AND LAB UTILIZATION)

The Power of a Test

Henry JB, Kurec AS. The clinical laboratory: Organization, purposes, and practice. In Henry JB (ed), Clinical Diagnosis and Management by Laboratory Methods, ed 19. Philadelphia: WB Saunders, 1996;76-77.
Annesley TM. Analytical test variables. In McClatchey KD (ed). Clinical Laboratory Medicine. Baltimore, Md: Williams and Wilkins, 1997;92-95.

Specimen Collection

Henry JB, Kurec AS. The clinical laboratory: Organization, purposes, and practice. In Henry JB (ed), Clinical Diagnosis and Management by Laboratory Methods, ed 19. Philadelphia: WB Saunders Co, 1996;1-24.

Chemistry

Lee-Lewandrowski E, Lewandrowski K. The plasma proteins. In McClatchey KD (ed). Clinical Laboratory Medicine. Baltimore: Williams and Wilkins, 1997;239-258.
Wiebe DA, Artiss JD. Lipids, lipoproteins, and apolipoproteins. In McClatchey KD (ed), Clinical Laboratory Medicine. Baltimore: Williams and Wilkins, 1997;287-302.
Moyer TP, Lawson GM. Theraputic drug monitoring. In McClatchey KD. Clinical Laboratory Medicine. Baltimore: Williams and Wilkins, 1997;445-468.
Kwong TC. Toxicology. In McClatchey KD (ed). Clinical Laboratory Medicine. Baltimore: Williams and Wilkins, 1997;469-490.
Gianni E, Botta F, Fasoli A, Ceppa P, Risso D, Lantieri B, Celle G, Testa R. Progressive liver functional impairment is associated with an increase in AST/ALT ratio. Dig Dis Sci 1999;6:1249-1253.
Mayfield ED. Endocrinology I and II, Acid-base and electrolytes, and Enzymes and liver, extracted from Osler Notes, 1997.
Aziz DC. Clinical use of tumor markers based on outcome analysis. Lab Med 1996;27:817-821.
Wu HB, Apple FS, Gibler WB, Jesse RL, Warshaw MM, Valdes R. National academy of clinical biochemistry standards of laboratory practice: Recommendations for the use of cardiac markers in coronary artery diseases. Clin Chem 1999:45:1104-1121.
Keffer JH. Myocardial markers of injury, evolution and insights. Clin Chem 199:105:305-315.
Check W. Reaching agreement on tumor markers. CAP Today 1998:36-52.

Henry JB, Kurec AS. The clinical laboratory: Organization, purposes, and practice. In Henry JB (ed), Clinical Diagnosis and Management by Laboratory Methods, ed 19. Philadelphia: WB Saunders Company, 1996;238-240.

Blood Bank

Chaffin DJ. Blood Bank I-III, extracted from Osler Notes, 1997.

Vengelen-Tyler V (ed). Technical Manuel, ed 12. American Association of Blood Banks. Bethesda, Md. 1996, 78-80, 86-101, 115-131, 136-156, 213-227, 255-275, 331-347, 379-459, 543-562.

Sazama K, DeChristopher PJ, Dodd R, Harrison C, Shulman I, Cooper S, Labotka RJ, Oberman HA, Zahn CM, Greenberg G, Stehling L, Lauenstein KJ, Price TH, Williams L. Practice parameter for the recognition, management, and prevention of adverse consequences of blood transfusion. Arch Pathol Lab Med 2000;124:61-70.

Immunology

Sinard JH. Outlines in Pathology, W.B Saunders Company. New Haven, Conn, 1996;6-11.

Robbins SL, Cotran RS, Kumar V. Pocket Companion to Robbins Pathologic Basis of Disease. Philadelphia: WB Saunders, 1995;86.

Carey III JL, Keren DF. Autoimmune disease and serology. In McClatchey KD (ed), Clinical Laboratory. Baltimore: Williams and Wilkins, 1997;1612.

Duquesnoy RJ. Histocompatibility testing in organ transplantation. Lab Med 1999;30:796-801.

Kavanaugh A, Tomar R, Reveille J, Soloman DH, Homburger HA. Guidelines for clinical use of the antinuclear antibody test and tests for specific autoantibodies to nuclear antigens. Arch Pathol Lab Med 2000;124:71-81.

Microbiology

Levinson W, Jawetz W. Medical Microbiology and Immunology, ed 5. Stanford, Conn: Appleton and Lange, 1998;1-313.

Molecular Pathology

Hanson CA. Clinical applications of molecular biology in diagnostic hematopathology. Lab Med 1995;24:562-573.

Medeiros LF, Carr J. Overview of the role of molecular methods in the diagnosis of malignant lymphoma. Arch Pathol Lab Med 1999;123:1189-1207.

Sreekantaiah C, Ladanyi M, Rodriguez E, Chaganti RS. Chromosomal aberrations in soft tissue tumors. Relevance to diagnosis, classification, and molecular mechanisms. Am J Pathol 1994;144:1121-1134.

Rabbits TH. Chromosomal translocations in human cancer. Nature 1994;372:143-149.

Cooper CS. Translocations in solid tumours. Cur Op Gen Develop 1996;6:71-75.

Wolman SR. Chromosomal markers: Signposts on the road to understanding neoplastic diseases. Diag Cytopathol 1998;18:18-23.

Dal Cin P, Van den Berghe V. Ten years if the cytogenetics of soft tissue tumors. Cancer Genet Cytogenet 1997;95:59-66.

Anatomic Pathology

Society for Ultrastructural Pathology, Handbook Committee. Handbook of Diagnostic Electron Microscopy for Pathologists-in-Training. New York NY, Igaku-Shoin Medical Publishers;1996:1-1 to 2-3.

Hasson J, Schneiderman H. Autopsy training programs; to Right a wrong. Arch Pathol Lab Med 1995:119:289-291.

Cote RJ, Taylor CR. Immunohistochemistry and related marking techniques. In: Anderson's Pathology, ed 10. Damjanov I, Linder J (eds), St. Louis: Mosby-Year Book: 1996;136-163.

Beckstead JH. Histochemistry. In: Anderson's Pathology, ed 10. Damjanov I, Linder J (eds), St. Louis: Mosby-Year Book, 1996;176-189.
Rosai J. Ackerman's Surgical Pathology. St. Louis: Mosby-Year Book, 1996.
Hanzlick R (ed). The Medical Cause of Death Manual. College of American Pathologists, Northfield Ill, 1994.

CHAPTER 29 PEDIATRICS

Behrman RE et al. Nelson's Textbook of Pediatrics, ed 16. Philadelphia: WB Saunders, 2000.
Ehrman WG, Matson SC. Approach to assessing adolescents on serious sensitive issues. Pediatr Clin North Am 1998;45:189-204.
Johnson KB, Oski FA. Oski's Essential Pediatrics. Philadelphia: Lippincott-Raven, 1997.
National High Blood Pressure Education Program, Working Group on Hypertension Control in Children and Adolescents. Update on the 1987 Task Force Report on High Blood Pressure in Children and Adolescents: A Working Group Report from the National High Blood Pressure Education Program. Pediatrics 1996;98:649-658.
Siberry GK, Iannone R. The Harriet Lane Handbook: A Manual for Pediatric House Officers, ed 15. St. Louis: Mosby; 2000.

CHAPTER 30 PREVENTIVE MEDICINE

American Academy of Pediatrics. Report of the Committee on Infectious Diseases. Elk Grove Village, Ill: AAP, 1991.
Centers for Disease Control and Prevention. Advisory Committee on Immunization Practices: Recommendations for use of haemophilus b conjugate vaccines and a combined diphtheria, tetanus, pertussis, and haemophilus b vaccine. Morbidity and Mortality Weekly Report 1993;42(RR-13):1-15, Centers for Disease Control and Prevention. Advisory Committee on Immunization Practices: General recommendations on immunizations. Morbidity and Mortality Weekly Report 1994;43(RR-1):1-38.
Centers for Disease Control and Prevention. Case Definitions for Infectious Conditions under Public Health Surveillance. Morbidity and Mortality Weekly Report 1997;46(RR-10):1-55.
Centers for Disease Control and Prevention. Health Information for International Travel, 2001-2002. U.S. Department of Health and Human Services. Public Health Service. Atlanta: National Center for Infectious Diseases, 2001.
Centers for Disease Control and Prevention. CDC Publishes Updated Poliomyelitis Prevention Recommendations for the U.S. Morbidity and Mortality Weekly Report 2000;49:1-22.
Centers for Disease Control and Prevention. Screening for Tuberculosis and Tuberculosis Infection in High-Risk Populations/Recommendations of the Advisory Council for the Elimination of Tuberculosis. Morbidity and Mortality Weekly Report 1995;44(RR-11):18-34.
Jekel JF, Katz DL. Epidemiology, Biostatistics, and Preventive Medicine, Saunders Text and Review Series. Philadelphia: WB Saunders, 1996.
U.S. Department of Health and Human Services. Clinician's Handbook of Preventive Services: Put Prevention into Practice. Washington DC: USDHHS, Office of Public Health and Science, Office of Disease Prevention and Health Promotion, 1998.
U.S. Preventive Services Task Force. Guide to Clinical Preventive Services. Baltimore: Williams and Wilkins, 1989.

CHAPTER 31 PSYCHIATRY

Dubovsky SL. Concise Guide to Clinical Psychiatry. Washington, DC: American Psychiatric Press, 1988.
Folstein MF, Folstein SE, McHugh PR. Mini-mental state: A practical method for grading the cognitive state of patients for the clinician, J Psych Res 1975;12:189-198.

Kaplan HI, Sadock BJ. Synopsis of Psychiatry. Behavioral Sciences, Clinical Psychiatry, ed 5. Baltimore: Williams and Wilkins, 1988.
Wise MG, Randall JR. Concise Guide to Consultation Psychiatry. Washington, DC: American Psychiatric Press, 1988; pp. 12-13.

CHAPTER 32 PULMONOLOGY

Bates B et al. A Guide to Physical Examination and History Taking, ed 6. Philadelphia: JB Lippincott, 1995.
Bennet P et al. Cecil's Textbook of Medicine, ed 20. Philadelphia: WB Saunders, 1996.
Braunwald E, Fanci AS, Hauser SL, Longo DL, Jameson JL (eds). Harrison's Principles of Internal Medicine, ed 15. New York: McGraw Hill Companies, 2001.
Marino P. The ICU Book, ed 2. Baltimore: Williams & Wilkins, 1998.
Murray JF, Nadel JA, Mason. Textbook of Respiratory Medicine, ed 3. Philadelphia: WB Saunders, 1998.
Rakel R. Textbook of Family Practice, ed 6. Philadelphia: WB Saunders, 2002.
Wilkins RK, Sheldon RL, Krider SJ. Clinical Assessment in Respiratory Care, ed 4. Philadelphia: Lippincott Williams & Wilkins, 2000.

CHAPTER 33 GENERAL SURGERY

Abernathy CM, Harken AH. Surgical Secrets. Philadelphia: Hanley and Belfus, 1991.
Bloomfield RL, Chandler ET. Pocket Mnemonics for Practitioners. Charlotte, NC: Delmar, 1983.
Clain A (ed). Hamilton Bailey's Demonstrations of Physical Signs in Clinical Surgery. Baltimore: Williams and Wilkins, 1967.
Condon RE, Nyhus LM (eds). Manual of Surgical Therapeutics. New York: Little, Brown, 1996.
DeGowin EL, DeGowin RL. Bedside Diagnostic Examination. New York: Macmillan, 1976.
Maingot R (ed). Abdominal Operations. New York: Appleton-Century-Crofts, 1980.
McEntyre RL. Practical Guide to the Care of the Surgical Patient. St. Louis: CV Mosby, 1980.
Morris PJ, Malt RA (eds). Oxford Textbook of Surgery. Oxford, England: Oxford University Press, 1994.
Schwartz SI, Shires GT, Spencer FC, Storer EH (eds). Principles of Surgery. New York: McGraw-Hill, 1984.
Silen W. Cope's Early Diagnosis of the Acute Abdomen. Oxford, England: Oxford University Press, 1996.
Taylor TV, Armstrong CP, Carroll RNP. Case Presentations in General Surgery. London: Butterworths, 1987.
Tenner SM, Masterson TM. Pocket Book of Eponyms and Subtle Signs of Disease. Alexandria, Va: International Medical Publishing, 1993.
Thorek P. Surgical Diagnosis. Philadelphia: JB Lippincott Company, 1965.

CHAPTER 34 UROLOGY

Carter BS, Bova GS, Beaty TH et al. Hereditary prostate cancer; Epidemiologic and clinical features. J Urol 1993;150:797-802.
Gillenwater JY, Grayhack JT, Howards SS, Duckett JW (eds). Adult and Pediatric Urology, ed 3. St Louis: Mosby, 1996.
MacFarlane MT. Urology, ed 2. Baltimore: Williams & Wilkins, 1995.
Messing EM, Young TB, Hunt VB et al: The significance of asymptomatic microhematuria in men 50 or more years old: Findings of a home screening study using urinary dipsticks. J Urol 1987;137:919.
Tanagho EA, McAninch JW (eds). Smith's General Urology, ed 14. Norwalk, NJ: Appleton & Lange, 1995.
Walsh PC, Retik AP, Vaughan ED, Wein AJ (eds). Campbell's Urology, ed 7. Philadelphia: WB Saunders, 1998.

SECTION III FOCUSED HISTORY AND PHYSICAL EXAMINATION

CHAPTER 35 ALCOHOL SCREENING

Bush B, Shaw S, Cleary P et al. Screening for alcohol abuse using the CAGE questionnaire. Am J Medicine 1987;82:231-235.
Criteria Committee NCA. Criteria for the diagnosis of alcoholism. Ann Internal Medicine 1972;77:249-258.
Lieber CS, Worner TM. Drug therapy for alcoholism and alcohol withdrawal. Int Med 1987; 8:148-158.
Mayfield D, McLeod G, Hall P. The CAGE questionnaire: Validation of a new alcoholism screening instrument. Am J Psychiatry 1974;131(10):1121-1123.
National Institute on Alcohol Abuse and Alcoholism. Alcohol Alert No. 8 PH285, Screening for alcoholism. Publication no. 1990-0-860-570. Washington, DC: U.S. Government Printing Office, 1990; pp. 1-4.
National Institute on Alcohol Abuse and Alcoholism. Alcohol Alert No. 12 PH294, Assessing alcoholism Publication no. 1991-522-479/40001. Washington, DC: U.S. Government Printing Office, 1991; pp. 1-4.
National Institute on Alcohol Abuse and Alcoholism. Alcohol Alert No. 49, New advances in alcoholism treatment. Washington, DC: NIAAA Publications, 2000;11-14.

General References

1. Harrison's Textbook of Internal Medicine
2. Cecil & Loeb Textbook of Internal Medicine
3. Stedman's Medical Dictionary
4. DeGowin & DeGowin, Bedside Diagnostic Examination, which was published by MacMillan (Library of Congress catalog card # 69-10931).
5. Mosby for some alcohol-related definitions

CHAPTER 36 EPIDEMIOLOGY

Essex-Sorlie DP. Medical Biostatistics and Epidemiology, A Lange Medical Book. Norwalk, Conn: Appleton and Lange, 1995.
Jekel JF, Katz DL. Epidemiology, Biostatistics, and Preventive Medicine, Saunders Text and Review Series. Philadelphia: WB Saunders, 1996.
Greenberg RS, Flanders WD, Eley JW, Boring III JR. Medical Epidemiology: A Lange Medical Book. Stamford, Conn: Appleton and Lange, 1996.
Schlesselman JJ. Case-Control Studies/Design, Conduct, Analysis. New York: Oxford University Press, 1982.
Susser ML. Causal Thinking in the Health Sciences. New York: Oxford University Press, 1973.
Norell SE. Workbook of Epidemiology. New York: Oxford University Press, 1995.
Hammond EC, Seidman H. Asbestos Exposure, Cigarette Smoking, and Death Rates. Annals of the New York Academy of Sciences, 1979;330:473-490.
Benenson AS. Control of Communicable Disease Manual. Washington, DC: American Public Health Association, 1995.

CHAPTER 37 ETHICAL CONSIDERATIONS

Informed Consent

Beachamp TL, Childress JF. Principles of Biomedical Ethics, ed 4. New York: Oxford University Press, 1994;132-172.
Braddock C, Edwards K, Hasenberg N et al. Informed decision-making in outpatient practice: Time to get back to basics. JAMA 1999;282(24):2313-2320.

Carney M, Neugroschl J, Morrison S et al. The development and piloting of a capacity assessment tool. J Clin Ethics 2001;12(1):17-23.

Culver CM, Gert B. The inadequacy of incompetence. Milbank Quarterly 1990;68(4):619-643.

Lo B. Assessing decision-making capacity. Law Med Health Care 1990;18(3):193-201.

Redelmeier DA, Rozin P, Kahneman D. Understanding patients' decisions: Cognitive and emotional perspectives. JAMA 1993;270(1):72-76.

Advanced Directives

Beachamp TL, Childress JF. Principles of Biomedical Ethics, ed 4. New York: Oxford University Press, 1994; pp. 170-181, 241-249.

Emanuel EJ, Emanuel L. Proxy decision making for incompetent patients; an ethical and empirical analysis. JAMA 1992;267(15):2067-2071.

Layde P, Beam C, Broste S et al. Surrogates' predictions of seriously ill patients' resuscitation preferences. Arch Fam Med 1995;4(6):503-504.

Morris CD et al. Determining the capability of individuals with mental retardation to give informed consent. Am J Ment Retard 1993;98(2):263-272.

Seckler AB et al. Substituted judgment: How accurate are proxy predictions? Ann Int Med 1991;115:92-98.

Sonnenblick M, Friedlander Y, Steinber A. Dissociation between the wishes of terminally ill patients and decisions by their offspring. J Amer Geriatric Soc 1993;41:599-604.

DNR References

Alpers A, Lo B. When is CPR futile? JAMA 1995;273(2):156-158.

ASA Committee on Ethics. Ethical guidelines for the anesthesia care of patients with do not resuscitate orders or other directives that limit treatment. In The American Society of Anesthesiologists Standards, Guidelines, and Statements, 2000; pp. 13-14.

Beachamp TL, Childress JF. Principles of Biomedical Ethics, ed 4. New York: Oxford University Press, 1994; pp. 196-206.

Schneiderman LJ, Jecker NS, Jonsen AR. Medical futility: Its meaning and ethical implications. Ann Int Med 1990;112:99-103.

The SUPPORT principle investigators. A controlled trial to improve care for seriously ill hospitalized patients. The Study to Understand Prognoses and Preferences for Outcomes and Risks of Treatments (SUPPORT). JAMA 1995;274(23):1839-1844.

Truog R, Waisel D. Do-not-resuscitate orders: From the ward to the operating room; from procedures to goals. International Anesth Clin 2001;39(3):53-65.

CHAPTER 38 NUTRITIONAL STATUS EVALUATION

Blackburn GL, Bistrian BR, Maini BS et al. Nutritional and metabolic assessment of the hospitalized patient. JPEN 1977;1:11-22.

Foxx-Orenstein A, Kirby DF. Understanding malnutrition and refeeding syndrome. In Kirby DF, Dudrick SJ (eds), Practical Handbook of Nutrition in Clinical Practice. Boca Raton, Fla: CRC Press, 1994;19-30.

Ireton-Jones CS. Evaluation of energy expenditures in obese patients. Nutr Clin Pract 1989;4(4):127-129.

Kirby DF, DeLegge MH. Nutritional assessment: The high tech and low tech tour. In Kirby DF, Dudrick SJ (eds), Practical Handbook of Nutrition in Clinical Practice. Boca Raton, Fla: CRC Press, 1994; pp. 1-18.

Levenhagen DK, Borel MJ, Welch DC et al. A comparison of air displacement plethysmography with three other techniques to determine body fat in healthy adults. JPEN 1999;23:293-299.

McClave SA, Snider HL. Use of indirect calorimetry in clinical medicine. Nutr Clin Pract 1992;7:207-221.

Misra S, Kirby DF. Micronutrient and trace element monitoring in adult nutrition support. Nutr Clin Pract 2000;15:120-126.

CHAPTER 39 TOBACCO SCREENING

Guide to Clinical Preventive Services, ed 2. Edition, Report of the U.S. Preventive Services Task Force. Baltimore: Williams and Wilkins, 1996.

Centers for Disease Control and Prevention. Cigarette smoking—attributable mortality and years of potential life lost—United States, 1990. MMWR 1993:42:645-649.

Department of Health and Human Services. Reducing the health consequences of smoking: 25 years of progress. A report of the Surgeon General. Rockville, MD; Department of Health and Human Services 1989. (Publication No. DHHS (CDC 89-8411).

Department of Health and Human Services. The health benefits of smoking cessation: a report of the Surgeon General. Rockville, MD: Department of Health and Human Services, 1990. (Publication No. DHHS (CDC) 90-8416.

Kottke TE, Williams DG, Solberg LI et al. Physician-delivered smoking cessation advice: issues identified during ethnographic interviews. Tobacco Control 1994;3:46-49.

Watson DL, Tharp RG. Self-Directed Behavior/Self-Modification for Personal Adjustment, ed 4. Monterey, Calif: Brooks/Cole Publishing, 1985.

Treating Tobacco Use and Dependence. Fact Sheet, June 2000. U.S. Public Health Service. www.surgeongeneral.gov/tobacco/smokfact.htm.

Targeting Tobacco Use: The Nation's Leading Cause of Death, At-A-Glance, 2000. U.S. Department of Health and Human Services, Centers for Disease Control and Prevention, www.cdc.gov/tobacco/issue.htm.

New Guidelines Challenge All Clinicians to Help Smokers Quit, Tobacco Information and Prevention Source, Centers for Disease Control and Prevention, www.cdc.gov/tobacco/guidline_new.htm.

Cancer Facts/Cancer Research Because Lives Depend on It/Questions and Answers About the Benefits of Smoking Cessation/ http://cis.nci.nih.gov/fact/8_11.htm.

QUITNET/Triggers and Cues/ http://www.quitnet.org/library/guides/Quitnet/g_triggr.jtml

Contributors

Amro Y. Al-Astal, MD
Senior Clinical Fellow, Pulmonary and Critical Care Medicine
Medical College of Ohio
Toledo, OH

James Eric Bermudez, MD
Captain, Medical Service
United States Air Force

Richard A. Bernert, MD
Staff Pathologist
Clin-Path Associates
Tempe, AZ

Jay T. Bishoff, MD, FACS
Director, Endourology Section
Department of Urology
59th Medical Wing
Wilford Hall Medical Center
Lackland Air Force Base, TX;
Associate Clinical Professor, Surgery
University of Texas Health Science Center
San Antonio, TX

Patricio G. Bruno, DO
Resident, Department of Family Medicine
Albert Einstein College of Medicine, Beth Israel Hospital, Institute for Urban Family Health
New York, NY

William P. Butler, MD, MTM&H, FACS
Squadron Commander
59th Aerospace Medicine Squadron
Lackland Air Force Base, TX

Jonathan W. Buttram, MD
Chief, Allergy and Immunology Services
81st Medical Group
Keesler Air Force Base, MS

Stephen J. Cina, MD
Clinical Associate Professor, Pathology
University of Colorado Health Sciences Center
Denver, CO;
Vice Chair, Pathology
McKee Medical Center
Loveland, CO;
Forensic Pathology Consultant
Colorado Pathology Association
Loveland, CO;
Coroner/Medical Examiner
Weld County, CO

William D. Clark, MD, DDS, FACS
Associate Professor, Otolaryngology
University of Florida College of Medicine;
Attending Staff, Shands Hospital at the University of Florida
Gainesville, FL

Roy J. DiLeo, Lt. Col, USAF, MC
Flight Commander/Medical Director
Emergency Services Flight
51st Medical Group
Osan Air Base, Republic of Korea

Irel Scott Eppich, MD
Commander, Nephrology Flight
Nephrology Consultant to the Surgeon General

Department of Nephrology
59th Medical Wing
Wilford Hall Medical Center
Lackland Air Force Base, TX

Jill Catalano Feig, MD, MPH
Preventive Medicine Consultant
Epidemiology Services Branch (RSRH)
Air Force Institute for Operational Health
United States Air Force
San Antonio, TX

Michael R. Foley, MD
Clinical Professor, Obstetrics/Gynecology, Division of Medical-Fetal Medicine
University of Arizona
Tucson, AZ;
Medical Director, Phoenix Perinatal Associates/Obstetrics Medical Group
Phoenix, AZ

Karrie Francois, MD
Associate Director
Phoenix Perinatal Associates;
Department of Maternal-Fetal Medicine
Good Samaritan Regional Medical Center
Phoenix, AZ

Samuel M. Galvagno Jr., DO
56 Medical Group,
56 Aerospace Medicine Squadron
United States Air Force
Luke Air Force Base, AZ;
Flight Surgeon/Squadron Medical Element
63rd Fighter Squadron
Luke Air Force Base, AZ

Roger L. Gibson
Program Director, Military Public Health
Office of the Assistant Secretary for Defense
Health Affairs
Washington, DC

Eric H. Hanson, MD, MPH
Headquarters United States Air Force
Office of the Surgeon General
Directorate of Modernization
Science and Technology Division
Division Chief, Science and Technology
Chief, Operational Biotechnology
Bolling Air Force Base, Washington, D.C.

Sharon G. Harris, MD
Associate Professor of Medicine
University of Texas at San Antonio, TX
and University of the Health Sciences.
Bethesda, MD;
Program Director
and Chairperson,
Department of Endocrinology
Wilford Hall Medical Center
Lackland Air Force Base, TX

Michael S. Jaffee, MD
Clinical Assistant Professor, Neurology and Psychiatry
University of Texas Health Sciences Center
San Antonio, TX;
Associate Program Director, Neurology
Wilford Hall Medical Center;
San Antonio, TX;
Assistant Professor, Neurology

Uniformed Services University of Health Sciences
Bethesda, MD

Christine L. Johnson, MD
LCDR, MC, USN
Assistant Professor of PediatricsDepartment of Pediatrics
Uniformed Services University of the Health Sciences
Bethesda, MD

Woodson Scott Jones, MD
Pediatric Clerkship Director,
Assistant Professor of Pediatrics
Uniformed Services University of the Health Sciences
Bethesda, MD

Bryan Kahl, MD
Staff Endocrinologist
Department of Endocrinology
59th Medical Wing
Wilford Hall Medical Center
Lackland Air Force Base, TX

Nina J. Karlin, MD
Geriatrics Fellow
UCLA School of Medicine
Los Angeles, CA

Patrick S. Kelley, MD
Staff Ophthalmologist
Chief, Ophthalmology and Refractive Surgery Services
Department of Ophthalmology
Keesler Medical Center
Keesler Air Force Base, MS

Donald F. Kirby, MD, FACP, FACN, FACG, CNSP, CPNS
Professor of Medicine, Psychiatry, Biochemistry and Molecular Physics
Department of Internal Medicine;
Chief, Section of Nutrition and Wellness
Division of Gastroenterology
Virginia Commonwealth University
Richmond, VA

Todd Kobayashi, MD
Chief, Dermatology Clinic
Department of Dermatology
965th Medical Dental Operations Squadron
Eglin Air Force Base, FL

Alan P. Marco, MD, MMM
Associate Professor, Department of Anesthesiology;
Quality Medical Liaison
Medical College of Ohio
Toledo, OH

R. Clay McDonohugh III, MD
Resident in Urology
Department of Urology
59th Medical Wing
Wilford Hall Medical Center
Lackland Air Force Base, TX

Patricia A. Meier, MD
Resident in Pathology
Department of Pathology
59th Medical Wing
Wilford Hall Medical Center
Lackland Air Force Base, TX

Daniel R. More, MD
Clinical Instructor of Medicine
Department of Internal Medicine
Uniformed Services University of the Health Sciences School of Medicine
Bethesda, MD;
Fellow
Department of Allergy and Immunology

Wilford Hall Medical Center
Lackland Air Force Base, TX

Jamal Mourad, DO
Assistant Professor of Clinical Education
Department of Obstetrics and Gynecology
Midwestern University–Arizona College of Osteopathic Medicine
Glendale, AZ;
Attending Physician, Obstetrics and Gynecology
Good Samaritan Regional Medical Center
Phoenix, AZ

Anne L. Naclerio, MD, MPH
Chief, Pediatric Critical Care Medicine
Department of Neonatology
59th Medical Wing
Wilford Hall Medical Center
Lackland Air Force Base, TX

Katerina M. Neuhauser, MD, PhD, MPH
Medical Epidemiologist
Epidemiology Services Branch
Air Force Institute for Operational Health
Brooks City-Base, TX

Thomas S. Neuhauser, MD
Staff Pathologist
Director of Hematology
Department of Pathology
59th Medical Wing
Wilford Hall Medical Center
Lackland Air Force Base, TX

Carey L. O'Bryan IV, MD
Assistant Professor of Medicine, Department of Medicine
Uniformed Services University of the Health Sciences
Bethesda, MD;
Staff Cardiologist, Cardiology
59th Medical Wing
Wilford Hall Medical Center
Lackland Air Force Base, TX

Dorene A. O'Hara, MD, MSE
Associate Professor, Anesthesia
New York Medical College
Valhalla, NY;
Anesthesiologist-Attending
Metropolitan Hospital Center
New York, NY

Michael Osswald, MD
Staff Oncologist
Fellowship Program Director
Department of Hematology-Oncology
59th Medical Wing
Wilford Hall Medical Center
Lackland Air Force Base, TX

Gregory R. Owens, MD
Assistant Flight Commander, Gastroenterology Staff
Department of Gastroenterology
59th Medical Wing
Wilford Hall Medical Center
Lackland Air Force Base, TX

Thomas Papadimos, MD, MPH
Assistant Professor
Department of Anesthesiology
Medical College of Ohio
Toledo, OH

Phillip E. Parker, MD, MPH
Chief, Aerospace and Occupational Medicine
Aerospace Medicine Squadron
325th Medical Group
Tyndall Air Force Base, FL

Theodore W. Parsons III, MD, FACS
Associate Dean for Graduate Medical Education
59th Medical Wing
Wilford Hall Medical Center
Lackland Air Force Base, TX;
Associate Professor, Orthopaedic Surgery
University of Texas Health Science Center
San Antonio, TX;
Associate Professor, Orthopaedic Surgery
Uniformed Services University of the Health Sciences
Bethesda, MD;
Chief, Orthopaedic Oncology Service
Orthopaedic Surgery
Wilford Hall Medical Center
Lackland Air Force Base, TX

James M. Quinn, MD
Assistant Clinical Professor, Medicine
Uniformed Services University of the Health Sciences
Bethesda, MD;
Chairman, Allergy/Immunology
59th Medical Wing
Wilford Hall Medical Center
Lackland Air Force Base, TX

Tom J. Sauerwein, MD
Staff Endocrinologist
Assistant Program Director
Department of Endocrinology
59th Medical Wing
Wilford Hall Medical Center
Lackland Air Force Base, TX

Gregory J. Sengstock, DC, MD, PhD
Neurologist
Neurology
Baptist Medical Center
Jacksonville, FL

Brian P. Skop, MD
Associate Clinical Professor Psychiatry
University of Texas Health Science Center
San Antonio, TX

Ingrid P. Skop, MD
Obstetrics and Gynecology Northeast Baptist Hospital San Antonio, TX

Gail A. van Norman, MD
Attending Anesthesiologist
St. Joseph's Medical Center
Tacoma, WA

Jorge L. Romeu Vélez, MD, MS
Neonatology Fellow
Department of Pediatrics
Tripler Army Medical Center
Honolulu, Hawaii

Theresa M. Worner, MD
Associate Professor Clinical Medicine
State University of New York
Health Science Center
Brooklyn, NY;
Clinical Associate Professor of Public Health,
Cornell University Medical College;
Consultant, American Medical Forensic Specialists;
President, Menachem Publishing

INDEX

Page numbers followed by *f* indicate figures; *t* indicate tables; and *b* indicate boxes.

C

D

N

P

X

Y

Z